Concepts of Fitness and Wellness

A COMPREHENSIVE LIFESTYLE APPROACH

Seventh Edition

Charles B. Corbin
Arizona State University

Gregory J. Welk
Iowa State University

William R. Corbin
Yale University

Karen A. Welk
Mary Greeley Medical Center
Ames, Iowa

Boston   Burr Ridge, IL   Dubuque, IA   New York   San Francisco   St. Louis
Bangkok   Bogotá   Caracas   Kuala Lumpur   Lisbon   London   Madrid   Mexico City
Milan   Montreal   New Delhi   Santiago   Seoul   Singapore   Sydney   Taipei   Toronto

The McGraw-Hill Companies

Mc Graw Hill **Higher Education**

CONCEPTS OF FITNESS AND WELLNESS: A COMPREHENSIVE LIFESTYLE APPROACH
Published by McGraw-Hill, an imprint of The McGraw-Hill Companies, Inc., 1221 Avenue
of the Americas, New York, NY 10020. Copyright © 2008, 2006, 2004, 2002, 2000, 1997, 1994
by The McGraw-Hill Companies, Inc. All rights reserved. No part of this publication may be
reproduced or distributed in any form or by any means, or stored in a database or retrieval
system, without the prior written consent of The McGraw-Hill Companies, Inc., including,
but not limited to, in any network or other electronic storage or transmission, or broadcast for
distance learning.

This book is printed on acid-free paper.

1 2 3 4 5 6 7 8 9 0 DOW/DOW 0 9 8 7 6

ISBN: 978-0-07-352359-0
MHID: 0-07-352359-3

Editor in Chief: *Emily Barrosse*
Publisher: *William Glass*
Executive Editor: *Christopher Johnson*
Executive Marketing Manager: *Pamela S. Cooper*
Director of Development: *Kathleen Engelberg*
Senior Developmental Editor: *Carlotta Seely*
Developmental Editor for Technology: *Julia D. Akpan*
Project Manager: *Jill Eccher*
Manuscript Editor: *Dale Boroviak*
Senior Designer/Cover Design: *Violeta Diaz*
Interior Design: *Jeanne Calabrese*
Photo Research: *Alex Ambrose/Emily Tietz*
Cover Photo: © *PhotoDisc/Getty Images*
Senior Production Supervisor: *Rich DeVitto*
Media Producer: *Michele Perez*
Media Project Manager: *Kate Boylan*

This book was set in 10/12 Janson by Precision Graphics and printed on 45# New Era Matte by R. R. Donnelley & Sons.

The credits section for this book begins on page C-1 and is considered an extension of the copyright page.

Library of Congress Cataloging-in-Publication Data

Concepts of fitness and wellness: a comprehensive lifestyle approach / Charles B. Corbin ... [et al.]—7th ed.
    p. cm.
Includes bibliographical references and index.
ISBN-13: 978-0-07-352359-0; ISBN-10: 0-07-352359-3 (softcover : alk. paper)
    1. Physical fitness. 2. Exercise. 3. Health. I. Corbin, Charles B.
RA781.C644 2008
613.7--dc22

2006088453

www.mhhe.com

Brief Contents

Contents

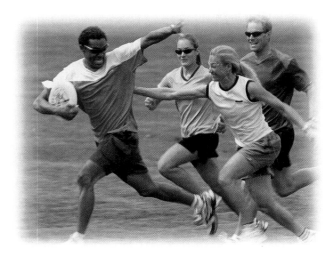

Section III

The Physical Activity Pyramid 97

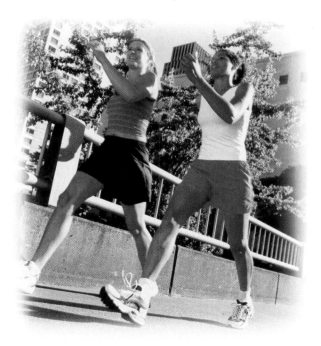

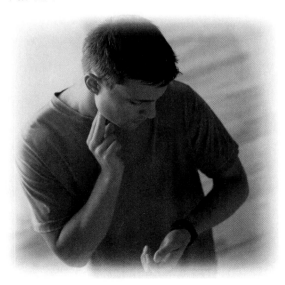

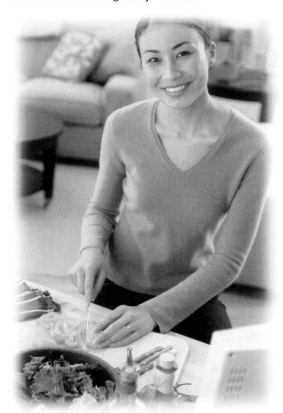

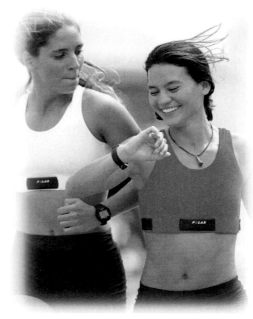

Technology Updates

In the News

Preface

Fitness and Wellness: Celebrating Four Decades of Success and Remembering Our Beloved Colleague and Co-Author

In 1968 our first *Concepts* book was published. It was the predecessor of this seventh edition of *Concepts of Fitness and Wellness*. The 2008 copyright date signals the end of the first four decades of book publication. It is with great joy that we celebrate our 40 years of success and look forward to continued success in our fifth decade. We think that the changes that we have made in this new edition will make it the best yet. But as we celebrate, we also reflect on the loss of our beloved colleague, Ruth Lindsey. As the memorial tribute on the opposite page attests, Ruth Lindsey played a significant role in the success of the *Concepts* books. We hope that you will join us in celebrating Ruth's life by reading the tribute and reflecting on her life's accomplishments.

The current author team has been together for two editions. Chuck Corbin, who has been lead author since the first edition, is now professor emeritus at Arizona State University and continues in the lead author role. Greg Welk, an associate professor at Iowa State University, increased his contributions with the retirement of Ruth Lindsey and continues to play a major role in total book development. Will Corbin, an assistant professor of clinical psychology at Yale University, focuses on topics related to stress, health behavior change, and destructive behaviors. Karen Welk, a physical therapist at Mary Greeley Medical Center, focuses on safe exercises, care of the back and neck, and correct technique for performing exercises.

As we move into our fifth decade of publication of books related to health, fitness, and wellness, we continue to focus on healthy lifestyles. In our early editions, we focused on trying to get people fit and well. To be sure, fitness is an important product, as is wellness, another product of healthy lifestyle change. But scientific advances have shown that health, wellness, and fitness (all products) are not things you can "do" to people. You have to help people help themselves. Educating them and giving them the self-management skills that help them adopt healthy lifestyles can do this.

The focus of the new millennium is on the *process*. Healthy lifestyles, or what a person does, rather than what a person can do, constitute process. If a person does the process (i.e., adopts a healthy lifestyle), positive changes will occur to the extent that change is possible for that person. As noted in the first concept of the book, lifestyles are the most important factors, influencing health, wellness, and fitness. Healthy lifestyles (the processes) are also within a person's individual control. *Any person* can benefit from lifestyle change, and any person can change a lifestyle. These lifestyle changes will make a difference in health, fitness, and wellness for all people.

The emphasis on lifestyle change in the seventh edition is consistent with the focus of national health objectives for the new millennium. Though the principal national health goals are to increase years and quality of life (products) for all people, the methods of accomplishing these goals focus on changing lifestyles. In this new century, we must adopt a new way of thinking to help all people change their lifestyles to promote health, fitness, and wellness.

Our Basic Philosophy

The HELP Philosophy

Over time, the features of our book have evolved. However, the HELP philosophy on which the book is based remains sound. We believe that the "new way of thinking" based on the HELP philosophy serves us, the faculty who choose our book, and the students who use it. **H** is for *health*. Health and its positive component—wellness—are central to the philosophy. Health, fitness, and wellness are for all people. **E** is for *everyone*. **L** is for *lifetime lifestyle change*, and **P** is for *personal*. The goal is to HELP

Ruth Lindsey 1926–2005
In Memoriam:
A Tribute to Our Co-author and Friend

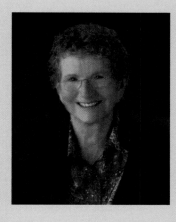

On May 29, 2005, we lost a great leader and an outstanding advocate for healthy lifestyles, physical activity, and physical education. Our long-time co-author and friend, Ruth Lindsey, will long be remembered for her contributions to the *Concepts* books and to our profession. Ruth was born in 1926 in Kingfisher, Oklahoma, and graduated from high school in Checotah. She earned her BS from Oklahoma State University in 1948, her MS from the University of Wisconsin in 1954, and her doctorate from Indiana University in 1965.

Ruth began her college teaching career at Oklahoma State University (OSU) in 1948, and after brief stints at Monticello College and DePauw University, she returned to OSU in 1956, where she advanced through the ranks to full professor. In 1976, she was a visiting professor at the University of Utah. Ruth then served as professor of physical education at California State University at Long Beach until her retirement in 1988. She continued to contribute as author of the *Concepts* books until 2003.

Ruth was a recognized scholar in physical education with special expertise in biomechanics, kinesiology, questionable exercises, nutrition, and physical activity for senior adults. She actively campaigned against consumer health fraud. She was the author of more than a dozen books, including *Body Mechanics, The Ultimate Fitness Book, Fitness for Life, Concepts of Physical Fitness,* and *Concepts of Fitness and Wellness.* Ruth published numerous papers and served as a leader in many professional organizations. She was an accomplished athlete who won the Oklahoma Women's Fencing Championship and was a low-handicap golfer.

Over the years, hundreds of thousands of students have read Ruth's writings. Her own students and her co-authors will remember her for her command of her subject matter, her attention to detail, the red ink on papers and manuscripts, her concern for her profession, and her personal concern for each individual. Ruth was a woman of principle and character. She will long be remembered for her contributions to our field and for being the kind and caring person that she was. We will miss our co-author, our colleague, and our friend.

---

all people make personal lifetime lifestyle changes that promote health, fitness, and wellness.

To ensure that the book is consistent with the HELP philosophy and that it is useful to everyone, we include discussions about how to adapt healthy lifestyles based on personal needs. Separate sections are *not* included for specific groups, such as older people, women, ethnic groups, or those with special needs. Rather, we focus on healthy lifestyles *for all people* throughout the book.

Meeting Higher-Order Objectives

The "new way of thinking" based on the HELP philosophy suggests that each person must make decisions about healthy lifetime lifestyles if the goals of longevity and quality of life are to be achieved. What one person chooses may be quite different from what another chooses. Accordingly, our goal in preparing this edition is to help readers become good problem solvers and decision makers. Rather than focusing on telling them what to do, we offer information to help readers make informed choices about lifestyles. The stairway to lifetime fitness and wellness that we present helps readers understand the importance of "higher-order objectives" devoted to problem solving and decision making.

Our Approach
Pedagogically Sound Organization

Planning and self-management strategies are presented early (Concept 2) to familiarize students with basic principles and guidelines that will be used in later planning. Preparation strategies and basic activity principles follow. Each type of health-related fitness and the type of activity that promotes it are included in the next section. This section is organized around the physical activity pyramid. Special considerations—including safe exercise, care of the back and neck, posture, and performance—are included in the next section. Other priority healthy lifestyles are the focus of nutrition, body composition, and stress-management sections. The next to last section includes extensive discussion of tobacco, alcohol, drugs, and STIs. The final section is designed to help students become good consumers and to learn to use self-management and self-planning skills to develop lifelong health, fitness, and wellness.

Concept Format

The content of this text is organized according to concepts rather than chapters. Each concept contains factual statements that follow concise informational paragraphs.

This approach has proven to be educationally sound and well received by both students and instructors.

Focus on Self-Management Skills

The educational effectiveness of a text depends on more than just presenting information. If lifestyle changes are to be implemented, there must be opportunities to learn how to make these changes. Research suggests that learning self-management skills is important to lifestyle change. A section on self-management skills is included early in the book, and recurring discussions of how to practice and implement these skills are presented throughout the text.

Coverage for North America

Statistics for all of North America are included, in addition to those typically presented for the United States. Several Canadian Web sites have been included, as have been new statistics and a color version of *Canada's Food Guide to Healthy Eating*.

Magazine Format

The attractive design supports student reading and studying with an appealing magazine format. This format has been shown to be educationally effective and has been well received by users.

Highlights of the New Edition

New Content

Much new information is included in the seventh edition of *Concepts of Fitness and Wellness*. A summary follows.

- The new, colorful design includes dozens of new photos and added artwork.
- Muscle illustrations have been added to help students learn more about the specific muscles used in important exercises.
- New lab worksheets have been added:
  - Stages of Change Questionnaire
  - Self-Management Skills Questionnaire
  - Physical Activity Attitudes
  - Environmental Questionnaire
  - Exercise Adherance
- Health and Wellness Model in Concept 1 has been expanded to emphasize the importance of personal and social choices.
- Concepts 2 and 6 were combined to integrate coverage of lifestyle change (former Concept 2) with program planning (former Concept 6). This facilitates the application of decision-making skills for different lifestyle behaviors.
- The Strategies for Action sections have been expanded throughout the text to help users apply the self-management skills they have learned.

- Coverage of environmental issues influencing health has been expanded. Examples include coverage of policies on nutrition and the development of more "walkable" communities.
- New Concept 11 (Body Mechanics: Posture, Questionable Exercises, and Care of the Back and Neck) combines coverage of safe exercise practice (former Concept 12) with information on body mechanics (former Concept 13). This provides for a more efficient presentation of these related concepts.
- The 2005 Dietary Guidelines for Americans and MyPyramid help students adopt and maintain healthier nutrition choices.
- New Technology Update and In the News sections help students understand and interpret new health-related information and resources.
- All concepts have been updated with the most recent statistics. New suggested readings and Web sites have been added.
- Updated or expanded discussions include metabolic syndrome, Alzheimer's disease, cancer, CPR, quackery, supplements, standards for blood pressure, and recommendations for effectively using the health-care system.
- Concept 24, the final concept in the book, includes many new Strategies for Action and activities for self-planning to aid students in using self-management skills to take personal control of health issues, to plan personal programs, and to make healthy lifestyle choices.

New Features

New Design

The new design for *Concepts of Fitness and Wellness* includes many new photos and illustrations. The new artwork is designed to aid visual learning of complex concepts, such as the metabolic syndrome and the benefits of physical activity related to the cardiovascular system. Many of the photos involve "text wrapping," which integrates them with the text discussion. Color bands are used throughout the text to make it easy to locate opening pages for concepts, lab resource materials, and lab worksheets.

Muscle Illustrations

Many of the exercise illustrations are accompanied by muscle illustrations that present a close-up view of the targeted muscle. This new feature is designed to focus attention on the mechanics of the muscle action. Examples of these muscle illustrations can be found in A Guided Tour of *Concepts of Fitness and Wellness* at the end of this Preface and in Concepts 9, 10, and 11.

Successful Features

This edition retains the following popular features, which made the previous editions so successful.

Web Icons

Newly designed Web icons are place throughout the text. These icons guide students in locating, at the point of use, relevant information on the Web. By accessing the On the Web feature at **www.mhhe.com/corbinweb**, students and instructors can click on the number shown in the Web icon to explore the concept topic in greater depth.

Health Goals for the Year 2010

The health goals featured in this text are based on the Health Goals for the Year 2010. These goals are highlighted at the beginning of each concept to help students relate the text content to these goals.

Technology Update

Each concept contains a technology feature, which describes technological advances relating to health, wellness, and fitness lifestyles.

In the News

This feature provides summaries of news reports, press releases, and research findings highlighted in the news, offering interesting topics for class discussion.

Activity Features

Exercises for each part of physical fitness are illustrated and described in easy-to-locate tables. Opportunities to perform the exercises are provided in the labs.

Terms at Point-of-Use

It greatly pleased us that the *Surgeon General's Report on Physical Activity and Health* adopted our physical fitness definitions. Just as we have led the way in defining fitness, we include state-of-the-art definitions related to wellness and quality of life. These (and all other definitions) appear at the first point-of-use to make them easy to find.

Strategies for Action

Strategies for Action are suggestions for putting content into action. Many of these strategies require readers to perform or practice self-assessment or other self-management techniques.

Easy-to-Use Labs

The attractive and popular labs are designed to motivate students to practice self-management skills that will promote healthy lifestyle change. New labs have been added to this edition to further enhance the utility of the materials for individual behavior change. The labs are presented in a bright, attractive, and educationally effective format.

They are easy to find and use. In many cases, lab resource materials that aid the student in performing lab activities precede them. The labs are designed to get students active early in the course and ultimately to allow each to plan his or her own personal activity program.

Web Resources

At the end of every concept, key Web sites are listed to provide students with additional online resources that supplement the content just learned.

Suggested Readings

Because students want to know more about a particular topic, a list of readings is given at the end of each concept. Most suggested readings are readily available at bookstores or public libraries. Also included is the Web address (URL) for additional references related to topics covered in each concept. This expanded reference list will help those interested in further study of specific topics.

New and Expanded Topics

1   Health, Wellness, Fitness, and Healthy Lifestyles: An Introduction

- Updated information and statistics about mid-decade progress toward *Healthy People 2010* goals for the nation
- Revised integrated wellness model
- Updated sections covering the impact of the aging population on health and the health-care system
- New coverage of impact of the environment on health

2   Self-Management and Self-Planning Skills for Health Behavior Change

- *New concept* integrating content from Concept 2 and Concept 6 in past editions; provides a broader coverage of planning for lifestyle behavior change
- New framework for healthy lifestyle behavior change
- Updated information on how knowledge of self-assessments can contribute to behavior change
- Updated information on the importance of various behavioral skills for promoting behavior change
- Updated sections on goal setting using the SMART goal-setting approach; expanded content short- and long-term goals as behavioral (process) and outcome (product) goals
- New content on monitoring and tracking personal health data, such as blood pressure
- New labs: Stages of Change Questionnaire (2A) and Self-Management Skills Questionnaire (2B)

3   Preparing for Physical Activity

- New shoe and clothing technology information
- Updated information on warm-up and cool-down
- Additional information on exercising in the cold

- New information about exercising in the heat and fluid replacement, including coverage of additional health problems, such as hyponatremia (water intoxication)
- Updated injury treatment information
- New section on attitudes toward physical activity and new lab: Physical Activity Attitude Questionnaire (3C)

4   The Health Benefits of Physical Activity

- New information on modifiable and nonmodifiable risk factors, including coverage of new emerging risk factors
- Revised health-risk screening profile (lab)

5   How Much Physical Activity Is Enough?

- Reorganized material on the principles of training
- New material on the meaning and interpretation of the fitness classifications used in the book
- New section on activity guidelines explaining differences between ACSM/CDC and recent Institute of Medicine guidelines
- New statistics on the percentage of people engaging in appropriate levels of physical activity
- New physical activity survey lab and revised fitness evaluation lab

6   Lifestyle Physical Activity: Being Active in Diverse Environments

- New content on impact of environment on activity
- New information on lifestyle physical activity, including coverage of active commuting, work-related activity, and active work at home
- New content on the possible benefits of accumulating light activity throughout the day, described along with research on nonexercise activity thermogenesis (NEAT)
- Updated content on health, wellness, and cardiovascular benefits of activity
- New information on pedometers and their role in self-monitoring of physical activity
- New lab, Planning and Self-Monitoring Your Lifestyle Physical Activity (6A), helps evaluate environmental impact

7   Cardiovascular Fitness

- Revised CV system illustrations and content
- New integrative figure that depicts the characteristics of a healthy cardiovascular system
- New table that compares cardiovascular parameters and measures during rest and exercise; helps explain how cardiovascular system works to increase oxygen delivery during exercise
- New presentation and graphics that depict different calculations of target heart rate for exercise
- New lab (7A) and new content allowing students to compare field estimates with non-exercise fitness estimates

8   Active Aerobics, Sports, and Recreational Activities

- Reorganized section on types of aerobic activities
- New results and graphs of activity patterns and trends (SGMA)
- New lab (8A) on Physical Activity Adherence

9   Flexibility

- New section on the popularity of movement disciplines
- Expanded sections on yoga, tai chi, and Pilates
- New section on flexibility exercise equipment

10   Muscle Fitness and Resistance Exercises

- New information on the importance of "core" strength for health and good muscular fitness
- New information on functional balance training
- New exercises for building core strength
- Additions to equipment section, including photos and descriptions of BOSU® Balance Trainer

11   Body Mechanics: Posture, Questionable Exercises, and Care of the Back and Neck

- *New concept* integrating information on back health (formerly Concept 11) with information on safe exercise (formerly Concept 13)
- New content on structure and function of back
- New information on the causes of back pain
- New content on proper body mechanics and explanations of factor's putting back at risk

12   Performance Benefits of Physical Activity

- Revised descriptions of anaerobic metabolism and lactic acid
- Revised sections on training for endurance sports
- Updated information on ergogenic aids

13   Body Composition

- Updated statistics on the prevalence of overweight
- Updated content on body composition including DXA and Bod Pod
- Additions to the section on the health risks of overweight and obesity
- New information on the bio/behavior model for the origin of body fatness, including updates on genetics and the role of leptin in the etiology of obesity

14   Nutrition

- New information on 2005 Dietary Guidelines for Americans
- New information on updated food labeling guidelines
- New information on the requirements for documenting the trans fat content of foods
- New model integrating MyPyramid and Physical Activity Pyramid; depicts integration of nutrition and activity behavior
- New sections that provide tips to help students follow and adhere to the 2005 Dietary Guidelines for Americans

Other Resources

Daily Fitness and Nutrition Journal (ISBN: 0-07-302988-2)

This logbook helps students track their diet and exercise programs. It can be packaged with any McGraw-Hill textbook for a small additional fee.

Health and Fitness Pedometer (ISBN: 0-07-320933-3)

An electronic digital pedometer (step counter) can be packaged with *Concepts of Fitness and Wellness*. This pedometer is useful in tracking walking steps, miles/kilometers, and kilocalories.

NutritionCalc Plus CD-ROM (ISBN: 0-07-319570-7)

NutritionCalc Plus is a powerful dietary self-assessment tool. Students can use it to analyze and monitor their personal diet and health goals. The program is based on the reliable ESHA database and has an easy-to-use interface.

HealthQuest 4.2 CD-ROM (ISBN: 0-07-295117-6)

This interactive CD helps students explore and change their wellness behavior. It includes tutorials, assessments, and behavior change guidelines in key areas such as nutrition, fitness, stress, cardiovascular disease, cancer, tobacco, and alcohol.

PageOut: The Course Web site Development Center: www.pageout.net

PageOut, available free to instructors who use a McGraw-Hill textbook, is an online program that lets them create their own course Web site. PageOut offers the following features: a course home page, an instructor home page, a syllabus (interactive and customizable, including quizzing, instructor notes, and links to the text's Online Learning Center), Web links, discussions (multiple discussion areas per class), an online gradebook, and links to student Web pages. Contact your McGraw-Hill sales representative to obtain a password.

Course Management Systems: www.mhhe.com/solutions

McGraw-Hill's Instructor Advantage program offers customers access to a complete online teaching Web site called the Knowledge Gateway, prepaid toll-free phone support, and unlimited e-mail support directly from WebCT and Blackboard. Instructors who use 500 or more copies of a McGraw-Hill textbook can enroll in the Instructor Advantage Plus program, which provides on-campus, hands-on training from a certified platform specialist. Consult your McGraw-Hill sales representative to learn what other course management systems are easily used with McGraw-Hill online materials.

Classroom Performance System: www.einstruction.com

Classroom Performance System (CPS) is a revolutionary system that brings ultimate interactivity to the lecture hall or classroom. CPS is a wireless response system that gives you immediate feedback from every student in the class. CPS units include easy-to-use software for creating and delivering questions and assessments to your class and are compatible with Macintosh or PC systems. With CPS you can ask subjective and objective questions. Then every student simply responds with his or her wireless response pad, providing instant results. CPS is the perfect tool for engaging students while gathering important assessment data. For your convenience, we have created CPS test and polling questions to accompany *Concepts of Fitness and Wellness*. To find out how you can use CPS in your classroom, please contact your sales representative.

Primis Online: www.mhhe.com/primis/online

Primis Online is a database-driven publishing system that allows instructors to create content-rich textbooks, lab manuals, or readers for their courses directly from the Primis Web site. The customized text can be delivered in print or electronic (eBook) form. A Primis eBook is a digital version of the customized text (sold directly to students as a file downloadable to their computer or accessed online by a password). *Concepts of Fitness and Wellness* is included in the database.

Acknowledgments

It hardly seems possible that the first edition of the *Concepts* book was published 40 years ago. As we enter our fifth decade of publication, we want to acknowledge the many people who have helped us along the way. Our success, and the success of the *Concepts* books, would not have been possible without their help. At the risk of inadvertently failing to mention someone, we want to acknowledge the following people for their role in the development of this book.

First, we would like to acknowledge a few people who have made special contributions over the years. Linus Dowell, Carl Landiss, and Homer Tolson, all of Texas A & M University, were involved in the development of the first *Concepts* book in 1968.

Other pioneers were Jimmy Jones of Henderson State University, who started one of the first *Concepts* classes in 1970 and has led the way in teaching fitness in the years that have followed; Charles Erickson, who started a quality program at Missouri Western; and Al Lesiter, a leader in the East at Mercer Community College in New Jersey. David Laurie and Barbara Gench at Kansas State University, as well as others on that faculty, were instrumental in developing a prototype concepts program, which research has shown to be successful.

A special thanks is extended to Andy Herrick and Jim Whitehead, who have contributed to much of the development of various editions of the book, including excellent suggestions for change. Mark Ahn, Keri Chesney, Chris MacCrate, Guy Mullins, Stephen Hustedde, Greg Nigh, Doreen Mauro, Marc vanHorne, Ken Rudich, and Fred Huff, along with other current or former employees of the Applied Learning Technologies Institute and the University Technology Office, deserve special recognition.

We wish to thank the following reviewers of *Concepts of Fitness and Wellness*, whose comments and suggestions were very helpful in making the seventh edition of this text as complete, accurate, and current as possible: Kym Y. Atwood, University of West Florida; Amy Bowersock, University of Tampa; Karla M. Bruntzel, Missouri Valley College; P. Greg Comfort, Missouri Baptist University; Betsy Danner, Ouachita Baptist University; Janelle Handlos, University of Montana–Western; Arthur A. Jones, St. Petersburg College; Richard Krejci, Columbia College; Alexis Hayes Lowe, Palo Alto Community College; Matthew Rhea, Southern Utah University; McKinley Thomas, Augusta State University; and Patricia A. Zezula, Huntington University.

We also want to thank the following people who reviewed the current edition of *Concepts of Physical Fitness*: Diane Bartholomew, Graceland University; J. Jesse DeMello, Louisiana State University-Shreveport; Linda Gazzillo Diaz, William Patterson University; Caprice Dodson, Houston Community College; Jeffrey T. Godin, Fitchburg State College; Amy Howton, Kennesaw State University; Wayne Jacobs, LeTourneau University; James E. Leone, Southern Illinois University-Carbondale; Paul Luebbers, Virginia Commmonwealth University; Kelly Quick, University of Sioux Falls; Christine Rockey, Coastal Carolina University; Garth D. Schoffman, University of Akron; and Louise Whitney; Lansing Community College.

For reviewing *Fundamental Concepts of Fitness and Wellness*, we wish to thank: Ann Bolton, Maranatha Baptist Bible College; Terry Dibble, Oakland Community College; Janet Hamilton, Clayton State University; William Kuehl, Grand Canyon University; Garry Ladd, Southwestern Illinois College; Charles Pelitera, Canisius College; and Wiley T. Piazza, Northern Kentucky University.

In addition, we want to acknowledge the following individuals who aided us in the preparation of earlier editions: Kelly Adam, Nena Amundson, James Angel, Vincent Angotti, Candi D. Ashley, Jeanne Ashley, Debra Atkinson, Mark Bailey, Carl Beal, Debra A. Beal, Roger Bishop, Eugene B. Blackwell, Laura L. Borsdorf, Marika Botha, David S. Brewster, Stanley Brown, Joseph W. Bubenas, Kenneth L. Cameron, Ronnie Carda, Bill Carr, Curt W. Cattau, Robert Clayton, Bridget Cobb, Ruth Cohoon, Sarah Collie, Cindy Ekstedt Connelly, Karen Cookson, John Dippel, Dennis Docheff, Joseph Donnelly, Paul Downing, J. Ellen Eason, Melvin Ezell Jr., Linda Farver, Bridget A. Finley, Pat Floyd, Diane Sanders Flickner,

Judy Fox, James A. Gemar, Ragen Gwin, Earlene Hannah, Carole J. Hanson, James Harvey, John Hayes, Lisa Hibbard, Virginia L. Hicks, Robin Hoppenworth, David Horton, Sister Janice Iverson, Tony Jadin, Martin W. Johnson, William B. Karper, Dawn Ketterman-Benner, Todd Kleinfelter, Larry E. Knuth, Jon Kolb, Craig Koppelman, Mary Jeanne Kuhar, Ron Lawman, Jennifer L. H. Lechner, Keri Lewis, James Marett, R. Cody McMurtry, Pat McSwegin, Betty McVaigh, John Merriman, Beverly F. Mitchell, Sandra Morgan, Robert J. Mravetz, J. Dirk Nelson, J. D. Parsley, George Perkins, Judi Phillips, Lindy S. Pickard, William Podoll, Karen (Pea) Poole, Robert Pugh, Harold L. Rainwater, Robert W. Rausch Jr., Larry Reagan, Peter Rehor, Stan Rettew, Mary Rice, Amy P. Richardson, Sharon Rifkin, Rose Schmitz, James Shebban, James J. Sheehan, Jan Sholes, Mary Slaughter, Robert L. Slevin, Laurel Smith, Dixie Stanforth, Robert Stokes, Jack Clayton Stovall, Dawn Strout, Frederick C. Surgent, Laura Switzer, Terry R. Tabor, Thomas E. Temples, Paul H. Todd, Susan M. Todd, Don Torok, Maridy Troy, Kenneth R. Turley, Karen Watkins, Kenneth E. Weatherman, John R. Webster, James R. Whitehead, Marjorie Avery Willard, Patty Williams, Tillman (Chuck) Williams, Newton Wilkes, Bruce Wilson, Dennis Wilson, and Ann Woodard.

Finally, we want to acknowledge others who have contributed, including Virginia Atkins, Charles Cicciarella, Donna Landers, Susan Miller, Robert Pangrazi, Karen Ward, Darl Waterman, and Weimo Zhu. Among other important contributors are former graduate students who have contributed ideas, made corrections, and contributed in other untold ways to the success of these books. We wish to acknowledge Jeff Boone, Laura Borsdorf, Lisa Chase, Tom Cuddihy, Darren Dale, Bo Fernhall, Ken Fox, Connie Fye, Louie Garcia, Steve Feyrer-Melk, Sarah Keup, Guy LeMasurier, James McClain, Kirk Rose, Jack Rutherford, Cara Sidman, Scott Slava, Dave Thomas, Min Qui Wang, Jim Whitehead, Bridgette Wilde, and Ashley Woodcock.

A very special thanks goes to David E. Corbin of the University of Nebraska at Omaha and Jodi Hickman LeMasurier. Dr. Corbin is a health educator who has provided valuable assistance. Jodi spent many hours researching photos for this book. We especially appreciate the Spanish translation of vocabulary terms by Julio Morales from Lamar University, as well as the thorough and excellent proofreading by Bob Widen. We also want to thank Cara Sidman and Michelle Ihmels for developing and coordinating all the supplemental materials. Finally, we want to thank Ron Hager and Lynda Ransdell for their assistance with the development of the Web resources and the development of the Test Bank materials for past editions.

We also would like to thank all past editors (there have been many), including Michelle Turenne, and our current editors, Christopher Johnson, Carlotta Seely, Jill Eccher, and Melissa Williams, who used their expertise to make the *Concepts* books outstanding.

Charles B. Corbin
Gregory J. Welk
William R. Corbin
Karen A. Welk

Dedication

The authors wish to dedicate this book in loving memory of **Charles Samuel "Charlie" Corbin** (April 22, 2004–July 18, 2004), son of Will and Suzi Corbin, grandson of Cathie and Chuck Corbin, and **Alyson Welk** (April 30, 1995–June 2, 2003), daughter of Karen and Greg Welk.

A Guided Tour of
Concepts of Fitness and Wellness

Looking for the latest information in health, wellness, and fitness? Making plans for a healthier lifestyle? Want to get the most out of this course? The special features in *Concepts of Fitness and Wellness* are designed to help you do all this and more! Let's take a look inside the book.

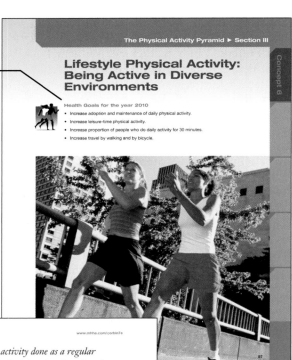

Health Goals

Each concept highlights certain national health goals presented in *Healthy People 2010.* As you plan your individual goals for optimal health, consider how they fit into the big picture.

Concept Statement

What's the theme for each concept in this book? The concept statement tells you in just one or two sentences. The content that follows builds on that theme, offering information that's clear, practical, and authoritative.

On the Web:
www.mhhe.com/corbinweb

On the Web is a valuable resource designed specially for *Concepts of Fitness and Wellness.* Focusing on fitness and wellness topics, this feature invites you to go beyond the pages of this text for different approaches, greater depth, and new ideas.

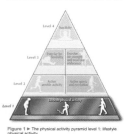

Web Icon

Used throughout each concept, this icon directs you to the On the Web feature. Take a minute to explore what it has to offer and learn more.

Illustration Program

The full-color illustrations in this text are both attractive and educational. With clarity and precision, they make the text discussions vivid, enhancing understanding and learning.

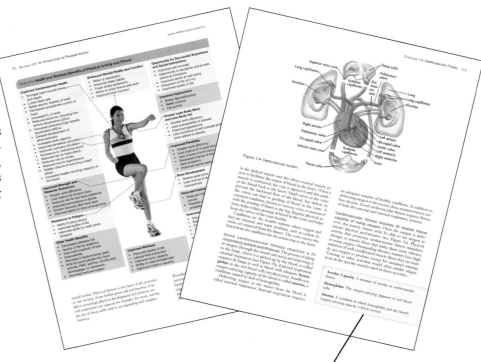

Definition Boxes

All key terms are set in **bold** type in the text discussions. The nearby definition box highlights these terms for easy reference and review.

Table of Exercises

Many of the concepts present tables of exercises for helping you improve your physical fitness, such as trunk stretching exercises. The illustrations, which demonstrate proper position and technique, are accompanied by step-by-step descriptions of what to do. Variations are suggested, and cautions are offered for safety.

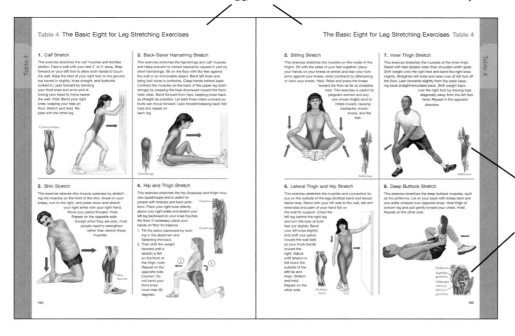

Muscle Illustrations

Many of the exercises presented in this book include an exciting new feature that highlights the main muscle at work in the exercise. The illustration showing how to perform the exercise is accompanied by an anatomic drawing of the musculature involved.

Strategies for Action

What steps do you need to take to achieve your healthy lifestyle goals? This feature offers practical advice on putting what you're learning into practice in your daily life.

Online Learning Center: www.mhhe.com/corbin7e

The Online Learning Center offers a wide range of resources that make learning interesting and effective: Video Activities, On the Web, Application Assignments, Concept Terms, Concept Outlines, Interactive Quizzes, and Downloadable Audio Summaries.

Suggested Readings

Recent readings are listed at the end of each concept for easy reference. You can also check the On the Web feature for more reading resources.

Web Resources

This feature presents a list of sites that include information on concept-related topics, making exploration easy and fun.

Technology Update

Need a little help on the road to better fitness and wellness? Read about the latest that technology has to offer—such as PDAs and the MyPyramid Tracker—to help you monitor your progress and keep on track.

In the News

What's the latest in health, wellness, and fitness information? This feature will keep you up-to-date on everything from organic foods to ecotourism.

Lab Resource Materials

Certain lab activities are preceded by a special page that explains exactly what you'll need to perform the lab. This helps you be prepared and saves time.

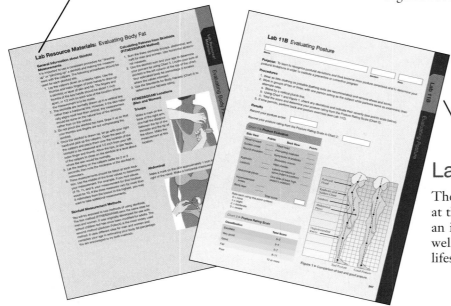

Labs (Tear-Out)

The lab activities are presented on tear-out pages at the end of each concept. These activities are an important way of assessing your fitness and wellness, planning your approach to a healthier lifestyle, and monitoring your progress.

Health, Wellness, Fitness, and Healthy Lifestyles: An Introduction

Health Goals for the year 2010

- Increase quality and years of healthy life.
- Eliminate health disparities.
- Increase incidence of people reporting "healthy days."
- Increase access to health information and services for all people.

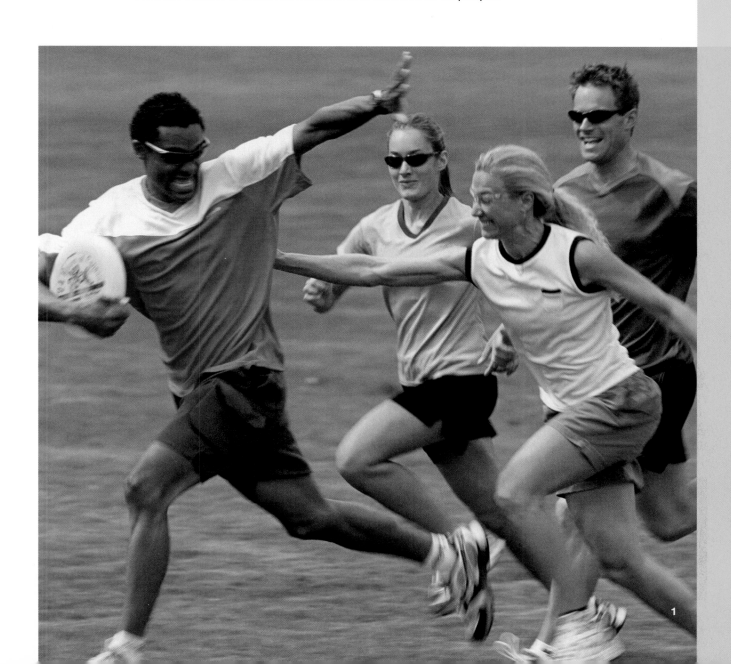

Good health, wellness, fitness, and healthy lifestyles are important for all people.

Internet Access

Web 01

There is a wealth of reliable health and wellness information that cannot be included in this text because of space limitations. The Internet provides an easy and effective method of delivering this extra content. Internet icons are located throughout this text to direct you to additional information related to topics at the site of the icon. To access this content:

1. Type in this URL: **www.mhhe.com/corbinweb**
2. See On the Web list of concepts.
3. Click on the concept number you want to view.

You can also access all Web icons shown in this text by visiting the Online Learning Center:

1. Type in this URL: **www.mhhe.com/corbin7e**
2. Choose "Student Edition."
3. Use the drop-down menu and select "On the Web."
4. Choose the concept you want to view.

The Online Learning Center provides you with much more than access to Internet icon content. Also included are video activities, Web links, interactive quizzes, concept outlines and terms, Web resources, and downloadable audio summaries.

National Health Goals

At the beginning of each concept in this book is a section containing abbreviated statements of the national health goals from the document *Healthy People 2010: National Health Promotion and Disease Prevention Objectives.* These statements, established by expert groups representing more than 350 national organizations, are intended as realistic national health goals to be

On the Web

Web 01
www.mhhe.com/corbinweb
Log on to this URL before reading this concept. See On the Web list of concepts. Click on the concept number you want to view. To access supplemental information, click on the number shown at each Web icon.

achieved by the year 2010. Health goals established two decades ago focused on disease treatment, while the current goals focus on disease prevention and health promotion. This book is written with the achievement of these important health goals in mind.

Web 01
For *Healthy People 2010,* achieving the vision of "healthy people in healthy communities" is paramount. There are two central goals. The first goal focuses on quality of life, well-being, and functional capacity—all important wellness considerations. This emphasis is consistent with the **World Health Organization**'s focus on quality of life and its efforts to break down the artificial divisions between physical and mental well-being. Second, the national health goals for 2010 take the "bold step" of trying to "eliminate" health disparities, as opposed to reducing them. In 2005, a midcourse review was conducted to determine the status of the 2010 health goals. New science and available data were used to modify goals and to eliminate goals for which there were insufficient data. More than 40 goals were eliminated and many more were revised. Consistent with the revised health goals for the new millennium, this book is designed to aid all people in adopting healthy lifestyles to achieve lifetime health, wellness, and fitness.

Health and Wellness

Good health is of primary importance to adults in our society. When polled about important social values, 99 percent of adults in the United States identified "being in good **health**" as one of their major concerns. The two other concerns expressed most often were good family life and good self-image. The 1 percent who did not identify good health as an important concern had no opinion on any social issues. Among those polled, none felt that good health was unimportant. Results of surveys in Canada and other Western nations show similar interests in good health.

Increasing the span of healthy life is a major health goal. The principal public health goal of Western nations is to increase the healthy life span of all individuals. Over the past 100 years the life expectancy of the average person has increased by 60 percent. Currently, life expectancy is at a record high of 77.6 for people in the United States. Increasing healthy life span means more than just living longer. It also means having fewer unhealthy years. Unhealthy years include those with illness, impaired function, and/or significantly
Web 02

reduced quality of life. Over the past decade the number of unhealthy years has decreased considerably from near 10 to approximately 8 years. As illustrated in Figure 1, average life expectancy in North America is related to the country in which you live, with Canadians living the longest and Mexicans having the lowest life expectancy. In the U.S., as well as in Canada and Mexico, women have a greater life expectancy than men, though men typically have fewer unhealthy years.

Eliminating health disparities is a major national health goal. Health varies greatly with ethnicity, income, gender, and age. For example, African Americans, Hispanics, and Native Americans have a shorter life expectancy than White non–Hispanics and men have a shorter life expectancy than women. Health disparities also exist in quality of life. One method of assessing disparities in quality of life is to compare the number of **healthy days** diverse groups experience each month. Minorities, including African Americans, Hispanics and Native Americans, experience about 24 healthy days each month compared to 25 for White non–Hispanics. People with very low income typically have 22 healthy days per month, compared with 26 days for those with high income. Men have a higher number of healthy days than women. Healthy days decrease as we age, with young adults experiencing more healthy days each month than older adults. Over the past two decades, there has been a steady decline in healthy days for the average person, no doubt because of the increase in the number of older adults in our society.

The relatively higher number of unhealthy days for women is, at least in part, because they live longer and

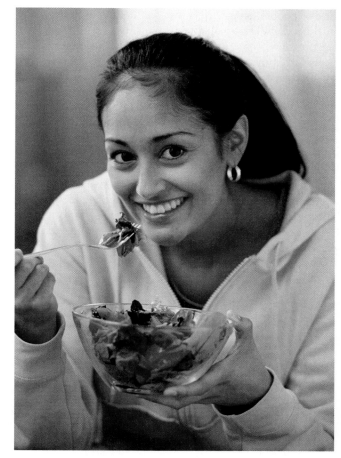

Healthy lifestyles are the principal contributor to health and wellness.

for this reason have more unhealthy years late in life. Number of healthy days takes its biggest drop after age 75. Disparities in healthy days by level of income may be due to environmental, social or cultural factors as well as less access to preventive care. Both physical and mental

World Health Organization (WHO) WHO is the United Nations' agency for health and has 192 member countries. Its principal goal is the attainment of the highest possible level of health for all people. WHO has been instrumental in making health policy and in implementing health programs worldwide since its inception in 1948.

Health Optimal well-being that contributes to one's quality of life. It is more that freedom from disease and illness, though freedom from disease is important to good health. Optimal health includes high-level mental, social, emotional, spiritual, and physical wellness within the limits of one's heredity and personal abilities.

Healthy Days A self-rating of the number of days (per week or month) a person considers himself or herself to be in good or better than good health.

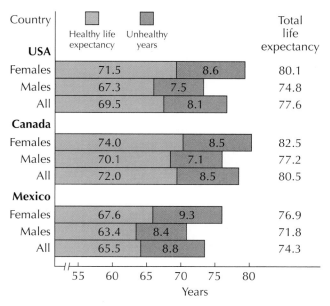

Country	Healthy life expectancy	Unhealthy years	Total life expectancy
USA			
Females	71.5	8.6	80.1
Males	67.3	7.5	74.8
All	69.5	8.1	77.6
Canada			
Females	74.0	8.5	82.5
Males	70.1	7.1	77.2
All	72.0	8.5	80.5
Mexico			
Females	67.6	9.3	76.9
Males	63.4	8.4	71.8
All	65.5	8.8	74.3

55 60 65 70 75 80
Years

Figure 1 ▶ Healthy life expectancy for North America.

Sources: World Health Organization and National Center for Health Statistics.

health problems are the most frequent reasons for unhealthy days. Physical illness, pain, depression, anxiety, sleeplessness, and limitations in ability to function or perform enjoyable activities are the problems most frequently reported.

Health is more than freedom from illness and disease. Over 50 years ago, the World Health Organization defined health as more than freedom from illness, disease, and debilitating conditions. Prior to that time, you were considered to be "healthy" if you were not sick. In recent years, health experts have expanded the definition of health to include wellness as exemplified by "quality of life" and "a sense of well-being."

Figure 2 illustrates the modern concept of health. This general state of being is characterized by freedom from disease and debilitating conditions (outer circle), as well as wellness (center circle).

Wellness is the positive component of optimal health. Death, disease, **illness,** and debilitating conditions are negative components that detract from optimal health. Death is the ultimate opposite of optimal health. Disease, illness, and debilitating conditions obviously detract from optimal health. **Wellness** has been recognized as the positive component of optimal health. It is characterized by a sense of well-being reflected in optimal functioning, health–related **quality of life,** meaningful work, and a contribution to society. Wellness allows the expansion of one's potential to live and work effectively and to make a significant contribution to society. *Healthy People 2010* objectives use the term *health-related quality of life* to describe a general sense of happiness and satisfaction with life.

Health and wellness are personal. Every individual is different from all others. Health and wellness depend on each person's unique characteristics. Making comparisons to other people on specific characteristics may produce feelings of inadequacy that detract from one's profile of total health and wellness. Each of us has personal limitations and strengths. Focusing on strengths and learning to accommodate weaknesses are essential keys to optimal health and wellness.

Health and wellness are multidimensional. The dimensions of health and wellness include the emotional–mental, intellectual, social, spiritual, and physical. Table 1 describes the various dimensions and Figure 3 illustrates the importance of each one for optimal health and wellness. Some people include environmental and vocational dimensions in addition to the five described in Figure 3. In this book, health and wellness are considered to be personal factors. While the environment and one's vocation can certainly influence the adoption and maintenance of healthy lifestyles, they are not viewed as independent (or personal) dimensions of wellness. The importance of environmental factors for health and wellness are described through the book—particularly in the last concept. Specific references are made to the dimensions described in Table 1 and Table 2.

Wellness reflects how one feels about life, as well as one's ability to function effectively. A positive total outlook on life is essential to each of the wellness dimensions. As illustrated in Table 2, a "well" person is satisfied in work, is spiritually fulfilled, enjoys leisure time, is physically fit, is socially involved, and has a positive emotional-mental outlook. He or she is happy and fulfilled.

The way one perceives each of the dimensions of wellness affects one's total outlook. Researchers use the term *self–perceptions* to describe these feelings. Many researchers

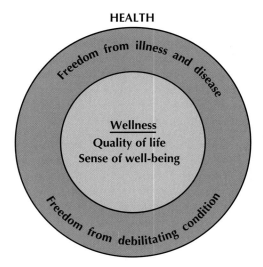

Figure 2 ▶ A model of optimal health, including wellness.

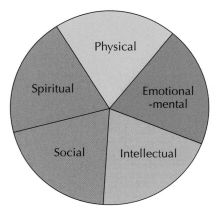

Figure 3 ▶ The dimensions of health and wellness.

Table 1 ▶ Definitions of Health and Wellness Dimensions

Emotional-mental health—A person with emotional health is free from emotional/mental illnesses such as clinical depression, and possesses emotional wellness. The goals for the nation's health refer to mental rather than emotional health and wellness. In this book, mental health and wellness are considered to be the same as emotional health and wellness.

Emotional/mental wellness—Emotional wellness is a person's ability to cope with daily circumstances and to deal with personal feelings in a positive, optimistic, and constructive manner. A person with emotional wellness is generally characterized as happy instead of depressed.

Intellectual health—A person with intellectual health is free from illnesses that invade the brain and other systems that allow learning. A person with intellectual health also possesses intellectual wellness.

Intellectual wellness—Intellectual wellness is a person's ability to learn and to use information to enhance the quality of daily living and optimal functioning. A person with intellectual wellness is generally characterized as informed instead of ignorant.

Physical health—A person with physical health is free from illnesses that affect the physiological systems of the body, such as the heart and the nervous system. A person with physical health possesses an adequate level of physical fitness and physical wellness.

Physical wellness—Physical wellness is a person's ability to function effectively in meeting the demands of the day's work and to use free time effectively. Physical wellness includes good physical fitness and the possession of useful motor skills. A person with physical wellness is generally characterized as fit instead of unfit.

Social health—A person with social health is free from illnesses or conditions that severely limit functioning in society, including antisocial pathologies.

Social wellness—Social wellness is a person's ability to interact with others successfully and to establish meaningful relationships that enhance the quality of life for all people involved in the interaction (including self). A person with social wellness is generally characterized as involved instead of lonely.

Spiritual health—Spiritual health is the one component of health that is totally comprised of the wellness dimension; for this reason, spiritual health is considered to be synonymous with spiritual wellness.

Spiritual wellness—Spiritual wellness is a person's ability to establish a values system and act on the system of beliefs, as well as to establish and carry out meaningful and constructive lifetime goals. Spiritual wellness is often based on a belief in a force greater than the individual that helps one contribute to an improved quality of life for all people. A person with spiritual wellness is generally characterized as fulfilled instead of unfulfilled.

Table 2 ▶ The Dimensions of Wellness

Wellness Dimension	Negative — — — — — — — Positive
Emotional-mental	Depressed — — — — — — Happy
Intellectual	Ignorant — — — — — — Informed
Physical	Unfit — — — — — — — — Fit
Social	Lonely — — — — — — — Involved
Spiritual	Unfulfilled — — — — — — Fulfilled
Total outlook	Negative — — — — — — Positive

believe that self-perceptions about wellness are more important than actual circumstances or a person's actual state of being. For example, a person who has an important job may find less meaning and job satisfaction than another person with a much less important job. Apparently, one of the important factors for a person who has achieved high-level wellness and a positive outlook on life is the ability to reward himself or herself. Some people, however, seem unable to give themselves credit for their successes. The development of a system that allows a person to perceive the self positively is important. Of course, the adoption of positive **lifestyles** that encourage improved self-perceptions is also important. The questionnaire in Lab 1A will help you assess your self-perceptions of the various wellness dimensions. For optimal wellness, it is important to find positive feelings about each dimension.

Illness The ill feeling and/or symptoms associated with a disease or circumstances that upset homeostasis.

Wellness The integration of many different components (social, emotional-mental, spiritual, and physical) that expand one's potential to live (quality of life) and work effectively and to make a significant contribution to society. Wellness reflects how one feels (a sense of well-being) about life, as well as one's ability to function effectively. Wellness, as opposed to illness (a negative), is sometimes described as the positive component of good health.

Quality of Life A term used to describe wellness. An individual with quality of life can enjoyably do the activities of life with little or no limitation and can function independently. Individual quality of life requires a pleasant and supportive community.

Lifestyles Patterns of behavior or ways an individual typically lives.

Health and wellness are integrated states of being. The segmented pictures of health and wellness shown in Figure 3 and Tables 1 and 2 are used only to illustrate the multidimensional nature of health and wellness. In reality, health and wellness are integrated states of being that can best be depicted as threads that are woven together to produce a larger, integrated fabric. Each dimension relates to each of the others and overlaps all the others. The overlap is so frequent and so great that the specific contribution of each thread is almost indistinguishable when looking at the total (Figure 4). The total is clearly greater than the sum of the parts.

It is possible to possess health and wellness while being ill or possessing a debilitating condition. Many illnesses are curable and may have only a temporary effect on health. Others, such as Type I diabetes, are not curable but can be managed with proper eating, physical activity, and sound medical treatment. Those with manageable conditions may, however, be at risk for other health problems. For example, unmanaged diabetes is associated with a high risk for heart disease and other health problems.

Debilitating conditions, such as the loss of a limb or loss of function in a body part, can contribute to a lower level of functioning or an increased risk for illness and thus to poor health. On the other hand, such conditions need not limit wellness. A person with a debilitating condition who has a positive outlook on life may have better overall health than a person with a poor outlook on life but no debilitating condition.

Just as wellness is possible among those with illness and disability, evidence is accumulating that people with a positive outlook are better able to resist the progress of disease and illness than are those with a negative outlook. Thinking positive thoughts has been associated with enhanced results from various medical treatments and surgical procedures.

Wellness is a useful term that may be used by the uninformed as well as experts. Unfortunately, some individuals and groups have tried to identify wellness with products and services that prom-

Web 04

ise benefits that cannot be documented. Because well-being is a subjective feeling, it is easy for unscrupulous people to make claims of improved wellness for their product or service without facts to back them up.

Holistic health is a term that is similarly abused. Optimal health includes many areas; thus, the term *holistic* (total) is appropriate. In fact, the word *health* originates from a root word meaning "wholeness." Unfortunately, questionable health practices are sometimes promoted under the guise of holistic health. Care should be used when considering services and products that make claims of wellness and/or holistic health to be sure that they are legitimate.

Physical Fitness

Physical fitness is a multidimensional state of being. **Physical fitness** is the body's ability to function efficiently and effectively. It is a state of being that consists of at least five health-related and six skill-related physical fitness components, each of which contributes to total quality of life. Physical fitness is associated with a person's ability to work effectively, enjoy leisure time, be healthy, resist **hypokinetic diseases or conditions,** and meet emergency situations. It is related to, but different from, health and wellness. Although the development of physical fitness is the result of many things, optimal physical fitness is not possible without regular physical activity.

The health-related components of physical fitness are directly associated with good health. The five components of health-related physical fitness are body composition, cardiovascular fitness, flexibility, muscular endurance, and strength (see Figure 5). Each health–related fitness characteristic has a direct relationship to good health and reduced risk for hypokinetic disease. It is for this reason that the five health-related physical fitness components are emphasized in this book.

Possessing a moderate amount of each component of health-related fitness is essential to disease prevention and health promotion, but it is not essential to have exceptionally high levels of fitness to achieve health benefits. High levels of health-related fitness relate more to performance than to health benefits. For example, moderate amounts of strength are necessary to prevent back and posture problems, whereas high levels of strength contribute most to improved performance in activities such as football and jobs involving heavy lifting.

The skill-related components of physical fitness are associated more with performance than with good health. The components of skill-related physical fitness are agility, balance, coordination, power, reaction time, and speed (see Figure 6). They are called skill-related

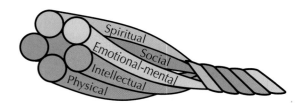

Figure 4 ▶ The integration of wellness dimensions.

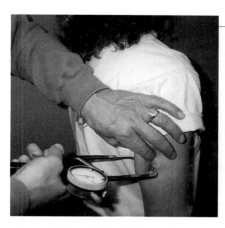

Body composition—The relative percentage of muscle, fat, bone, and other tissues that comprise the body. A fit person has a relatively low, but not too low, percentage of body fat (body fatness).

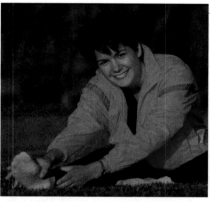

Flexibility—The range of motion available in a joint. It is affected by muscle length, joint structure, and other factors. A fit person can move the body joints through a full range of motion in work and in play.

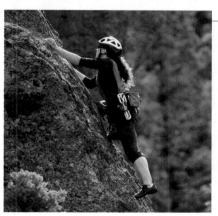

Strength—The ability of the muscles to exert an external force or to lift a heavy weight. A fit person can do work or play that involves exerting force, such as lifting or controlling one's own body weight.

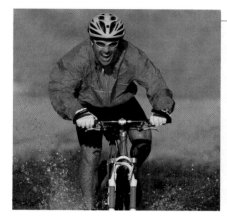

Cardiovascular fitness—The ability of the heart, blood vessels, blood, and respiratory system to supply nutrients and oxygen to the muscles and the ability of the muscles to utilize fuel to allow sustained exercise. A fit person can persist in physical activity for relatively long periods without undue stress.

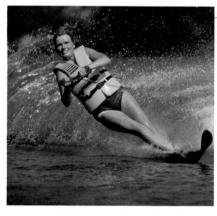

Muscular endurance—The ability of the muscles to exert themselves repeatedly. A fit person can repeat movements for a long period without undue fatigue.

Figure 5 ▶ Components of health-related physical fitness.

because people who possess them find it easy to achieve high levels of performance in motor skills, such as those required in sports and in specific types of jobs. Power is sometimes referred to as a combined component of fitness, since it requires both strength (a health-related component) and speed (a skill-related component). Because most experts consider power to be associated more with performance than with good health, it is classified as a skill-related component of fitness in this book.

Physical Fitness The body's ability to function efficiently and effectively. It consists of health-related physical fitness and skill-related physical fitness, which have at least 11 components, each of which contributes to total quality of life. Physical fitness also includes metabolic fitness and bone integrity. Physical fitness is associated with a person's ability to work effectively, enjoy leisure time, be healthy, resist hypokinetic diseases, and meet emergency situations. It is related to, but different from, health, wellness, and the psychological, sociological, emotional-mental, and spiritual components of fitness. Although the development of physical fitness is the result of many things, optimal physical fitness is not possible without regular exercise.

Hypokinetic Diseases or Conditions *Hypo-* means "under" or "too little," and *-kinetic* means "movement" or "activity." Thus, *hypokinetic* means "too little activity." A hypokinetic disease or condition is one associated with lack of physical activity or too little regular exercise. Examples include heart disease, low back pain, adult-onset diabetes, and obesity.

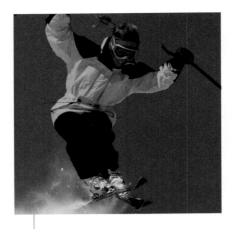

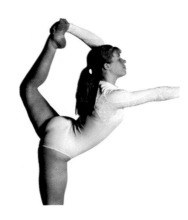

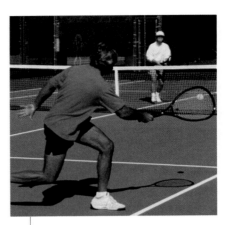

Agility—The ability to rapidly and accurately change the direction of the movement of the entire body in space. Skiing and wrestling are examples of activities that require exceptional agility.

Balance—The maintenance of equilibrium while stationary or while moving. Water skiing, performing on the balance beam, and working as a riveter on a high-rise building are activities that require exceptional balance.

Coordination—The ability to use the senses with the body parts to perform motor tasks smoothly and accurately. Juggling, hitting a tennis ball, and kicking a ball are examples of activities requiring good coordination.

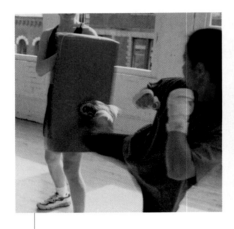

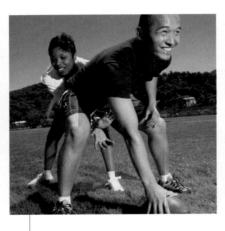

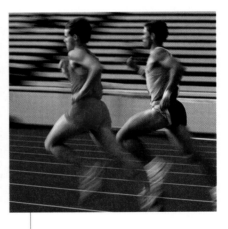

Power—The ability to transfer energy into force at a fast rate. Throwing the discus and putting the shot are activities that require considerable power.

Reaction time—The time elapsed between stimulation and the beginning of reaction to that stimulation. Driving a racing car and starting a sprint race require good reaction time.

Speed—The ability to perform a movement in a short period of time. Sprinters and wide receivers in football need good foot and leg speed.

Figure 6 ▶ Components of skill-related physical fitness.

Skill–related fitness is sometimes called sports fitness or motor fitness.

There is little doubt that other abilities could be classified as skill-related fitness components. Also, each part of skill-related fitness is multidimensional. For example, coordination could be hand-eye coordination, such as batting a ball; foot-eye coordination, such as kicking a ball; or any of many other possibilities. The six parts of skill-related fitness identified here are those commonly associated with successful sports and work performance. Each could be measured in ways other than those presented in this book.

Measurements are provided to help you understand the nature of total physical fitness and to help you make important decisions about lifetime physical activity.

Metabolic fitness is a nonperformance component of total fitness. Physical activity can provide health benefits that are independent of changes in traditional health-related fitness measures. Physical activity promotes good **metabolic fitness,** a state associated with reduced risk for many chronic diseases. People with a cluster of low metabolic fitness characteristics are said to have metabolic symndrome (also known as Syndrome X). Metabolic syndrome is discussed in more detail in Concept 4.

Bone integrity is often considered to be a nonperformance measure of fitness. Traditional definitions do not include **bone integrity** as a part of physical fitness, but some experts feel that they should. Like metabolic fitness, bone integrity cannot be assessed with performance measures the way most health-related fitness parts can. Regardless of whether bone integrity is considered a part of fitness or a component of health, strong, healthy bones are important to optimal health and are associated with regular physical activity and sound diet.

The many components of physical fitness are specific but are also interrelated. Physical fitness is a combination of several aspects, rather than a single characteristic. A fit person possesses at least adequate levels of each of the health-related, skill-related, and metabolic fitness components. Some relationships exist among various fitness characteristics, but each of the components of physical fitness is separate and different from the others. For example, people who possess exceptional strength may not have good cardiovascular fitness, and those who have good coordination do not necessarily possess good flexibility.

Good physical fitness is important, but it is not the same as physical health and wellness. Good physical fitness contributes directly to the physical component of good health and wellness and indirectly to the other four components. Good fitness has been shown to be associated with reduced risk for chronic diseases, such as heart disease, and has been shown to reduce the consequences of many debilitating conditions. In addition, good fitness contributes to wellness by helping us look our best, feel good, and enjoy life. Other physical factors can also influence health and wellness. For example, having good physical skills enhances quality of life by allowing us to participate in enjoyable activities, such as tennis, golf, and bowling. Although fitness can assist us in performing these activities, regular practice is also necessary. Another example is the ability to fight off viral and bacterial infections. Although fitness can promote a strong immune system, other physical factors can influence our susceptibility to these and other conditions.

A Model for Achieving and Maintaining Lifelong Health, Wellness, and Fitness

Many factors are important in developing lifetime health, wellness, and fitness, and some are more in your control than others. Figure 7 provides a model for describing many of the factors that contribute to health,

wellness, and fitness. Central to the model are health, wellness, and fitness because these are the states of being (shaded in green and yellow) that each of us wants to achieve. Around the periphery are the factors that influence these states of being. Those shaded in blue are the factors over which you have the least control (heredity, age, and disability). Those shaded in light blue (health care and environmental factors) are factors over which you have some control but are those that you have less ability to change than the factors shaded in red. Those shaded in red are the factors over which you have greater control (healthy lifestyles and personal actions/interactions, cognitions and emotions).

Factors Influencing Health, Wellness, and Fitness

Heredity (human biology) is a factor over which we have little control. Experts estimate that human biology, or heredity, accounts for 16 percent of all health problems, including early death. Heredity influences each of the parts of health-related physical fitness, including our tendencies to build muscle and to deposit body fat. Each of us reaps different benefits from the same healthy lifestyles, based on our hereditary tendencies. Even more important is that predispositions to diseases are inherited. For example, some early deaths are a result of untreatable hereditary conditions (e.g., congenital heart defects). Obviously, some inherited conditions are manageable (e.g., diabetes) with proper medical supervision and appropriate lifestyles. Heredity is a factor over which we have little control and is, therefore, illustrated in dark blue in Figure 7. Each of us can limit the effects of heredity by being aware of our personal family history and by making efforts to best manage those factors over which we do have control.

In the concepts that follow, you will learn more about heredity and how it affects health, wellness, and fitness.

Web 05 **Health, wellness, and fitness are influenced by the aging of our population.** As noted previously, the average life expectancy in Western cultures has increased dramatically in recent decades. By

---

Metabolic Fitness Metabolic fitness is a positive state of the physiological systems commonly associated with reduced risk for chronic diseases such as diabetes and heart disease. Metabolic fitness is evidenced by healthy blood fat (lipid) profiles, healthy blood pressure, healthy blood sugar and insulin levels, and other nonperformance measures.

Bone Integrity Soundness of the bones is associated with high density and absence of symptoms of deterioration.

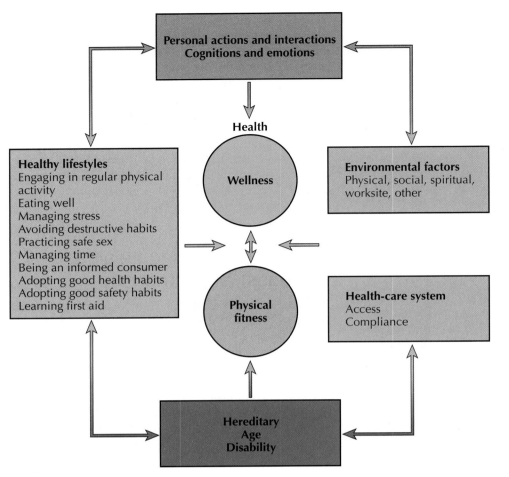

Figure 7 ▶ Factors influencing health, wellness, and physical fitness.

Age is shaded in dark blue in Figure 7 because it is a factor that you cannot control. However, healthy lifestyles can reduce the effects of aging on health, wellness, and fitness. As detailed later in this book, healthy lifestyles can extend life and have a positive effect on quality of life.

Disabilities can affect, but do not necessarily limit, health, wellness, and fitness. Disabilities typically result from factors beyond control (shaded in blue in Figure 7). Many types of disabilities affect health, fitness, and wellness. An objective disability (e.g., loss of a limb, impaired intellectual functioning) can make it difficult to function in certain circumstances but need not limit health, wellness, and fitness. All people have a limitation of one kind or another. Societal efforts to help all people function within their limitations can help everyone, including people with disabilities, have a positive outlook on life and experience a high quality of life. With assistance from an instructor, it is possible for all people to adapt the information in this book for use in promoting heath, wellness, and fitness.

the year 2040, the number of Americans over age 65 will double, accounting for more than 20 percent of the total population. By the year 2010, more than 100,000 people will be over 100. The definition of old is changing, with most people believing that a person is not old until age 71 or older. Nearly a quarter of the population believes that being old begins at 81.

Whatever the standard for being old, age is a factor over which we have no control. The major health and wellness concerns of older adults include losing health, losing the ability to care for oneself, losing mental abilities, running out of money, being a burden to family, and being alone. Chronic pain is also a major problem among older adults. Nearly 30 percent of adults over 65 experience chronic pain, as opposed to 3 percent of those under 30. Nearly 60 percent of older adults experience frequent pain, as opposed to 17 percent of those under 30. Older adults have 36 percent more unhealthy days than young adults.

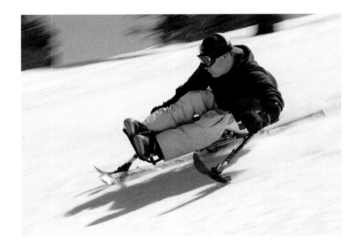

Physical activity is for everyone.

Web 07 **The health-care system affects our ability to overcome illness and improve our quality of life.** Approximately 10 percent of unnecessary deaths occurs as a result of disparities in the health-care system. The quality of life for those who are sick and those who tend to be sick is influenced greatly by the type of medical care they receive. Access to health care is not equally available to all. A recent study by the Institute of Medicine, entitled "Insuring America's Health," indicates that 18,000 people die unnecessarily in the United States each year because they lack health insurance. Those without health insurance are more likely to go to, but are less likely to be admitted to, emergency rooms; are less likely to get high-quality medical care than those with insurance. Many of those without insurance have chronic conditions that go undetected and as a result become untreatable. One of the great health inequities is that those with lower income are less likely to be insured.

Many people fail to seek medical help even though care is accessible. Others seek medical help but fail to comply with medical advice. For example, they do not take prescribed medicine or do not follow up with treatments. Men are less likely to seek medical advice than women. For this reason, treatable conditions sometimes become untreatable. Once men seek medical care, evidence reveals, they get better care than women. Also, more of the medical research has been done on men. This is of concern, since treatments for men and women often vary for similar conditions.

Wellness as evidenced by quality of life is also influenced by the health-care system. Traditional medicine, sometimes referred to as the **medical model,** has focused primarily on the treatment of illness with medicine, rather than illness prevention and wellness promotion. Efforts to educate health-care personnel about techniques for promoting wellness have been initiated in recent years. Still, it is often up to the patient to find information about health promotion. For example, a patient with risk factors for heart disease might be advised to eat better or to exercise more, but little specific information may be offered. In Figure 7, the health-care system is colored in a light shade of blue to illustrate the fact that it is a factor over which you may have limited control.

Web 08 **The environment is a major factor affecting our health, wellness, and fitness.** Environmental factors account for nearly one-fourth of all early deaths and affect quality of life in many ways. We do have more control over environmental factors than heredity, but they are not totally under our control. For this reason, the environmental factors box is depicted in Figure 7 with a lighter shade of blue than the heredity, age, and disability box.

You can exert personal control by selecting healthy environments rather than by exposing yourself to unhealthy or unsafe environments. This includes your choice of living and work location, as well as the social, spiritual, and intellectual environments. On the other hand, circumstances may make it impossible for you to make the choices you would prefer. Important environmental factors are discussed throughout the text, particularly in Concept 6 and the final concept in the book. Some suggestions for how you can work to alter the environment in a positive way are also discussed in the last concept.

Web 09 **Personal actions, interactions, cognitions, and emotions all have an effect on health, wellness, and fitness.** Some people think that good health, wellness, and fitness are totally out of personal control. Others think that they are totally in control. Neither statement is entirely true. While heredity, age, and disability are factors you cannot control and health care and the environment are factors over which you have limited control, there are things that you can do relating to these factors. You can use your cognitive abilities to learn about your family history and use that information to limit the negative influences of heredity. You can learn how to adapt to disabilities and personal limitations, as well as to the aging process. You can do research about the health-care system and the environment to minimize the problems associated with them.

Your personal interactions also influence your health, wellness, and fitness. You are not alone in this world. Your various environments, and how you interact with them, influence you greatly. You have a choice about the environments in which you place yourself and the people with whom you interact in these environments.

Humans have the ability to think (cognitions) and to use critical thinking to make choices and to determine the actions they take and the interactions they make. Emotions also affect personal actions and interactions. A major goal of this book is to help you learn self-management skills designed to help you use your cognitive abilities to solve problems and make good decisions about good health, wellness, and fitness, as well as to help you to be in control of your emotions when taking action and making decisions that affect your health.

None of us makes perfect decisions all of the time. Sometimes we take actions and make choices based on inadequate information, faulty thinking, pressure from others, or negative influences from our emotions. While the focus of this book is on healthy lifestyles, all of the factors that influence health, wellness, and fitness will

---

Medical Model The focus of the health-care system on treating illness with medicine, with little emphasis on prevention or wellness promotion.

be discussed in greater detail in the concepts that follow. The goal is to help you consider all factors and to make informed decisions that will lead to healthful behaviors. Some strategies for action for each of the factors are presented in the final concept of this book.

Healthy Lifestyles

Lifestyle change, more that any other factor, is considered to be the best way to prevent illness and early death in our society. When people in Western society die before the are of 65, the death is considered to be early. Statistics show that more than half of early deaths are caused by unhealthy lifestyles. Based on the "leading health indicators" in *Healthy People 2010*, 11 healthy lifestyles have been associated with reduced disease risk and increased wellness. As shown in Figure 7, these lifestyles affect health, wellness, and physical fitness. The double-headed arrow between heath/wellness and physical fitness illustrates the interaction between these factors. Physical fitness is important to health and wellness development and vice versa.

Web 10

The major causes of early death have shifted from infectious diseases to chronic lifestyle–related conditions. Scientific advances and improvements in medicine and health care have dramatically reduced the incidence of infectious diseases over the past 100 years (see Table 3). Diphtheria and polio, both major causes of death in the 20th century, have been virtually eliminated in Western culture. Smallpox was globally eradicated in 1977.

Web 11

Infectious diseases have been replaced with chronic lifestyle-related conditions as the major causes of death. Four of the top six current causes of death (heart disease, cancer, stroke, and diabetes) fall into this category. The *Healthy People 2010* midcourse (2005) review indicates significant reductions in death rates from the top three causes of death over the past decade. It is interesting that the most recent data from the National Center for Health Statistics list heart disease as the leading cause of death (see Table 3). Recently, newspaper headlines proclaimed cancer to be the number 1 killer in the United States. In fact, American Cancer Society statistics indicate that cancer is the leading cause of death for those under the age of 85, while heart disease remains the leading cause of death for people of all ages. Regardless, continued progress in reducing deaths from these two conditions is critical.

HIV/AIDS, formerly in the top 10, has dropped well down the list, primarily because of the development of treatments to increase the life expectancy of those infected. Many among the top 10 are referred to as chronic lifestyle–related conditions because alteration of lifestyles can result in reduced risk for these conditions.

Table 3 ▶ Major Causes of Death

Current Rank	Cause	1900 Rank	Cause
1	Heart disease	1	Pneumonia
2	Cancer	2	Tuberculosis
3	Stroke	3	Diarrhea/enteritis
4	Bronchitis/emphysema	4	Heart disease
5	Injuries/accidents	5	Stroke
6	Diabetes	6	Liver disease
7	Pneumonia/influenza	7	Injuries
8	Alzheimer's disease	8	Cancer
9	Kidney disease	9	Senility
10	Septicemia	10	Diphtheria

Source: National Center for Health Statistics.

Healthy lifestyles are critical to wellness. Just as unhealthy lifestyles are the principal causes of modern–day illnesses, such as heart disease, cancer, and diabetes, healthy lifestyles can result in the improved feeling of wellness that is critical to optimal health. In recognizing the importance of "years of healthy life," the Public Health Service also recognizes what it calls "measures of well-being." This well-being, or wellness, is associated with social, emotional–mental, spiritual, and physical functioning. Being physically active and eating well are two healthy lifestyles that can improve well-being and add years of quality living. Many of the healthy lifestyles associated with good physical fitness and optimal wellness will be discussed in detail later in this book. The Healthy Lifestyle Questionnaire at the end of this concept gives you the opportunity to assess your current lifestyles.

Regular physical activity, sound nutrition, and stress management are considered to be priority healthy lifestyles. Three of the lifestyles listed in Figure 7 are considered to be priority healthy lifestyles. These are engaging in regular **physical activity** or **exercise,** eating well, and managing stress. There are several reasons for placing priority on these lifestyles. First, they affect the lives of all people. Second, they are lifestyles in which large numbers of people can make improvement. Finally, modest changes in these behaviors can make dramatic improvements in individual and public health. For example, statistics suggest that modest changes in physical activity patterns and nutrition can prevent more than 400,000 deaths annually. Stress also has a major impact on drug, alcohol, and smoking behavior, so managing stress can help individuals minimize or avoid those behaviors.

The other healthy lifestyles shown in Figure 7 are also very important for good health. The reason that they are not emphasized as priority lifestyles is that not all people have problems in these areas. Many healthy lifestyles will be discussed in this book, but the focus is on the priority healthy lifestyles because virtually all people can achieve positive wellness benefits if they adopt them.

The "actual causes" of most deaths are due to unhealthy lifestyles. As illustrated in Table 3, chronic diseases (e.g., heart diseases, cancer) are the direct causes of most deaths in our society. Public health experts have used epidemiological statistics to show that unhealthy lifestyles such as tobacco use, inactivity, and poor eating actually cause the chronic diseases and for this reason are referred to as the "actual causes of death." Tobacco is the leading actual cause of death, but inactivity and poor diet account for the next largest percentage of deaths (see Table 4). The percentage of deaths attributed to inactivity and poor diet has recently been questioned, but their overall influence on health is indisputable. The information presented throughout this book is designed to help you change behaviors to reduce your risk for early death from the actual causes listed in Table 4.

The HELP Philosophy

The HELP philosophy can provide a basis for making healthy lifestyle change possible. The four-letter acronym HELP summarizes the overall philosophy used in this book. Each letter in HELP characterizes an important part of the philosophy (*Health* is available to

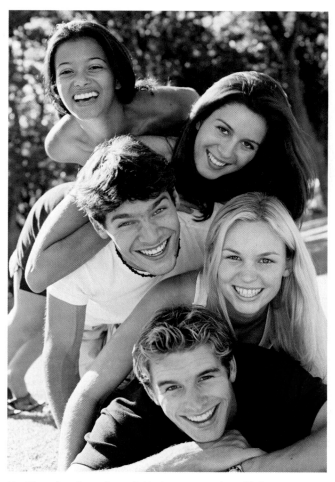

Health and wellness is available to everyone for a lifetime.

Everyone for a *Lifetime*—and it's *Personal*). The concepts in the book provide important principles and guidelines that help you adopt positive lifestyles. The labs provide experiences that help you build the behavioral skills needed to learn and maintain these lifestyles.

A personal philosophy that emphasizes health can lead to behaviors that promote it. The *H* in HELP stands for *health*. One theory that has been extensively tested indicates that people who believe in the benefits of healthy lifestyles are more likely to engage in healthy behaviors. The theory also suggests that people who state

Table 4 ▶ Actual Causes of Death in the United States		
Rank	**Actual Cause**	**Percent of Deaths**
1	Tobacco use	18.1
2	Inactivity/poor diet	16.6
3	Alcohol consumption	3.5
4	Microbial agents (flu, pneumonia)	3.1
5	Toxic agents	2.3
6	Motor vehicles	1.8
7	Firearms	1.2
8	Sexual behavior	0.8
9	Illicit drug use	0.7
10	Other	<.05

Source: Mokdad et al.

Physical Activity Generally considered to be a broad term used to describe all forms of large muscle movements, including sports, dance, games, work, lifestyle activities, and exercise for fitness. In this book, exercise and physical activity will often be used interchangeably to make reading less repetitive and more interesting.

Exercise Physical activity done for the purpose of getting physically fit.

intentions to put their beliefs into action are likely to adopt behaviors that lead to health, wellness, and fitness.

Everyone can benefit from healthy lifestyles. The *E* in HELP stands for *everyone.* Accepting the fact that anyone can change a behavior or lifestyle means that *you* are included. Nevertheless, many adults feel ineffective in making lifestyle changes. Physical activity is not just for athletes—it is for all people. Eating well is not just for other people—you can do it, too. All people can learn stress-management techniques. Healthy lifestyles can be practiced by everyone. As noted earlier in this concept, important health goals include eliminating health disparities and promoting "health for all."

Healthy behaviors are most effective when practiced for a lifetime. The *L* in HELP stands for *lifetime.* Young

people sometimes feel immortal because the harmful effects of unhealthy lifestyles are often not immediate. As we grow older, we begin to realize that we are not immortal and that unhealthy lifestyles have cumulative negative effects. Starting early in life to emphasize healthy behaviors results in long-term health, wellness, and fitness benefits. One study showed that, the longer healthy lifestyles are practiced, the greater the beneficial effects. This study also demonstrated that long-term healthy lifestyles can even overcome hereditary predisposition to illness and disease.

Healthy lifestyles should be based on personal needs. The *P* in HELP stands for *personal.* No two people are exactly alike. Just as no single pill cures all illnesses, no single lifestyle prescription exists for good health, wellness, and fitness. Each person must assess personal needs and make lifestyle changes based on those needs.

 ## Strategies for Action

Self-assessments of lifestyles will help you determine areas in which you may need changes to promote optimal health, wellness, and fitness. As you begin your study of health, wellness, fitness, and healthy lifestyles, it is wise to make a self-assessment of your current behaviors. The Healthy Lifestyle Questionnaire in the lab resource materials will allow you to assess your current lifestyle behaviors to determine if they are contributing positively to your health, wellness, and fitness. Because this questionnaire contains some very personal information, answering all the questions honestly will help you get an accurate assessment. As you continue your study, you may want to refer back to this questionnaire to see if your lifestyles have changed.

Initial self-assessments of wellness and fitness will provide information for self-comparison.
Web 12 ♥ The Healthy Lifestyle Questionnaire allows you to assess your lifestyles or behaviors. It is also important to assess your wellness and fitness at an early stage. These early assessments will only be estimates. As you continue your study, you will have the opportunity to do more

comprehensive self-assessments that will allow you to see how accurate your early estimates were.

In Lab 1A, you will estimate your wellness using a Wellness Self-Perceptions questionnaire, which assesses five wellness dimensions. Remember, wellness is a state of being that is influenced by healthy lifestyles. Because other factors, such as heredity, environment, and health care, affect wellness, it is possible to have good wellness scores even if you do not do well on the lifestyle questionnaire. However, over a lifetime, unhealthy lifestyles will catch up with you and have an influence on your wellness and fitness.

The World Health Organization (WHO) has developed a wellness instrument called the WHO Quality of Life Assessment (WHOQOL). There is a long version, with 100 items, and a shorter, 16-item version that assess physical, psychological, social, and spiritual factors, as well as general quality of life status. Some of the factors in the assessment include energy and fatigue, pain and comfort, sleep and rest, self-esteem, work capacity, effective daily living, personal relationships, and spirituality. You can learn more about this assessment by accessing the WHO website (see Web Resources) and searching for WHOQOL.

 ## Online Learning Center

www.mhhe.com/corbin7e
The Online Learning Center contains a variety of Web-based resources that will help you get the most out of this book and your course. In addition to the On the Web pages, there are video activities, interactive quizzes, application assignments, and a variety of other useful study aids. Log on to the URL above to access these resources.

Web Resources

 American Medical Association (AMA)
www.ama-assn.org
Web 13 ♥ Centers for Disease Control and Prevention (CDC)
www.cdc.gov
CDC Behavioral Risk Factor Surveillance System
www.cdc.gov/brfss

Health Canada **www.healthcanada.ca**
Healthfinder **www.healthfinder.gov**
Healthier United States **www.healthierus.gov**
Healthy People 2010 **www.health.gov/healthypeople**
Healthy People 2010 Midcourse Review
    www.healthypeople.gov/data/midcourse
Institute of Medicine **www.iom.edu**
National Center for Chronic Disease Prevention and Health
    Promotion Publications **www.cdc.gov/nccdphp/publicat.htm**
National Center for Health Statistics **www.cdc.gov/nchs/**
National Institutes of Health (NIH) **www.nih.gov**
President's Council on Physical Fitness and Sports
    www.fitness.gov
World Health Organization **www.who.int**

Suggested Readings

Additional reference materials for Concept 1 are available at Click 14.

Web 14

American Heart Association. 2005. *Metabolic Syndrome.* Dallas, TX: American Heart Association. Available at www.americanheart.org/presenter.jhtml?identifier=4756.

Booth, F. W., and M. V. Chakravarthy. 2004. Cost and consequences of sedentary living: New battleground for an old enemy.

Brown, D. W., et al. 2004. Associations between physical activity dose and health-related quality of life. *Medicine and Science in Sports and Exercise* 36(5):890–896.

Centers for Disease Control and Prevention. 2000. *Measuring Healthy Days.* Atlanta: CDC.

Chenoweth, D. et al. 2006. The cost of sloth: Using a tool to measure the cost of physical inactivity. *ACSM's Health and Fitness Journal.* 10(2), 8–13.

Corbin, C. B., et al. 2004. Toward a uniform definition of wellness: A commentary. In C. B. Corbin et al. *Toward a Better Understanding of Physical Fitness and Activity, Selected Topics,* Volume II. Scottsdale, AZ: Holcomb Hathaway.

Corbin, C. B., et al. 2004. Definitions: Health, Fitness and Physical Activity. In C.B. Corbin et al. *Toward a Better Understanding of Physical Fitness and Activity, Selected Topics,* Volume II. Scottsdale, AZ: Holcomb Hathaway.

Federal Interagency Forum on Age-Related Statistics. 2004. *Older Americans 2004: Key Indicators of Well-Being.* Washington, DC: United States Government Printing Office. Also available at www.agingstats.gov/chartbook2004/default.htm.

Gorman, C., and A. Park. 2005. New heart scanning technology could save your life. *Time* 166(10):58–71.

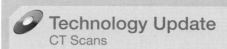

Technology Update
CT Scans

One of the principal reasons for the increase in longevity in Western society is improvement in medical care. One such technological development is the CT scan. A CT (computerized axial tomography) scan is an X-ray procedure that uses a computer to combine many X-ray images to generate cross-sectional and three-dimensional views of the internal organs and other parts of the body. One of the most recent applications is the cardiac CT scan that produces a computer image of the heart. The CT scan procedure is not a replacement for other assessment techniques, but can sometimes be used instead of more invasive tests to more accurately diagnose and treat heart disease. Other types of CT scan procedures are not new and have been used to assess conditions of the head (e.g., traumatic skull injuries, blood clots, stroke), and spine (spinal cord and disk problems), as well as other conditions, such as tumors and infections.

Hoyert, D. L., H. Kung, and B. L. Smith. 2005. Deaths: Preliminary data for 2003. *National Vital Statistics Reports* 53(15):1–32.

Institute of Medicine. 2004. *Insuring Our Health.* Washington, DC: National Academies Press.

Jha, A. 2006. Measuring hospital quality: What physicians do? How patients fare? Or both? *Journal of the American Medical Association.* 296(1):95–97.

Mokdad, A. H., et al. 2004. Actual causes of death in the United States. *Journal of the American Medical Association* 291(10):1238–1246.

Noonan, P. J. 2004. Do you suffer from Syndrome X? *USA Weekend* (April):23–35.

Payne, W. A., and D. B. Hahn, and E.B. Lucas. 2007. *Understanding Your Health.* 9th ed. New York: McGraw-Hill.

Sanmartin, C., et al. 2004. *Joint Canada/United States Survey of Health, 2002–2003.* Atlanta: Centers for Disease Control and Prevention.

U.S. Department of Health and Human Services. 1996. *Physical Activity and Health: A Report of the Surgeon General.* Atlanta: U.S. Department of Health and Human Services.

U.S. Department of Health and Human Services. Nov. 2000. *Healthy People 2010.* 2nd ed. With *Understanding and Improving Health* and *Objectives for Improving Health.* 2 vols. Washington, DC: U.S. Government Printing Office.

World Health Organization. 2005. *World Health Report 2005: Make Every Mother and Child Count.* Geneva: World Health Organization. Available at www.who.int/whr/en.

In the News

Health, Wellness, and Fitness: The Good News

Reports of bad news are common in the media. The tragic events of September 11, the horrors of ongoing wars, and the continuing threat of terrorism have added considerable stress to our lives. These events also cause us all to pause and consider what is truly important in our lives. The importance of family, friends, good health, and personal safety are certainly high on most people's list of priorities. It is our hope that the information in this book will help you focus on wellness and quality of life issues that are important to you, your friends, and your loved ones.

The reports of bad news in the media may lead some people to conclude that events are out of our personal control. However, information from a variety of recent studies indicates that there is considerable good news about health, wellness, and fitness. Some examples of the general good news are

- Life expectancy, including years with good quality of life, is at an all-time high (review Figure 1).
- Life expectancy for men has increased, resulting in a smaller gap in death rates between men and women.
- African American men and women are living longer than ever before.
- Most people in the United States (85 percent) and Canada (88 percent) report having good, very good, or excellent health. One in four reports having excellent health.
- At the time of the midcourse review of the *Healthy People 2010* goals, death rates for 8 of the 15 leading causes of death had declined.
- Heart disease deaths are down 3.6 percent, cancer deaths are down 2.2 percent, and stroke deaths decreased by 4.6 percent.
- Deaths from HIV, firearms, and suicide have decreased in recent years.

- Most adults say that they are taking steps now to ensure health later in life.
- Medical care, for those who seek it and can afford it, is better than at any other time in history.
- More adults have had exams, such as mammograms, than in previous decades.
- Infant mortality rates have fallen by 75 percent since 1950.
- Youth deaths (12 months to 24 years) have decreased 50 percent since 1950.
- More than 78 percent of adults are satisfied with their standard of living.
- Health and fitness club membership increased 100 percent from 1980 to 1990 and 63 percent to the present.
- Over 50 percent of all adults own home exercise equipment.
- We have more vacation time than previous generations.
- Smoking has decreased by 50 percent over the past five decades.

The Centers for Disease Control and Prevention (CDC) recently identified 10 major achievements, including vaccinations, safer workplaces, safer and healthier foods, and decline in heart disease deaths to name but a few. Evidence suggests that many similar positive developments will occur in this century.

This "good news" provides optimism that we can overcome threats to our safety and health and make progress in meeting the national health goals outlined in this book. We have placed special emphasis on the *Healthy People 2010* vision of helping "us all to make healthy lifestyle choices for ourselves and our families." For more details see the *On the Web* feature for this concept.

Lab Resource Materials: The Healthy Lifestyle Questionnaire

The purpose of this questionnaire is to help you analyze your lifestyle behaviors and to help you make decisions concerning good health and wellness for the future. Information on this Healthy Lifestyle Questionnaire is of a personal nature. For this reason, this questionnaire is not designed to be submitted to your instructor. **It is for your information only.** Answer each question as honestly as possible and use the scoring information to help you assess your lifestyle.

Directions: Place an X over the "yes" circle to answer yes. If you answer "no," make no mark. Score the questionnaire using the procedures that follow.

(yes) 1. I accumulate 30 minutes of moderate physical activity most days of the week (brisk walking, stair climbing, yard work, or home chores).

(yes) 2. I do vigorous activity that elevates my heart rate for 20 minutes at least 3 days a week.

(yes) 3. I do exercises for flexibility at least 3 days a week.

(yes) 4. I do exercises for muscle fitness at least 2 days a week.

(yes) 5. I eat three regular meals each day.

(yes) 6. I select appropriate servings from the major food groups each day.

(yes) 7. I restrict the amount of fat in my diet.

(yes) 8. I consume only as many calories as I expend each day.

(yes) 9. I am able to identify situations in daily life that cause stress.

(yes) 10. I take time out during the day to relax and recover from daily stress.

(yes) 11. I find time for family, friends, and things I especially enjoy doing.

(yes) 12. I regularly perform exercises designed to relieve tension.

(yes) 13. I do not smoke or use other tobacco products.

(yes) 14. I do not abuse alcohol.

(yes) 15. I do not abuse drugs (prescription or illegal).

(yes) 16. I take over-the-counter drugs sparingly and use them only according to directions.

(yes) 17. I abstain from sex or limit sexual activity to a safe partner.

(yes) 18. I practice safe procedures for avoiding sexually transmitted infections (STI).

(yes) 19. I use seat belts and adhere to the speed limit when I drive.

(yes) 20. I have a smoke detector in my house and check it regularly to see that it is working.

(yes) 21. I have had training to perform CPR if called on in an emergency.

(yes) 22. I can perform the Heimlich maneuver effectively if called on in an emergency.

(yes) 23. I brush my teeth at least two times a day and floss at least once a day.

(yes) 24. I get an adequate amount of sleep each night.

(yes) 25. I do regular self-exams, have regular medical checkups, and seek medical advice when symptoms are present.

(yes) 26. When I receive advice and/or medication from a physician, I follow the advice and take the medication as prescribed.

(yes) 27. I read product labels and investigate their effectiveness before I buy them.

(yes) 28. I avoid using products that have not been shown by research to be effective.

(yes) 29. I recycle paper, glass, and aluminum.

(yes) 30. I practice environmental protection, such as carpooling and energy conservation.

[ ] **Overall Score—Total "Yes" Answers**

Scoring: Give yourself 1 point for each "yes" answer. Add your scores for each of the lifestyle behaviors. To calculate your overall score, sum the totals for all lifestyles.

Physical Activity

1. ☐
2. ☐
3. ☐
4. ☐
☐ Total +

Nutrition

5. ☐
6. ☐
7. ☐
8. ☐
☐ Total +

Managing Stress

9. ☐
10. ☐
11. ☐
12. ☐
☐ Total +

Avoiding Destructive Habits

13. ☐
14. ☐
15. ☐
16. ☐
☐ Total +

Practicing Safe Sex

17. ☐
18. ☐
☐ Total +

Adopting Safety Habits

19. ☐
20. ☐
☐

Knowing First Aid

21. ☐
22. ☐
☐ Total +

Personal Health Habits

23. ☐
24. ☐
☐ Total +

Using Medical Advice

25. ☐
26. ☐
☐ Total +

Being an Informed Customer

27. ☐
28. ☐
☐ Total +

Protecting the Environment

29. ☐
30. ☐
☐ Total =

Sum All Totals for Overall Score

☐

Interpreting Scores: Scores of 3 or 4 on the four-item scales are indicative of generally positive lifestyles. For the two-item scales, a score of 2 indicates the presence of positive lifestyles. An overall score of 26 or more is a good indicator of healthy lifestyle behaviors. It is important to consider the following special note when interpreting scores.

Special Note: Your scores on the Healthy Lifestyle Questionnaire should be interpreted with caution. There are several reasons for this. First, all lifestyle behaviors do not pose the same risks. For example, using tobacco or abusing drugs has immediate negative effects on health and wellness, whereas others, such as knowing first aid, may have only occasional use. Second, you may score well on one item in a scale but not on another. If one item indicates an unhealthy lifestyle in an area that poses a serious health risk, your lifestyle may appear to be healthier than it really is. For example, you could get a score of 3 on the destructive habits scale and be a regular smoker. For this reason, the overall score can be particularly deceiving.

Strategies for Change: In the space to the right, you may want to make some notes concerning the healthy lifestyle areas in which you could make some changes. You can refer to these notes later to see if you have made progress.

Healthy Lifestyle Ratings

Rating	Two-Item Scores	Four-Item Scores	Overall Scores
Positive lifestyles	2	3 or 4	26 to 30*
Consider changes	Less than 2	Less than 3	Less than 26

*See Special Note.

Lab 1A Wellness Self-Perceptions

Name		Section	Date

Purpose: To assess self-perceptions of wellness

Procedures

1. Place an X over the appropriate circle for each question (4 = strongly agree, 3 = agree, 2 = disagree, 1 = strongly disagree).
2. Write the number found in that circle in the box to the right.
3. Sum the three boxes for each wellness dimension to get your wellness dimension totals.
4. Sum all wellness dimension totals to get your comprehensive wellness total.
5. Use the rating chart to rate each wellness area.
6. Complete the Results section and the Conclusions and Implications section.

Question	Strongly Agree	Agree	Disagree	Strongly Disagree	Score
1. I am happy most of the time.	4	3	2	1	
2. I have good self-esteem.	4	3	2	1	
3. I do not generally feel stressed.	4	3	2	1	
			Emotional Wellness Total	**=**	
4. I am well informed about current events.	4	3	2	1	
5. I am comfortable expressing my views and opinions.	4	3	2	1	
6. I am interested in my career development.	4	3	2	1	
			Intellectual Wellness Total	**=**	
7. I am physically fit.	4	3	2	1	
8. I am able to perform the physical tasks of my work.	4	3	2	1	
9. I am physically able to perform leisure activities.	4	3	2	1	
			Physical Wellness Total	**=**	
10. I have many friends and am involved socially.	4	3	2	1	
11. I have close ties with my family.	4	3	2	1	
12. I am confident in social situations.	4	3	2	1	
			Social Wellness Total	**=**	
13. I am fulfilled spiritually.	4	3	2	1	
14. I feel connected to the world around me.	4	3	2	1	
15. I have a sense of purpose in my life.	4	3	2	1	
			Spiritual Wellness Total	**=**	
			Comprehensive Wellness (Sum of five wellness scores)		

In the results below, record your scores from the previous page; then determine your ratings for each score using the Wellness Rating Chart. Record your ratings in the Results section.

Results

Wellness Dimension	Score	Rating
Emotional-mental		
Intellectual		
Physical		
Social		
Spiritual		
Comprehensive		

Wellness Rating Chart

Rating	Wellness Dimension Scores	Comprehensive Wellness Scores
High-level wellness	10–12	50–60
Good wellness	8–9	40–49
Marginal Wellness	6–7	30–39
Low-level wellness	Below 6	Below 30

Conclusions and Implications: In the space provided below, use several paragraphs to describe your current state of wellness. Do you think the ratings are indicative of your true state of wellness? Are there areas in which there is room for improvement?

Self-Management and Self-Planning Skills for Health Behavior Change

Health Goals for the year 2010

- Increase quality and years of healthy life.
- Increase incidence of people reporting "healthy days."
- Increase adoption and maintenance of daily physical activity.
- Increase proportion of all people who eat well.
- Decrease personal stress levels and mental health problems.
- Modify determinants of good health.

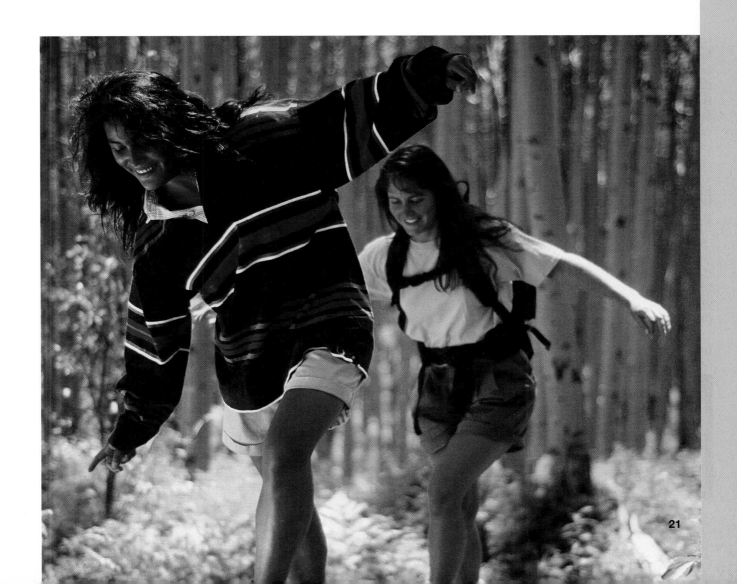

Learning and regularly using self-management skills can help you adopt and maintain healthy lifestyles throughout life.

Reducing illness and debilitating conditions and promoting wellness and fitness are important public health goals. As noted in Concept 1, adopting healthy lifestyles is a key factor in health, wellness, and fitness promotion but evidence suggests that many people are not able to make changes, even when they want to do so. Experts have determined that people who practice healthy lifestyles possess certain characteristics. These characteristics, including personal responsibility, can be modified to improve the health behaviors of all people. Researchers have also identified several special skills, referred to as **self-management skills,** that can be useful in helping you alter factors related to adherence and ultimately help you make lifestyle changes. Like any skill, self-management skills must be practiced if they are to be useful. The factors relating to adherence and the self-management skills described in this concept can be applied to a wide variety of healthy lifestyles. In early sections of this book, the focus is on using self-management skills to become and stay active throughout life. In the later sections of the book, the focus is on using these skills to adopt other healthy lifestyles that promote good health and wellness. In the final section, you get an opportunity to use the skills to make informed choices and plan for healthy living.

Making Lifestyle Changes

Many adults want to make lifestyle changes but are unable to do so. The majority of adults (66 percent) would prefer to alter their diet to improve health rather than take medicine. Nine out of 10 people indicate that regular physical activity is important to their health, but only 1 in 3 does enough exercise to benefit health. Approximately two-thirds of adults feel "great stress" at least 1 day a week and would like to reduce their stress levels. In spite of these statistics, those who profess interest in

On the Web

www.mhhe.com/corbinweb

Web 01 Log on to this URL before reading this concept. See On the Web list of concepts. Click on the concept number you want to view. To access supplemental information, click on the number shown at each Web icon.

dietary change are often unsuccessful in making lasting changes. Those who say they value physical activity often fail to adhere to even modest activity schedules. Though stress reduction is important, nearly half of all adults still feel that there is a stigma associated with seeking help for an emotional problem. Changes in other lifestyles are frequently desired but often not accomplished.

Practicing one healthy lifestyle does not mean you will practice another, though adopting one healthy behavior often leads to the adoption of another. College students are more likely to participate in regular physical activity than older adults. However, they are also much more likely to eat poorly and abuse alcohol. Many young women adopt low-fat diets to avoid weight gain and smoke because they have the mistaken belief that smoking will contribute to long-term weight maintenance. These examples illustrate the fact that practicing one healthy lifestyle does not ensure **adherence** to another. However, there is evidence that making one lifestyle change often makes it easier to make other changes. For example, smokers who have started regular physical activity programs often see improvements in fitness and general well-being and decide to stop smoking.

People do not make lifestyle changes overnight. Rather, people progress forward and backward through several stages of change. When asked about a specific healthy lifestyle, people commonly respond with yes or no answers. If asked, "Do you exercise regularly?" the answer is yes or no. When asked, "Do you eat well?" the answer is yes or no. We know that there are many different stages of lifestyle behavior.

Prochaska (a well known health psychology expert) and his colleagues developed a model for classifying **stage of change** as part of their transtheoretical model. They suggest that lifestyle changes occur in at least five different stages. These stages are illustrated in Figure 1. The stages were originally developed to help clarify negative lifestyles. Smokers were among the first studied. Smokers who are not considering stopping are at the stage of precontemplation. Those who are thinking about stopping are classified in the contemplation stage. Those who have bought a nicotine patch or a book about smoking cessation are classified in the preparation stage. They have moved beyond contemplation and are preparing to take action. The action stage occurs when the smoker makes a change in behavior, even a small one. Cutting back on the number of cigarettes smoked is an example. The fifth stage is maintenance. When a person finally stops smoking for a relatively long period of time (e.g., 6 months), this stage has been reached.

The stages of change model (as illustrated in Figure 1) has been applied to positive lifestyles as well as negative ones. Those who are totally sedentary are considered to be in the precontemplation stage. Contemplators are thinking about becoming active. A person at the preparation stage may have bought a pair of walking shoes and appropriate clothing for activity. Those who have started activity, even if infrequent, are considered to be at the stage of action. Those who have been exercising regularly for at least 6 months are at the stage of maintenance.

Whether the lifestyle is positive or negative, people move from one stage to another in an upward or a downward direction. Individuals in action may move on to maintenance or revert back to contemplation. Smokers who succeed in quitting permanently report having stopped and started dozens of times before reaching lifetime maintenance. Similarly, those attempting to adopt positive lifestyles, such as eating well, often move back and forth from one stage to another, depending on their life circumstances.

Once maintenance is attained, relapse is less likely to occur. Although it is possible to relapse completely, it is generally less likely after the maintenance stage is reached. At this point, the behavior has been integrated into a personal lifestyle and it becomes easier to sustain. For example, a person who has been active for years does not have to undergo the same thought processes as a beginning exerciser—the behavior becomes automatic and habitual. Similarly, a nonsmoker is not tempted to smoke in the same way as a person who is trying to quit. Some people have termed the end of this behavior change process as termination.

Factors That Promote Lifestyle Change

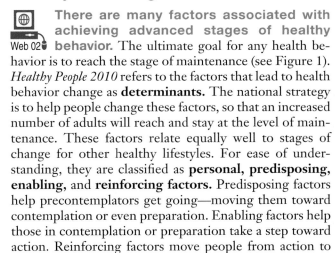

There are many factors associated with achieving advanced stages of healthy behavior. The ultimate goal for any health behavior is to reach the stage of maintenance (see Figure 1). *Healthy People 2010* refers to the factors that lead to health behavior change as **determinants.** The national strategy is to help people change these factors, so that an increased number of adults will reach and stay at the level of maintenance. These factors relate equally well to stages of change for other healthy lifestyles. For ease of understanding, they are classified as **personal, predisposing, enabling,** and **reinforcing factors.** Predisposing factors help precontemplators get going—moving them toward contemplation or even preparation. Enabling factors help those in contemplation or preparation take a step toward action. Reinforcing factors move people from action to maintenance and help those in maintenance stay there.

Personal factors affect health behaviors but are often out of your personal control. Your age, gender, heredity, social status, and current health and fitness levels are all personal factors that affect your health behaviors. For example, there are significant differences in health behaviors among people of various ages. According to one

Self-Management Skills Skills that you learn to help you adopt healthy lifestyles and adhere to them.

Adherence Adopting and sticking with healthy behaviors, such as regular physical activity or sound nutrition, as part of your lifestyle.

Stage of Change The level of motivational readiness to adopt a specific health behavior.

Determinants Factors identified by health experts as responsible for healthy and unhealthy behaviors.

Personal Factors Factors, such as age or gender, related to healthy lifestyle adherence but not typically under personal control.

Predisposing Factors Factors that make you more likely to adopt a healthy lifestyle, such as participation in regular physical activity, a part of your normal routine.

Enabling Factors Factors that help you carry out your healthy lifestyle plan.

Reinforcing Factors Factors that provide encouragement to maintain healthy lifestyles, such as physical activity, for a lifetime.

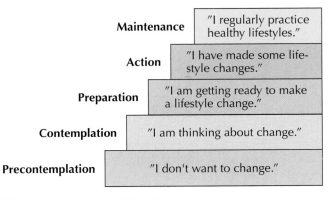

Maintenance	"I regularly practice healthy lifestyles."
Action	"I have made some lifestyle changes."
Preparation	"I am getting ready to make a lifestyle change."
Contemplation	"I am thinking about change."
Precontemplation	"I don't want to change."

Figure 1 ► Stages of lifestyle change.

survey, young adults between the ages of 18 and 34 are more likely to smoke (30 percent) than those 65 and older (13 percent). On the other hand, young adults are much more likely to be physically active than older adults.

Gender differences are illustrated by the fact that women use health services more often than men. Women are more likely than men to have identified a primary care doctor and are more likely to participate in regular health screenings. As you will discover in more detail later in this book, heredity plays a role in health behaviors. For example, some people have a hereditary predisposition to gain weight, and this may affect their eating behaviors.

Age, gender, and heredity are factors you cannot control. Other personal factors that relate to health behaviors include social status and current health and fitness status. Evidence indicates that people of lower socioeconomic status and those with poor health and fitness are less likely to contemplate or participate in activity and other healthy behaviors. No matter what personal characteristics you have, you can change your health behaviors. If you have several personal factors that do not favor healthy lifestyles, it is important to do something to change your behaviors.

Making an effort to modify the factors that predispose, enable, and reinforce healthy lifestyles is essential.

Predisposing factors are important in getting you started with the process of change. There are many predisposing factors that help you move from contemplation to preparation and taking action with regard to healthy behavior. A person who possesses many of the predisposing factors is said to have self-motivation (also called intrinsic motivation). If you are self-motivated, you will answer positively to two basic questions: "Am I able?" and "Is it worth it?"

"Am I able to do regular activity?" "Am I able to change my diet or to stop smoking?" Figure 2 includes a list of four factors that help you say, "Yes, I am able." Two of these factors are **self-confidence** and **self-efficacy.** Both have to do with having positive perceptions about your own ability. People with positive self-perceptions are more self-motivated and feel they are capable of making behavior changes for health improvement. Other factors that help you feel you are able to do a healthy behavior include easy access and a safe environment. For

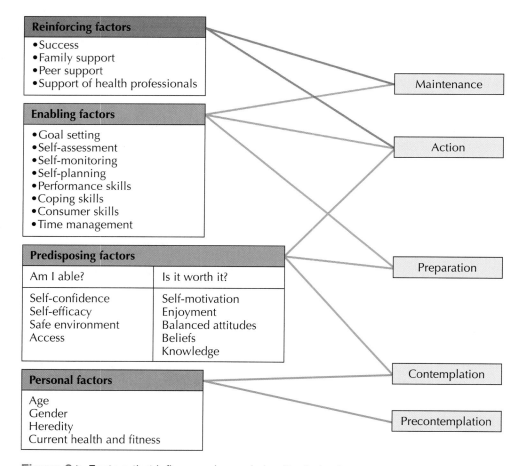

Figure 2 ▶ Factors that influence change in healthy behaviors.

Table 1 ▶ Self-Management Skills for Changing Predisposing Factors

Self-Management Skill	How Is It Useful?
Overcoming Barriers	**Lifestyle Example**
This involves developing skills that allow you to overcome problems, such as lack of facilities, lack of equipment, and inconvenience. People who develop skills to overcome barriers can learn to rearrange schedules and acquire personal equipment and other skills to overcome these barriers.	People at work are often exposed to snack foods high in empty calories. For this reason, their nutrition is not what it could be. Skills in overcoming barriers include planning, preparing, and selecting good foods.
Building Self-Confidence and Motivation	**Lifestyle Example**
This involves taking small steps that allow success. With each small step, confidence and motivation increase and you develop the feeling "I can do that."	A person says, "I would like to be more active, but I have never been good at physical activities." Starting with a 10-minute walk, the person sees that "I can do it." Over time, the person becomes confident and motivated to do more physical activity.
Balancing Attitudes	**Lifestyle Example**
This involves learning to balance positive and negative attitudes. To adhere to a healthy lifestyle, it is important to develop positive attitudes and reduce the negative attitudes.	A person does not do activity because he or she lacks support from friends, has no equipment, and does not like to get sweaty. These are negatives. Shifting the balance to positive things, such as fun, good health, and good appearance, can help promote activity.
Building Knowledge and Changing Beliefs	**Lifestyle Example**
An educated person knows the truth and builds his or her beliefs on sound information. Knowledge does not always change beliefs, but awareness of the facts can play an important role in achieving good health.	A person says, "I don't think what I eat has much to do with my health and wellness." Acquiring knowledge is fundamental to being an educated person. Studying the facts about nutrition can provide the basis for changes in beliefs and lifestyles.

example, people who have easy access to exercise equipment at home or the workplace or who have a place to exercise within 10 minutes of home are more likely to be active than those who do not. A safe environment, such as safe neighborhoods or parks, increases the chances that a person will be active.

"Is it worth it?" People who say yes to this question are willing to make an effort to change their behaviors. Predisposing factors that make it worth it to change behaviors include enjoying the activity, balancing attitudes, believing in the benefits of a behavior, and having knowledge of the health benefits of a behavior (see Figure 2). If you enjoy something and feel good about it (have positive attitudes and beliefs), you will be self-motivated to do it. It will be worth it. Taking steps to change the predisposing factors will help you become self-motivated and move toward effectively changing your health behaviors.

Enabling factors are important in moving you from the beginning stages of change to action and maintenance. Enabling factors include a variety of skills that help people follow through with decisions to make changes in behaviors. Eight of these important skills are listed in Figure 2. A few examples of the skills that enable healthy lifestyle change include goal setting, self-assessment, and self-monitoring.

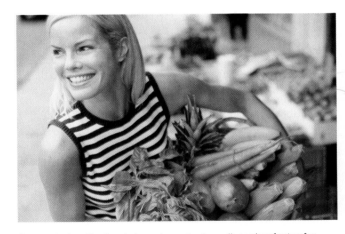

Access to healthy foods is an important predisposing factor for good nutrition.

Self-Confidence The belief that you can be successful at something (for example, the belief that you can be successful in sports and physical activities and can improve your physical fitness).

Self-Efficacy Confidence that you can perform a specific task (a type of specific self-confidence).

Table 2 ▶ Self-Management Skills for Changing Enabling Factors

Self-Management Skill	How Is It Useful?
Goal-Setting Skills	**Lifestyle Example**
This involves learning how to establish things that you want to achieve in the future. It is important that goals be realistic and achievable. Learning to set goals for behavior change is especially important for beginners.	A person wants to lose body fat. If he or she sets a goal of losing 50 pounds, success is unlikely. Setting a process goal of restricting 200 calories a day or expending 200 more a day for several weeks makes success more likely.
Self-Assessment Skills	**Lifestyle Example**
This involves how to assess your own fitness, health, and wellness. In addition, it requires you to learn to interpret your own self-assessment results. It takes practice to become good at doing self-assessments.	A person wants to know his or her health strengths and weaknesses. The best procedure is to select good tests and self-administer them. Practicing the assessments in this book will help you become good at self-assessment.
Self-Monitoring Skills	**Lifestyle Example**
This involves monitoring behavior and recordkeeping. Many people think that they adhere to healthy lifestyles, but they do not. They have a distorted view of what they actually do. Self-monitoring helps give you a true picture of your own behavior and progress.	A person can't understand why he or she is not losing weight, even though he or she is restricting calories. Keeping records may show that the person is eating more than he or she thinks. Learning to keep records of progress is also important to adherence.
Self-Planning Skills	**Lifestyle Example**
This involves learning how to plan for yourself rather than having others do all the planning for you. Knowledge and practice in planning can help you develop these skills.	A person wants to be more active, to eat better, and to manage stress. Self-planning skills will help him or her plan a personal activity, nutrition, or stress-management program.
Performance Skills	**Lifestyle Example**
This involves learning the skills necessary for performing specific tasks, such as sports or relaxation. These skills can help you feel confident and enjoy activities.	A person avoids physical activity because he or she does not have the physical skills equal to those of peers. Learning sports or other motor skills allows this person to choose to be active, anyway.
Coping Skills	**Lifestyle Example**
This involves developing a new way of thinking about things. People with this skill can see situations in more than one way and learn to think more positively about life situations.	A person is stressed and frequently anxious. Learning stress-management skills, such as relaxation, can help a person cope. Like all skills, stress-management skills must be practiced to be effective.
Consumer Skills	**Lifestyle Example**
This involves gaining knowledge about products and services. It also may require rethinking untrue beliefs that may lead to poor consumer decisions.	A person avoids seeking medical help when sick. Instead, the person takes an unproven remedy. Learning consumer skills provides knowledge for making sound medical decisions.
Time-Management Skills	**Lifestyle Example**
This involves recordkeeping similar to self-monitoring. It relates to total time use rather than the monitoring of specific behaviors. Skillful monitoring of time can help you plan and adhere to healthy lifestyles.	A person wants more quality time with family and friends. Monitoring time can help a person reallocate time to spend it in ways that are more consistent with personal priorities.

Reinforcing factors are important in adhering to lifestyle changes. Once a person has reached the action or maintenance stage, it is important to stay at this high level. Reinforcing factors help people stick with a behavior change (see Figure 2).

As illustrated in Figure 2, perhaps the most important reinforcing factor is success. If you change a behavior and have success, it makes you want to keep doing the behavior. If you fail, you may conclude that the behavior does not work and give up on it. Planning for success is essential for adhering to healthy lifestyle changes. Using the self-management skills described in this concept and throughout this book can help you plan effectively and achieve success.

Social support from family, peers, and health professionals can also be reinforcing. There are, however, different kinds of support and some are more helpful than others. Support for well-informed personal choices is referred to as support of autonomy. One example is the encouragement of family, friends, or a doctor for starting and sticking to a nutritious diet. The supporting person might ask, "How can I help you meet your goals?" One of the goals of this book is to help you take control of your own behaviors concerning your personal health, fitness, and wellness.

Not all feedback is perceived as reinforcing and supportive. Although the people providing the feedback may feel that they are being helpful and supportive, some feedback may be perceived as applying pressure or as an attempt to control behavior. For example, scolding a person for not sticking to his or her diet, or even offering the suggestion that "you are not going to get anywhere if you don't stick to your diet," will often be perceived as applying pressure. Research suggests that support of autonomy, providing support for personal choices, is most effective in enabling and reinforcing behavior change. Those who want to help friends and family make behavior changes should be careful to avoid applying pressure and attempt to provide positive support for well-informed choices.

Self-Management Skills

Learning self-management skills can help you alter factors that lead to healthy lifestyle change. Personal, predisposing, enabling, and reinforcing factors influence the way you live. These factors are of little practical significance, however, unless they can be altered to promote healthy lifestyles. Learning self-management skills (sometimes called self-regulation skills) can help you change the predisposing, enabling, and reinforcing factors described in Tables 1 (page 25), 2 (page 26), and 3. In fact, some of the enabling factors are self-management skills. It takes practice to learn these skills, but with effort anyone can learn them. There are many opportunities to learn self-management skills in this book. Many of the labs allow you to practice these skills.

It takes time to change unhealthy lifestyles. People in Western cultures are used to seeing things happen quickly. We flip a switch, and the lights come on. We want food quickly, and thousands of fast-food restaurants provide it. The expectation that we should have what we want when we want it has led us to expect instantaneous changes in health, wellness, and fitness. Unfortunately, there is no quick way to health. There is no pill that can reverse the effects of a lifetime of sedentary living, poor eating, or tobacco use. Changing your lifestyle is the key. But lifestyles that have been practiced for years are not easy to change. As you progress through this book, you will have the opportunity to learn how to implement self-management skills. Learning these skills is the surest way to make permanent lifestyle changes.

Self-Planning for Healthy Lifestyles

Self-planning is a particularly important self-management skill. A goal of this book is to help you develop a personal plan for adopting and maintaining healthy lifestyles, beginning with a six-step self-planning process. In the last concept in this book, after you have studied a variety of concepts and self-management skills, you will have the opportunity to develop a personal plan for several healthy lifestyles. Several self-management skills, including self–assessment, self-monitoring, and goal-setting, are used in the self-planning process (see Table 4).

Step 1: Clarifying Reasons

Clarifying your reasons for behavior change is an important first step in program planning. Web 03 People at precontemplation stage are not considering change in behavior; they see no need. When they reach the contemplation stage, they are considering changes in behavior. One of the most common and most

Table 3 ▶ Self-Management Skills for Changing Reinforcing Factors	
Self-Management Skill	**How Is It Useful?**
Social Support	**Lifestyle Example**
This involves learning how to get the support of others for healthy lifestyles. You learn how to get support from family and friends for your autonomous decisions. Support of a doctor can help.	A person has gradually developed a plan to be active. Friends and loved ones encourage activity and help the person develop a schedule that will allow and encourage regular activity.
Relapse Prevention	**Lifestyle Example**
This involves staying with a healthy behavior once you have adopted it. It is sometimes easy to relapse to an unhealthy lifestyle. There are skills, such as avoiding high-risk situations and learning how to say no, that can help you avoid relapse.	A person stops smoking. To stay at maintenance, the person can learn to avoid situations where there is pressure to smoke. The person can learn methods of saying no to those who offer tobacco.

Table 4 ▶ Self-Planning Skills

Self-Planning	Description	Self-Management Skill
1. Clarifying Reasons	Knowing the general reasons for changing a behavior helps you determine the type of behavior change that is most important for you at a specific point in time. If losing weight is the reason for wanting to change behavior, altering eating and activity patterns will be emphasized.	Results of the Self-Management Skills Questionnaire (Lab 2B) will help you determine which self-management skills you use regularly and the ones you might need to develop.
2. Identifying needs	If you know your strengths and weaknesses, you can plan to build on your strengths and overcome weaknesses.	Self-assessment: In the concepts that follow, you will learn how to assess different health, wellness and fitness characteristics. Learning these self-assessments will help you identify needs.
3. Setting personal goals	Goals are more specific than reasons (see #1). Establishing specific things that you want to accomplish can provide a basis for feedback that your program is working.	Goal setting: Guidelines in this concept will help you set goals. In subsequent concepts, you will establish goals for different lifestyles.
4. Selecting program components	A personal plan should include the specific program components that will meet your needs and goals based on steps 1–3. Examples include meal plans for nutrition and specific activities for your physical activity plan.	Many self-management skills, including time management, consumer, and performance skills, are useful in developing plans for a variety of healthy behaviors.
5. Writing your plan	Once program components, such as meal plans for nutrition and specific activities for physical activity, have been determined, you should put your plan in writing. This establishes your intentions and increases your chances of adherence.	Self-planning: This includes writing down the time of day, day of the week, and other details you will include in your plan.
6. Evaluating progress	Once you have used your plan, you will know what works and what does not. Periodic self-assessments can help you modify the plan to make it better.	Self-monitoring: This skill is used in keeping records (logs) and determining if goals are met. Self-assessment: This skill is used to help you determining if goals are met.

powerful reasons for contemplating a change in a lifestyle is the recommendation of a doctor, often after a visit associated with an illness. Other common reasons are to improve personal appearance, lose weight, increase energy levels, improve the ability to perform daily tasks, and improve quality of life (wellness). Identifying your reasons for wanting to change will help you determine which behaviors you want to change first and will help you establish specific goals. It is important to reflect on your reasons for wanting to make lifestyle changes before moving on to step 2.

Step 2: Identifying needs

Self-assessments are useful in establishing personal needs, planning your program, and evaluating your progress. You have already done some self-assessments of wellness, current activity levels, and current lifestyles. In the labs for this concept and others that follow, you will make additional assessments. The results of these

assessments help you build personal profiles for a variety of health behaviors that can be used as the basis for program planning. With practice, self-assessments become more accurate. It is for this reason that it is important to repeat self-assessments and to pay careful attention to the procedures for performing them. If questions arise, get a professional opinion rather than making an error.

Periodic self-assessments can aid in determining if a person is meeting health, wellness, and fitness standards and is making progress toward personal health goals. Self-assessments, when performed properly, can help you determine if you have met your goals and if you are meeting health standards (e.g., meeting health fitness standards, eating appropriate amounts of nutrients). Self-assessments also provide a measure of independence and can help you avoid unnecessary and expensive tests. Because self-assessments may not be as accurate as tests by health and medical professionals, it is wise to have periodic tests by an expert to see if your self-assessments are accurate. In some cases, your self-assessments may be used as a type of screening procedure to determine if you need professional assistance. In the final concept in this book, you will have an opportunity to use the many self-assessments you have learned to build a health, wellness, and fitness profile.

Self-assessments have the advantage of consistent error rather than variable error. The best type of assessments are done by highly qualified experts using precise instruments. Eliminating error is always desirable. Following directions and practicing assessment techniques will reduce error significantly. Still, errors will occur. One advantage of a self-assessment is that the person doing the assessment is always the same—you. Even if you make an error in a self-assessment, it is likely to be consistent over time, especially if you use the same equipment each time you make the assessment. For example, scales have limitations for monitoring changes in weight (and fat). But, if you measure your own weight using a home scale and your measurement always shows your weight to be 2 pounds higher than it really is, you have made a consistent error. You can determine if you are improving because you know the error exists. Variable errors are likely when different instruments are used, when different people make the assessments and when procedures vary from test to test. Differences in scores are harder to explain with variable forms of error because they are not consistent.

Step 3: Setting Personal Goals

Learning to set realistic goals is useful as a basis for self-planning. If any lifestyle change is to be of value, it is important to determine—ahead of time—what you hope to accomplish. Effective goals have several important characteristics. The acronym SMART can help you remember several of these characteristics. Goals are objectives that you hope to accomplish as a result of lifestyle changes. They should be specific *(S)*. Many individuals make the mistake of setting vague goals, such as "be more active" or "eat less." These are really the reasons you want to set goals. A specific goal provides details such as limiting calories to a specific number each day. Goals should be measurable *(M)*. Assessments should be performed before establishing goals and again after a lifestyle change is made to see if the goals were met. Goals should also be attainable *(A)* and realistic *(R)*, neither too hard nor too easy. If the goal is too hard, failure is likely. Failure is discouraging. By setting a goal that is realistic and attainable, you have a greater chance of success. Finally, a goal should be timely *(T)*. Timely goals are especially relevant to you at the present time. If you set too many goals, you may not reach any of them. Choosing goals that are timely can help you decide on which goals you should focus your current efforts.

Beginners are encouraged to focus on short-term goals. Short-term goals are easier to accomplish than **long-term goals.** Realistic short-term goals make you successful because one success leads to another. When you meet short-term goals, establish new ones. Long-term goals take a long time to accomplish and may be discouraging to beginners. After a series of short-term goals have been successfully accomplished, set long-term goals. In fact, setting and achieving a series of short-term goals is the best way to achieve long-term goals.

Short-term goals should be behavioral goals rather than outcome goals. A **behavioral goal** is associated with something you do. An example of a specific short-term behavioral goal is "to perform 30 minutes of brisk walking 6 days a week for the next 2 weeks." It is a behavioral goal because it refers to a behavior (something you do). It is a SMART goal because it is specific, measurable, attainable, realistic, and timely. The principal factor associated with success is your willingness to give effort. No matter who you are, you can accomplish this behavioral goal if you give a daily effort. In addition, behavioral goals are easy to self–monitor. Keeping an activity log of your weekly

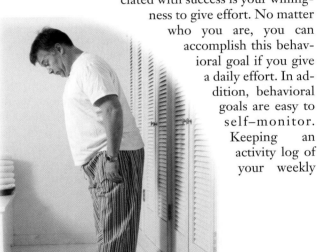

A consistent self-assessment error is better than a variable error.

Short-Term Goals Statements of intent to change a behavior or achieve an outcome in a period of days or weeks.

Long-Term Goals Statements of intent to change behavior or achieve a specific outcome in a period of months or years.

Behavioral Goal A statement of intent to perform a specific behavior (changing a lifestyle) for a specific period of time. An example is "I will walk for 15 minutes each morning before work."

participation in brisk walking will help you comply with the walking goal.

An **outcome goal** is associated with a physical characteristic (e.g., lowering your body weight or lowering your blood pressure) or something that you can do (e.g., perform 10 pushups or perform CPR). Outcome goals are not recommended for beginners.

- *Typically, it takes time (weeks or months) to reach outcome goals.* For this reason, short-term fitness goals are not recommended for beginners because they are often not achieved in the designated time, resulting in a perception of failure.
- *Outcome goals depend on many things other than your lifestyle behavior.* For example, your heredity affects your body fat and muscle development. Setting a goal of achieving a certain percentage of body fat or lifting a certain weight is influenced by heredity as well as your physical activity program. This makes it hard for beginners to set realistic goals. Too often the tendency is to set the goal based on a comparative standard rather than on a standard that is possible for the individual to achieve in a short period of time. As you become more experienced, you learn to set more realistic outcome goals and learn that these goals often take time to achieve.
- *Different people progress at different rates.* The same lifestyle change program may produce different results for different people. For this reason, goals, especially outcome goals, must vary from person to person. For example, two people may establish an outcome goal of losing 5 pounds over a 6-week period. Because we inherit predispositions to body composition, one person may meet the goal, while another may not, even if both strictly adhere to the same diet.

A similar example can be used for fitness and physical activity. People not only inherit a predisposition to fitness but also inherit a predisposition to benefit from training. In other words, if 10 people do exactly the same physical activities, there will be 10 different results. One person may improve performance by 60 percent, while another might improve only 10 percent. Experience will help you learn how to establish outcome goals that are realistic for you.

Long-term goals can be either behavioral or outcome goals. Long-term goals can be either outcome or behavioral. For example, a person who has high blood pressure (160 systolic) may set an outcome goal of lowering systolic blood pressure to 120 over a period of 6 months. Several behavioral goals can be established for the 6-month period, including taking blood pressure medication (daily), performing 30 minutes of moderate physical activity each day, and limiting salt in the diet to less than 100 percent of the recommended dietary allowance. If the outcome goal is realistic, adhering to the behavioral goals will result in achieving the outcome goal.

It is appropriate to consider maintenance goals. Outcome goals have their limits. For example, the person who lowers systolic blood pressure from 160 to 120 need not continue to lower the new healthy blood pressure. Once a healthy outcome goal has been achieved, a new outcome goal of maintaining a systolic blood pressure of 120 is appropriate. Behavioral goals will also have to be modified. For the person who has reduced blood pressure to a healthy level, medication levels might be reduced for maintenance.

Maintenance goals are appropriate in other areas as well. For example, dietary restriction and extra exercise for weight maintenance will likely be different from those used to lose weight. When a person reaches a healthy level of fitness, maintenance may be the goal rather than continued improvement. You cannot improve forever; at some point, attempting to do so may be counterproductive to health.

Making improvement can motivate you to reach long-term goals. As noted earlier, setting short-term goals that are both attainable and realistic will help you reach your long-term goals. Meeting short-term goals encourages and motivates you to continue with your healthy lifestyle plan. It is not always possible to set goals that are perfect. No matter how much self-assessing and self-monitoring a person does, sometimes goals are set too low or too high. If the goal is set too low, it is easily achieved and a new, higher goal can be established. If the goal was set too high, you may fail to reach it, even though you have made considerable progress toward the goal.

Rather than becoming discouraged when a goal is not met, consider the improvement you have made. Improvement, no matter how small, means that you are moving toward your goal. Also, you can measure your improvement

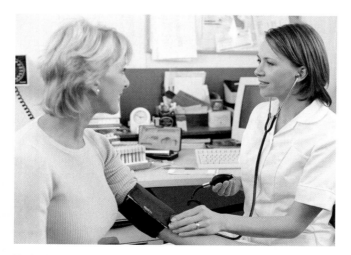

Reducing blood pressure is an example of an outcome goal.

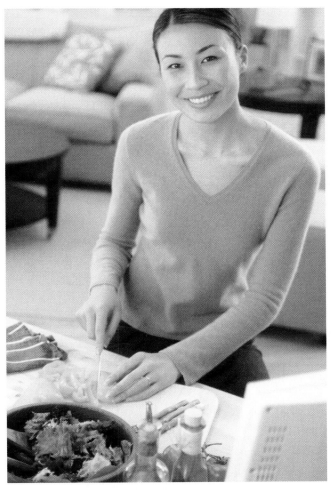

Reducing calories in your diet is an example of a behavioral goal.

and use it to help you set future goals. Of course, periodic self-assessments and good recordkeeping (self-monitoring) are necessary to keep track of improvements accurately.

Putting your goals in writing helps formalize them. Put your goals in writing. Otherwise, your goals will be easy to forget. Writing them helps establish a commitment to yourself and clearly establishes your goals. You can revise them if necessary. Written goals are not cast in concrete.

Step 4: Selecting Program Components

There are many different program components from which you can choose to meet your goals. Many different components can be included in a lifestyle change program. Eleven types of lifestyle change were described in Concept 1 (see Figure 7, page 10), ranging from priority lifestyles (physical activity, nutrition, and stress management) to avoiding destructive habits and

adopting positive safety and personal health habits. The components depend on the goals of the program. For example, if the goal is to become more fit and physically active, the program components will be the activities you choose. You will want to identify activities that match your abilities and that you enjoy. You will want to select activities that build the type of fitness you want to improve.

Other examples of program components are preparing menus for healthy eating, participating in stress-management activities, planning to attend meetings to help avoid destructive habits, and attending a series of classes to learn CPR and first aid. Preparing a list of program components that will help you meet your specific goals will prepare you for step 5, writing your plan.

Step 5: Writing Your Plan

Preparing a written plan can improve your adherence to the plan. A written plan is a pledge, or a promise, to be active. Research shows that intentions to be active are more likely to be acted on when put in writing. In the concepts that follow, you will be given the opportunity to prepare written plans for all of the activities in the physical activity pyramid, as well as for other healthy lifestyles. A good written plan includes daily plans with scheduled times and other program details. For example, the daily written plan for stress management could include the time of day when specific program activities are conducted (e.g., 15-minute quiet time at noon, yoga class from 5:30 to 6:30). An activity plan would include a schedule of the activities for each day of the week, including starting and finishing time and specific details concerning the activities to be performed. A dietary plan would include specific menus for each meal and between-meal snacks.

In the labs that accompany the final concept of this book, you will write plans for several different lifestyles. By then you will have learned a variety of self-management skills that will assist you. You will also have learned more about a variety of self-management skills that will assist you.

Step 6: Evaluating Progress

Web 05 **Self-assessment and self-monitoring can help you evaluate progress.** Once you have written a plan, it is important to determine your effectiveness in sticking with your plan. Keeping written records is one type of self-monitoring.

Outcome Goal A statement of intent to achieve a specific test score (attainment of a specific standard) associated with good health, wellness, or fitness. An example is "I will lower my body fat by 3 percent."

Self-monitoring is a good way to assess success in meeting behavioral goals. Keeping a dietary log or using a pedometer to keep track of steps are examples of self-monitoring. Self-assessments are a good way to see if you have met outcome goals.

Throughout this book, you will learn to self-assess a variety of outcomes (e.g., fitness, body fatness) and self-monitor behaviors (e.g., diet, physical activities, stress-management activities). In the second step in program planning, you used self-assessments to determine your needs and to help you plan your goals (step 3). Once you have tried your program, you can use the same self-assessments and self-monitoring strategies to evaluate the effectiveness of your program. You can see if you have met the goals you established for yourself.

Strategies for Action

Many people feel that factors influencing health and wellness are out of their control. A recent poll indicates that 91 percent of adults would like to change their lifestyles to make their lives more enjoyable and to change factors associated with wellness. Unfortunately, many people feel that they do not have personal control over good health and wellness. For example, one survey suggests that most of the lifestyle changes deemed important in our society remain in the realm of fantasy, just beyond realization. Experts have shown that people who feel that health is beyond personal control express such ideas as "Bad things [illness] can't happen to me and good things [wellness] are beyond my reach."

With practice, you can improve self-management skills that lead to acquiring and maintaining healthy lifestyles. Many opportunities are provided in this book for you to practice and learn self-management skills. Table 5 refers you to labs in the text designed to enhance specific self-management skills.

You can benefit from a critical analysis of the theories and models that help us understand the factors that lead to healthy living. Much of the information presented in this concept is based on theories and models used by researchers to study the factors associated with healthy living. Table 6 provides brief descriptions of several of the most widely accepted theories and models. You do not have to have a thorough understanding of health behavior theory to use the self-management skills (see Tables 1–3). The brief descriptions in Table 6 are intended to give you a brief overview, rather than a comprehensive understanding, of the theories and models. These brief descriptions, as well as the suggested readings at the end of the concept, should be useful to those seeking more information concerning health behavior change theory.

Many people can benefit from a new way of thinking about health, wellness, and fitness. Many people have unrealistic expectations about health and fitness. They compare their fitness with that of athletes and their appearance with that of models and movie stars, often setting standards for themselves that are impossible to achieve. Some say, "I could never do that," when considering becoming physically active, altering eating patterns, or learning to manage stress. Many lack information about what is really possible concerning healthy lifestyles. Those who feel a lack of control set unrealistic standards for themselves and lack confidence in their own abilities to change.

Table 5 ▶ Opportunities for Learning Self-Management Skills

Self-Management Skill	Lab Number
Overcoming barriers	6B, 15A, 17A, 24B
Building self-confidence and motivation	2A, 2B
Balancing attitudes	1A, 2A, 2B, 3C, 8A, 19B
Building knowledge and beliefs	1A, 4A, 7A, 12B, 14A, 15A, 15B, 18A, 18B, 19A, 19B, 20A, 21A, 22A, 22B, 23A, 23B
Goal setting	6A, 8B, 9B, 10C, 10D, 11C, 14B, 24B, 24C
Self-assessment	1A, 2A, 3A, 3C, 4A, 5A, 5B, 6B, 7B, 8A, 9A, 10A, 10B, 10D, 11A, 11B, 12A, 12B, 13A, 13B, 13C, 14A, 15B, 16A, 16B, 22A, 22B, 23B, 24A, 24B, 24C
Self-monitoring	2A, 5A, 6A, 7A, 8A, 8B, 9B, 10C, 11C, 17A, 17D, 19A, 22B, 24B, 24C
Self-planning	6A, 8B, 9B, 10C, 10D, 11C, 14B, 24B, 24C
Performance skills	3B, 12A, 17C
Adopting coping skills	16A, 16B, 17A, 17B, 17C, 17D
Learning consumer skills	14B, 15A, 18A, 20A, 23A, 23B, 24B, 24C
Managing time	17A
Finding social support	17D
Preventing relapse	15A, 19B, 24B, 24C

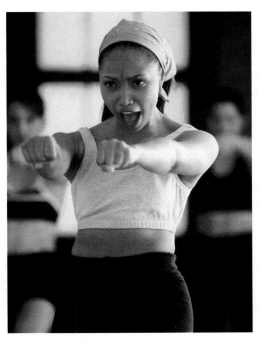

A new way of thinking can help you adopt healthy lifestyles.

Adopting a new way of thinking can have dramatic implications. A major purpose of this text is to help you

Assessing self-management skills that influence healthy lifestyles provides a basis for changing your health, wellness, or fitness. Self-assessments of your current health, wellness, and fitness status, as well as self-monitoring of your current lifestyles, can help you determine your reasons and establish reasonable goals for healthy lifestyle change. The Healthy Lifestyle Questionnaire and the Wellness Self-Perceptions Questionnaire you took in Concept 1 got you started. In this concept you can use The Stage of Change Questionnaire (Lab 2A) to help you decide which lifestyles you might need to modify. You can use the Self-Management Skills Questionnaire (Lab 2B) to determine which self–management skills you may need to improve to help you make effective changes in your lifestyles. In later concepts, you will have the opportunity to make self-assessments for a variety of lifestyles.

Table 6 ▶ Theories and Models Associated with Healthy Lifestyle Adoption

Transtheoretical Model

This model is also referred to as the stages of change model. This model suggests five stages of change that characterize various health behaviors. The model suggests that doing the correct things (processes) at the right time (stage of change) is important to self-change in health behaviors.

Social Cognitive Theory

Social cognitive theory is also referred to as social learning theory. Central to this theory are self-efficacy and positive expectations about behavior change. Also, the theory suggests that a person must value the outcomes of a behavior if he or she is likely to do that behavior.

Health Beliefs Model

This model suggests that a person's health behavior is related to the following five factors: the belief that a health problem will have harmful effects, the belief that a person is susceptible to the problem, the perceived benefits of changing a lifestyle to prevent the problem, the perceived barriers to overcoming the problem, and the confidence that he or she can do what is necessary to prevent it.

Theory of Planned Behavior

This theory is often combined with the theory of reasoned action. It has the same basic tenets but adds the concept of "perceived control" over the environment. The person must believe that he or she has some control over the factors that allow the performance of that behavior. Perceived control is in many ways similar to self-efficacy in social cognitive theory.

Social Ecological Model

The social ecological model is based on the notion that health behavior change is influenced by the interactions of intrapersonal, social, cultural, and physical environmental factors. For example, when people smoke, they affect the environment, which in turn affects the health of others in the environment. While this model does not focus on individual behavior change, it is included here to emphasize the importance of a multitude of social and environmental factors on public health.

Self-Determination Theory

Central to self-determination theory is the importance of choice in a person's life (autonomy). Perceptions of competence at mastering life's tasks are also critical to the theory. Making personal choices in an attempt to master the tasks of daily living are emphasized rather than making choices based on external pressures to comply. Self-determination theory and cognitive evaluation theory (its subtheory) emphasize intrinsic motivation. The intrinsic motivation inherent in behaviors that are exciting and/or fulfilling is important in making activity choices.

Theory of Reasoned Action

This theory suggests that a person's behavior is most associated with the person's intention to do the behavior. The two factors most likely to influence a person's intentions are attitudes (beliefs) and the social environment (opinions of others).

Online Learning Center

www.mhhe.com/corbin7e
The Online Learning Center contains a variety of Web-based resources that will help you get the most out of this book and your course. In addition to the On the Web pages, there are video activities, interactive quizzes, application assignments, and a variety of other useful study aids. Log on to the URL above to access these resources.

Web Resources

ACSM's Fit Society Page
www.acsm.org/health+fitness/ fit_society.htm
Web 09 ACSM's Health and Fitness Journal
www.acsm.org/publications/health_fitness_journal.htm
American Heart Association Health and Fitness Center
www.justmove.org
American Red Cross
www.redcross.org
Journal of Sport and Exercise Psychology
www.humankinetics.com/products/journals/ journal.cfm?id=JSEP
The Sport Psychologist
www.humankinetics.com/products/ journals/ journal.cfm?id=TSP

Technology Update
Personal Digital Assistant (PDA)

Web 08 Self-monitoring is an important self-management skill that can help people determine how many calories they eat and how much physical activity they perform. Software is available to use handheld computers, or personal digital assistants (PDAs), to track healthy behaviors and record exercise. The MySportTraining software tool (see illustration) is one of the more robust and comprehensive tools available. It can transfer exercise data from your PDA to a desktop computer for long-term tracking. Data from Polar Heart Rate monitors can also be directly downloaded using the infrared sensors on the PDA. Information on this tool can be found at the Vida One website: **www.VidaOne.com**. To see links to other PDA software for health fitness and diet refer to Web08.

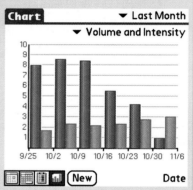

Suggested Readings

Additional reference materials for Concept 2 are available at Web 10.

Web 10

American Heart Association. 2005. American Heart Association guidelines for cardiopulmonary resuscitation and emergency cardiovascular care. *Circulation* 112 (24 supplement): 1–203 (a series of articles).

Bandura, A. 1986. *Social Foundations of Thought and Action: A Social-Cognitive Theory.* Englewood Cliffs, NJ: Prentice-Hall.

Bandura, A. 2004. Health promotion by social cognitive means. *Health Education and Behavior* 31(2):143–164.

Brannon, L., and J. Feist. 2006. *Health Psychology—An Introduction to Behavior and Health.* 5th ed. Stamford, CT: Wadsworth.

Breslow, L. 2006. Health measurement in the third era of health. *American Journal of Public Health* 96(1):17–19

Burgard, M., and K. I. Gallagher. 2006. Self-monitoring: Influencing effective behavior change in your clients. *ACSM's Health and Fitness Journal* 10(1):14–19.

The Communication Initiative. 2006. Change theories: Descriptions of various theories of behavior change. www.comminit.com/changetheories.html.

Deci, E. L., and R. M. Ryan (eds.). 2002. *Handbook of Self-Determination Research.* Rochester, NY: University of Rochester Press.

Dunsmore, S., and P. Goodson. 2006. Motivation for healthy behavior: A review of health promotion research. *American Journal of Health Promotion.* 37(3):170–183.

Janz, N. K., et al. 2002. The health belief model. In K. Glanz et al. (eds.). *Health Behavior and Health Education: Theory, Research and Practice.* 3rd ed. San Francisco: Jossey-Bass.

Levy, S. S. 2004. Effects of a self-determination theory-based mail-mediated intervention on adults' exercise behavior. *American Journal of Health Promotion* 18(5):345–349.

Maddux, J. E. 2002. Self-efficacy: The power of believing you can. In C. R. Snyder and S. J. Lopez (eds.). *Handbook of Positive Psychology.* Oxford, UK: Oxford University Press.

Marcus, B. H., and B. A. Lewis. 2003. Physical activity and the stages of change motivational readiness for change model. *President's Council on Physical Fitness and Sports Research Digest* 4(1):1–8.

Montano, D. E., and D. Kasperzyk. 2002. The theory of reasoned action and theory of planned behavior. In K. Glanz et al. (eds.). *Health Behavior and Health Education: Theory, Research and Practice.* 3rd ed. San Francisco: Jossey-Bass.

Prochaska, J. O., et al. 2002. The transtheoretical model and stages of change. In K. Glanz et al. (eds.). *Health Behavior and Health Education: Theory, Research and Practice*. 3rd ed. San Francisco: Jossey-Bass.

Rhodes, R. E., et al. 2002. Extending the theory of planned behavior to the exercise domain. *Research Quarterly for Exercise and Sport* 73(2):193–199.

Ryan, R. M., and E. L. Deci. 2000. Self-determination theory and the facilitation of intrinsic motivation, social development, and well-being. *American Psychologist* 55:68–78.

Sallis, J. F., and N. Owen. 2002. Ecological models. In K. Glanz et al. (eds.). *Health Behavior and Health Education: Theory, Research and Practice*. 3rd ed. San Francisco: Jossey-Bass.

Stewart, D. E. 2004. What about men's health? Women's perspectives of men's health and gender medicine. *Journal of Men's Health and Gender* 1(1):20–21.

Stone, W. J., and D. A. Klein. 2004. Long-term exercisers: What can we learn from them? *ACSM's Health and Fitness Journal* 8(2):11–14.

Taylor, S. 2006. *Health Psychology*. 6th ed. New York: McGraw-Hill.

 In the News

Challenges in Adopting Healthy Lifestyles

A recent Research American Health Poll (Taking Our Pulse) indicates that Americans generally accept responsibility for their health. Over 80 percent of Americans reported taking some action to improve their health (being more active and eating healthier were the top choices), 86 percent reported that it is important for people to do more to prevent their own health problems, and 70 percent indicated that personal habits and choices are more important than genetics and family traits for determining health. The survey also revealed some interesting results about why people don't do what they should to maintain health. The most common reason reported in the survey was "being too busy" (43 percent), but the second most common reason was that "people enjoy unhealthy behaviors and don't want to change" (28 percent). Only 3 percent felt that lack of knowledge or lack of awareness explained our nation's poor lifestyle habits. The survey reveals that people generally know what to do to improve their health but find it hard to follow through and maintain healthy lifestyles. Much of the problem stems from the unhealthy environment in which we live. To adopt and maintain healthy lifestyles, it is often necessary to fight against the forces (and environments) in our society that limit activity and encourage overeating.

Lab Resource Materials

Use the diagram below in answering the questions in Lab 2A. It is a reproduction of Figure 7 from Concept 1 and includes factors that influence change in healthy behaviors.

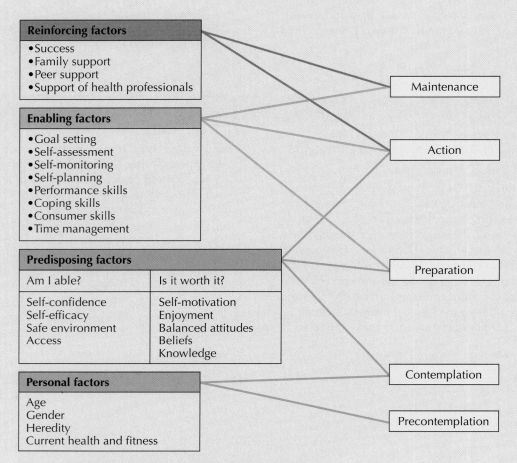

Factors that influence change in healthy behaviors.

Lab 2A The Stage of Change Questionnaire

Name	**Section**	**Date**

Purpose: To help assess your current level in the stage of change hierarchy for a variety of health behaviors

Procedures

1. For each health behavior listed in The Stage of Change Questionnaire, assess your current "stage" in the stage of change hierarchy. Circle the stage that you think best represents your current stage.
2. Answer the questions in the Conclusions and Implications section.

Results: Complete the Stage of Change Questionnaire on back of this page.

Conclusions and Implications: When making health behavior change, it may be difficult to make change as quickly as you might like. You may have better luck if you try to move from one stage to the next higher stage. Look at the figure in the Lab Resource Materials on page 36. It will help you determine which factors (personal, predisposing, enabling, and reinforcing) will be of the most help in moving from your current stage to the next higher stage, and ultimately to the stage of maintenance. You have different stages for each health behavior and will need to consider different factors for each.

Identify two health behaviors expecially in need of change (from the first six in the questionnaire on the front of this sheet). Identify your current stage for each and discuss the factors that you will consider when attempting to make a change. Write one paragraph of several sentences for each of the two behaviors.

Stage of Change Questionnaire (choose one choice for each question)

1. **Physical Activity**
   Precontemplation—I am not active and I do not plan to start.
   Contemplation—I am not active but I am thinking about starting.
   Preparation—I am getting ready to become active.
   Action—I do some activity but need to do more.
   Maintenance—I have been active regularly for several months.

2. **Eating Well (Nutrition)**
   Precontemplation—I do not eat well and don't plan to change.
   Contemplation—I do not eat well but am thinking about change.
   Preparation—I am planning to change my diet.
   Action—I sometimes eat well but need to do more.
   Maintenance—I have eaten well regularly for several months.

3. **Managing Stress**
   Precontemplation—I do not manage stress well and plan no changes.
   Contemplation—I am thinking about making changes to manage stress.
   Preparation—I am planning to change to manage stress better.
   Action—I sometimes take steps to manage stress better but need to do more.
   Maintenance—I have used good stress-management techniques for several months.

4. **Adopting Good Safety Habits (e.g., Seat Belt Use, Safe Storage of Medicine)**
   Precontemplation—I have at least one unsafe habit but plan no changes.
   Contemplation—I am thinking about making changes regarding a safety habit.
   Preparation—I am planning to make change regarding a safety habit.
   Action—I have taken action concerning a habit but need to do more.
   Maintenance—I have no safety habits that need to change (I practice good safety).

5. **Adopting Good Personal Health Habits (e.g., Brushing and Flossing, Adequate Sleep)**
   Precontemplation—I have at least one health habit that needs change but plan no changes.
   Contemplation—I am thinking about making changes related to a health habit.
   Preparation—I am planning to make change regarding a health habit.
   Action—I have taken action concerning a habit but need to do more.
   Maintenance—I have no health habits that need to change.

6. **Learning First Aid (e.g., CPR/First Aid)**
   Precontemplation—I do not know CPR/first aid and do not plan to learn.
   Contemplation—I am thinking about learning CPR/first aid.
   Preparation—I have made plans to learn CPR/first aid.
   Action—I once knew CPR/first aid but need an update.
   Maintenance—I am up-to-date on my CPR/first aid and will keep updated.

Questions 7 and 8 are highly personal. Answer for your own use, but do not record answers on this sheet.

7. **Avoiding destructive Habits (e.g., Tobacco, Drugs, Alcohol)**
   Precontemplation—I have a least one destructive habit but plan no change.
   Contemplation—I am thinking about making changes related to a destructive habit.
   Preparation—I am planning to make change regarding a destructive habit.
   Action—I have taken action concerning a habit but need to do more.
   Maintenance—I have no destructive habits or have stopped the habit for months.

8. **Practicing Safe Sex**
   Precontemplation—I have practiced unsafe sex and plan no change.
   Contemplation—I am thinking about making changes in an unsafe habit.
   Preparation—I am planning to make change regarding an unsafe habit.
   Action—I have taken action concerning a habit but need to do more.
   Maintenance—I do not practice unsafe sex or have stopped the habit for months.

Lab 2B The Self-Management Skills Questionnaire

Name		Section	Date

Purpose: To help you assess your self-management skills that are important for three priority lifestyles (physical activity, healthy nutrition, stress management)

Procedures

1. Each question in the questionnaire on page 41 and 42 reflects one of the self-management strategies described in this text. Each of the 12 questions requires an answer about 3 different healthy behaviors. Answer each question using a 3 for very true, 2 for somewhat true, or 1 for not true. Record the number of your answer in the appropriate box for each of the 3 healthy lifestyles.
2. After you have answered all 12 questions for each of the 3 lifestyles, total the 3 columns to get a total score for physical activity, nutrition, and stress management.
3. Determine your rating for each lifestyle using the Self-Management Skills Rating Chart. Record your rating in the Results section.
4. Answer the questions in the Conclusions and Implications section.

Results: Record your rating for each of 3 healthy lifestyles in the chart below.

Self-Management Skills Rating Chart	
Rating	**Score**
Good	30–36
Marginal	24–29
Needs improvement	<24

Self-Management Skills Results	Rating
Physical activity	
Nutrition	
Stress management	

Conclusions and Implications: In several sentences, discuss your ratings regarding self-management skills related to physical activity. You may have a good total score but still have several self-management skills on which you need improvement. Comment on your overall scores and those individual self-management skills on which you had scores of 1 (not true).

In several sentences, discuss your ratings regarding self-management skills related to nutrition. You may have a good total score but still have several self-management skills on which you need improvement. Comment on your overall scores and those individual self-management skills on which you had scores of 1 (not true).

In several sentences, discuss your ratings regarding self-management skills related to stress management. You may have a good total score but still have several self-management skills on which you need improvement. Comment on your overall scores and those individual self-management skills on which you had scores of 1 (not true).

The Self-Management Skills Questionnaire

	Very true	Somewhat true	Not true	Activity Score	Nutrition Score	Stress Score
1. I regularly self-asses: (self-assessment)						
personal physical fitness and physical activity levels	3	2	1			
the contents of my diet	3	2	1			
personal stress levels	3	2	1			
2. I self-monitor and keep records concerning: (self-monitoring)						
physical activity	3	2	1			
diet	3	2	1			
stress in my life	3	2	1			
3. I set realistic and attainable goals for: (goal setting)						
physical activity	3	2	1			
eating behaviors	3	2	1			
reducing stress in my life	3	2	1			
4. I have a personal written or formal plan for: (self-planning)						
regular physical activity	3	2	1			
what I eat	3	2	1			
managing stress in my life	3	2	1			
5. I possess the skills to: (performance skills)						
perform a variety of physical activities	3	2	1			
analyze my diet	3	2	1			
manage stress (e.g., progressive relaxation)	3	2	1			
6. I have positive attitudes about: (balancing attitudes)						
my ability to stick with an activity plan	3	2	1			
my ability to stick to a nutrition plan	3	2	1			
my ability to manage stress in my life	3	2	1			
7. I can overcome barriers that I encounter: (overcoming barriers)						
in my attempts to be physically active	3	2	1			
in my attempts to stick to a nutrition plan	3	2	1			
in my attempts to manage stress in my life	3	2	1			

The Self-Management Skills Questionnaire

	Very true	Somewhat true	Not true	Activity Score	Nutrition Score	Stress Score
8. I know how to identify misinformation: (consumer skills)						
relating to fitness and physical activity	3	2	1	☐		
relating to nutrition	3	2	1		☐	
relating to stress management	3	2	1			☐
9. I am able to get social support for my efforts to: (social support)						
be active	3	2	1	☐		
stick to a healthy nutrition plan	3	2	1		☐	
manage stress in my life	3	2	1			☐
10. When I have problems, I can get back to: (relapse prevention)						
my regular physical activity	3	2	1	☐		
my nutrition plan	3	2	1		☐	
my plan for managing stress	3	2	1			☐
11. I am able to adapt my thinking to: (coping strategies)						
stick with my activity plan	3	2	1	☐		
stick with my nutrition plan	3	2	1		☐	
stick with my stress-management plan	3	2	1			☐
12. I am able to manage my time to: (time management)						
stick with my physical activity plan	3	2	1	☐		
shop for and prepare nutritious food	3	2	1		☐	
perform stress-management activities	3	2	1			☐
Total Activity Score				☐		
Total Nutrition Score					☐	
Total Stress Score						☐

Preparing for Physical Activity

Health Goals for the year 2010

• Improve health, fitness, and quality of life through daily physical activity.

• Increase leisure-time physical activity.

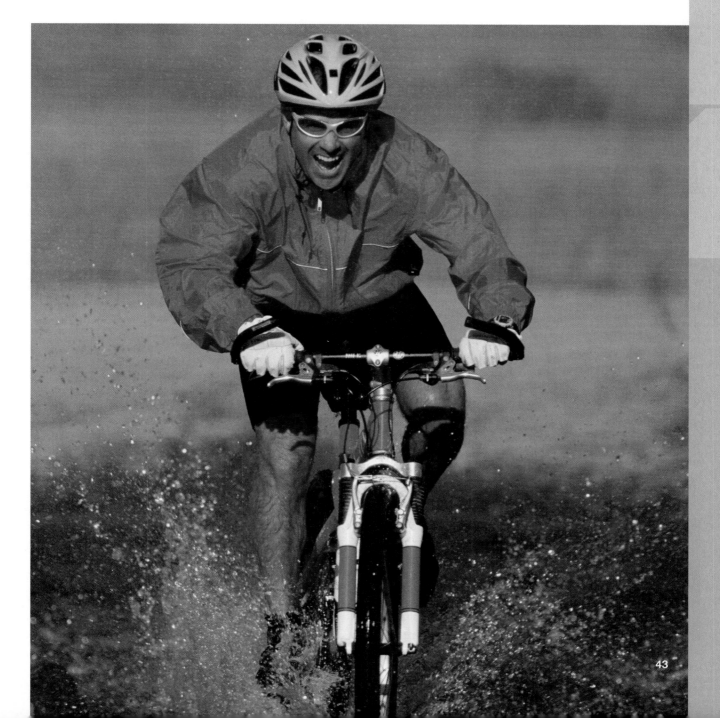

Proper preparation can help make physical activity enjoyable, effective, and safe.

For people just beginning a physical activity program, adequate preparation may be the key to persistence. For those who have been regularly active for some time, sound preparation can help reduce risk of injury and make activity more enjoyable. It is hoped that a person armed with good information about preparation will become involved and stay involved in physical activity for a lifetime. For long-term maintenance, physical activity must be something that is a part of a person's normal lifestyle. Some factors that will help you prepare for and make physical activity a part of your normal routine are presented in this concept.

Factors to Consider Prior to Physical Activity

Before beginning regular physical activity, it is important to establish medical readiness. Physical activity requires the cardiovascular system to work harder. While this level of stress can promote positive adaptations, the stress on the heart can be unsafe and dangerous for certain individuals. The British Columbia (Canada) Ministry of Health conducted extensive research to devise a procedure that will help people to know when it is advisable to seek medical consultation prior to beginning or altering an exercise program. The goal is to prevent unnecessary medical examinations, while helping people be reasonably assured that regular exercise was appropriate. The research resulted in the development of the Physical Activity Readiness Questionnaire **(PAR-Q).** The most recent revision of the PAR-Q consists of seven simple questions you can ask yourself to determine if medical consultation is necessary prior to exercise involvement.

The American College of Sports Medicine (ACSM) has developed additional guidelines to help determine if medical consultation or a **clinical exercise test** is necessary prior to participation in physical activity programs. The ACSM divides people into three general categories

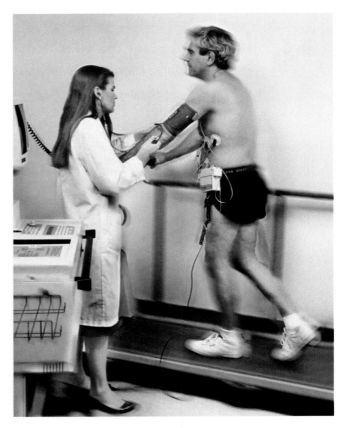

A clinical exercise test is recommended to those at high risk.

(Table 1). Young adults classified as apparently healthy with low risk, and who answer "NO" to all PAR-Q questions, are generally cleared for moderate and vigorous physical activity without a medical exam or clinical exercise test. For those with moderate risk, moderate exercise is generally appropriate without a medical exam or an exercise test, but both are recommended prior to undertaking vigorous physical activity. For those in the high risk category, a medical exam and exercise testing are recommended for moderate and vigorous activity. For those just beginning a program or those resuming physical activity after an injury or illness, consultation with a physician is always wise, no matter what your age or medical condition.

Consideration should also be given to altering exercise patterns if you have an illness or a temporary sickness, such as a cold or the flu. The immune system and other body systems may be weaker at this time and medicines (even over-the-counter ones) may alter responses

---

On the Web
www.mhhe.com/corbinweb
Log on to this URL before reading this concept. See On the Web list of concepts. Click on the concept number you want to view. To access supplemental information, click on the number shown at each Web icon.

Table 1 ▶ American College of Sports Medicine Risk Stratification Categories and Criteria

Stratification Category	Criteria
Low risk	Younger people (less than 45 for men and 55 for women) who have no heart disease symptoms and have no more than one of the risk factors listed below
Moderate risk	People without heart disease symptoms but who are older (men 45 or more and women 55 and older) OR who have 2 or more of the risk factors listed below
High risk	People with 1 or more of the signs or symptoms listed below OR who have known cardiovascular, pulmonary, or metabolic disease

Risk Factors

Family history of heart disease; smoker; high blood pressure (hypertension); high cholesterol; abnormal blood glucose levels; obesity (high BMI, excess waist girth); sedentary lifestyle; low HDL cholesterol level

Signs and Symptoms

Chest, neck, or jaw pain from lack of oxygen to the heart; shortness of breath at rest or in mild exercise; dizziness or fainting; difficult or labored breathing when lying, sitting, or standing; ankle swelling; fast heartbeat or heart palpitations; pain in the legs from poor circulation; heart murmur; unusual fatigue or shortness of breath with usual activities

Source: American College of Sports Medicine.

to exercise. It is best to work back gradually to your normal routine after illness.

There is no way to be absolutely sure that you are medically sound to begin a physical activity program. Even a thorough exam by a physician cannot guarantee that a person does not have some limitations that may cause a problem during exercise. Use of the PAR-Q and adherence to the ACSM guidelines are advised to help minimize the risk while preventing unnecessary medical cost. However, if you are unsure about your readiness for activity, a medical exam and a clinical exercise test are the surest ways to make certain that you are ready to participate.

Those who plan to do intensive training (particularly for sports) may want to answer some additional questions concerning whether a medical exam is necessary before beginning (see Lab 3A).

Shoes are an important consideration for safe and effective exercise. Decisions about Web 02 shoes should be based on intended use (e.g., running, tennis), shoe and foot characteristics, and comfort rather than looks or cosmetics. Shoes are designed for specific activities and comfort and performance will typically be best if you select and use them for their intended purpose. Hybrid shoes, known as a "cross-trainers," can be a versatile option, but they typically don't provide the needed features for specific activities. For example, they may lack the cushioning and support needed for running and the ankle support for activities such as basketball. Features of common activity shoes are highlighted in Figure 1.

Most shoes have very thin sockliners, but supplemental inserts can be purchased to provide more cushioning and support. Custom orthotics can also be used to correct alignment problems or minimize foot injuries (e.g., plantar fasciitis). A very important, and frequently neglected, consideration is to replace shoes after extended use. Runners typically replace shoes every 4 to 6 months (or 400 to 600 miles), even if the outer appearance of the shoe is still good. The main functions of athletic shoes are to reduce shock from impact and protect the foot—one of the best prevention strategies for avoiding injuries is to replace your shoes on a regular basis.

It is important to keep up with advancing technology in shoes and sports equipment. Recently, two new innovations in running shoes were introduced. The first innovation is a shoe with an "all-air" sole. A "partial-air" sole has been used for several years. This feature eliminated foam from the outsole but had a midsole that included ¼ inch of foam. The Nike 360 is the first to eliminate foam completely. The shoe is lighter and uses a pocket of air from the heel to the front of the shoe based on relative need for cushioning in various parts of the shoe. The second innovation is the "smart shoe." This new shoe, made by Adidas, uses a small computer chip to automatically adjust for the runner's body weight, changes in stride caused by fatigue, terrain, and pace. The processor is lightweight but does add weight to the shoe because a battery is required. It is too early to tell how these technologies will shape the athletic shoe market. Additional detail on shoe technology is provided on the Web (click on Web02). Information about becoming a wise consumer is presented later in the book.

PAR-Q An acronym for Physical Activity Readiness Questionnaire; designed to help determine if you are medically suited to begin an exercise program.

Clinical Exercise Test A test, typically administered on a treadmill, in which exercise is gradually increased in intensity while the heart is monitored by an EKG. Symptoms not present at rest, such as an abnormal EKG, may be present in an exercise test.

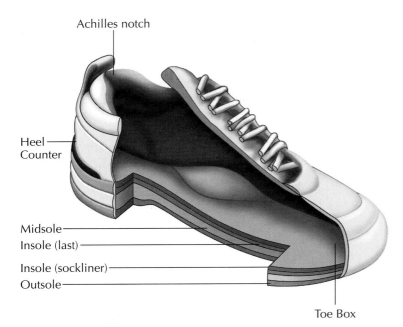

Achilles notch

Heel Counter

Midsole
Insole (last)
Insole (sockliner)
Outsole

Toe Box

Achilles notch: Protects tendon

Arch support: Supports arch; height and shape of arch should vary with foot characteristics

Heel counter: Provides movement control; a stiff counter helps with pronation (toes turn in) but can cause problems for those who do not pronate

Insole (last): Refers to shoe shape; curved (more flexible for those with rigid arches who pronate), straight (good for heavier or flat-footed people), or semi-curved (moderate flexibility and stability)

Insole (sockliner): Removable layer for additional shock and sweat absorption; can be replaced periodically and /or customized

Material: Light, porous materials that can breathe are recommended

Midsole: Provides cushion, stability, and motion control; important for shock absorption

Outsole: Provides traction; determines shoe flexibility; type depends on intended purpose of shoe

Toe box: Should have adequate height to wiggle toes and prevent rubbing on top of toes and adequate length so toes do not contact front of shoe

Figure 1 ▶ Anatomy of an activity shoe.

It is important to dress properly for physical activity. Clothing should be appropriate for the Web 03 type of activity being performed and the conditions in which you are participating. Similar to shoes, comfort is a much more important consideration than looks. Table 2 provides guidelines for dressing for activity.

Factors to Consider during Daily Physical Activity

There are three components of the daily activity program: the warm-up, the workout, and the cool-down. The key component of a fitness program is the daily workout. Experts agree, however, that the workout should be preceded by a warm-up and followed by a cool-down. The **warm-up** prepares the body for physical activity, and the **cool-down** returns the body to rest and promotes effective recovery by aiding the return of blood from the working muscles to the heart (see Figure 2).

A warm-up prior to exercise is recommended. There are two compo-Web 04 nents of an effective warm-up. The first (a general cardiovascular warm-up) is intended to prepare the heart and the circulatory system for exercise. When you start physical activity, blood flow is not immediately available to the heart and muscles. A proper warm-up decreases the risk of irregular heartbeats associated with poor coronary circulation.

The American College of Sports Medicine (ACSM) recommends 5 to 10 minutes of low-intensity large muscle activity, such as walking for the first phase of the warm-up. The second phase of the warm-up involves static stretching of the major large muscle groups. This phase is recommended after the general cardiovascular warm-up.

Table 2 ▶ Selecting Appropriate Clothing for Activity

General Guidelines
- Avoid clothing that is too tight or that restricts movement.
- Material in contact with skin should be porous.
- Clothing should protect against wind and rain but allow for heat loss and evaporation—e.g., Gortex, Coolmax.
- Wear layers so that a layer can be removed if not needed.
- Wear socks for most activities to prevent blisters, abrasions, odor, and excessive shoe wear.
- Socks should be absorbent and fit properly.
- Do not use nonporous clothing that traps sweat in an attempt to lose weight; these garments prevent evaporation and cooling.

Special Considerations
- Women should wear an exercise bra for support.
- Men should consider an athletic supporter for support.
- Wear helmets and padding for activities with risk of falling, such as biking or inline skating.
- Wear reflective clothing for night activities.
- Wear water shoes for some aquatic activities.
- Consider lace-up ankle braces to prevent injury.
- Consider a mouthpiece for basketball and other contact sports.

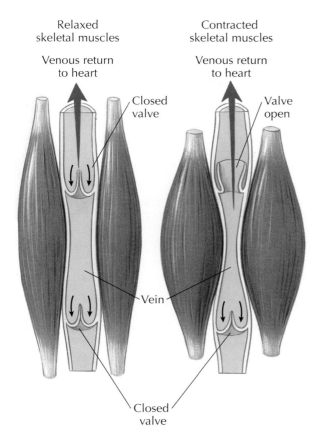

Figure 2 ▶ Muscle contractions aid the veins in returning blood to the heart.

A warm-up that is suitable for walking, jogging, running, cycling, and even basketball is presented in Lab 3B (page 60). This warm-up can be used for other activities, provided stretching exercises for the major muscle groups involved in the activities are added. The ACSM indicates that dynamic forms of stretching (e.g., ballistic and proprioceptive neuromuscular facilitation—PNF) can be incorporated into the later stages of a warm-up, depending on the nature of the activity. Information concerning these types of stretching exercises is included in Concept 9. The cardiovascular warm-up is suitable for most activities, but other mild exercise (such as a slow swim for swimmers or a slow ride for cyclists) can be substituted.

The most common reasons for recommending a stretching warm-up are to reduce risk of injury and to enhance performance. It should be noted that the evidence is mixed concerning the benefits of the stretching warm-up for injury prevention. Also, there is some evidence that excessive stretching may affect some types of performances (e.g., strength and power) by reducing force production. Future research will likely help clarify some of these issues.

In summary, there is good evidence that a general cardiovascular warm-up is important before performing vigorous physical activity. When performing a stretching warm-up, make certain that you use gentle, static stretch. The stretching warm-up is not intended to substitute for a regular program of stretching exercises designed to improve flexibility. (See Web04 and Concept 9 for more information on warm-ups and stretching.)

A cool-down after the workout is important to promote an effective recovery from physical activity. A cool-down allows for a gradual recovery immediately after a workout. The ACSM indicates that the cool-down is "a critical ingredient of a comprehensive, safe program for both healthy participants as well as patients with disease." Similar to warm-up, a two-phase cool-down is recommended.

The first phase of the cool-down includes low-intensity activity (e.g., walking, slow jogging, or cycling) for approximately 5 minutes. This cool-down phase allows a gradual slowing of the metabolic and cardiovascular systems.

During physical activity, the heart pumps a large amount of blood to supply the working muscles with the oxygen necessary to keep moving. The muscles squeeze the veins (see Figure 2),

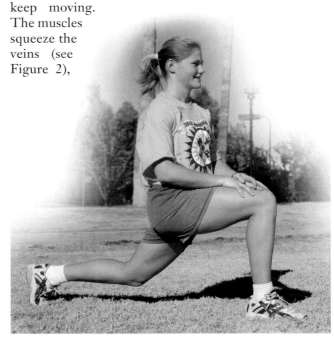

A warm-up before and a cool-down after a workout is recommended.

Warm-Up Light to moderate activity done prior to a workout. Its purpose is to reduce the risk of injury and soreness and possibly improve performance in a physical activity.

Cool-Down Light to moderate activity done after a workout to help the body recover; often consisting of the same exercises used in the warm-up.

which forces the blood back to the heart. Valves in the veins prevent the blood from flowing backward. As long as exercise continues, muscles move the blood back to the heart, where it is once again pumped to the body. If exercise is stopped abruptly, the blood is left in the area of the working muscles and has no way to get back to the heart. In the case of a runner, the blood pools in the legs. Because the heart has less blood to pump, blood pressure may drop. This can result in dizziness and can even cause a person to pass out. The best way to prevent this problem is to slow down gradually after exercise and keep moving until blood pressure and heart rate have returned to near resting values. This phase is especially important for those with cardiovascular risk factors or disease.

The second phase of the cool-down involves stretching exercises. Stretching after exercise may be more important than stretching before exercise because it may help relieve spasms in fatigued muscles. Stretching as part of the cool-down may also be more effective for lengthening the muscles than is stretching at other times because the muscle temperature is elevated and the muscles are more capable of being stretched. The cool-down stretch should last 5 minutes or more. The ACSM indicates that activities such as yoga, Tai Chi, and relaxation exercises can also be used as part of the second phase of the cool-down.

Physical Activity in the Heat and Cold

Web 05 **Physical activity in hot and humid environments challenges the body's heat loss mechanisms.** During vigorous activity, the body produces heat, which must be dissipated to regulate body temperature. The body has several ways to dissipate heat. *Conduction* is the transfer of heat from a hot body to a cold body. *Convection* is the transfer of heat through the air or any other medium. Fans and wind can facilitate heat loss by convection and help regulate temperature. The primary method of cooling is through *evaporation* of sweat. The chemical process involved in evaporation transfers heat from the body and reduces the body temperature. When conditions are humid, the effectiveness of evaporation is reduced, since the air is already saturated with moisture. This is why it is difficult to regulate body temperature when conditions are hot and humid.

Heat-related illness can occur if proper hydration is not maintained. Maximum sweat rates during physical activity in the heat can approach 1–2 liters per hour. If this fluid is not replaced, **dehydration** can occur. If dehydration is not corrected with water or other fluid-replacement drinks, it becomes increasingly more difficult for the body to maintain normal body temperatures. At some point, the rate of sweating decreases as the body begins to conserve

Table 3 ▶ Types of Heat-Related Problems

Problem	Symptoms	Severity
Heat cramps	Muscle cramps, especially in muscles most used in exercise	Least severe
Heat exhaustion	Muscle cramps, weakness, dizziness, headache, nausea, clammy skin, paleness	Moderately severe
Heat stroke	Hot, flushed skin; dry skin (lack of sweating); dizziness; fast pulse; unconsciousness; high temperature	Extremely severe

its remaining water. It shunts blood to the skin to transfer excess heat directly to the environment, but this is less effective than evaporation. **Hyperthermia** and associated heat-related problems can result (see Table 3).

One way to monitor the amount of fluid loss is to monitor the color of your urine. The American College of Sports Medicine indicates that clear (almost colorless) urine produced in large volumes indicates that you are hydrated. As water in the body is reduced the urine becomes more concentrated and is a darker yellow color. This indicates dehydration and a need for fluid replacement. Dietary supplements that contain amphetamine derivatives and/or creatine may contribute to undetected dehydration among some individuals.

Acclimatization improves the body's tolerance in the heat. Individuals with good fitness will respond better to activity in the heat than individuals with poor fitness. With regular exposure, the body adapts to the heat. The majority of the adaptation to hot environments occurs in 7 to 14 days but complete acclimatization can take up to 30 days. As you adapt to the heat, your body becomes conditioned to sweat earlier, to sweat more profusely, and to distribute the sweat more effectively around the body, and the composition of sweat is altered. This process makes it easier for your body to maintain a safe body temperature.

Web 06 **Precautions should be taken when doing physical activity in hot and humid environments.** The combination of high-heat and humidity presents the greatest risk for heat-related problems during exercise. The **apparent temperature** (also referred to as the heat index) is an index that combines temperature and humidity. Physical activity is safe when the apparent temperature is below 80°F (26.7°C). Above this temperature, there are four zones (see Table 4) that illustrate the danger of doing activity when the apparent temperature is high. Consider the following

Table 4 ▶ Exercise in the Heat (Apparent Temperatures)

To read the table, find air temperature on the top; then find the humidity on the left. Find the apparent temperature where the columns meet.

Relative Humidity (%)	Air Temperature (Degrees F)										
	70	75	80	85	90	95	100	105	110	115	120
100	72	80	91	108	132						
95	71	79	89	105	128						
90	71	79	88	102	122						
85	71	78	87	99	117	141					
80	71	78	86	97	113	136					
75	70	77	86	95	109	130					
70	70	77	85	93	106	124	144				
65	70	76	83	91	102	119	138				
60	70	76	82	90	100	114	132	149			
55	69	75	81	89	98	110	126	142			
50	69	75	81	88	96	107	120	135	150		
45	68	74	80	87	95	104	115	129	143		
40	68	74	79	86	93	101	110	123	137	151	
35	67	73	79	85	91	98	107	118	130	143	
30	67	73	78	84	90	96	104	113	123	135	148
25	66	72	77	83	88	94	101	109	117	127	139
20	66	72	77	82	87	93	99	105	112	120	130
15	65	71	76	81	86	91	97	102	108	115	123
10	65	70	75	80	85	90	95	100	105	111	116
5	64	69	74	79	84	88	93	97	102	107	111
0	64	69	73	78	83	87	91	95	99	103	107

"Apparent Temperatures" (Heat Index)

= Exreme danger zone
= Danger zone
= Extreme caution zone
= Caution zone
= Safe

Source: Data from National Oceanic and Atmospheric Administration.

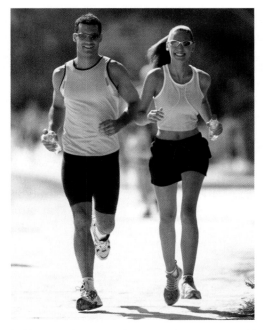

Proper clothing, sunglasses, and water are important considerations for exercise in the heat.

guidelines for performing exercise in the heat and humidity.

- Limit or cancel activity if the apparent temperature reaches the danger zone (see Table 4).
- Drink fluids before, during, and after activity. Guidelines suggest about 2 cups before activity and about 1 cup for each 15–20 minutes during activity. After activity, drink about 2 cups for each pound of weight lost. The thirst mechanism lags behind the body's actual need for fluid, so drink even if you don't feel thirsty. Fluid-replacement

Dehydration Excessive loss of water from the body, usually through perspiration, urination, or evaporation.

Hyperthermia Excessively high body temperature caused by excessive heat production or impaired heat loss capacity. Heat stroke is a hyperthermic condition.

Apparent Temperature A combination of temperature and humidity, used to determine if it is dangerous to perform physical activity (also called heat index).

beverages (e.g., Gatorade, Power-Aid) are designed to provide added energy (from carbohydrates) without impeding hydration. If you choose to use one of these beverages, select one that contains electrolytes and no more than 4 to 8 percent carbohydrates.

- Avoid extreme fluid intake. Drinking too much water can cause a condition called **hyponatremia,** sometimes referred to as "water intoxication." It occurs when you drink too much water, resulting in the dilution of the electrolytes in the blood; interestingly, it has symptoms similar to those of dehydration. If left untreated, in can result in loss of consciousness and even death. (See Web06 for details).
- Gradually expose yourself to physical activity in hot and humid environments to facilitate acclimatization.
- With extreme care, experienced exercisers who have become acclimatized to the heat may be able to perform at higher apparent temperatures than those who are less experienced. However, care should be used by all people who perform physical activity in hot and humid environments.
- Dress properly for exercise in the heat and humidity. Wear white or light colors that reflect rather than absorb heat. Select wickable clothes instead of cotton to aid evaporative cooling. Rubber, plastic, or other nonporous clothing is especially dangerous. A porous hat or cap can help when exercising in direct sunlight.
- Watch for signs of heat stress (see Table 3). If signs are present, stop immediately, get out of the heat, remove excess clothing, and drink cool water. Seek medical attention if symptoms progress.

 Physical activity in exceptionally cold and windy weather can be dangerous. Activity in the cold presents the opposite problems as exercise in the heat. In the cold, the primary goal is to retain the body's heat and avoid **hypothermia** and frostbite. Early signs of hypothermia include shivering and cold extremities caused by blood shunted to the body core to conserve heat. As the core temperature continues to drop, heart rate, respiration, and reflexes are depressed. Subsequently, cognitive functions decrease, speech and movement become impaired, and bizarre behavior may occur. Frostbite results from water crystallizing in the tissues, causing cell destruction.

When doing activity in cold, wet, and windy weather, precautions should be taken. A combination of cold and wind (windchill) poses the greatest danger for cold-related problems during exercise. Research conducted in Canada, in cooperation with the U.S. National Weather Service, produced tables for determining **windchill factor** and the time of exposure necessary to get frostbite (see Table 5). The old method of measurement overestimated the impact of cold weather. Consider the following guidelines for performing physical activity in cold and wind:

- Limit or cancel activity if the windchill factor reaches the danger zone (see Table 5).
- Dress properly. Wear light clothing in several layers rather than one heavy garment. The layer of clothing closest to the body should transfer (wick) moisture away from the skin to a second, more absorbent layer.

Table 5 ▶ Windchill Factor Chart

Actual Temperature Reading (Degrees F)	Estimated Wind Speed (mph)									Minutes to Frostbite
	Calm	5	10	15	20	25	30	35	40	
40	40	36	34	32	30	29	28	27	27	
30	30	25	21	19	17	16	15	14	13	
20	20	13	9	6	4	3	1	0	-1	
10	10	1	-4	-7	-9	-11	-12	-14	-15	
0	0	-11	-16	-19	-22	-24	-26	-27	-29	30
-10	-10	-22	-28	-32	-35	-37	-39	-41	-43	10
-20	-20	-34	-41	-45	-48	-51	-53	-55	-57	5
-30	-30	-46	-53	-58	-61	-64	-67	-69	-71	
-40	-40	-57	-66	-71	-74	-78	-80	-82	-84	

Source: National Weather Service.

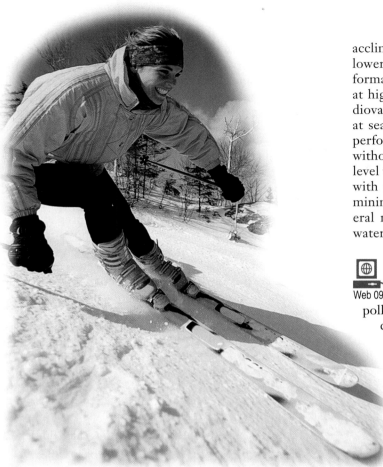

Wind, cold and altitude present some additional challenges for winter exercise.

Polypropylene and capilene are examples of wickable fabrics. A porous windbreaker will keep wind from cooling the body and will allow the release of body heat. The hands, feet, nose, and ears are most susceptible to frostbite, so they should be covered. Wear a hat or cap, mask, and mittens. Mittens are warmer than gloves. A light coating of petroleum jelly on exposed body parts can be helpful.

• Keep from getting wet in cold weather

Physical Activity in Other Environments

High altitude may limit performance and require adaptation of normal physical activity. Web 08 The ability to do vigorous physical tasks is diminished as altitude increases. Breathing rate and heart rates are more elevated at high altitude. With proper acclimation (gradual exposure), the body adjusts to the lower oxygen pressure found at high altitude, and performance improves. Nevertheless, performance ability at high altitudes, especially for activities requiring cardiovascular fitness, is usually less than would be expected at sea level. At extremely high altitudes, the ability to perform vigorous physical activity may be impossible without an extra oxygen supply. When moving from sea level to a high altitude, vigorous exercise should be done with caution. Acclimation to high altitudes requires a minimum of 2 weeks and may not be complete for several months. Care should be taken to drink adequate water at high altitude.

Exposure to air pollution should be limited. Web 09 Various pollutants can cause poor performance and, in some cases, health problems. Ozone, a pollutant produced primarily by the sun's reaction to car exhaust, can cause symptoms, including headache, coughing, and eye irritation. Similar symptoms result from exposure to carbon monoxide, a tasteless and odorless gas, caused by combustion of oil, gasoline, and/or cigarette smoke. Most news media in metropolitan areas now provide updates on ozone and carbon monoxide levels in their weather reports. When levels of these pollutants reach moderate levels, some people may need to modify their exercise. When levels are high, some may need to postpone exercise. Exercisers wishing to avoid ozone and carbon monoxide may want to exercise indoors early in the morning or later in the evening. It is wise to avoid areas with a high concentration of traffic.

Pollens from certain plants may cause allergic reactions for certain people. Some people are allergic to dust or other particulates in the air. Weather reports of pollens and particulates may help exercisers determine the best times for their activities and when to avoid vigorous activities.

Hyponatremia A condition caused by excess water intake, sometimes referred to as "water intoxication," that can cause loss of electrolytes, leading to serious medical complications.

Hypothermia Excessively low body temperature (less than 95°F), characterized by uncontrollable shivering, loss of coordination, and mental confusion.

Windchill Factor An index that uses air temperature and wind speed to determine the chilling effect of the environment on humans.

Soreness and Injury

Web 10 **Understanding soreness can help you persist in physical activity and avoid problems.** A common experience for many exercisers is a certain degree of muscle soreness that occurs 24–48 hours after intense exercise. This soreness, termed delayed-onset muscle soreness **(DOMS),** typically occurs when muscles are exercised at levels beyond their normal use. Some people mistakenly believe that lactic acid is the cause of muscle soreness. Lactic acid (a byproduct of anaerobic metabolism) is produced during vigorous exercise, but levels return to normal within 30 minutes after exercise, while DOMS occurs 24 hours after exercise. DOMS is caused by microscopic muscle tears which result from the excessive loads on the muscles. Soreness is not a normal part of the body's response to exercise but occurs if an individual violates the principle of progression and does more exercise than the body is prepared for. While it may be uncomfortable to some, it has no long-term consequences and does not predispose one to muscle injury. To reduce the likelihood of DOMS, it is important to progress your program gradually. Additional detail and images of muscle tears are provided at *On the Web* 10.

Web 11 **The most common injuries incurred in physical activity are sprains and strains.** A strain occurs when the fibers in a muscle are injured. Common activity-related injuries are hamstring strains that occur after a vigorous sprint. Other commonly strained muscles include the muscles in the front of the thigh, the low back, and the calf.

A sprain is an injury to a ligament—the connective tissue that connects bones to bones. The most common sprain is to the ankle; frequently, the ankle is rolled to the outside (inversion) when jumping or running. Other common sprains are to the knee, the shoulder, and the wrist.

Tendonitis is an inflammation of the tendon; it is most often a result of overuse rather than trauma. Tendonitis can be painful but often does not swell to the extent that sprains do. For this reason, elevation and compression are not as effective as ice and rest. Information about other common injuries is included on the Web but a physician should be consulted for an appropriate diagnosis.

Being able to treat minor injuries will help reduce their negative effects. Minor injuries, such as muscle strains and sprains, are common to those who are persistent in their exercise. If a serious injury should occur or if symptoms persist, it is important to get immediate medical attention. However, for minor injuries, following the **RICE** formula will help you reduce the pain and speed recovery. In this acronym, *R* stands for *rest.*

Muscle sprains and strains heal best if the injured area is rested. Rest helps you avoid further damage to the muscle. *I* stands for *ice.* The quick application of cold (ice or ice water) to a minor injury minimizes swelling and speeds recovery. Cold should be applied to as large a surface area as possible (soaking is best). If ice is used, it should be wrapped to avoid direct contact with the skin. Apply cold for 20 minutes, three times a day, allowing 1 hour between applications. *C* stands for *compression.* Wrapping or compressing the injured area also helps minimize swelling and speeds recovery. Elastic bandages or elastic socks are good for applying compression. Care should be taken to avoid wrapping an injury too tightly because this can result in loss of circulation to the area. *E* stands for *elevation.* Keeping the injured area elevated (above the level of the heart) is effective in minimizing swelling. If pain or swelling does not diminish after 24 to 48 hours, or if there is any doubt about the seriousness of an injury, seek medical help. Some experts recommend adding a *P* to RICE (PRICE) to indicate that prevention (P) is as important as treatment of injuries. Building strength and flexibility, warming up, beginning gradually when starting a new activity, and wearing protective equipment, such as lace-up ankle braces, are simple methods of prevention.

Taking over-the-counter pain remedies can help reduce the pain of muscle strains and sprains. Aspirin and ibuprofen (e.g., Excedrin, Motrin) have anti-inflammatory properties. However, acetaminophen (e.g., Tylenol) does not. It may reduce the pain but will not reduce inflammation.

Muscle cramps can be relieved by statically stretching a muscle. Muscle cramps are pains in the large muscles that result when the muscles contract vigorously for a continued period of time. Muscle cramps are usually not considered to be an injury, but they are painful and may seem like an injury. They are usually short in duration and can often be relieved with proper treatment. Cramps can result from lack of fluid replacement (dehydration), from fatigue, and from a blow directly to a muscle. Static stretching can help relieve some cramps. For example, the calf muscle, which often cramps among runners and other sports participants, can be relieved using the calf stretcher exercise, which is part of the warm-up in this concept.

Attitudes about Physical Activity

Knowing the most common reasons for inactivity can help you avoid sedentary living. Most people want to be active but find many barriers get in the way. The most commons reasons given by people who do not do regular physical activity are listed in Table 6. Experts consider many of these attitudes to be barriers that can

Table 6 ► Common Reasons People Give for Not Being Active

Reason	Description	Strategy for Change
I don't have the time.	This is the number one reason people give for not exercising. Invariably, those who feel they don't have time know they should do more exercise. They say they plan to do more in the future when "things are less hectic." Young people say that they will have more time to exercise in the future. Older people say that they wish they had taken the time to be active when they were younger.	Planning a daily schedule can help you find the time for activity and avoid wasting time on things that are less important. Learning the facts in the concepts that follow will help you see the importance of activity and how you can include it in your schedule with a minimum of effort and with time efficiency.
It's too inconvenient.	Many who avoid physical activity do so because it is inconvenient. They are procrastinators. Specific reasons for procrastinating include "It makes me sweaty" and "It messes up my hair."	If you have to travel more than 10 minutes to do activity or if you do not have easy access to equipment, you will avoid activity. Locating facilities and finding a time when you can shower is important.
I just don't enjoy it.	Many do not find activity to be enjoyable or invigorating. These people may assume that all forms of activity have to be strenuous and fatiguing.	There are many activities to choose from. If you don't enjoy vigorous activity, try more moderate forms of activity, such as walking.
I'm no good at physical activity.	"People might laugh at me," "Sports make me nervous," and "I am not good at physical activities" are reasons some people give for not being active. Some people lack confidence in their own abilities. This may be because of past experiences in physical education or sports.	With properly selected activities, even those who have never enjoyed exercise can get hooked. Building skills can help, as can changing your way of thinking. Avoiding comparisons with others can help you feel successful.
I am not fit, so I avoid activity.	Some people avoid exercise because of health reasons. Some who are unfit lack energy. Starting slowly can build fitness gradually and help you realize that you can do it.	There are good medical reasons for not doing activity, but many people with problems can benefit from exercise if it is properly designed. If necessary, get help adapting activity to meet your needs.
I have no place to be active, especially in bad weather.	Regular activity is more convenient if facilities are easy to reach and the weather is good. Opportunities have increased considerably in recent years. Some of the most popular activities require little equipment, can be done in or near home, and are inexpensive.	If you cannot find a place, if it is not safe, or if it is too expensive, consider using low-cost equipment at home, such as rubber bands or calisthenics. Lifestyle activity can be done by anyone at almost any time.
I am too old.	As people grow older, many begin to feel that activity is something they cannot do. For most people, this is simply not true! Properly planned exercise for older adults is not only safe but also has many health benefits—e.g., longer life, fewer illnesses, an improved sense of well-being, and optimal functioning.	Older people who are just beginning activity should start slowly. Lifestyle activities are a good choice. Setting realistic goals can help, as can learning to do resistance training and flexibility exercises.

be overcome. In fact, a key self-management skill that predicts long-tern behavior change is the ability to overcome barriers. The strategies in Table 6 can help inactive people become more active.

Knowing the reasons people give for being active can help you adopt positive attitudes toward activity. To enhance the promotion of physical activity in society, many researchers have sought to determine why some people choose to be active and others do not. The most common reasons for physical activity are highlighted in Table 7. The table also offers strategies for changing behaviors.

DOMS An acronym for delayed-onset muscle soreness, a common malady that follows relatively vigorous activity, especially among beginners.

RICE An acronym for rest, ice, compression, and elevation; a method of treating minor injuries.

Table 7 ▶ Common Reasons for Doing Regular Physical Activity

Reason	Description	Strategy for Change
I do activity for my health, wellness, and fitness.	Surveys show this is the number one reason for doing regular physical activity. Unfortunately, many adults say that a "doctor's order to exercise" would be the most likely reason to get them to begin a program. For some, however, waiting for a doctor's order may be too late.	Gaining information contained in this book will help you see the value of regular physical activity. Performing the self-assessments in the various concepts will help you determine the areas in which you need personal improvement.
I do activity to improve my appearance.	In our society, looking good is highly valued; thus, physical attractiveness is a major reason people participate in regular exercise. Regular activity can contribute to looking your best.	Some people have failed in past attempts to change their appearance through activity. Setting realistic goals and avoiding comparisons with others can help you be more successful.
I do activity because I enjoy it.	A majority of adults say that enjoyment is of paramount importance in deciding to be active. Statements include experiencing the "peak experience," the "runner's high," or "spinning free." The sense of fun, well-being, and general enjoyment associated with physical activity are well documented.	People who do not enjoy activity often lack performance skills or feel that they are not competent in activity. Improving skills with practice, setting realistic goals, and adopting a new way of thinking can help you be successful and enjoy activities.
I do activity because it relaxes me.	Relaxation and release from tension rank high as reasons people do regular activity. It is known that activity in the form of sports and games provides a catharsis, or outlet, for the frustrations of daily activities. Regular exercise can help reduce depression and anxiety.	Activities such as walking, jogging, or cycling are ways of getting some quiet time away from the job or the stresses of daily living. In a later concept, you will learn about exercises that you can do to reduce stress.
I like the challenge and sense of personal accomplishment I get from physical activity.	A sense of personal accomplishment is frequently a reason for people doing activity. In some cases, it is learning a new skill, such as racquetball or tennis; in other cases, it is running a mile or doing a certain number of crunches. The challenge of doing something you have never done before is apparently a powerful experience.	Some people get little sense of accomplishment from activity. Taking lessons to learn skills or attempting activities new to you can provide the challenge that makes activity interesting. Also, adopting a new way of thinking allows you to focus on the task rather than on competition with others.
I like the social involvement I get from physical activities.	"Why am I physically active?" "It is a good way to spend time with members of my family." "It is a good way to spend time with close friends." "Being part of the team is satisfying." Activity settings can also provide an opportunity for making new friends.	If you find activity to be socially unrewarding, you may have to find activities that you, your family, or your friends enjoy. Taking lessons together can help. Also, finding a friend with similar skills can help. Focus on the activity rather than the outcome.
Competition is the main reason I enjoy physical activity.	"The thrill of victory" and "sports competition" are two reasons given for being active. For many, the competitive experience is very satisfying.	Some people simply do not enjoy competing. If this is the case for you, select noncompetitive individual activities.
Physical activity helps me feel good about myself.	For many people, participation in physical activity is an important part of their identity. They feel better about themselves when they are regularly participating.	Physical activity is something that is self-determined and within your control. Participation can help you feel good about yourself, build your confidence, and increase your self-esteem.
Physical activity provides opportunities to get fresh air.	Being outside and experiencing nature are reasons that some people give for being physically active.	Many activities provide opportunities to be outside. If this is an important reason for you, seek out parks and outdoor settings for your activities.

Strategies for Action

Screening for risks can help make activity safer. Athletes in competitive sports often undergo preparticipation physical examinations to screen for potential cardiac arrhythmias or conditions known to increase risks during exercise. Recreational athletes may not take the same precautions. The best advice is to get a physical prior to beginning serious training. This is especially critical if you have a family history of heart problems. Lab 3A will help you determine if you should consult a physician.

A proper warm-up and cool-down can make activity more effective and more enjoyable. A proper warm-up can prepare your body for activity and a gradual cool-down can improve recovery. Lab 3B provides a sample flexibility-based warm-up and cool-down routine that may be helpful. Determine what works best for your needs.

When preparing for physical activity, assessing your attitudes can be helpful. Active people generally have more positive attitudes than negative ones. This is referred to as a "positive balance of attitudes." The questionnaire in Lab 3C gives you the opportunity to assess your balance of attitudes. If you have a "negative balance" score, you can analyze your attitudes and determine how you can change them to view activity more favorably.

Technology Update
Automatic External Defibrillators (AEDs)

 Web 12

The automatic external defibrillator (AED) is a computerized device similar in size to a laptop. It is used to revive people who have suffered from sudden cardiac arrest. The AED has a heart rhythm analysis system, which advises the operator when to deliver a "shock" to the heart. Each year about 60,000 people suffer from a heart problem that could benefit from an AED. When the heart is "shocked" within 6 minutes of the event, the person usually lives. With longer waits, odds decrease dramatically.

Originally, defibrillators were used only by professionals. When defibrillators were automated, they became commonplace in airports and other public locations. In recent years, the AED has been authorized for use by nonprofessionals. The most recent AED has a voice prompt, which cues the user concerning operation. Recently, the Food and Drug Administration (FDA) approved over-the-counter sales of the AED. However, a doctor's prescription is needed to get an AED for home use. The FDA is now considering approval for a French pocket-sized defibrillator named FRED. It weighs only 1 pound.

A recent position statement from ACSM and American Heart Association advises health and fitness clubs to have an AED system available and a staff trained to use them. Federal law and "good Samaritan" laws in 47 states extend protection to AED users. See Web12 for more information.

Online Learning Center

www.mhhe.com/corbin7e
The Online Learning Center contains a variety of Web-based resources that will help you get the most out of this book and your course. In addition to the On the Web pages, there are video activities, interactive quizzes, application assignments, and a variety of other useful study aids. Log on to the URL above to access these resources.

Web Resources

 Web 13

ACSM's Fit Society Page
   www.acsm.org/health+fitness/ fit_society.htm
ACSM's Health and Fitness Journal **www.acsm.org/ publications/health_fitness_journal.htm**
American College of Sports Medicine **www.acsm.org**
American Red Cross (AED information) **www.redcross.org**
National Athletic Trainers Association **www.nata.org**
Med Watch **www.fda.gov/medwatch**
The Physician and Sportsmedicine **www.physsportsmed.com**

Suggested Readings

Web 14

Additional reference materials for Concept 3 are available at Web14.

Almond, C. S. D., et al. 2005. Hyponatremia among runners in the Boston Marathon. *New England Journal of Medicine* 352(15):1550–1556.

American College of Sports Medicine. 2006. *ACSM's Guidelines for Exercise Testing and Prescription*. 7th ed. Philadelphia: Lippincott, Williams and Wilkins.

American College of Sports Medicine and American Heart Association. 2002. Automated external defibrillators in health/fitness facilities. *Medicine and Science in Sports and Exercise* 34(3):561–564.

Asplund, C. A., and D. L. Brown. 2005. The running shoe prescription: Fit for performance. *The Physician and Sportsmedicine* 33(1):17–24.

Bracko, M. R. 2002. Can stretching prior to exercise and sports improve performance and prevent injury? *ACSM's Health and Fitness Journal* 6(5):17–22.

Hootman, J. M., et al. 2002. Epidemiology of musculoskeletal injuries among sedentary and physically active adults. *Medicine and Science in Sports and Exercise* 34(5):838–844.

Inter-Association Task Force on Exertional Heat Illnesses. 2003. Inter-Association Task Force on Exertional Heat Illnesses consensus statement. *National Athletic Trainers Association Newsletter* June:24–29. Also available online at **www.nata.org**.

Montain, S. J., et al. 2006. Exercise associated hyponatremia: Quantitative analysis to understand the aetiology. *British Journal of Sports Medicine* 40:98–105.

Noakes, T. D. 2005. Mind over matter: Deducing heatstroke pathology. *The Physician and Sportsmedicine* 33(10):39–58.

Noakes, T. D. 2006. Sports Drinks: Prevention of "voluntary dehydration" and development of exercise-associated hyponatremia. *Medicine and Science in Sports & Exercise* 38(1):193.

Shrier, I. 2005. An intervention program to reduce hamstring injuries. *The Physician and Sportsmedicine* 33(12):8–8.

Shrier, I. 2005. When and how to stretch? *The Physician and Sportsmedicine* 33(3):22–26.

 In the News

New CPR Guidelines

The American Heart Association has recently made dramatic changes in its CPR guidelines. The changes were made partly based on new information concerning the most effective techniques and partly to increase the likelihood that bystanders will give help when needed. When confronted with a person who needs help, less than one-third of all bystanders give help, even those who have been trained. The reason for lack of willingness to use CPR include fear of getting a disease from mouth-to-mouth contact (research indicates the risk is low), lack of knowledge about what to do, and fear of using an incorrect technique.

To overcome the barriers for laypeople, the guidelines have been simplified. There has been a shift in emphasis from mouth-to-mouth contact to chest compression. The goal is to get laypeople to dare to help—some CPR is better than no CPR.

For laypeople who do not want to apply mouth-to-mouth the recommendations are to

- Quickly check for responsiveness (shake the victim).
- Call for help as you continue.
- Begin compression immediately at a rate of 100–120 per minute.

- Minimize interruptions in compression.
- Continue compression until help arrives.
- Perform compressions "hard and fast," but allow the chest to recoil. It is better to press too hard than not to press hard enough. Lock the elbows and keep the arms straight, place one hand over the other, and compress the center of the chest with the heel of the hand.

The layperson who wants to apply mouth-to-mouth should provide 2 rescue breaths lasting 1 second each before beginning compression—look for the chest to rise. If 2 laypeople are willing to give mouth-to-mouth, give 2 rescue breaths; then apply compression. Continue at a rate of 2 breaths and 30 compressions (same rate for children and adults).

The rules for health-care providers are different from those for laypeople. Health-care providers must have certification. Certification is recommended for laypeople, but the guidelines were revised to get more people to help even when not certified. A kit called *CPR Anytime for Family and Friends* is available to train family members of all ages. It contains a DVD, a booklet, and a manikin. The kit may be ordered at **www.cpranytime.org**.

Lab 3A Readiness for Physical Activity

Name	**Section**	**Date**

Purpose: To help you determine your physical readiness for participation in a program of regular exercise

Procedures

1. Read the directions on the "PAR-Q & You" on page 58.
2. Answer each of the seven questions on the form.
3. If you answered "yes" to one or more of the questions, follow the directions just below the PAR-Q questions regarding medical consultation.
4. If you answered "no" to all seven questions, follow the directions at the lower left-hand corner of the PAR-Q.
5. Answer the five questions about physical readiness for sports or vigorous training in Chart 1 below.
6. Record your score below and answer the question in the Conclusions and Implications section.

Results

Chart 1 ▶ Physical Readiness for Sports or Vigorous Training

Answer the PAR-Q before using this chart. If your answer to any of these questions is "yes," then you should consult with your personal physician by telephone or in person to determine if you have a potential problem with sports or vigorous training.

Yes	No	
☐	☐	1. Do you plan to participate on an organized team that will play intense competitive sports (e.g., varsity team, professional team)?
☐	☐	2. If you plan to participate in a collision sport (even on a less organized basis), such as football, boxing, rugby, or ice hockey, have you been knocked unconscious more than one time?
☐	☐	3. Do you currently have symptoms from a previous muscle injury?
☐	☐	4. Do you currently have symptoms from a previous back injury, or do you experience back pain as a result of involvement in physical activity?
☐	☐	5. Do you have any other symptoms during physical activity that give you reason to be concerned about your health?

Determine your PAR-Q score. Place an X over the circle that includes the number of "yes" answers that you had for the PAR-Q (see page 58).

⓪ ① ② ③ ④ ⑤ ⑥ ⑦

Determine your readiness for sports or rigorous training (see Chart 1 above). Place an X over the number of "yes" answers that you had for the Physical Readiness for Sports or Vigorous Training chart.

⓪ ① ② ③ ④ ⑤

Conclusions and Implications: In several sentences, discuss your readiness for physical activity. Base your comments on your questionnaire results and the types of physical activities you plan to perform in the future.

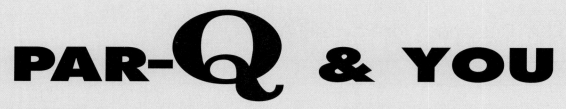

PAR-Q & YOU

Regular physical activity is fun and healthy, and increasingly more people are starting to become more active every day. Being more active is very safe for most people. However, some people should check with their doctor before they start becoming much more physically active.

If you are planning to become much more physically active than you are now, start by answering the seven questions in the box below. If you are between the ages of fifteen and sixty-nine, the PAR-Q will tell you if you should check with your doctor before you start. If you are over sixty-nine years of age, and you are not used to being very active, check with your doctor.

Common sense is your best guide when you answer these questions. Please read the questions carefully and answer each one honestly: check YES or NO.

YES	NO	
☐	☐	1. Has your doctor ever said that you have a heart condition <u>and</u> that you should only do physical activity recommended by a doctor?
☐	☐	2. Do you feel pain in your chest when you do physical activity?
☐	☐	3. In the past month, have you had chest pain when you were not doing physical activity?
☐	☐	4. Do you lose your balance because of dizziness or do you ever lose consciousness?
☐	☐	5. Do you have a bone or joint problem that could be made worse by a change in your physical activity?
☐	☐	6. Is your doctor currently prescribing drugs (for example, water pills) for your blood pressure or heart condition?
☐	☐	7. Do you know of <u>any other reason</u> you should not do physical activity?

If you answered

Yes

YES to one or more questions

Talk with your doctor by phone or in person BEFORE you start becoming much more physically active or BEFORE you have a fitness appraisal. Tell your doctor about the PAR-Q and which questions you answered YES.

- You may be able to do any activity you want—as long as you start slowly and build up gradually. Or you may need to restrict your activities to those that are safe for you. Talk with your doctor about the kinds of activities you wish to participate in and follow his or her advice.
- Find out which community programs are safe and helpful for you.

No

NO to all questions

If you answered NO honestly to <u>all</u> PAR-Q questions, you can be reasonably sure that you can

- Start becoming much more physically active—begin slowly and build up gradually. This is the safest and easiest way to go.
- Take part in a fitness appraisal—this is an excellent way to determine your basic fitness so that you can plan the best way for you to live actively.

DELAY BECOMING MUCH MORE ACTIVE:

- If you are not feeling well because of a temporary illness, such as a cold or a fever—wait until you feel better or
- If you are or may be pregnant—talk to your doctor before you start becoming more active.

Please note: If your health changes so that you then answer YES to any of the above questions, tell your fitness or health professional. Ask whether you should change your physical activity plan.

<u>Informed Use of the PAR-Q:</u> The Canadian Society for Exercise Physiology, Health Canada, and their agents assume no liability for persons who undertake physical activity, and if in doubt after completing this questionnaire, consult your doctor prior to physical activity.

You are encouraged to copy the PAR-Q but only if you use the entire form

*Developed by the British Columbia Ministry of Health.
Produced by the British Columbia Ministry of Health and the Department of National Health & Welfare

Physical Activity Readiness
Questionnaire • PAR-Q
(revised 2002)

Note: It is important that you answer all questions honestly. The PAR-Q is a scientifically and medically researched pre-exercise selection device. It complements exercise programs, exercise testing procedures, and the liability considerations attendant with such programs and testing procedures. PAR-Q, like any other preexercise screening device, will misclassify a small percentage of prospective participants, but no preexercise screening method can entirely avoid this problem.

Lab 3B The Warm-Up and Cool-Down

Name		Section	Date

Purpose: To familiarize you with a sample group of warm-up and cool-down exercises

Procedures

1. Perform a 2- to 5-minute cardiovascular warm-up (walk, jog, slow jump rope, swim).
2. Perform the exercises in Chart 1, including the alternative exercises, on the back of this lab page three times each. Hold the stretch for 15 to 30 seconds.
3. Complete the Results section below and answer the questions in the Conclusions and Implications section.

Results: In the following, put an X over the circle that represents the amount of tightness you felt when performing each of the stretching warm-up and cool-down exercises. Tightness indicates that you may have shortness of a specific muscle group and that stretching exercises at times other than the warm-up or cool-down are needed.

	None	Moderate	Severe
Calf stretch	◯	◯	◯
Hamstring stretch	◯	◯	◯
Leg hug	◯	◯	◯
Sitting side stretch	◯	◯	◯
Zipper	◯	◯	◯

Alternative Exercises

	None	Moderate	Severe
Side stretch	◯	◯	◯
One-leg stretch	◯	◯	◯
Hip and thigh stretch	◯	◯	◯

Conclusions and Implications: In several sentences, discuss the warm-up and cool-down. Include in the discussion your feelings about the adequacy of the warm-up and cool-down for you personally. Those who plan to do vigorous sports will need to supplement this group of exercises.

Chart 1 ▶ Sample warm-up and cool-down exercises

The exercises shown here can be used before a moderate workout as a warm-up or after a workout as a cool-down. Perform these exercises slowly, preferably after completing a cardiovascular warm-up. Do not bounce. Hold each stretch for at least 15-30 seconds. Perform each exercise at least once and up to three times. Other stretching exercises are presented in the concept on flexibility and they can be used in a warm-up or cool-down.

Cardiovascular Exercise

Before you perform a vigorous workout, walk or jog slowly for 2 minutes or more. After exercise, do the same. Do this portion of the warm-up prior to muscle stretching.

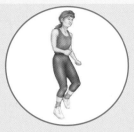

Calf Stretcher

This exercise stretches the calf muscles (gastrocnemius and soleus). Face a wall with your feet 2 or 3 feet away. Step forward on your left foot to allow both hands to touch the wall. Keep the heel of your right foot on the ground, toe turned in slightly, knee straight, and buttocks tucked in. Lean forward by bending your front knee and arms and allowing your head to move nearer the wall. Hold. Repeat with the other leg.

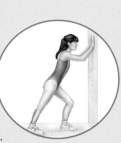

Hamstring Stretcher

This exercise stretches the muscles of the back of the upper leg (hamstrings) as well as those of the hip, knee, and ankle. Lie on your back. Bring the right knee to your chest and grasp the toes with the right hand. Place the left hand on the back of the right thigh. Pull the knee toward the chest, push the heel toward the ceiling, and pull the toes toward the shin. Attempt to straighten the knee. Stretch and hold. Repeat with the other leg.

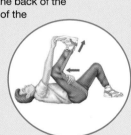

Leg Hug

This exercise stretches the hip and back extensor muscles. Lie on your back. Bend one leg and grasp your thigh under the knee. Hug it to your chest. Keep the other leg straight and on the floor. Hold. Repeat with the opposite leg.

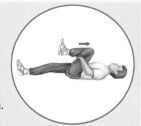

Seated Side Stretch

This exercise stretches the muscles of the trunk. Begin in a seated position with the legs crossed. Stretch the left arm over the head to the right. Bend at the waist (to right), reaching as far as possible to the left with the right arm. Hold. Do not let the trunk rotate. Repeat to the opposite side. For less stretch, the overhead arm may be bent. This exercise can be done in the standing position but is less effective.

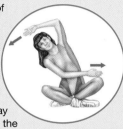

Zipper

This exercise stretches the muscle on the back of the arm (triceps) and the lower chest muscles (pecs). Lift the right arm and reach behind the head and down the spine (as if pulling up a zipper). With the left hand, push down on the right elbow and hold. Reverse arm position and repeat.

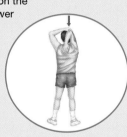

ALTERNATE EXERCISES

Because of location (wet or hard surface), you may choose to substitute exercises that do not require you to lie down. The side stretch (standing) can be substituted for the seated side stretch, the one-leg stretch (standing) for the hamstring stretch, and the hip and thigh stretch for the leg hug (does not stretch the exact same muscles).

Side Stretch

This exercise stretches the trunk lateral flexors. Stand with feet shoulder-width apart. Stretch left arm overhead to right. Bend to right at waist reaching as far as possible with left arm; reach as far as possible with right arm. Hold. Do not let trunk rotate or lower back arch. Repeat on opposite side. Note: This exercise is made more effective if a weight is held down at the side in the hand opposite the side being stretched. More stretch will occur if the hip on the stretched side is dropped and most of the weight is borne by the opposite foot.

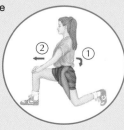

Hip and Thigh Stretch

This exercise stretches the hip (iliopsoas) and thigh muscles (quadriceps) and is useful for people with lordosis and back problems. Place right knee directly above right ankle and stretch left leg backward so knee touches floor. If necessary, place hands on floor for balance.
1. Tilt the pelvis backward by tucking in the abdomen and flattening the back.
2. Then shift the weight forward until a stretch is felt on the front of the thigh: hold. Repeat on opposite side. Caution: Do not bend front knee more than 90 degrees.

One-Leg Stretch

This exercise stretches the lower back muscles. Stand with one foot on a bench, keeping both legs straight. Contract the hamstrings and gluteals by pressing down on bench with the heel for three seconds; then relax and bend the trunk forward, toward the knee. Hold for 10–15 seconds. Return to starting position and repeat with opposite leg. As flexibility improves, the arms can be used to pull the chest toward the legs. Do not allow either knee to lock. This exercise is useful in relief of backache and correction of swayback.

Lab 3C Physical Activity Attitude Questionnaire

Name _____ **Section** _____ **Date** _____

Purpose: To evaluate your feelings about physical activity and to determine the specific reasons you do or do not participate in regular physical activity

Directions: The term *physical activity* in the following statements refers to all kinds of activities, including sports, formal exercises, and informal activities, such as jogging and cycling. Make an X over the circle that best represents your answer to each question.

	Strongly Disagree	Disagree	Undecided	Agree	Strongly Agree	Item Score		Attitude Score
1. I should do physical activity regularly for my health.	①	②	③	④	⑤			Health and Fitness Score
2. Doing regular physical activity is good for my fitness and wellness.	①	②	③	④	⑤	+	=	
3. Regular exercise helps me look my best.	①	②	③	④	⑤			Appearance Score
4. I feel more physically attractive when I do regular physical activity.	①	②	③	④	⑤	+	=	
5. One of the main reasons I do regular physical activity is that it is fun.	①	②	③	④	⑤			Enjoyment Score
6. The most enjoyable part of my day is when I am exercising or doing a sport.	①	②	③	④	⑤	+	=	
7. Taking part in physical activity helps me relax.	①	②	③	④	⑤			Relaxation Score
8. Physical activity helps me get away from the pressures of daily living.	①	②	③	④	⑤	+	=	
9. The challenge of physical training is one reason I do physical activity.	①	②	③	④	⑤			Challenge Score
10. I like to see if I can master sports and activities that are new to me.	①	②	③	④	⑤	+	=	
11. I like to do physical activity that involves other people.	①	②	③	④	⑤			Social Score
12. Exercise offers me the opportunity to meet other people.	①	②	③	④	⑤	+	=	
13. Competition is a good way to make physical activity fun.	①	②	③	④	⑤			Competition Score
14. I like to see how my physical abilities compare with those of others.	①	②	③	④	⑤	+	=	
15. When I do regular exercise, I feel better than when I don't.	①	②	③	④	⑤			Feeling Good Score
16. My ability to do physical activity is something that makes me proud.	①	②	③	④	⑤	+	=	
17. I like to do outdoor activities.	①	②	③	④	⑤			Outdoor Score
18. Experiencing nature is something I look forward to when exercising.	①	②	③	④	⑤	+	=	

Procedures

1. Read and answer each question in the questionnaire.
2. Write the number in the circle of your answer in the box labeled "Item Score."
3. Add scores for each pair of scores and record in the "Attitude Score" box.
4. Record each attitude score and a rating for each score (use Rating Chart) in the chart below.
5. Record the number of good and excellent scores in the box provided. Use the score in the box to determine your rating using the Balance of Feelings Rating Chart.

Results: Record your results as indicated in the Procedures section.

Physical Activity Attitude Questionnaire Results

Attitude	Score	Rating
Health and fitness		
Appearance		
Enjoyment		
Relaxation		
Challenge		
Social		
Competition		
Feeling good		
Outdoor		

Attitude Rating Chart

Rating Category	Attitude Score
Excellent	9–10
Good	7–8
Fair	5–6
Poor	3–4
Very poor	2

How many good or excellent scores do you have?

Balance of Feeling Score

Having 5 or more in the box above indicates that you have a positive balance of feelings (more positive than negative attitudes).

Balance of Feelings Rating Chart

Excellent	6–9
Good	5
Fair	4
Poor	2–3
Very poor	0–1

In a few sentences, discuss your "balance of feelings" rating. Having more positive than negative scores (positive balance of feelings) increases the probability of being active. Include comments on whether you think your ratings suggest that you will be active or inactive and whether your ratings are really indicative of your feelings. Do you think that the scores on which you were rated poor or very poor might be reasons you would avoid physical activity? Explain.

The Health Benefits of Physical Activity

Health Goals for the year 2010

- Increase quality and years of healthy life.
- Increase incidence of "healthy days."
- Increase daily physical activity.
- Increase prevalence of a healthy weight and reduce prevalence of overweight.
- Reduce days with pain for those with arthritis, osteoporosis, and chronic back problems.
- Reduce activity limitations, especially among older adults.
- Reduce incidence of and deaths from cancer.
- Increase diagnosis of and reduce incidence of Type II diabetes.
- Decrease incidence of depression.
- Decrease incidence of heart diseases, including stroke and high blood pressure.
- Decrease incidence of high cholesterol levels among adults.

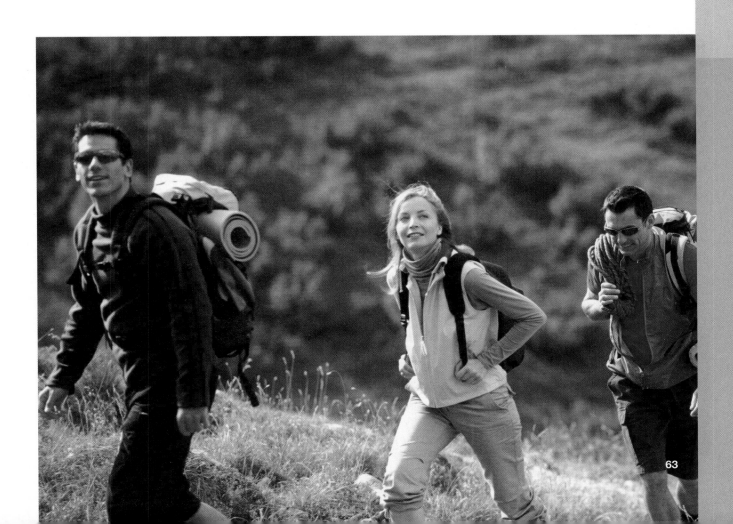

Physical activity and good physical fitness can reduce risk of illness and contribute to optimal health and wellness.

The *Surgeon General's Report on Physical Activity and Health* was an especially important document that informed the general public of the risks of sedentary living and the health benefits of physical activity. Since that document was published, more evidence has accumulated supporting the health benefits of an active lifestyle. One recent study has shown that physical fitness measured using a treadmill test is a more powerful predictor of longevity than any other risk factor, including smoking, heart problems, high blood pressure, high cholesterol, and diabetes. The evidence has led to reports, such as *Healthy People 2010* in the United States and *Achieving Health for All* in Canada, that establish health goals designed to promote active healthy living in the 21st century. In this concept, the health benefits of regular physical activity and good fitness will be summarized.

Physical Activity and Hypokinetic Diseases

Web 01 **Regular physical activity and good fitness can promote good health, help prevent disease, and be a part of disease treatment.** There are three major ways in which regular physical activity and good fitness can contribute to optimal health and wellness. First, they can aid in disease/illness prevention. There is considerable evidence that the risk of **hypokinetic diseases or conditions** can be greatly reduced among people who do regular physical activity and achieve good physical fitness. Virtually all **chronic diseases** that plague society are considered to be hypokinetic, though some relate more to inactivity than others. Nearly three-quarters of all deaths among those 18 and older are a result of chronic diseases. Leading public health officials have suggested that physical activity reduces the risk for several of these diseases. Physical activity also stimulates

positive changes with respect to other risk factors and may produce a shortcut for the control of chronic diseases, much as immunization controls infectious diseases.

Second, physical activity and fitness can be significant contributors to disease/illness treatment. Even with the best disease prevention practices, some people will become ill. Regular exercise and good fitness have been shown to be effective in alleviating symptoms and aiding rehabilitation after illness for such hypokinetic conditions as diabetes, heart disease, and back pain.

Finally, physical activity and fitness are methods of health and wellness promotion. They contribute to quality living associated with wellness, the positive component of good health. In the process, they aid in meeting many of the nation's health goals.

Web 02 **Too many adults suffer from hypokinetic disease and the economic cost is high.** In 1961, Kraus and Raab coined the term *hypokinetic disease* to describe health problems associated with lack of physical activity. They showed how sedentary living, or, as they called it "take it easy" living, contributes to the leading killer diseases in our society.

A public advocacy group has recently coined the term **sedentary death syndrome (SeDS)** to describe inactive living and associated hypokinetic disease risk factors. They indicate that SeDS is responsible for the epidemic of chronic disease in our society and resulting increases in health costs. It is expected that, in the next few years, expenditures for health care will account for one-fifth of all spending in the United States.

Regular physical activity over a lifetime may overcome the effects of inherited risk. Some people with a family history of disease may conclude they can do nothing because their heredity works against them. There is no doubt that heredity significantly affects risk for early death from hypokinetic diseases. New studies of twins, however, suggest that active people are less likely to die early than inactive people with similar genes. This suggests that long-term adherence to physical activity can overcome other risk factors, such as heredity.

Hypokinetic diseases and conditions have many causes. Regular physical activity and good physical fitness are only two of the preventive factors associated with the conditions described in this concept as hypokinetic diseases. Other healthy lifestyle factors, such as nutrition and stress management, cannot be overlooked.

Web 01 **On the Web**
www.mhhe.com/corbinweb
Log on to this URL before reading this concept. See On the Web list of concepts. Click on the concept number you want to view. To access supplemental information, click on the number shown at each Web icon.

Physical Activity and Cardiovascular Diseases

The many types of cardiovascular diseases are the leading killers in automated societies. There are many forms of **cardiovascular disease (CVD).** Some are classified as **coronary heart disease (CHD)** because they affect the heart muscle and the blood vessels that supply the heart. **Coronary occlusion** (heart attack) is a type of CHD. **Atherosclerosis** and **arteriosclerosis** are two conditions that increase risk for heart attack and are considered to be types of CHD. **Angina pectoris** (chest or arm pain), which occurs when the oxygen supply to the heart muscle is diminished, is sometimes considered to be a type of CHD, though it is really a symptom of poor circulation.

Hypertension (high blood pressure), **stroke** (brain attack), **peripheral vascular disease,** and **congestive heart failure** are other forms of CVD. Inactivity relates in some way to each of these types of disease.

In the United States, CHD accounts for approximately 31 percent of all premature deaths. Stroke accounts for an additional 7 percent. Men are more likely to suffer from heart disease than women, although the differences have narrowed in recent years. African American, Hispanic, and Native American populations are at higher than normal risk. Heart disease and stroke death rates are similar in the United States, Canada, Great Britain, Australia, and other automated societies.

There is a wealth of statistical evidence that physical inactivity is a primary risk factor for CHD. Much of the research relating inactivity to heart disease has come from occupational studies that show a high incidence of heart disease in people involved only in sedentary work. Even with the limitations inherent in these types of studies, the findings of more and more occupational studies present convincing evidence that the inactive individual has an increased risk for coronary heart disease. A study summarizing all of the important occupational studies shows a 90 percent reduced risk for coronary heart disease for those in active versus inactive occupations.

The American Heart Association, after carefully examining the research literature, elevated sedentary living from a secondary to a primary risk factor, comparable to high blood pressure, high blood cholesterol, obesity, and cigarette smoke. The reason for this change is that inactivity increases risk in multiple ways and large numbers of adults are sedentary and vulnerable to these risks. After reviewing hundreds of studies on exercise and heart disease, the *Surgeon General's Report on Physical Activity and Health* concluded that "physical inactivity is causally linked to atherosclerosis and coronary heart disease."

Physical Activity and the Healthy Heart

Regular physical activity will increase the heart muscle's ability to pump oxygen-rich blood. A fit heart muscle can handle extra demands placed on it. Through regular exercise, the heart muscle gets stronger, contracts more forcefully, and therefore pumps more

Hypokinetic Diseases or Conditions *Hypo-* means "under" or "too little" and *-kinetic* means "movement" or "activity." Thus, *hypokinetic* means "too little activity." A hypokinetic disease or condition is associated with lack of physical activity or too little regular exercise. Examples include heart disease, low back pain, and Type II diabetes.

Chronic Diseases Diseases or illnesses associated with lifestyle or environmental factors, as opposed to infectious diseases; hypokinetic diseases are considered to be chronic diseases.

Sedentary Death Syndrome (SeDS) A group of symptoms associated with sedentary living, including low health-related fitness (low cardiovascular fitness and weak muscles), low bone density, and the presence of metabolic syndrome (poor metabolic fitness).

Cardiovascular Disease (CVD) A broad classification of diseases of the heart and blood vessels that includes CHD, high blood pressure, stroke, and peripheral vascular disease.

Coronary Heart Disease (CHD) Diseases of the heart muscle and the blood vessels that supply it with oxygen, including heart attack.

Coronary Occlusion The blocking of the coronary blood vessels; sometimes called heart attack.

Atherosclerosis The deposition of materials along the arterial walls; a type of arteriosclerosis.

Arteriosclerosis Hardening of the arteries due to conditions that cause the arterial walls to become thick, hard, and nonelastic.

Angina Pectoris Chest or arm pain resulting from reduced oxygen supply to the heart muscle.

Hypertension High blood pressure; excessive pressure against the walls of the arteries that can damage the heart, kidneys, and other organs of the body.

Stroke A condition in which the brain, or part of the brain, receives insufficient oxygen as a result of diminished blood supply; sometimes called apoplexy or cerebrovascular accident (CVA).

Peripheral Vascular Disease A lack of oxygen supply to the working muscles and tissues of the arms and legs, resulting from decreased blood flow.

Congestive Heart Failure The inability of the heart muscle to pump the blood at a life-sustaining rate.

blood with each beat. The heart is just like any other muscle—it must be exercised regularly to stay fit. The fit heart also has open, clear arteries free of atherosclerosis (see Figure 1).

The hypothetical "normal" resting heart rate is said to be 72 beats per minute (bpm). However, resting rates of 50 to 85 bpm are common. People who regularly do physical activity typically have lower resting heart rates than people who do no regular activity. Some endurance athletes have heart rates in the 30 and 40 bpm range, which is considered healthy or normal. Although resting heart rate is *not* considered to be a good measure of health or fitness, decreases in individual heart rate following training reflect positive adaptations. Low heart rates in response to a standard amount of physical activity *are* a good indicator of fitness. The bicycle and step tests presented later in this book use your heart rate response to a standard amount of exercise to estimate your cardiovascular fitness.

Physical Activity and Atherosclerosis

Atherosclerosis, which begins early in life, is implicated in many cardiovascular diseases. Web 03 Atherosclerosis is a condition that contributes to heart attack, stroke, hypertension, angina pectoris, and peripheral vascular disease. Deposits on the walls of arteries restrict blood flow and oxygen supply to the tissues. Atherosclerosis of the coronary arteries, the vessels that supply the heart muscle with oxygen, is particularly harmful. If these arteries become narrowed, the blood supply to the heart muscle is diminished, and angina pectoris may occur. Atherosclerosis increases the risk of heart attack because a fibrous clot is more likely to obstruct a narrowed artery than a healthy, open one.

Current theory suggests that atherosclerosis begins when damage occurs to the cells of the inner wall, or intima, of the artery (see Figure 2). Substances associated with blood clotting are attracted to the damaged area. These substances seem to cause the migration of smooth muscle cells, commonly found only in the middle wall of the artery (media), to the intima. In the later stages, fats (including cholesterol) and other substances are thought to be deposited, forming plaques, or protrusions, that diminish the internal diameter of the artery. Research indicates that the first signs of atherosclerosis begin in early childhood.

Regular physical activity can help prevent atherosclerosis by lowering blood lipid levels. There are several kinds of **lipids** (fats) in the bloodstream, including **lipoproteins**, phospholipids, triglycerides, and cholesterol. Cholesterol is the most well known, but it is not the only culprit. Many blood fats are manufactured by the body itself, whereas others are ingested in high-fat foods, particularly saturated fats (fats that are solid at room temperature).

As noted earlier, blood lipids are thought to contribute to the development of atherosclerotic deposits on the inner walls of the artery. One substance, called **low-density lipoprotein (LDL),** is considered to be a major culprit in the development of atherosclerosis. LDL is basically a core of cholesterol surrounded by protein and another substance that makes it water soluble. The benefit of regular exercise is that it can reduce blood lipid levels, in-

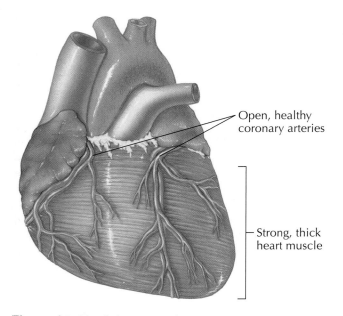

Figure 1 ▶ The fit heart muscle.

Open, healthy coronary arteries

Strong, thick heart muscle

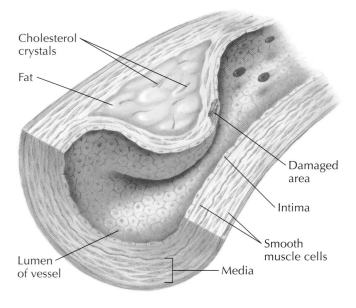

Figure 2 ▶ Atherosclerosis.

Cholesterol crystals

Fat

Damaged area

Intima

Smooth muscle cells

Lumen of vessel

Media

cluding LDL-C (the cholesterol core of LDL). People with high total cholesterol and LDL levels have been shown to have a higher than normal risk for heart disease (see Table 1). New evidence indicates that there are subtypes of LDL cholesterol (characterized by their small size and high density) that pose even greater risks. These subtypes are hard to measure and not included in most current blood tests, but future research will no doubt help us better understand and measure them. Recently, the FDA approved a skin cholesterol test that, when combined with traditional tests, may help in predicting future heart disease.

Triglycerides are another type of blood lipid. Elevated levels of triglycerides are related to heart disease. Triglycerides lose some of their ability to predict heart disease with the presence of other risk factors, so high levels are more difficult to interpret than other blood lipids. Normal levels are considered to be 150 mg/dL or less. Values of 151 to 199 are borderline, 200 to 499 are high, and above 500 are very high. It would be wise to include triglycerides in a blood lipid profile. Physical activity is often prescribed as part of a treatment for high triglyceride levels.

Whereas LDLs carry a core of cholesterol that is involved in the development of atherosclerosis, **high-density lipo-protein (HDL)** picks up cholesterol and carries it to the liver, where it is eliminated from the body.

Regular physical activity can help prevent atherosclerosis by increasing HDL in the blood. For this reason, it is often called the "good cholesterol." High levels of HDL are considered to be desirable. When you have a blood test, it is wise to ask for information about total cholesterol, LDL, and HDL levels. A recent report has provided new information about healthy levels for each (see Table 1). Individuals who do regular physical activity have lower total cholesterol, lower LDL, and higher HDL levels. For this reason, a total blood lipid profile should be considered rather than using a single indicator when calculating risk.

Regular physical activity can help prevent atherosclerosis by reducing blood coagulants. Fibrin and platelets (types of cells involved in blood coagulation) deposit at the site of an injury on the wall of the artery, contributing to the process of plaque build-up, or atherosclerosis. Regular physical activity has been shown to reduce fibrin levels in the blood. The breakdown of fibrin seems to reduce platelet adhesiveness and the concentration of platelets in the blood.

Other indicators of inflammation of the arteries are predictive of atherosclerosis. Web 04 Recently, a number of other constituents in the blood have been shown to be associated with risk for cardiovascular disease. Among these are indicators of inflammation inside the arteries, such as C-reactive protein (CRP), interleukin-6 (IL-6), Chlamydia pneumonia heat shock protein (Cp-HSP60), and tumor necrosis factor-a (TNF-a). These compounds are not necessarily causes of atherosclerosis, but they are indicators of inflammatory processes that lead to plaque formation. Inflammatory processes also soften existing plaque and increase the likelihood of plaque rupture or the formation of clots, which can directly precipitate heart attacks.

CRP is the most commonly used indicator of inflammation. Testing for CRP is increasingly being conducted to provide more effective screening for patients at risk for heart disease. Preliminary standards from the American Heart Association suggest that levels below 1 mg/L indicate low risk, levels between 1 mg/K and 3 mg/L indicate moderate risk and above 3 mg/L indicate high risk.

High levels of the amino acid homocysteine have also been associated with increased risk for heart disease, though the American Heart Association says it is too early to begin screening for it. Tentative fasting values have been established at 5 to 15 millimoles per liter of blood for the normal range, 16 to 30 as moderate, 31 to 100 as intermediate, and above 100 as high. Adequate levels of folic acid, vitamin B-6 and B-12 help prevent high blood

Table 1 ▶ Cholesterol Classifications (mg/dL)

	Total (TC)	LDL-C	HDL-C	TC/HDL-C
Optimal	– – –	<100	– – –	
Near optimal	– – –	100–129	– – –	– – –
Desirable	<200	– – –	>60	– – –
Borderline	200–239	130–159	39–59	3.6–5.0
High risk	>240	160–189	<40	5.0+
Very high Risk	– – –	>190	– – –	– – –

Source: Third Report of the National Cholesterol Education Program.

Lipids All fats and fatty substances.

Lipoproteins Fat-carrying proteins in the blood.

Low-Density Lipoprotein (LDL) A core of cholesterol surrounded by protein; the core is often called "bad cholesterol."

Triglycerides A type of blood fat associated with increased risk for heart disease.

High-Density Lipoprotein (HDL) A blood substance that picks up cholesterol and helps remove it from the body; often called "good cholesterol."

homocysteine levels, so eating foods that ensure adequate daily intake of these vitamins is recommended.

Physical Activity and Heart Attack

Web 05
Regular physical activity reduces the risk for heart attack, the most prevalent and serious of all cardiovascular diseases. A heart attack (coronary occlusion) occurs when a coronary artery is blocked (see Figure 3). A clot, or thrombus, is the most common cause, reducing or cutting off blood flow and oxygen to the heart muscle. If the blocked coronary artery supplies a major portion of the heart muscle, death will occur within minutes. Occlusions of lesser arteries may result in angina pectoris or a nonfatal heart attack.

People who perform regular sports and physical activity have half the risk for a first heart attack, compared with those who are sedentary. Possible reasons are less atherosclerosis, greater diameter of arteries, and less chance of a clot forming.

Regular exercise can improve coronary circulation and, thus, reduce the chances of a heart attack or dying from one. Within the heart, many tiny branches extend from the major coronary arteries. All of these vessels supply blood to the heart muscle. Healthy arteries can supply blood to any region of the heart as it is needed. Active people are likely to have greater blood-carrying capacity in these vessels, probably because the vessels are larger and more elastic. Also, the active person may have a more profuse distribution of arteries within the heart muscle (see Figure 4), which results in greater blood flow. A few studies show that physical activity may promote the growth of "extra" blood vessels, which are thought to open up to provide the heart muscle with the necessary blood and oxygen when the oxygen supply is diminished, as in a heart attack. Blood flow from extra blood vessels is referred to as **coronary collateral circulation.**

Improved coronary circulation may provide protection against a heart attack because a larger artery would require more atherosclerosis to occlude it. In addition, the development of collateral blood vessels supplying the heart may diminish the effects of a heart attack if one does occur. These extra (or collateral) blood vessels may take over the function of regular blood vessels during a heart attack.

The heart of an inactive person is less able to resist stress and is more susceptible to an emotional storm that may precipitate a heart attack. The heart is rendered inefficient by one or more of the following circumstances: high heart rate, high blood pressure, and excessive stimulation. All of these conditions require the heart to use more oxygen than is normal and decrease its ability to adapt to stressful situations.

The inefficient heart is one that beats rapidly because it is dominated by the **sympathetic nervous system,** which speeds up the heart rate. Thus, the heart continuously beats rapidly, even at rest, and never has a true rest period. High blood pressure also makes the heart work harder and contributes to its inefficiency.

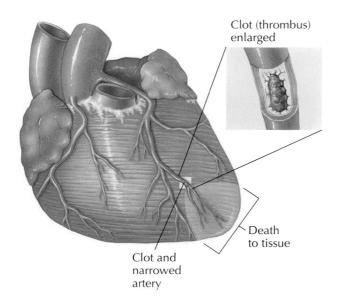

Figure 3 ▶ Heart attack.

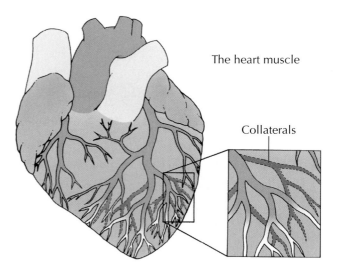

Figure 4 ▶ Coronary collateral circulation.

Research indicates five things concerning physical activity and the inefficient heart:

1. Regular activity leads to dominance of the **parasympathetic nervous system,** which slows heart rate and helps the heart work efficiently.
2. Regular activity helps the heart rate return to normal faster after emotional stress.
3. Regular activity strengthens the heart muscle, making it better able to weather an **emotional storm.**
4. Regular activity reduces hormonal effects on the heart, thus lessening the chances of the circulatory problems that accompany this state.
5. Regular activity reduces the risk of sudden death from ventricular fibrillation (arrhythmic heartbeat).

Regular physical activity is one effective means of rehabilitation for a person who has coronary heart disease or who has had a heart attack. Not only does regular physical activity seem to reduce the risk of developing coronary heart disease, but those who already have the condition may reduce the symptoms of the disease through regular exercise. For people who have had heart attacks, regular and progressive exercise can be an effective prescription when carried out under the supervision of a physician. Remember, however, that exercise is not the treatment of preference for all heart attack victims. In some cases, it is harmful.

Physical Activity and Other Cardiovascular Diseases

Regular physical activity is associated with a reduced risk for high blood pressure (hypertension). "Normal" **systolic blood pressure** is 120 mmHg or less and normal **diastolic blood pressure** is 80 mm Hg or less. Prehypertension is a condition that exists when your blood pressure is higher than normal but not high enough to be considered hypertension (see Table 2). Prehypertension has been linked to higher than normal risk of heart attack and, though not as serious as hypertension, should be taken seriously. Values for the two stages of hypertension are shown in Table 2. Nearly one-third of American adults have high blood pressure. High blood pressure is associated with heart disease, stroke, diabetes and many other diseases, described in this concept. African Americans, Hispanics, and Native Americans have higher incidence than White non-Hispanics. Older people have higher incidence than younger people.

High blood pressure is sometimes referred to as the "silent killer" because nearly one-third of people with elevated blood pressure do not know they have it. For early detection and chronic disease prevention, it is important to monitor your blood pressure on a regular basis. You can learn to monitor your own pressure, and with practice and good equipment your measurements can be quite accurate. It is important to measure your blood pressure when in a resting, nonstressed state because blood pressure can be elevated by emotions and circumstances of measurement. Self-assessments are not meant to be a substitute for recommended periodic blood pressure assessment by a qualified medical person. Exceptionally low blood pressures (below 100 systolic and 60 diastolic) do not pose the same risks to health as high blood pressure but can cause dizziness, fainting, and lack of tolerance to change in body positions. Learn more about blood pressure and how to measure it at Web06 (also see Technology Update, page 78).

Table 2 ► Blood Pressure Classifications for Adults*		
Category	Systolic Blood Pressure (mm Hg)	Diastolic Blood Pressure (mm Hg)
Normal	<120	<80
Prehypertensive	130–139	80–89
Stage 1 hypertension	140–159	90–99
Stage 2 hypertension	>160	>100

Source: National Institutes of Health.

*Not taking antihypertensive drugs and not acutely ill. When the systolic and diastolic blood pressure categories vary, the higher reading determines the blood pressure classification.

Fibrin A sticky, threadlike substance that, in combination with blood cells, forms a blood clot.

Coronary Collateral Circulation Circulation of blood to the heart muscle associated with the blood-carrying capacity of a specific vessel or development of collateral vessels (extra blood vessels).

Sympathetic Nervous System The branch of the autonomic nervous system that prepares the body for activity by speeding up the heart rate.

Parasympathetic Nervous System The branch of the autonomic nervous system that slows the heart rate.

Emotional Storm A traumatic emotional experience that is likely to affect the human organism physiologically.

Systolic Blood Pressure The upper blood pressure number, often called working blood pressure. It represents the pressure in the arteries at its highest level just after the heart beats.

Diastolic Blood Pressure The lower blood pressure number, often called "resting pressure." It is the pressure in the arteries at its lowest level occurring just before the next beat of the heart.

A recent research summary indicates that the effects of physical activity on blood pressure are more dramatic than previously thought and are independent of age, body fatness, and other factors. Inactive, less fit individuals have a 30 to 50 percent greater chance of being hypertensive than active, fit people. Regular physical activity can also be one effective method of reducing blood pressure for those with prehypertension or hypertension. Physical inactivity in middle age is associated with risk for high blood pressure later in life. The most plausible reason is a reduction in resistance to blood flow in the blood vessels, probably resulting from dilation of the vessels.

Regular physical activity can help reduce the risk for stroke. Stroke is a major killer of adults. People with high blood pressure and atherosclerosis are susceptible to stroke. Since regular exercise and good fitness are important to the prevention of high blood pressure and atherosclerosis, exercise and fitness are considered helpful in the prevention of stroke.

Regular physical activity is helpful in the prevention of peripheral vascular disease. People who exercise regularly have better blood flow to the working muscles and other tissues than inactive, unfit people. Since peripheral vascular disease is associated with poor circulation to the extremities, regular exercise can be considered one method of preventing this condition.

Physical activity is associated with metabolic syndrome. Metabolic syndrome is the opposite of poor metabolic fitness, as discussed in Concept 1. It is sometimes referred to as Syndrome X. Several groups, including the American Heart Association and the American Medical Association, have defined the characteristics of metabolic syndrome (see Figure 5). People with at least three of the following characteristics have metabolic syndrome: blood pressure above 135/85, a fasting blood sugar level of 110 or higher, blood triglycerides of 150 or above, a low blood HDL level (less than 40), and/or a high abdominal circumference (equal to or above 40 inches for men or 35 inches for women).

People with metabolic syndrome have a higher than normal risk of chronic diseases, such as diabetes, heart disease, and stroke. A questionnaire (see Web03) developed by researchers who conducted the Framingham Heart Study uses metabolic measures and several other measures to predict heart disease. This questionnaire is better at predicting heart disease than metabolic syndrome alone, but metabolic syndrome is a better predictor of diabetes. Lab 4A at the end of the concept can be used by those who do not have the necessary metabolic syndrome measures, though having a metabolic fitness assessment is advised periodically, especially as you grow older.

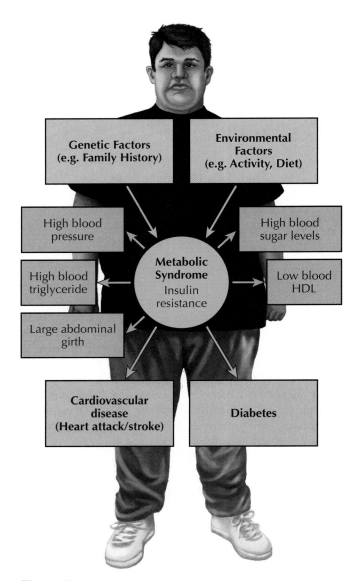

Figure 5 ▶ Mechanism and effects of metabolic syndrome.

Many factors in addition to healthy lifestyle have led to a significant reduction in cardiovascular disease deaths in recent years. The focus of this book is on healthy lifestyle changes. While lifestyle changes such as being active, eating well, managing stress, and abstaining from tobacco use are important in the prevention and treatment of cardiovascular diseases, a variety of other factors have contributed to the recent decrease in deaths associated with the diseases. Heart disease is still the leading killer of both men and women, killing nearly 1 million Americans each year. However, over the past 15 years deaths from heart disease have decreased by 22 percent. Some of the reasons for that decline, other than healthy lifestyle change, in-

Web 07

clude earlier and better detection (e.g., exercise tests, angiograms, CT scans) and better emergency care. Improved medications for lowering blood fat levels (e.g., blood thinners, including aspirin), and lowering blood pressure levels have also played a role. Improved and less invasive surgical methods (e.g., angioplasty, stents) and improvements in postcoronary care have also contributed to reducing death rates.

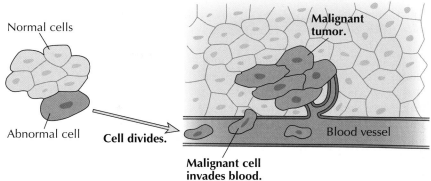

Figure 6 ▶ The spread of cancer (metastasis).

Physical Activity and Other Hypokinetic Conditions

Physical activity reduces the risk of some forms of cancer. According to the American Cancer Society, cancer is a group of many different conditions characterized by abnormal, uncontrolled cell growth. As illustrated in Figure 6, the abnormal cells divide, forming **malignant tumors (carcinomas).** If the abnormal cells reach the blood, they can spread, causing tumors elsewhere in the body. **Benign tumors** are generally not considered to be cancerous because their growth is restricted to a specific area of the body by a protective membrane. The first editions of this book did not include any form of cancer as a hypokinetic disease. We now know, however, that overall death rates from cancer are lower among active people than among those who are sedentary (50 to 250 percent) and that some specific forms of cancer are related to sedentary living. These cancers are described in Table 3 with possible reasons for the

cancer/inactivity link (if known). The entries in Table 3 are listed in order based on the strength of evidence supporting the cancer/inactivity link. As noted in Concept 1, cancer is the second leading cause of death for people under the age of 85.

The American Cancer Society recently released guidelines designed to help reduce risk for cancer as a result of eating well and doing regular activity. The document places a special emphasis on maintaining a healthy body fatness level as one method of reducing cancer risk. Physical activity is also considered to be important to the wellness of the cancer patient. Patients can benefit from activity in many ways, including improved quality of life, physical functioning, and self-esteem, as well as less dependence on others, reduced risk for other diseases, and reduced fatigue from disease or disease therapy.

Physical activity plays a role in the management and treatment of Type II diabetes. Diabetes mellitus (diabetes) is a group of disorders that results when there is too much sugar in the blood. It occurs when the body does not make enough **insulin** or when the body is not able to use insulin effectively.

Type I diabetes, or insulin-dependent diabetes, accounts for a relatively small number of the diabetes cases and is not considered to be a hypokinetic condition. Type

Table 3 ▶ Physical Activity and Cancer

Cancer Type	Effect of Physical Activity
Colon	Exercise speeds movement of food and cancer-causing substances through the digestive system, and reduces prostaglandins (substances linked to cancer in the colon).
Breast	Exercise decreases the amount of exposure of breast tissue to circulating estrogen. Lower body fat is also associated with lower estrogen levels. Early life activity is deemed important for both reasons. Fatigue from therapy is reduced by exercise.
Rectal	Similar to colon cancer, exercise leads to more regular bowel movements and reduces "transit time."
Prostate	Fatigue from therapy is reduced by exercise.

Malignant Tumors (carcinomas) An uncontrolled and dangerous growth capable of spreading to other areas; a cancerous tumor.

Benign Tumors An abnormal growth of tissue confined to a particular area; not considered to be cancer.

Insulin A hormone secreted by the pancreas that regulates levels of sugar in the blood.

II diabetes (often not insulin-dependent) was formerly called "adult-onset diabetes." In recent years, Type II diabetes has become common in children and is associated with high levels of body fat

Diabetes is the seventh leading cause of death among people over 40. It accounts for at least 10 percent of all short-term hospital stays and has a major impact on health-care costs in Western society. According to the American Diabetes Association (ADA), there are 20.8 million people in the United States who have diabetes. Unfortunately, 6.2 million of those don't know it. An estimated additional 10 million are prediabetic; they have metabolic profiles characteristic of those with diabetes (see *Web Resources*, ADA or Canadian Diabetes Association, for more statistics).

People who perform regular physical activity are less likely to suffer from Type II diabetes than sedentary people. For people with Type II diabetes, regular physical activity can help reduce body fatness, decrease **insulin resistance,** improve **insulin sensitivity,** and improve the body's ability to clear sugar from the blood in a reasonable time. All of these factors contribute to controlling the disease. With sound nutritional habits and proper medication, physical activity can be useful in the management of both types of diabetes.

Regular physical activity is important to maintaining bone density and decreasing risk for osteoporosis. As noted in Concept 1, some experts consider bone integrity to be a health-related component of physical fitness. Bone density cannot be self-assessed. It is measured using a dual X-ray absorptiometry (DXA) machine, an expensive and sophisticated form of X-ray machine that can also be used to measure body fatness (see Technology Update in Concept 13). Healthy bones are dense and strong. When bones lose calcium and become less dense, they become porous and are at risk for fracture. The bones of young children are not especially dense, but during adolescence (see Figure 7) bone density increases to a level higher than at any other time in life (peak bone density). Though bone density often begins to decrease in young adulthood, it is not until older adulthood that bone loss becomes dramatic. As illustrated in Figure 7, many older adults have lost enough bone density to have a condition called **osteoporosis** (when bone density drops below the osteoporosis threshold). Some will have crossed the fracture threshold, putting them at risk for fractures, especially to the hip, vertebrae, and other "soft" or "spongy" bones of the skeletal system. Active people have a higher peak bone mass and are more resistant to osteoporosis (see blue line in Figure 7) than sedentary people (see red line in Figure 7).

Women, especially postmenopausal women, have a higher risk of osteoporosis than men, but it is a disease of

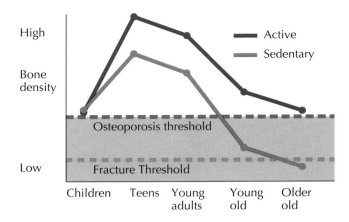

Figure 7 ▶ Changes in bone density with age.

both sexes. Males typically have a higher peak bone mass than females, and for this reason, can lose more bone density over time without reaching the osteoporosis or fracture threshold. More women reach the osteoporosis and fracture thresholds at earlier ages than men. Other risk factors for osteoporosis are northern European ancestry, smoking, caffeine use, alcohol use, current or previous eating disorders, early menstruation, low dietary calcium intake, low body fat, amenorrhea, and extended bed rest.

Guidelines for building bone integrity and preventing osteoporosis include the following:

- Do regular weight-bearing exercise and resistance training that stresses the bones of the body. The load bearing and pull of the muscles in these types of exercises build bone density.
- Eat a diet rich in calcium. Calcium is necessary to build strong bones. At-risk groups should consider a calcium supplement.
- Postmenopausal women, after consultation with a physician, should consider a calcium supplement and medications, such as raloxifene (sold as Evista) and alendronate (sold as Fosomax), that help prevent bone loss. Another drug, zoledronic acid, which was originally approved to stop calcium loss from the bones of cancer patients, shows promise for the treatment of osteoporosis in the future. It should also be noted that there are significant side effects of several of these medications, preventing some people from using them.
- Hormone replacement therapy (HRT), also called estrogen replacement therapy (ERT), has been shown to reduce risk for osteoporosis among postmenopausal women. One study (Women's Health Initiative) suggests that HRT can increase risk for breast cancer, stroke, and heart disease among older women, but another study did not show increased risk for younger women. Medical consultation based on individual factors is recommended.

- Start early in life to build strong bones because peak bone mass is developed in the teen years. It is never too late to start. Following these guidelines has been shown to help people of all ages, including those 80 and over.
- Older people with osteoporosis should consider protective hip pads, worn to prevent fractures from falls.

Active people who possess good muscle fitness are less likely to have back and musculoskeletal problems than are inactive, unfit people. Because few people die from it, back pain does not receive the attention given to such medical problems as heart disease and cancer. But back pain is considered to be the second leading medical complaint in the United States, second only to headaches. Only the common cold and the flu cause more days lost from work. At some point in our lives, approximately 80 percent of all adults experience back pain that limits their ability to function normally. In National Safety Council data, the back was the most frequently injured of all body parts, and the injury rate was double that of any other part of the body.

Many years ago, medical doctors began to associate back problems with the lack of physical fitness. It is now known that the great majority of back ailments are the result of poor muscle strength, low levels of endurance, and poor flexibility. Tests on patients with back problems show weakness and lack of flexibility in key muscle groups.

Though lack of fitness is probably the leading reason for back pain in Western society, there are many other factors that increase the risk of back ailments, including poor posture, improper lifting and work habits, heredity, and disease states such as scoliosis and arthritis.

Physical activity is important in maintaining a healthy body weight and avoiding the numerous health conditions associated with obesity. Recently, the surgeon general issued a *Call to Action to Prevent and Decrease Overweight and Obesity*. This report notes that one-third of adults are obese and nearly two-thirds are classified as overweight based on the body mass index. Approximately 19 percent of children and 17 percent of teens are classified as obese, dramatically up from 20 years ago. Obesity is not a disease state in itself but is a hypokinetic condition associated with a multitude of far-reaching complications. Research has shown that fat people who are fit are not at especially high risk for early death. However, when high body fatness is accompanied by low cardiovascular and low metabolic fitness, risk for early death increases substantially. Obesity contributes to sedentary death syndrome, described earlier in this concept.

Physical activity reduces the risk and severity of a variety of common mental (emotional) health disorders. Such disorders can be considered hypokinetic conditions. Some mental (emotional) health conditions are prevalent in modern society. Nearly one-half of adult Americans will report having a mental health disorder at some point in life. A recent summary of studies revealed that there are several emotional/mental disorders that are associated with inactive lifestyles.

Depression is a stress-related condition experienced by many adults. Thirty-three percent of inactive adults report that they often feel depressed. For some, depression is a serious disorder that physical activity alone will not cure; however, research indicates that activity, combined with other forms of therapy, can be effective.

Anxiety is an emotional condition characterized by worry, self-doubt, and apprehension. More than a few studies have shown that symptoms of anxiety can be reduced by regular activity. Low-fit people who do regular aerobic activity seem to benefit the most. In one study, one-third of active people felt that regular activity helped them cope better with life's pressures.

Physical activity is also associated with better and more restful sleep. People with insomnia (the inability to sleep) seem to benefit from regular activity if it is not done too vigorously right before going to bed. A recent study indicates that 52 percent of the population feel that physical activity helps them sleep better. Regular aerobic activity is associated with reduced brain activation, which can result in greater ability to relax or fall asleep.

Even more common than depression and insomnia is the condition called Type A behavior. Type A personalities are stress-prone individuals with a greater than normal incidence of diseases. A Type A person is tense, overcompetitive, and worried about meeting time schedules. Apparently, all Type A personalities are not equally stressed. It has been suggested that aggressive Type A personalities are most likely to be prone to negative consequences of stress. Regular physical activity can benefit the Type A person, especially the aggressive Type A. Noncompetitive activities are best for this personality type.

A final benefit of regular exercise is increased self-esteem. Improvements in fitness, appearance, and the ability to perform new tasks can improve self-confidence and self-esteem.

Insulin Resistance A condition that occurs when insulin becomes ineffective or less effective than necessary to regulate sugar levels in the blood.

Insulin Sensitivity A person with insulin resistance (see previous definition) is said to have decreased insulin sensitivity. The body's cells are not sensitive to insulin, so they resist it and sugar levels are not regulated effectively.

Osteoporosis A condition associated with low bone density and subsequent bone fragility, leading to high risk for fracture.

Physical activity can help the immune system fight illness. Until recently, infectious disease and other diseases of the immune system were not considered to be hypokinetic. Recent evidence indicates that regular moderate to vigorous activity can actually aid the immune system in fighting disease. Each of us is born with "an innate immune system," which includes anatomical and physiological barriers, such as skin, mucous membranes, body temperature, and chemical mediators that help prevent and resist disease. We also develop an "acquired immune system" in the form of special disease-fighting cells that help us resist disease. Figure 8 shows a J-shaped curve that illustrates the benefits of exercise to acquired immune function. Sedentary people have more risk than those who do moderate activity, but with very high and sustained vigorous activity, such as extended high performance training, immune system function actually decreases.

Regular moderate and reasonable amounts of vigorous activity have been shown to reduce incidence of colds and days of sickness from infection. The immune system benefit may extend to other immune system disorders as well. There is evidence that regular physical activity can enhance treatment effectiveness and improve quality of life for those with HIV/AIDS. However, as Figure 8 indicates, too much exercise may cause problems rather than solve them.

New evidence indicates that Alzheimer's disease and dementia are hypokinetic conditions. More than a few studies indicate that factors relating to heart health also contribute to brain health. The studies indicate that physical activity and challenging mental activities are especially important among the lifestyle factors involved in maintaining brain health and preventing Alzheimer's disease and dementia. See *In the News* for details on this research.

Regular physical activity can have positive effects on some nonhypokinetic conditions. Some nonhypokinetic conditions that can benefit from physical activity are

- *Arthritis.* Many, if not most, arthritics are in a deconditioned state resulting from a lack of activity. The traditional advice that arthritics should avoid physical activity is now being modified in view of the findings that carefully prescribed exercise has a variety of benefits. Common problems for both those with rheumatoid arthritis (RA) and osteoarthritis (OA) are decreased strength, loss of range of motion, and poor cardiovascular endurance. Well-planned exercise, designed to meet the needs of the specific type of arthritis of the individual, can be beneficial in preventing and treating impairments, enhancing function, and enhancing general fitness and well-being.
- *Asthma.* Asthmatics often have physical activity limitations. New evidence suggests that, with proper management, activity can be part of their daily life. In fact, when done properly, activity can reduce airway reactivity and medication use. Because exercise can trigger bronchial constriction, it is important to choose appropriate types of activity and to use inhaled medications to prevent bronchial constriction caused by exercise or other triggers, such as cold weather. Asthmatics should avoid cold weather exercise.
- *Premenstrual syndrome (PMS).* PMS, a mixture of physical and emotional symptoms that occurs prior to menstruation, has many causes. However, current evidence suggests that changes in lifestyle, including regular exercise, may be effective in relieving PMS symptoms.
- *Other conditions.* Low- to moderate-intensity aerobic activity and resistance training are currently being prescribed for some people who have chronic pain (persistent pain without relief) and/or fibromyalgia (chronic muscle pain). Evidence also suggests that active people have a 30 percent less chance of having gallstones than inactive people, and activity may decrease risk of impotence.

Physical Activity and Aging

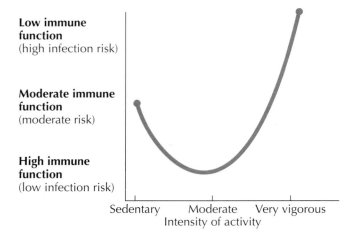

Regular physical activity can improve fitness and functioning among older adults. Approximately 30 percent of adults age 70 and over have difficulty with one or more activities of daily living. Women have more limitations than men, and low-income groups have more limitations than higher-income groups. Nearly one-half get no assistance with the activity in which they are limited.

The inability to function effectively as you grow older is associated with lack of fitness and inactive lifestyles. This loss of function is sometimes referred to as "acquired aging," as opposed to "time-dependent" aging.

Low immune function
(high infection risk)

Moderate immune function
(moderate risk)

High immune function
(low infection risk)

Sedentary   Moderate   Very vigorous
Intensity of activity

Figure 8 ▶ Physical activity and immune function.

Because so many people experience limitations in daily activities and find it difficult to get assistance, it is especially important for older people to stay active and fit. In Africa, Asia, and South America, where older adults maintain an active lifestyle, individuals do not acquire many of the characteristics commonly associated with aging in North America.

In general, older adults are much less active than younger adults. Losses in muscle fitness are associated with loss of balance, greater risk of falling, and less ability to function independently. Studies also show that exercise can enhance cognitive functioning and perhaps reduce risk for dementia. Though the amount of activity performed must be adapted as people grow older, fitness benefits discussed in the next section and throughout this book apply to people of all ages.

Regular physical activity can compress illness into a shorter period of our life. An important national health goal is to increase the years of healthy life. Living longer is important, but being able to function effectively during all years of life is equally—if not more—important. *Compression of illness*, also called compression of morbidity, refers to shortening the total number of years that illnesses and disabilities occur. Healthy lifestyles, including regular physical activity, have been shown to compress illness and increase years of effective functioning. Inactive people not only have a shorter life span, but have more years of illness and disability than active people.

Physical Activity, Health, and Wellness

Good health-related physical fitness and regular physical activity are important for optimal wellness. Regular physical activity and good fitness not only help prevent illness (see Table 4) and disease but also promote quality of life and wellness. Good health-related physical fitness can help you look good, feel good, and enjoy life. Some of the specific benefits of wellness that are associated with good fitness are the following:

- *Good physical fitness can help an individual enjoy leisure time.* A person who is lean, has no back problems, does not have high blood pressure, and has reasonable skills in a lifetime of sports is more likely to get involved and stay regularly involved in leisure-time activities than one who does not have these characteristics. Enjoying your leisure time may not add years to your life but can add life to your years.
- *Good physical fitness can help an individual work effectively and efficiently.* A person who can resist fatigue, muscle soreness, back problems, and other

symptoms associated with poor health-related fitness is capable of working productively and having energy left over at the end of the day. Surveys of employees who are involved with employee fitness programs indicate that 75 percent have an improved sense of well-being. Employers indicate that absenteeism decreases by up to 50 percent among program participants. People with good skill-related fitness may be more effective and efficient in performing specific motor skills required for certain jobs.

- *Good physical fitness is essential to effective living.* Although the need for each component of physical fitness is specific to each individual, every person requires enough fitness to perform normal daily activities without undue fatigue. Whether it be walking, performing household chores, or merely feeling good and enjoying the simple things in life without pain or fear of injury, good fitness is important to all people.
- *Physical fitness is the basis for dynamic and creative activity.* Though the following quotation by former President John F. Kennedy is more than 40 years old, it clearly points out the importance of physical fitness:

The relationship between the soundness of the body and the activity of the mind is subtle and complex. Much is not yet understood, but we know what the Greeks knew: that intelligence and skill can only function at the peak of their capacity when the body is healthy and strong, and that hardy spirits and tough minds usually inhabit

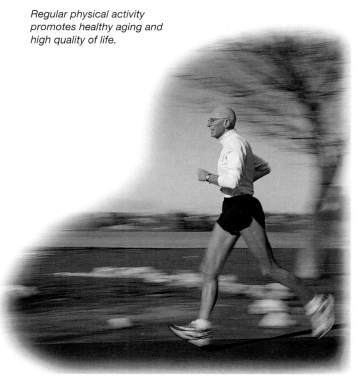

Regular physical activity promotes healthy aging and high quality of life.

Table 4 ▶ Health and Wellness Benefits of Physical Activity and Fitness

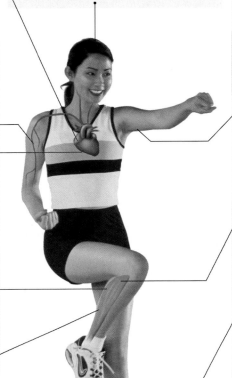

Improved Cardiovascular Health
- Stronger heart muscle fitness and health
- Lower heart rate
- Better electric stability of heart
- Decreased sympathetic control of heart
- Increased O_2 to brain
- Reduced blood fat, including low-density lipoproteins (LDLs)
- Increased protective high-density lipoproteins (HDLs)
- Delayed development of atherosclerosis
- Increased work capacity
- Improved peripheral circulation
- Improved coronary circulation
- Resistance to "emotional storm"
- Reduced risk for heart attack
- Reduced risk for stroke
- Reduced risk for hypertension
- Greater chance of surviving a heart attack
- Increased oxygen-carrying capacity of the blood

Improved Strength and Muscular Endurance
- Greater work efficiency
- Less chance for muscle injury
- Reduced risk for low back problems
- Improved performance in sports
- Quicker recovery after hard work
- Improved ability to meet emergencies

Resistance to Fatigue
- Ability to enjoy leisure
- Improved quality of life
- Improved ability to meet some stressors

Other Health Benefits
- Decreased diabetes risk
- Quality of life for diabetics
- Improved metabolic fitness
- Extended life
- Decrease in dysfunctional years
- Aids for some people who have arthritis, PMS, asthma, chronic pain, fibromyalgia, or impotence
- Improved immune system

Enhanced Mental Health and Function
- Relief of depression
- Improved sleep habits
- Fewer stress symptoms
- Ability to enjoy leisure and work
- Improved brain function

Improved Wellness
- Improved quality of life
- Leisure-time enjoyment
- Improved work capacity
- Ability to meet emergencies
- Improved creative capacity

Opportunity for Successful Experience and Social Interactions
- Improved self-concept
- Opportunity to recognize and accept personal limitations
- Improved sense of well-being
- Enjoyment of life and fun
- Improved quality of life

Improved Appearance
- Better figure/physique
- Better posture
- Fat control

Greater Lean Body Mass and Less Body Fat
- Greater work efficiency
- Less susceptibility to disease
- Improved appearance
- Less incidence of self-concept problems related to obesity

Improved Flexibility
- Greater work efficiency
- Less chance of muscle injury
- Less chance of joint injury
- Decreased chance of developing low back problems
- Improved sports performance

Bone Development
- Greater peak bone density
- Less chance of developing osteoporosis

Reduced Cancer Risk
- Reduced risk for colon and breast cancer
- Possible reduced risk for rectal and prostate cancers

Reduced Effect of Acquired Aging
- Improved ability to function in daily life
- Better short-term memory
- Fewer illnesses
- Greater mobility
- Greater independence
- Greater ability to operate an automobile
- Lower risk for dementia

sound bodies. Physical fitness is the basis of all activities in our society; if our bodies grow soft and inactive, if we fail to encourage physical development and prowess, we will undermine our capacity for thought, for work, and for the use of those skills vital to an expanding and complex America.

President Kennedy's belief that activity and fitness are associated with intellectual functioning has now been backed up with research. A recent research summary suggests that, though modest, the effect of activity and fitness on intellectual functioning is positive. One study shows activity to foster new brain cell growth.

Time taken to be active during the day has been shown to help children learn more, even though less time is spent in intellectual pursuits.

- *Good physical fitness may help you function safely and assist you in meeting unexpected emergencies.* Emergencies are never expected, but, when they do arise, they often demand performance that requires good fitness. For example, flood victims may need to fill sandbags for hours without rest, and accident victims may be required to walk or run long distances for help. Also, good fitness is required for such simple tasks as safely changing a spare tire or loading a moving van without injury.

Physical activity is a major part of most employee health promotion programs. Web 12 ✎ Companies have come to understand the importance of promoting healthy lifestyles among their employees. Worksite health promotion programs typically use a broad focus on promoting a variety of healthy lifestyles, but physical activity is considered the mainstay of most programs. To facilitate active lifestyles in employees, many companies build their own fitness centers inside the workplace or provide free or reduced-cost memberships for employees. Worksite programs that promote activity can reduce risk factors in employees and help companies control the high cost of health care. Studies have consistently documented that the cost of these programs more than offsets the expense. Companies that offer comprehensive programs frequently save more than $4 for each dollar invested. The expansion of worksite health programs is viewed as a critical public health priority and one of the most promising approaches for controlling health-care costs. See Web12 for more information.

There are many positive lifestyles that can reduce the risk for disease and promote health and wellness. Many of the factors that contribute to optimal health and quality of life are also considered risk factors. Changing these risk factors can dramatically reduce the risk for hypokinetic diseases. Inactivity, poor nutrition, smoking, and inability to cope with stress are all risk factors associated with various diseases (see Table 5). It is important to recognize that three risk factors (age, heredity, and gender) are not within your control.

By altering the controllable risk factors, you can reduce the risk for several hypokinetic conditions. For example, controlling body fatness reduces the risk for diabetes, hypertension, and back problems. Altering your diet can reduce the chances of developing high levels of blood lipids and reduce the risk for atherosclerosis. Being active and adopting healthy lifestyles is a proactive approach to health and wellness. While reducing risk can

Table 5 ▶ Hypokinetic Disease Risk Factors

Factors That Cannot Be Altered

1. *Age.* As you grow older, your risk of contracting hypokinetic diseases increases. For example, the risk for heart disease is approximately three times as great after 60 as before. The risk of back pain is considerably greater after 40.
2. *Heredity.* People who have a family history of hypokinetic disease are more likely to develop a hypokinetic condition, such as heart disease, hypertension, back problems, obesity, high blood lipid levels, and other problems. African Americans are 45 percent more likely to have high blood pressure than Caucasians; therefore, they suffer strokes at an earlier age with more severe consequences.
3. *Gender.* Men have a higher incidence of many hypokinetic conditions than women. However, differences between men and women have decreased recently. This is especially true for heart disease, the leading cause of death for both men and women. Postmenopausal women have a higher heart disease risk than premenopausal women.

Factors That Can Be Altered

4. *Regular physical activity.* As noted throughout this book, regular exercise can help reduce the risk for hypokinetic disease.
5. *Diet.* A clear association exists between hypokinetic disease and certain types of diets. The excessive intake of saturated fats, such as animal fats, is linked to atherosclerosis and other forms of heart disease. Excessive salt in the diet is associated with high blood pressure.
6. *Stress.* People who are subject to excessive stress are predisposed to various hypokinetic diseases, including heart disease and back pain. Statistics indicate that hypokinetic conditions are common among those in certain high-stress jobs and those having Type A personality profiles.
7. *Tobacco use.* Smokers have five times the risk of heart attack as nonsmokers. Most striking is the difference in risk between older women smokers and nonsmokers. Tobacco use is also associated with the increased risk for high blood pressure, cancer, and several other medical conditions. Apparently, the more you use, the greater the risk. Stopping tobacco use even after many years can significantly reduce the hypokinetic disease risk.
8. *Body (fatness).* Having too much body fat is a primary risk factor for heart disease and is a risk factor for other hypokinetic conditions as well. For example, loss of fat can result in relief from symptoms of Type II diabetes, can reduce problems associated with certain types of back pain, and can reduce the risks of surgery.
9. *Blood lipids, blood glucose, and blood pressure levels.* High scores on these factors are associated with health problems, such as heart disease and diabetes. Risk increases considerably when several of these measures are high.
10. *Diseases.* People who have one hypokinetic disease are more likely to develop a second or even a third condition. For example, if you have diabetes,* your risk of having a heart attack or stroke increases dramatically. Although you may not be entirely able to alter the extent to which you develop certain diseases and conditions, reducing your risk and following your doctor's advice can improve your odds significantly.

*Some types of diabetes cannot be altered.

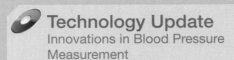

Technology Update
Innovations in Blood Pressure Measurement

In recent years, there have been many spectacular technological innovations that have benefited people with the hypokinetic conditions described in this concept. Though less dramatic than other more costly innovations, technology that allows easily administered and accurate self-assessment of blood pressure have great potential for preventing and treating hypertension and related conditions. The American Heart Association recently issued a statement that "blood pressure readings taken at home with approved devices can be a useful addition to blood pressure management, and may even predict cardiovascular disease (CVD) risk better than readings from the doctor's office alone" (www.aha.org). The AHA Web site provides information concerning effective home monitoring of blood pressure, as well as information about new blood pressure measurement technology. Examples include self-inflating cuffs, digital vs. more traditional monitors, and wrist cuff measurement devices. (See Web06 for more details).

alter the probability of disease, it does not assure disease immunity.

Too much activity can lead to hyperkinetic conditions. The information presented in this concept points out the health benefits of physical activity performed in appropriate amounts. When done in excess or incorrectly, physical activity can result in **hyperkinetic conditions.** The most common hyperkinetic condition is overuse injury to muscles, connective tissue, and bones. Recently, anorexia nervosa and body neurosis have been identified as conditions associated with inappropriate amounts of physical activity. These conditions will be discussed in the concept on performance.

Strategies for Action

A self-assessment of risk factors can help you modify your lifestyle to reduce risk for heart disease. The Heart Disease Risk Factor Questionnaire in Lab 4A will help you assess your personal risk for heart disease. Although the questionnaire is educationally useful in making you aware of risk factors, it is not a substitute for a regular medical exam. A medical exam that includes an assessment of blood lipids as described in this concept is recommended. This will allow you to use more sophisticated and accurate risk factor assessments, such as the Framingham Risk Score (see Web13).

Web 13

Selecting physical activities from the physical activity pyramid can help you achieve the health benefits described in this concept. The physical activity pyramid provides a conceptual model of the relative importance of different types of physical activity. Subsequent concepts in the book will cover the different components of health-related fitness and the type and amount of activity needed to improve these components. The lab activities in each of these concepts and the culminating lab activity at the end of the book are designed to help you plan for lifelong physical activity.

Online Learning Center

www.mhhe.com/corbin7e
The Online Learning Center contains a variety of Web-based resources that will help you get the most out of this book and your course. In addition to the On the Web pages, there are video activities, interactive quizzes, application assignments, and a variety of other useful study aids. Log on to the URL above to access these resources.

Web Resources

Alzheimer's Association **www.alz.org**
American Cancer Society **www.cancer.org**
American Diabetes Association **www.diabetes.org**
American Heart Association **www.americanheart.org**
American Lung Association **www.lungusa.org**
Arthritis Foundation **www.arthritis.org**
Canadian Diabetes Association **www.diabetes.ca**

Web 14

Centers for Disease Control and Prevention **www.cdc.gov**
Healthy People 2010 **www.health.gov/healthypeople**
National Osteoporosis Foundation **www.nof.org**
National Stroke Association **www.stroke.org**
Worksite Wellness Information
   http://healthproject.stanford.edu/koop/work.html

Suggested Readings

Additional reference materials for Concept 4 are available at Web15.

Web 15

American College of Sports Medicine. 2006. *ACSM's Guidelines for Exercise Testing and Prescription.* 7th ed. Philadelphia: Lippincott, Williams and Wilkins.

American Heart Association. 2005. *Metabolic Syndrome.* Dallas, TX: American Heart Association. Available at www.americanheart.org/presenter.jhtml?identifier=4756

Atlantis, E., et al. 2004. An effective exercise-based intervention for improving mental health and quality of life measures: A randomized controlled trial. *Preventive Medicine* 39(2):424–434.

Bassuck, S. S., and J. E. Manson. 2004. Preventing cardiovascular disease in women: How much physical activity is "good enough"? *President's Council on Physical Fitness and Sports Research Digest* 5(4):1–8.

Bernstein, L. 2005. Lifetime recreational exercise activity and breast cancer risk among Black women and White women. *Journal of the National Cancer Institute* 97(22):1–9.

Booth, F. W., and M. W. Chakravarthy. 2004. Cost and consequences of sedentary living: New battleground for an old enemy. In C. B. Corbin et al. (eds.). *Toward a Better Understanding of Physical Fitness and Activity: Selected Topics, Volume Two,* 63–72. Scottsdale, AZ: Holcomb-Hathaway.

Bouchard, C. and T. Rankinen. 2006. Are people physically active because of their genes? *President's Council on Physical Fitness and Sports Research Digest* 7(2):1–8.

Brown, D. W., et al. 2004. Associations between physical activity dose and health-related quality of life. *Medicine and Science in Sports and Exercise* 36(5):890–896.

Carnethon, M. R., et al. 2005. Prevalence and cardiovascular disease correlates of low cardiorespiratory fitness in adolescents and adults. *Journal of the American Medical Association* 294(23):2981–2988.

Chenoweth, D., et al. 2006. The cost of sloth: Using a tool to measure the cost of physical activity. *ACSM's Health and Fitness Journal* 10(2):8–13.

Divine, J. G. 2006. *ACSM's Action Plan for High Blood Pressure* Champaign, IL: Human Kinetics.

Durston, J. L. 2006. *ACSM's Action Plan for High Cholesterol* Champaign, IL: Human Kinetics.

Fitzgerald, S. J., et al. 2004. Muscular fitness and all-cause mortality: Prospective observations. *Journal of Physical Activity and Health* 1(1):7–18.

Franco, O. H., et al. 2005. Effects of physical activity on life expectancy with cardiovascular disease. *Archives of Internal Medicine* 165:2355–2360.

Greene, B., and S. S. Lim. 2004. The role of physical therapy in management of patients with osteoarthritis and rheumatoid arthritis. *Bulletin on the Rheumatic Diseases* 52(4):1+. Available online at http://www.arthritis.org/research/bulletin/archives.asp

Jonker, J. T., et al. 2006. Physical activity and life expectancy with and without diabetes: Life table analysis of the Framingham Heart Study. *Diabetes Care* 29(1):38–43.

Jurea, R., et al. 2005. Physical activity and nontraditional CHD risk factors. *President's Council on Physical Fitness and Sports Research Digest* 6(4):1–8.

Kohli, P., and P. Greenland. 2006. Role of the metabolic syndrome in risk assessment for coronary heart disease. *Journal of the American Medical Association* 295(7):819–821.

Larson, E. B., et al. 2006. Exercise associated with reduced risk of dementia in older sedentary counterparts. *Annals of Internal Medicine* 144(2):73–81.

McGill, S. M. 2001. Low back stability. *Exercise and Sports Sciences Reviews* 29(1):26–31.

Medical News Today. 2005. Exercise reduces breast cancer risk, even a little bit helps. *Medical News Today.* November 22, www.medicalnewstoday.com.

National Cholesterol Education Program. 2001. Executive summary of the third report of the National Cholesterol Education Program expert panel on detection, evaluation, and treatment of high blood cholesterol in adults. *Journal of the American Medical Association* 285:2486–2497.

National Cholesterol Education Program. 2004. Implications of recent clinical trials for the National Cholesterol Education Program Adult Treatment Panel III Guidelines. *Circulation* 110(2):227–239.

National Institutes of Health. 2002. Osteoporosis prevention, diagnosis, and therapy. *NIH Consensus Statements* 17(1):1–45.

Nieman, D. C. 2004. Does exercise alter immune function and respiratory infections? In C. B. Corbin, et al. (eds.). *Toward a Better Understanding of Physical Fitness and Activity: Selected Topics, Volume Two,* Scottsdale, AZ: Holcomb-Hathaway. 81–88.

Ogden, C. L., et al. 2006. Prevalence of overweight and obesity in the United States. *Journal of the American Medical Association* 295(13):1539–1548.

Schwartz, A. L. 2004. *Cancer Fitness* New York: Simon & Schuster.

Hyperkinetic Conditions Diseases/illnesses or health conditions caused, or contributed to, by too much physical activity.

Slattery, M. L., and J. D. Potter. 2002. Physical activity and colon cancer. *Medicine and Science in Sports and Exercise* 34(6):913–919.

Turner, C. H., and A. G. Robling. 2003. Designing exercise regimens to increase bone strength. *Exercise and Sports Sciences Reviews* 31(1):40–44.

U.S. Census Bureau. 2006. *Statistical Abstract.* Washington, DC: U.S. Census Bureau.

U.S. Department of Health and Human Services. 1996. *Physical Activity and Health: A Report of the Surgeon General.* Atlanta: U.S. Department of Health and Human Services.

U.S. Department of Health and Human Services. 2003. *Prevention Makes Common "Cents."* Washington, DC: U.S. Department of Health and Human Services.

U.S. Deparment of Health and Human Services. 2004. *Bone Health and Osteoporosis: A Report of the Surgeon General.* Rockville, MD: U.S.D, H.H.S., Office of Surgeon General.

Wannamethee, S. G., et al. 2005. Metabolic syndrome vs. Framingham risk score for prediction of coronary heart disease, stroke and type 2 diabetes mellitus. *Archives of Internal Medicine* 165(22):2644–2650.

Winters-Stone, K. 2005. *ACSM's Action Plan for Osteoporosis.* Champaign, IL: Human Kinetics.

 In the News

Exercise Shown to Reduce Risks for Alzheimer's Disease

Physical activity is know to reduce risks for many conditions and to improve overall mental health. New research (see Larson et al., 2006 in *Suggested Readings*) has revealed that regular physical activity can reduce the risks for Alzheimer's disease and other mental disorders in the elderly. Scientists in this large study tracked a sample of 1,740 people (ages >65) over a 6-year time span to look for factors that may be associated with incidence of dementia. Individuals who exercised three or more times a week had a 32 percent lower risk of developing Alzheimer's, compared with individuals who exercised fewer than 3 days a week. The participants were not cognitively impaired at the start of the study, and the analyses controlled for other conditions or variables that may have influenced the results. While additional research is needed to confirm these findings, this study provides important news for public health officials and physicians looking for ways to reduce the prevalence and impact of Alzheimer's disease. Approximately 4.5 million people in the United States have Alzheimer's and the prevalence is expected to increase in the future as people live longer. The fact that exercise can reduce the risks for this condition provides an additional justification for being a physically active person.

Lab 4A   Assessing Heart Disease Risk Factors

Name	**Section**	**Date**

Purpose: To assess your risk of developing coronary heart disease

Heart Disease Risk Factor Questionnaire
Risk Points

	①	②	③	④	Score
Unalterable Factors					
1. How old are you?	30 or less	31–40	41–54	55+	
2. Do you have a history of heart disease in your family?	None	Grandparent with heart disease	Parent with heart disease	More than one with heart disease	
3. What is your gender?	Female		Male		
				Total Unalterable Risk Score	
Alterable Factors					
4. Do you get regular physical activity?	4–5 days a week	3 days a week	Fewer than 3 days a week	No	
5. Do you have a high-fat diet?	No	Slightly high in fat	Above normal in fat	Eat a lot of meat and fried and fatty foods	
6. Are you under much stress?	Less than normal	Normal	Slightly above normal	Quite high	
7. Do you use tobacco?	No	Cigar or pipe	Less than 1/2 pack a day or use smokeless tobacco	More than 1/2 pack a day	
8. What is your percent of body fat?	F = 17–28% M = 10–20%	29–31% 21–23%	32–35% 24–30%	35+% 30+%	
9. What is the systolic number in your blood pressure?	120	121–140	141–160	160+	
10. Do you have other diseases?	No	Ulcer	Diabetes*	Both	

Extra Points: Add points for as many of the following test results as you have available: 1 point for CRP above 3, 1 point for homocysteine above 100, 3 points for LDL above 130, 3 points for TC/HDL-C above 4. If only total cholesterol is available, add 1 point for a score of 200 to 240 or 3 points for scores above 240.

Total Alterable Risk Score	
Extra Points	
Grand Total Risk Score	

Adapted from CAD Risk Assessor, William J. Stone. Reprinted by permission.

*Diabetes is a risk factor that is often not alterable.

Procedures

1. Complete the 10 questions and the extra points, if available, on the Heart Disease Risk Factor Questionnaire by circling the answer that is most appropriate for *you* (see front of this lab).
2. Look at the top of the column for each of your answers. In the box provided at the right of each question, write down the number of risk points for that answer.
3. Determine your unalterable risk score by adding the risk points for questions 1, 2, and 3.
4. Determine your alterable risk score by adding the risk points for questions 4 through 10.
5. Determine your total heart disease risk score by adding the scores obtained in steps 3 and 4.
6. Look up your risk ratings on the Heart Disease Risk Rating Scale and record them in the Results section. Answer the questions in the Conclusions and Implications section.

Results: Write your risk scores and risk ratings in the appropriate boxes below.

Heart Disease Risk Scores and Ratings

	Score	Rating
Unalterable risk		
Alterable risk		
Total heart disease risk		

Heart Disease Risk Rating Chart

Rating	Unalterable Score	Alterable Score	Total Score
Very high	9 or more	9–10	31 or more
High	7–8	15–20	26–30
Average	5–6	11–14	16–25
Low	4 or less	10 or less	15 or less

Conclusions and Implications: The higher your score on the Heart Disease Risk Factor Questionnaire, the greater your heart disease risk. In several sentences, discuss your risk for heart disease. Which of the risk factors do you need to control to reduce your risk for heart disease? Why?

How Much Physical Activity Is Enough?

Health Goals for the year 2010

- Improve health, fitness, and quality of life of all people through the adoption and maintenance of regular, daily physical activity.

- Increase proportion of people who do moderate daily activity for 30 minutes.

- Increase proportion of people who do vigorous physical activity 3 days a week.

- Increase proportion of people who do regular exercises for muscle fitness.

- Increase proportion of people who do regular exercise for flexibility.

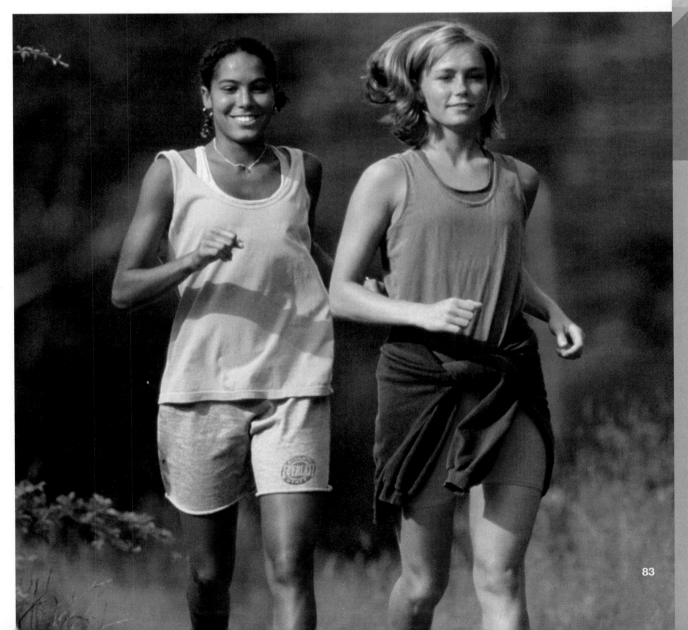

There is a minimal and an optimal amount of physical activity necessary for developing and maintaining good health, wellness, and fitness.

The authors would like to dedicate this chapter to the memory of Michael L. Pollock (1936–1998). Dr. Pollock, a past president of the American College of Sports Medicine, was a pioneer in the development of physical activity guidelines for building good health and fitness and determining how much fitness and activity are enough.

Just as there is a correct dosage of medicine for treating an illness, there is a correct dosage of physical activity for promoting health benefits and developing physical fitness. Several important principles of physical activity provide the basis for determining the correct dose or amount of physical activity. In this concept, a formula for implementing the important physical activity principles will be presented. This formula and the concepts of "threshold of training" and "target zones" will be described to help you determine how much physical activity is enough. New evidence indicates that the amount of physical activity necessary for developing metabolic fitness, and its associated health benefits, is different from the amount of physical activity necessary for developing health-related fitness and other performance benefits. Research also shows that the amount of activity or exercise necessary for maintaining fitness may differ from the amount needed to develop it. The guidelines presented in this concept, and throughout this book, are consistent with the most recent guidelines of the American College of Sports Medicine (ACSM)(see *Suggested Readings*).

The Principles of Physical Activity

Overload is necessary to achieve the health, wellness, and fitness benefits of physical activity. The **overload principle** is the most basic of all physical activity principles. This principle indicates that doing

On the Web
www.mhhe.com/corbinweb

Web 01 Log on to this URL before reading this concept. See On the Web list of concepts. Click on the concept number you want to view. To access supplemental information, click on the number shown at each Web icon.

"more than normal" is necessary if benefits are to occur. In order for a muscle (including the heart muscle) to get stronger, it must be overloaded, or worked against a load greater than normal. To increase flexibility, a muscle must be stretched longer than is normal. To increase muscular endurance, muscles must be exposed to sustained exercise for a longer than normal period. The health benefits associated with metabolic fitness seem to require less overload than for health-related fitness improvement, but overload is required, just the same.

Physical activity should be increased progressively for safe and effective results. The **principle of progression** indicates that overload should occur in a gradual progression rather than in major bursts. Failure to adhere to this principle can result in excess soreness or injury. While some tightness or fatigue is common after exercise, it is not necessary to feel sore in order to improve. Training is most effective when the sessions become progressively more challenging over time.

The benefits of physical activity are specific to the form of activity performed. The **principle of specificity** states that, to benefit from physical activity, you must overload specifically for that benefit. For example, strength-building exercises may do little for developing cardiovascular fitness, and stretching exercises may do little for altering body composition or metabolic fitness.

Overload is also specific to each body part. If you exercise the legs, you build fitness of the legs. If you exercise the arms, you build fitness of the arms. Some gymnasts, for example, have good upper body development but poor leg development, whereas some soccer players have well-developed legs but lack upper body development.

Specificity is important in designing your warm-up, workout, and cool-down programs for specific activities. Training is most effective when it closely resembles the activity for which you are preparing. For example, if your goal is to improve performance in putting the shot, it is not enough to strengthen the arm muscles. You should train using exercises that require overload of all muscles used and that require motions similar to those used in putting the shot.

The benefits achieved from overload last only as long as overload continues. The **principle of reversibility** is basically the overload principle in reverse.

To put it simply, if you don't use it, you will lose it. It is an important principle because some people have the mistaken impression that, if they achieve a health or fitness benefit, it will last forever. This, of course, is not true. There is evidence that you can maintain health benefits with less physical activity than it took to achieve them. Still, if you do not adhere to regular physical activity, any benefits attained will gradually erode.

In general, the more physical activity you do, the more benefits you receive. However, there are exceptions to this rule. A considerable body of research has demonstrated that improvements from physical activity follow a **dose-response relationship**—the more physical activity that you perform, the more you benefit. The overall patterns of improvements are summarized in Figure 1.

The red bar in Figure 1 indicates that inactive or sedentary people have a high risk for hypokinetic diseases and early death. A modest increase in physical activity, such as the 30 minutes of daily moderate lifestyle activity recommended by the surgeon general, results in a substantial decrease in risk and early death (green bar). Additional activity (blue bar) has extra benefits, but the benefits are not as great as those that come from making the change from being inactive to doing some activity. As the black bar (right) indicates, very high levels of activity produce little additional health benefit.

As you learned in Concept 4, and as will be pointed out in the concepts that follow, the "dose" of activity necessary to get one benefit is not the same as the "dose" for another. For example, changes in cholesterol levels resulting from physical activity may change at a different rate than changes in blood pressure. The greatest improvements in health, wellness, and fitness are obtained with moderate amounts of activity, so the key is to be at least active enough to obtain these benefits.

The rate of improvement levels off as you become fitter, and at some point maintenance is an appropriate goal. It is important to recognize that more is not always better. As the principle of progression indicates, beginners will benefit most from small doses of activity. For them, doing too much too soon is a bad idea. Also, the **principle of diminished returns** indicates that, as you get fitter and fitter, you may not get as big a benefit for each additional amount of activity that you perform. When improvements become more difficult and performance levels off, maintenance may become most important. In some cases, excessive amounts of activity can be counterproductive.

Health, wellness, and fitness benefits occur as you increase your physical activity. But it is important to understand that, if you keep increasing physical activity by equal increments, each additional amount of activity will yield less benefit. At some point, improvements will plateau and, if activity is overdone, may actually decrease.

Rest is needed to allow the body to adapt to exercise. The **principle of rest and recovery** indicates that it is important to allow time for recuperation after

Overload Principle The basic principle that specifies that you must perform physical activity in greater than normal amounts (overload) to get an improvement in physical fitness or health benefits.

Principle of Progression The corollary of the overload principle that indicates the need to gradually increase overload to achieve optimal benefits.

Principle of Specificity The corollary of the overload principle that indicates a need for a specific type of exercise to improve each fitness component or fitness of a specific part of the body.

Principle of Reversibility The corollary of the overload principle that indicates that disuse or inactivity results in loss of benefits achieved as a result of overload.

Dose-Response Relationship A term adopted from medicine. With medicine, it is important to know what response (benefit) will occur from taking a specific dose. When studying physical activity, it is important to know what dose provides the best response (most benefits). The contents of this book are designed to help you choose the best doses of activity for the responses (benefits) you desire.

Principle of Diminished Returns The corollary of the overload principle indicating that, the more benefits you gain as a result of activity, the harder additional benefits are to achieve.

Principle of Rest and Recovery The corollary of the overload principle that indicates that adequate rest is needed to allow the body to adapt to and recover from exercise.

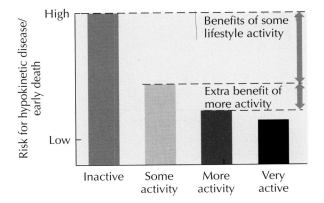

Figure 1 ▶ The health benefits from different levels of physical activity.

overload. Proper rest is needed within intense periods of activity, and appropriate rest is needed between training sessions. Rest provides time for the body to adapt to the stimulus provided during the workout. Failure to take sufficient rest can lead to overuse injuries, fatigue, and reduced performance. For recreational exercisers, rest generally implies taking a day off between bouts of exercise or alternating hard and easy days of exercise.

All people benefit from physical activity, but the benefits are unique for each person. Heredity, age, gender, ethnicity, lifestyles, current fitness and health status, and a variety of other factors make each person unique at any point in time. The **principle of individuality** indicates that the benefits of physical activity vary from individual to individual based on each person's unique characteristics.

The FIT Formula

The acronym FIT can help you remember the three important variables for applying the overload principle and its corollaries. For physical activity to be effective, it must be done with enough frequency and intensity and for a long enough time. The first letter from these three words spells **FIT** and can be considered as the formula for achieving health, wellness, and fitness benefits:

*F*requency (how often)—Physical activity must be performed regularly to be effective. The number of days a person does activity in a week is used to determine frequency. Most benefits require at least 3 days and up to 6 days of activity per week, but frequency ultimately depends on the specific benefit desired.

*I*ntensity (how hard)—Physical activity must be intense enough to require more exertion (overload) than normal to produce benefits. The method for determining appropriate intensity varies with the desired benefit. For example, metabolic fitness and associated health benefits require only moderate intensity; cardiovascular fitness for high-level performance requires vigorous activity that elevates the heart rate well above normal.

*T*ime (how long)—Physical activity must be done for an adequate length of time to be effective. The length of the activity session depends on the type of activity and the expected benefit.

Some health professionals add a second *T* to create the acronym FITT. This is done to illustrate the fact that there is a FIT formula for each different *T*ype, or mode, of physical activity. In this book, the acronym FIT formula will be used to describe the amount of activity necessary to produce benefits for each type of activity from the physical activity pyramid described later in this concept.

The FIT formula provides a practical means of applying the overload principle progressively for each specific type of activity and for each of the specific benefits expected.

The threshold of training and target zone concepts help you use the FIT formula. The **threshold of training** is the minimum amount of activity (frequency, intensity, and time) necessary to produce benefits. Depending on the benefit expected, slightly more than normal activity may not be enough to promote health, wellness, or fitness benefits. The **target zone** begins at the threshold of training and stops at the point where the activity becomes counterproductive. Figure 2 illustrates the threshold of training and target zone concepts.

Some people incorrectly associate the concepts of threshold of training and target zones with only cardiovascular fitness. As the principle of specificity suggests, each component of fitness, including metabolic fitness, has its own FIT formula and its own threshold and target zone. The target and threshold levels for **health benefits** are different from those for achieving **performance benefits** associated with high levels of physical fitness. Details of the different FIT formulas, threshold levels, and target zones for the various benefits of activity are presented later in this book.

It takes time for activity to produce health, wellness, and fitness benefits, even when the FIT formula is properly applied. Sometimes people just beginning a physical activity program expect to see immediate results. They expect to see large losses in body fat or great increases in muscle strength in just a few days. Evidence shows, however, that improvements in health-related physical fitness and the associated health benefits take several weeks to become apparent. Though some people report psychological benefits, such as "feeling better" and a "sense of personal accomplishment" almost immediately after beginning regular exer-

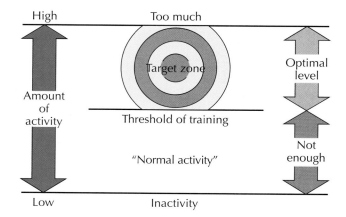

Figure 2 ▶ Physical activity target zone.

cise, the physiological changes take considerably longer to be realized. Proper preparation for physical activity includes learning not to expect too much too soon and not to do too much too soon. Attempts to try to get fit fast will probably be counterproductive, resulting in soreness and even injury. The key is to start slowly, stay with it, and enjoy yourself. Benefits will come to those who persist.

The Physical Activity Pyramid

The physical activity pyramid classifies activities by type and associated benefits. The **physical activity pyramid** (see Figure 3) is a good way to illustrate different types of activities and how each contributes to the development of health, wellness, and physical fitness. Each level includes one or two types of activity and characterizes the "portions" of physical activity necessary to produce different health, wellness, and fitness benefits.

The four levels of the pyramid are based on the beneficial health outcomes associated with regular physical activity. Activities having broad general health and wellness benefits for the largest number of people are placed at the base of the pyramid. Significant national health and economic benefits will occur if we can get inactive people, especially those who are totally sedentary, to do some type of activity. The activities at the higher levels provide additional benefits for health and wellness and are recommended in addition to the activities at the base of the pyramid.

Lifestyle activities are at the base of the physical activity pyramid. Lifestyle physical activity is encouraged as a part of everyday living and can contribute significantly to good health, wellness, and fitness. Lifestyle activities include walking to or from work, climbing the stairs rather than taking an elevator, working in the yard, and doing any other type of exercise as part of your normal daily activities. The national health strategy, as outlined in *Healthy People 2010*, suggests the accumulation of 30 minutes of physical activity equal to brisk walking on most, if not all, days of the week (see Figure 3, level 1).

Research has clearly documented that lifestyle activities can yield important health benefits even if the person does no other forms of activity. For example, studies have demonstrated that individuals with active jobs have reduced risks for many chronic conditions. Individuals who use active commuting (biking or walking) to get to work or to run errands have also been found to have better health profiles. The regular accumulation of activity as a part of one's lifestyle is sufficient to promote positive improvements in metabolic fitness, and these improvements can positively impact health. Additional activity from the other layers of the pyramid are strongly recommended, and additional benefits occur from involvement in these activities. Lifestyle activity can be viewed as the

baseline, or minimal, activity that should be performed. A summary of the FIT formula for this type of activity is illustrated in level 1 of Figure 3.

Active aerobics and sports and recreation are at the second level of the pyramid. Aerobic activities (level 2) include those that are of such an intensity that they can be performed for relatively long periods of time without stopping, but that also elevate the heart rate significantly. Lifestyle activities (level 1), also known as **moderate activity,** are technically aerobic but are not especially vigorous and are, therefore, not considered to be "active aerobics." More **vigorous activities,** such as jogging, biking, and aerobic dance, are commonly classified as "active aerobic" activities. This type of activity is included in the second level of the pyramid because benefits can be accomplished in as few as 3 days a week and is especially good for building cardiovascular fitness and helping to control body fat. This type of activity can provide metabolic fitness and health benefits similar to lifestyle activities.

Principle of Individuality The corollary of the overload principle that indicates that overload provides unique benefits to each individual based on the unique characteristics of that person.

FIT A formula used to describe the frequency, intensity, and length of time for physical activity to produce benefits. (When FITT is used, the second *T* refers to the type of physical activity you perform.)

Threshold of Training The minimum amount of physical activity that will produce health and fitness benefits.

Target Zone The amounts of physical activity that produce optimal health and fitness benefits.

Health Benefits The results of physical activity that provide protection from hypokinetic disease or early death.

Performance Benefits The results of physical activity that improve physical fitness and physical performance capabilities.

Physical Activity Pyramid A pyramid that illustrates how different types of activities contribute to the development of health and physical fitness. Activities lower in the pyramid require more frequent participation, whereas activities higher in the pyramid require less frequency.

Moderate Activity For the purposes of this book, activity equal in intensity to a brisk walk. Level 1 activities from the activity pyramid are included in this category.

Vigorous Activities For the purposes of this book, activities that elevate the heart rate and are greater in intensity than brisk walking; also referred to as moderate to vigorous activities. These activities from level 2 of the pyramid are included in this category.

Active sports and recreation are also included at level 2 of the pyramid. Examples of active sports include basketball, tennis, and racquetball, and active recreation includes hiking, backpacking, skiing, and rock climbing. Many of these activities involve short and intense bursts of physical activity followed by intermittent rest. They are typically performed longer than the continuous forms of active aerobic activities and can provide similar benefits. Some sports, such as golfing, may be better classified as a lifestyle activity, since they are done at a lower intensity and typically not for aerobic benefits. In general, activities at level 2 of the pyramid may substitute for activities at level 1 if done according to the FIT formula, but many experts encourage activities from both levels. They reason that people who develop active lifestyles from level 1 will be more likely to stay active later in life when they are less likely to participate in activities from level 2. Others argue that, if you are active at level 2, you will be fit enough to continue active aerobics and sports as you grow older. A summary of the FIT formula for level 2 activities is included in Figure 3.

Flexibility and muscle fitness exercises are at level 3 of the pyramid. Flexibility (stretching) exercises are a type of physical activity that is planned specifically to develop flexibility. This type of exercise is necessary because many of the activities lower in the pyramid do not contribute to flexibility development. The muscle fitness category includes exercises that are planned specifically to build strength and muscular endurance. This type of exercise is necessary because many of the activities lower in the pyramid do not contribute to these parts of fitness. A general description of the FIT formula for level 3 exercises is included in Figure 3.

Long periods of inactivity are discouraged. Rest is important to good health. Some "time-off" just to relax is important to us all, and, of course, proper amounts of rest and 8 hours of uninterrupted sleep help us recuperate. But sedentary living (too much inactivity) results in low fitness as well as poor health and wellness. Examples include excessive television viewing, web surfing or game playing. Inactivity is placed at the top of the pyramid because it should be minimized (see Figure 3).

Physical activity from any of the first three levels of the pyramid can help maintain a healthy body composition. Weight maintenance requires that energy intake be matched by energy expenditure. While 30 minutes of daily physical activity is recommended for general health benefits, it is not adequate

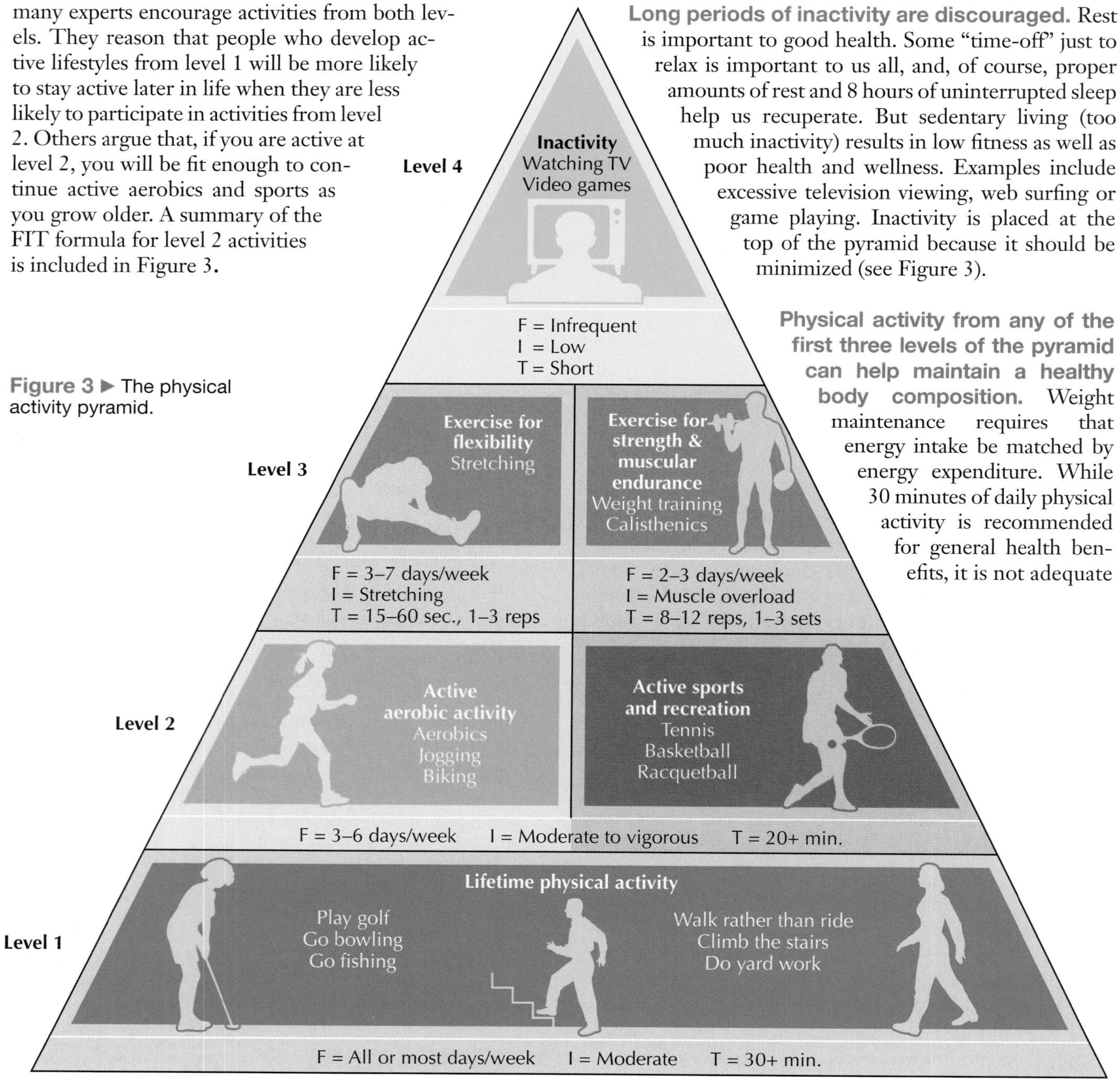

Figure 3 ▶ The physical activity pyramid.

Level 4
Inactivity
Watching TV
Video games

F = Infrequent
I = Low
T = Short

Level 3
Exercise for flexibility
Stretching

Exercise for strength & muscular endurance
Weight training
Calisthenics

F = 3–7 days/week
I = Stretching
T = 15–60 sec., 1–3 reps

F = 2–3 days/week
I = Muscle overload
T = 8–12 reps, 1–3 sets

Level 2
Active aerobic activity
Aerobics
Jogging
Biking

Active sports and recreation
Tennis
Basketball
Racquetball

F = 3–6 days/week   I = Moderate to vigorous   T = 20+ min.

Level 1
Lifetime physical activity
Play golf
Go bowling
Go fishing

Walk rather than ride
Climb the stairs
Do yard work

F = All or most days/week   I = Moderate   T = 30+ min.

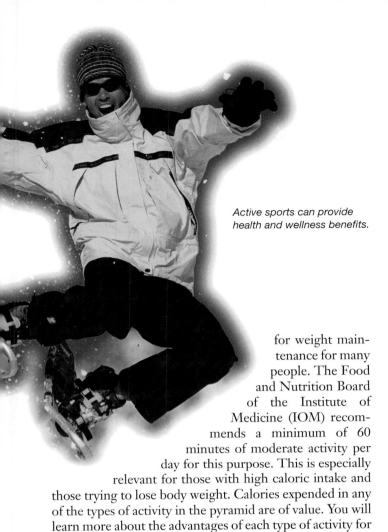

Active sports can provide health and wellness benefits.

for weight maintenance for many people. The Food and Nutrition Board of the Institute of Medicine (IOM) recommends a minimum of 60 minutes of moderate activity per day for this purpose. This is especially relevant for those with high caloric intake and those trying to lose body weight. Calories expended in any of the types of activity in the pyramid are of value. You will learn more about the advantages of each type of activity for healthy body composition maintenance later in this book.

Some important factors should be considered when using the physical activity pyramid. The physical activity pyramid is a useful model for describing different types of activity and their benefits. The pyramid is also useful in summarizing the FIT formula for each of the benefits of activity. However, as the American College of Sports Medicine pointed out, physical activity guidelines "cannot be implemented in an overly rigid fashion and recommendations presented should be used with careful attention to the goals of the individual." The following guidelines for using the pyramid should also be considered:

- *No single activity provides all of the benefits.* Many people have asked the question "What is the perfect form of physical activity?" It is evident that there is no single activity that can provide all of the health, wellness, and fitness benefits. For optimal benefits to occur, it is desirable to perform activities from all levels of the pyramid because each type of activity has different benefits.
- *In some cases, one type of activity can substitute for another.* Activities in level 1 of the pyramid provide general health benefits, such as reduced risk for heart disease, cancer, and other chronic conditions. Activities in level

2 provide many of the same benefits as well as the added health and performance benefits (see Concept 8). For this reason, a person who meets the FIT formula for level 2 activities does not necessarily need to perform activities at level 1. Nevertheless, participation in activity as part of your lifestyle is strongly recommended.

- *Something is better than nothing.* Some people may look at the pyramid and say, "I just don't have time to do all of these activities." This could lead some to throw up their hands in despair, concluding, "I just won't do anything at all." The best evidence indicates that something is better than nothing. If you do nothing or feel that you can't do it all, performing a lifestyle physical activity is a good place to start. Additional activities from different levels of the pyramid can be added as time allows.
- *Activities from level 3 are useful even if you are limited in performing activities at other levels.* Though flexibility and muscle fitness exercises do not produce all of the benefits associated with regular physical activity, they will produce benefits even if you are unable to perform as much activity from other levels as you like.
- *Good planning will allow you to schedule activities from all levels in a reasonable amount of time.* In subsequent concepts, you will learn more about each level of the pyramid, as well as more information about planning a total physical activity program.
- *Work-related activity counts.* The types of activities you do at work may not fit the categories of the pyramid exactly, but they count. People in active occupations do a variety of activities than can contribute to health and fitness. For example, warehouse work involves walking, lifting, and other activities and waiting tables involves walking and lifting. Of course, it is important that the guidelines discussed in this book are followed when doing work-related activities to prevent injury and to get optimal benefits. It is also important to note that work-related activities, depending on the activities performed, may need to get supplemented to get all of the benefits that accompany regular exercise. Work-related activities may not provide the enjoyment and wellness benefits associated with self-selected leisure-time activities.

Understanding Physical Activity Guidelines

There are multiple sets of guidelines for physical activity designed to help you achieve specific benefits. The joint recommendation of the ACSM and the Centers for Disease Control & Prevention (CDC) calls for adults to accumulate 30 minutes of moderate activity per day. This recommendation is consistent with recommendations in the *Surgeon General's*

Report on Physical Activity and Health, which call for the accumulation of approximately 1,000 kcal of physical activity a week—a level that can be achieved with 30 minutes of walking each day. These guidelines have been in place for over 10 years and provide threshold values for the physical activity target zone.

As mentioned, the IOM recently recommended that adults obtain 60 minutes of activity per day. This recommendation focuses on the activity required for the maintenance of a healthy body weight rather than general health benefits. While the recommendations differ, the recommendation of one group does not supercede that of the other group. In this case, the recommendations are complementary, emphasizing different goals.

It is equally important to understand that not all guidelines are correct. Visit the *On the Web* feature for additional information about the evolution of physical activity guidelines.

Specific activity recommendations exist for children. Children are different from adults and Web 05 they have different needs for activity. The National Association for Sports and Physical Education (NASPE) and the CDC have developed activity recommendations that are specific to children. According to these guidelines, children should accumulate at least 60 minutes, and up to several hours, of age-appropriate physical activity on most, if not all, days of the week. This daily accumulation should include participation in a variety of age-appropriate activities (both moderate and vigorous) with the majority of the time being spent in activity that is intermittent. The guidelines also recommend minimizing periods of inactivity (periods of 2 or more hours). Adults play a major role in shaping children's activity patterns. Helping children meet these guidelines may help reduce the prevalence of inactive and overweight adults in future years.

Physical Activity Patterns

The proportion of adults meeting national health goals varies with activity type and gender. National health goals have been established for each of the types of activity illustrated in the physical activity pyramid. The percentages of adults 18 and over who meet health goals for moderate activity (at least 5 days a week), vigorous activity (at least 3 days a week), muscle fitness exercise (no frequency specified), and flexibility (at least 3 days a week) are presented in Table 1. Also presented in Table 1 are the percentages of people who are totally inactive (no leisure-time bouts of activit).

More people reach the vigorous physical activity than reach the moderate activity criteria. With the exception of flexibility activity, more males than females achieve the various activity criteria. Only 14 percent of adults meet the moderate activity standard (equal to the surgeon gen-

Table 1 ▶ Percentage of Adults Who Meet Activity Goals and Who Do No Leisure Activity

	Male	Female	All
Gender			
Moderate	16	13	14
Vigorous	25	22	23
Muscle fitness	27	23	19
Flexibility	29	31	30
No leisure activity	35	41	38

	18–24	25–44	45–65
Age			
Moderate	14	16	13
Vigorous	28[a]	28[a]	22
Muscle fitness	19	27	23
Flexibility	30	29	31
No leisure activity	38	35	41

	Low	Medium	High
Income			
Moderate	11	14	17
Vigorous	16	20	25
Muscle fitness	18	22	36
Flexibility	— — —	— — —	— — —
No leisure activity	57	41	24

	White[b]	Hispanic[c]	Black[d]	Asian[e]
Ethnicity				
Moderate	16	10	10	23
Vigorous	24	17	19	20
Muscle fitness	28	21	30	28
Flexibility	31	22	26	34
No leisure activity	35	53	50	38

	With	Without
Disability		
Moderate	12	16
Vigorous	13	25
Muscle fitness	14	20
Flexibility	29	31
No leisure activity	56	36

Values represent percentages of adults who reach national goals for each of four types of activity and percentages of adults who get no leisure activity.
[a]Data available for 18–44, same statistic used for both.
[b]Non-Hispanic.
[c]Hispanic/Latino.
[d]African American.
[e]Or Pacific Islander.
Source: National Health Interview Survey.

eral's recommendation). However, one-third of adults can be considered "active enough" because they meet either the moderate or the vigorous standard. Unfortunately, 38 percent of all adults not only fail to get enough exercise but also get no leisure activity of any kind.

On a positive note, modest decreases in totally sedentary behavior have occurred since the 2010 health goals were written, and modest increases in vigorous and muscle fitness activities have occurred. A survey conducted by the Sporting Goods Manufacturers Association found that the percentage of people reporting "frequent" exercise has increased by 7.8 percent—the first increase noted in this study in more than a decade.

 The proportion of people meeting national health goals varies based on age. Children are the most active group in Western society. During adolescence activity starts to decrease but teens still do more activity than young adults. Activity levels of all types decrease from young adulthood to ages 65 and over.

Web 07

The proportion of adults meeting national health goals varies based on income, education, and disability status. People at or near poverty level are more than twice as likely to be totally inactive during leisure time, compared to those with high income. Though not illustrated in Table 1, evidence shows that high school dropouts are three times more likely to be inactive than college grads. Minority groups have high rates of inactivity, but this is likely associated with educational and economic factors. Adults identified as having one or more physical disabilities have a high probability of being inactive.

Physical Fitness Standards

Health-based criterion-referenced standards are recommended for rating your fitness. This concept has focused on the amount of physical activity necessary to get health and fitness benefits. Another question to be answered is "How much physical fitness is enough?" Most experts recommend **health-based criterion-referenced standards** to rate your current fitness. These standards are based on how much fitness is needed for good health. Other standards use norms or percentiles that compare a person's fitness against a reference population. Knowing how you compare with other people is not that important. In fact, such comparisons have been shown to be discouraging to many people. Determining if your fitness is adequate to enhance your health and wellness is more relevant.

Web 08

In this book, the health-related standard is referred to as the *good fitness zone* (see Table 2). With reasonable amounts of physical activity, most people should be able to improve their fitness enough to make it into this range. For personal reasons, some may wish to aim for a higher level, referred to as the *high performance zone*. Attaining this level does not provide many additional health benefits but may be important for those interested in performance. The *low fit zone* and the *marginal zone* are levels of fitness that are not sufficient for optimal health benefits. If you score in these ranges, you should try to improve your level of fitness.

Table 2 ▶ The Four Fitness Zones

High Performance Zone
It is not necessary to reach this level to experience good health benefits. Achievement of high performance scores has more to do with performance than it does with good health. In some cases, extreme fitness scores can increase health risk—e.g., very low body fatness.

Good Fitness Zone
If you reach the good fitness zone, you have enough of a specific fitness component to help reduce health risk. However, even reaching the good fitness zone may not result in optimal health benefits for inactive people.

Marginal Zone
Marginal scores indicate that some improvement is in order, but you are nearing minimal health standards set by experts.

Low-Fit Zone
If you score low in fitness, you are probably less fit than you should be for your own good health and wellness.

Technology Update
Using Technology to Track Activity Trends

Advances in technology have made it easier to monitor population levels of physical activity. Scientists frequently link data from national surveys with other data obtained from geodemographic information systems (GIS) and global positioning systems (GPS) to understand factors that may explain patterns and trends. Much of the data compiled by the CDC and National Center for Health Statistics are available online. Scientists and professionals can access data for research and presentations, and laypeople can access data for personal information. An interesting site to explore is the interactive Behavioral Risk Factor Surveillance System site, which allows you to see current levels (prevalence statistics) or trend graphs over time for a variety of health-related variables. The system allows you to make comparisons between states. It even has detailed statistics for some of the larger cities compared to averages in the state. Visit the website at **www.cdc.gov/brfss/**.

Health-Based Criterion-Referenced Standards
The amount of a specific type of fitness necessary to gain a health or wellness benefit.

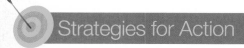
A self-assessment of your current activity at each level of the pyramid can help you determine future activity goals. Lab 5A provides you with the opportunity to assess your physical activity at each level of the pyramid. Lab 5B offers a general assessment of fitness. Later you will develop a program of activity, and these assessments will provide a basis for program planning.

Self-assessments of physical fitness can help you prepare a fitness profile that can be used in program planning. In the concepts that follow, you will learn to perform a variety of self-assessments of fitness and will learn the scores that are necessary on these assessments to reach the good fitness zone as described in Table 2. In the meantime, you can complete Lab 5B. This lab will help you understand the nature of each part of fitness and estimate your current fitness level for each type of fitness. When you complete the more accurate self-assessments later in the book, you will be able to determine the accuracy of your estimates.

Online Learning Center

www.mhhe.com/corbin7e
The Online Learning Center contains a variety of Web-based resources that will help you get the most out of this book and your course. In addition to the On the Web pages, there are video activities, interactive quizzes, application assignments, and a variety of other useful study aids. Log on to the URL above to access these resources.

Web Resources

Web 09

American College of Sports Medicine **www.acsm.org**
Centers for Disease Control and Prevention (CDC) **www.cdc.gov**
Health Canada **www.healthcanada.ca**
Healthy People 2010 **www.health.gov/healthypeople**
Morbidity and Mortality Weekly Reports **www.cdc.gov/mmwr**
Surgeon General's Report on Physical Activity and Health **www.cdc.gov/nccdphp/sgr/sgr.htm**

Suggested Readings

Web 10

Additional reference materials for Concept 5 are available at Web10.

American College of Sports Medicine. 2006. *ACSM's Guidelines for Exercise Testing and Prescription.* 7th ed. Philadelphia, PA: Lippincott, Williams and Wilkins.

Bassuk, S. S., and J. E. Manson, 2004. Preventing cardiovascular disease in women: How much physical activity is "good enough"? *President's Council on Physical Fitness and Sports Research Digest* 5(4):1–8.

Blair, S. N. 2004. The evolution of physical activity recommendations: How much is enough? *American Journal of Clinical Nutrition* 79(5):913A–920S.

Corbin, C. B., et al. 2004. Making sense of multiple physical activity recommendations. In C. B. Corbin et al. (eds). *Toward a Better Understanding of Physical Fitness and Activity, Selected Topics, Volume II,* 37–46. Scottsdale, AZ: Holcomb Hathaway.

Corbin, C. B., et al. 2004. Physical activity for children: Current patterns and guidelines. *President's Council on Physical Fitness and Sports Research Digest* 4(6):1–8.

Crespo, C. J. 2005. Physical activity in minority populations: Overcoming a health challenge. *President's Council on Physical Fitness and Sports Research Digest* 6(2):1–8.

National Association for Sports and Physical Education. 2004. *Physical Activity for Children: A Statement of Guidelines.* Reston, VA: National Association for Sports and Physical Education.

Rankinen, T., and C. Bouchard. 2004. Dose-response issues concerning relations between regular physical activity and health. In C.B. Corbin et al. (eds). *Toward a Better Understanding of Physical Fitness and Activity, Selected Topics, Volume II,* 73–80. Scottsdale, AZ: Holcomb Hathaway.

Strong, W. B., et al. 2005. Evidence-based physical activity for school-age youth. *Journal of Pediatrics* 146(6):732–737.

U.S. Department of Health and Human Services. 2005. Summary of health statistics for U.S. adults: National Health Interview Survey. *Vital and Health Statistics* 10(228):1–282.

In the News

Physical Activity Guidelines for Youth

As previously noted in this concept, less than one-third of American adults meet the physical activity guidelines for the major types of activity described in the physical activity pyramid. Forty percent do no regular leisure-time activity. As people age, the amount of activity that they get decreases. Of concern is that the decrease in activity begins during the school years. Consider the following statistics:

- Elementary school children are more active than secondary school youth.
- Activity levels decrease after the school years.
- The activity levels of young people decrease when they get out of school.
- Physical education in high schools decreased by nearly 30 percent over the last decade.
- Sedentary behavior during the school years tracks to adulthood.

Lab 5A Self-Assessment of Physical Activity

Name	**Section**	**Date**

Purpose: To estimate your current levels of physical activity from each category of the physical activity pyramid

Procedures

1. Place an X over the circle that characterizes your participation in each category in the pyramid.
2. Determine if you met the national goal for each type of activity. Place an X over the "yes" circle if you met the goal in each area (see Results). In the chart on the next page, place an X over the "yes" circle if you meet the goal in each area or an X over the "no" circle if you do not meet the goal.

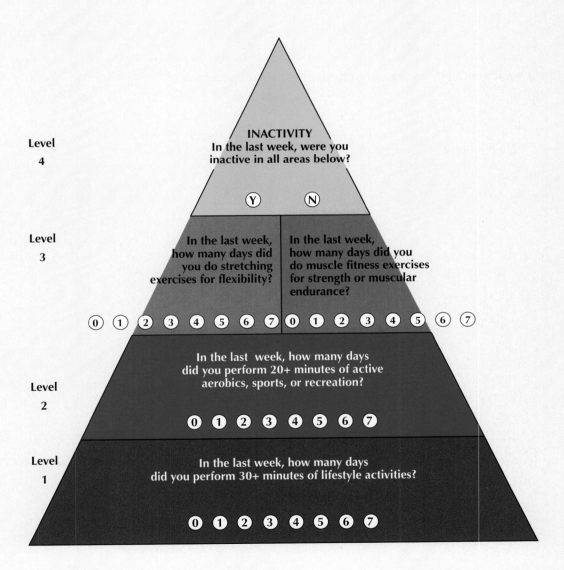

Level 4

INACTIVITY
In the last week, were you inactive in all areas below?

Ⓨ   Ⓝ

Level 3

In the last week, how many days did you do stretching exercises for flexibility?

In the last week, how many days did you do muscle fitness exercises for strength or muscular endurance?

⓪ ① ② ③ ④ ⑤ ⑥ ⑦   ⓪ ① ② ③ ④ ⑤ ⑥ ⑦

Level 2

In the last week, how many days did you perform 20+ minutes of active aerobics, sports, or recreation?

⓪ ① ② ③ ④ ⑤ ⑥ ⑦

Level 1

In the last week, how many days did you perform 30+ minutes of lifestyle activities?

⓪ ① ② ③ ④ ⑤ ⑥ ⑦

Results

Activity Type	Level	National Goal	Did You Meet the National Health Goal?	
Lifestyle activity	1	5 days or more	Yes	No
Active aerobics/sports	2	3 days or more	Yes	No
Flexibility exercises	3	3 days or more	Yes	No
Muscle fitness	3	2 days or more	Yes	No
Inactivity	4	Avoid total inactivity	Yes	No

Conclusions and Implications: In the space below, write a brief paper describing your current physical activity patterns. Do you meet the national health goals in all areas? If not, in what types of activity from the pyramid do you need to improve? Are the answers you gave for the past week typical of your regular activity patterns? If you meet all national health goals, explain why you think this is so. Do you think that meeting the goals in the pyramid on the previous page indicates good activity patterns for you?

Write your physical activity assessment paper in the space below.

Lab 5B Estimating Your Fitness

Name	Section	Date

Purpose: To help you better understand each of the 11 components of health-related and skill-related physical fitness and to help you estimate your current levels of physical fitness.

Special Note: The activities performed in the lab are *not intended as valid tests of physical fitness.* It is hoped that completing the activities will help you better understand each component of fitness and help you estimate your current fitness levels. You should not rely primarily on the results of the activities to make your estimates. Rather, you should rely on previous fitness tests you have taken and your own best judgment of your current fitness. Later in this book, you will learn how to perform accurate assessments of each fitness component and determine the accuracy of your estimates.

Procedures

1. Warm up. Perform each of the activities described in Chart 1 on page 96. Cool down.
2. Use past fitness test performances and your own judgment to estimate your current levels for each of the health-related and skill-related physical fitness parts. Low fitness = improvement definitely needed, marginal fitness = some improvement necessary, good fitness = adequate for healthy daily living.
3. Place an X in the appropriate circle for your fitness estimate in the Results section.

Results

Fitness Component	Low Fitness	Marginal Fitness	Good Fitness
Body composition	◯	◯	◯
Cardiovascular fitness	◯	◯	◯
Flexibility	◯	◯	◯
Muscular endurance	◯	◯	◯
Strength	◯	◯	◯
Agility	◯	◯	◯
Balance	◯	◯	◯
Coordination	◯	◯	◯
Power	◯	◯	◯
Reaction time	◯	◯	◯
Speed	◯	◯	◯

Conclusions and Implications: In several sentences, discuss the information you used to make your estimates of physical fitness. How confident are you that these estimates are accurate?

Directions: Attempt each of the activities in Chart 1. Place an X in the circle next to each component of physical fitness to indicate that you have attempted the activity.

Chart 1 ▶ Physical Fitness Activities

Balance

1. *One-foot balance.* Stand on one foot; press up so that the weight is on the ball of the foot with the heel off the floor. Hold the hands and the other leg straight out in front for 10 seconds.

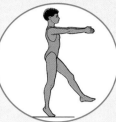

Power

2. *Standing long jump.* Stand with the toes behind a line. Using no run or hop step, jump as far as possible. Men must jump their height plus 6 inches. Women must jump their height only.

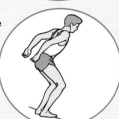

Agility

3. *Paper ball pickup.* Place two wadded paper balls on the floor 5 feet away. Run until both feet cross the line, pick up the first ball, and return both feet behind the starting line. Repeat with the second ball. Finish in 5 seconds.

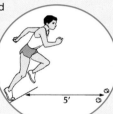

Reaction Time

4. *Paper drop.* Have a partner hold a sheet of notebook paper so that the side edge is between your thumb and index finger, about the width of your hand from the top of the page. When your partner drops the paper, catch it before it slips through the thumb and finger. Do not lower your hand to catch the paper.

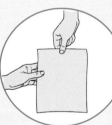

Speed

5. *Double-heel click.* With the feet apart, jump up and tap the heels together twice before you hit the ground. You must land with your feet at least 3 inches apart.

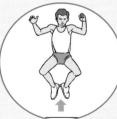

Coordination

6. *Paper ball bounce.* Wad up a sheet of notebook paper into a ball. Bounce the ball back and forth between the right and left hands. Keep the hands open and palms up. Bounce the ball three times with each hand (six times total), alternating hands for each bounce.

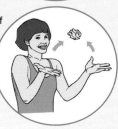

Cardiovascular Fitness

7. *Run in place.* Run in place for 1 ½ minutes (120 steps per minute). Rest for 1 minute and count the heart rate for 30 seconds. A heart rate of 60 (for 30 sec.) or lower passes. A step is counted each time the right foot hits the floor.

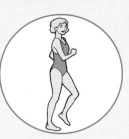

Flexibility

8. *Backsaver toe touch.* Sit on the floor with one foot against a wall. Bend the other knee. Bend forward at the hips. After three warm-up trials, reach forward and touch your closed fists to the wall. Bend forward slowly; do not bounce. Repeat with the other leg straight. Pass if fists touch the wall with each leg straight.

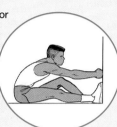

Body Composition

9. *The pinch.* Have a partner pinch a fold of fat on the back of your upper arm (body fatness), halfway between the tip of the elbow and the tip of the shoulder.

Men: no greater than 3/4 inch

Women: no greater than 1 inch

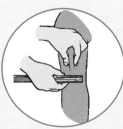

Strength

10. *Push-up.* Lie face down on the floor. Place the hands under the shoulders. Keeping the legs and body straight, press off the floor until the arms are fully extended. Women repeat once; men, three times.

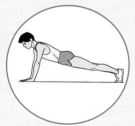

Muscular Endurance

11. *Side leg raise.* Lie on the floor on your side. Lift your leg up and to the side of the body until your feet are 24 to 36 inches apart. Keep the knee and pelvis facing forward. Do not rotate so that the knees face the ceiling. Perform 10 with each leg.

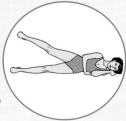

Lifestyle Physical Activity: Being Active in Diverse Environments

Health Goals for the year 2010

- Increase adoption and maintenance of daily physical activity.

- Increase leisure-time physical activity.

- Increase proportion of people who do daily activity for 30 minutes.

- Increase travel by walking and by bicycle.

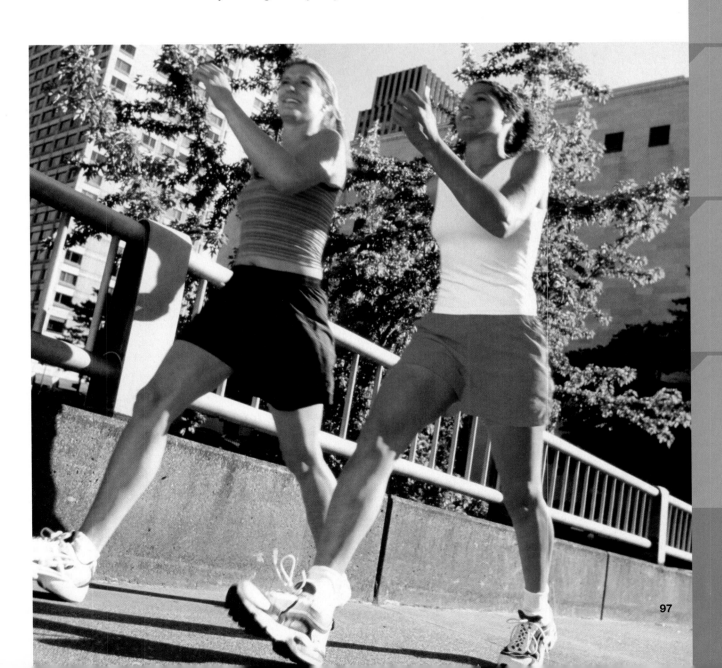

Concept 6

97

Moderate intensity physical activity done as a regular part of daily living has many health and wellness benefits.

Humans are clearly meant to move, but the nature of our society has made it difficult for many people to lead active lifestyles. Cars, motorized golf carts, snowblowers, elevators, remote control devices, and email are just some of the modern conveniences that have reduced the amount of activity in our daily lives. While most people appreciate the benefits of labor-saving technology, it is also important to consider the impact that these tools have on our activity patterns. Adding small amounts of physical activity back into your daily routine can help you develop and maintain a more active lifestyle. This concept will describe the importance of lifestyle physical activity for optimal health and wellness and provide strategies that will help you lead an active life in an inactive world.

Adopting an Active Lifestyle

Lifestyle activities include activities of daily living, as well as some less intense sports and recreational activities. Lifestyle physical activity is the foundation of an active lifestyle. Many people report that they don't enjoy structured forms of exercise. Others may enjoy exercise but feel unskilled or lack the time or motivation to keep up a regular program. While it is possible to meet physical activity guidelines by participating regularly in structured exercise, it is easier for most people to meet the guidelines if they perform some activity throughout the day. Lifestyle physical activities are activities that can be done as part of one's normal daily routine. They are at the base of the physical activity pyramid because they provide valuable benefits, require little skill, and can be easily performed by most people (see Figure 1). Involvement in lifestyle activity also provides a strong foundation for other forms of physical activity. Common examples of lifestyle activities include daily tasks, such as walking to work or to the store, doing housework, gardening, and climbing stairs. Some light- to moderate-intensity sports can be classified as lifestyle physical activities. Golf, shuffleboard, bocci ball, table tennis, and bowling are examples.

Recreational activities of light and moderate intensity can also be classified as lifestyle physical activities. Examples are fishing, canoeing, horseback riding, and gardening.

For children, play is considered a lifestyle physical activity because play is a normal activity for this age group. For retired adults, light- to moderate-intensity sports and recreational activities are lifestyle activities because they are a part of normal daily living.

Lifestyle physical activities should expend more energy than normally expended at rest. Scientists have devised a method to classify levels of activity by intensity. With this system, all activities are compared against the amount of activity needed at rest. The amount of energy expended at rest is referred to as one metabolic equivalent (1 **MET**). Activities listed as 2 METs require twice the energy of rest, and activities listed as 4 METs require four times the energy required for rest. Table 1 defines different intensity levels, so that you can distinguish among the various terms used later in this book.

Current physical activity recommendations have emphasized the importance of moderate-intensity physical activity. For a person with good cardiovascular fitness, moderate-intensity activities typically require 4.7–7.0 METs. Moderate-intensity activities are often referred

On the Web

Web 01

www.mhhe.com/corbinweb

Log on to this URL before reading this concept. See On the Web list of concepts. Click on the concept number you want to view. To access supplemental information, click on the number shown at each Web icon.

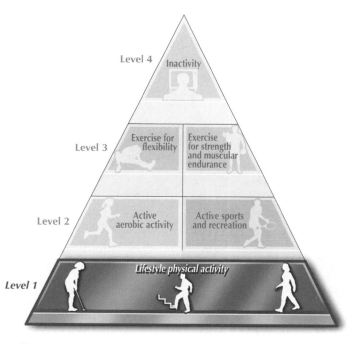

Figure 1 ▶ The physical activity pyramid level 1: lifestyle physical activity.

Table 1 ▶ Classification of Physical Activity Intensities for a Person with Good Cardiovascular Fitness

Classification	Description	Examples
Maximum	Activities more than 12 times as intense as rest (12+ METs)	Running (10 mph, 6 min. mile)
Very hard	Activities more than 10 and up to 12 times as intense as rest (10 to 12 METs)	Running (8.5 mph, 7 min. mile), handball, full-court competitive basketball
Hard	Activities more than 7 and up to 10 times as intense as rest (7 to 10 METs)	Digging, level jogging (5 mph, 12 min. mile), cycling (13 mph), skiing, fencing
Moderate	Activity about 4 2/3 to 7 times as intense as rest (4.7 to 7 METs)	Brisk walking, lawn mowing, shoveling, social dancing
Light	Activity that is 2 1/2 to 4 2/3 times as intense as rest (2.5 to 4.7 METs)	Normal walking, walking downstairs, bowling, mopping
Very light	Activity about 2 to 2 1/2 times as intense as lying or sitting at rest (2 to 2.5 METs)	Washing your face, dressing yourself, typing, driving a car

to as **aerobic physical activities** because the aerobic metabolism can meet the energy demand of the activity. Aerobic activities can be performed comfortably for extended periods of time by most people.

Anaerobic physical activities are so vigorous that your body cannot supply adequate oxygen to meet the energy demand using the aerobic system. The body must rely on short-term energy provided by the anaerobic metabolic system. Activities classified in Table 1 as hard, very hard, or maximum may be anaerobic, or at least partially anaerobic, and are not considered lifestyle physical activities.

Because lifestyle activities are relatively easy to perform, they are popular among adults. Walking is the most popular of all leisure-time activities among adults 18 years of age and over. About 40 percent of men and nearly 50 percent of women report walking for exercise. The percentages are slightly higher for older adults but walking is still a very popular activity among 18 to 29 year-olds. Approximately 33 percent of young males and about 47 percent of young females report walking for activity.

Web 02

Involvement in other lifestyle activities tends to vary more widely with age. While overall activity levels tend to decline with age, involvement in lifestyle activity actually tends to increase. This is because many older adults move away from vigorous sports and recreation and prefer to spend more time in lifestyle activity. Gardening and lifestyle sports, such as golf, are two activities that increase in popularity with age. Older adults tend to have more time and money for these types of recreational activities and the lower intensity may be appealing.

The advantage of lifestyle activity is that there are many opportunities to be active. Finding enjoyable activities that fit into your daily routine is the key to adopting a more active lifestyle.

Activity classifications vary, depending on one's level of fitness. Normal walking is considered light activity for a person with good fitness (see Table 1), but for a person with low to marginal fitness the same activity is considered moderate. For a very low-fit person, brisk walking is considered to be hard. Table 2 helps you determine the type of lifestyle activity considered moderate for you. Beginners with low fitness should start with normal rather than brisk walking, for example. Older people often have lower fitness levels than younger people and may find Table 2 useful in selecting appropriate lifestyle physical activities. For example, activities considered very light to light for young fit people are equal to moderate activity for many people 80 and over. For many people over 65, activities typically classified as light are equal to moderate activities.

Web 03

The Health Benefits of Lifestyle Physical Activity

Many health benefits can be achieved as a result of participation in lifestyle physical activities. Studies have clearly indicated that modest amounts of lifestyle activity can have important **health benefits.** One early epidemiology study reported that postal workers who delivered mail had fewer health

Web 04

MET One MET equals the amount of energy a person expends at rest. METs are multiples of resting activity (2 METS equals twice the resting energy expenditure).

Aerobic Physical Activities *Aerobic* means "in the presence of oxygen." Aerobic activities are activities or exercise for which the body is able to supply adequate oxygen to sustain performance for long periods of time.

Anaerobic Physical Activities *Anaerobic* means "in the absence of oxygen." Anaerobic activities are performed at an intensity so great that the body's demand for oxygen exceeds its ability to supply it.

Health Benefits Reductions in hypokinetic disease risk and risk for early death.

Table 2 ▶ Classification of Lifestyle Physical Activities for People of Different Fitness Levels

Sample Lifestyle Activities	Activity Classification by Fitness Level			
	Low Fitness	Marginal Fitness	Good Fitness	High Performance
Washing your face, dressing, typing, driving a car	Light	Very light/light	Very light	Very light
Normal walking, walking downstairs, bowling, mopping	Moderate	Moderate	Light	Light
Brisk walking, lawn mowing, shoveling, social dancing	Hard	Moderate/hard	Moderate	Light/moderate

problems than workers who sorted mail. Another study reported that drivers of double-decker buses in England had more health problems than conductors who climbed the stairs during the day to collect tickets. Other population studies have demonstrated that simple activities, such as gardening and active commuting, can provide important health benefits.

To better understand the mechanisms associated with this effect, several studies have directly compared lifestyle physical activity with more traditional exercise regimens. The results have indicated that regular brisk walking (or other moderate activities similar in intensity to brisk walking) can lead to improvements in fitness and reductions in risk factors—particularly among previously sedentary adults.

Sustained light-intensity activity may provide health benefits and promote weight control. Public health guidelines for physical activity have recommended that activities be at least moderate in intensity. However, evidence suggests that the accumulation of light intensity activity can have benefits, especially in those who are sedentary. Researchers at the Mayo Clinic, led by Dr. Jim Levine, have coined a term called *Non-Exercise Activity Thermogenesis (NEAT)* to refer to the substantial number of calories that can be burned by performing light-intensity activity.

Lifestyle activity builds some components of fitness more than others. Metabolic fitness is fitness of the systems that provide the energy for effective daily living. Indicators of good metabolic fitness include normal blood lipid levels, normal blood pressure, normal blood sugar levels, and healthy body fat levels. Though lifestyle physical activity does not promote high-level cardiovascular fitness, commonly referred to as a **performance benefit,** it effectively promotes metabolic fitness. The overall impact of lifestyle activity on individual fitness depends on a person's current level of fitness. Individuals with good levels of fitness will receive primarily metabolic benefits, but those with low fitness will likely receive metabolic and **cardiovascular fitness benefits.** Lifestyle activity is particularly important for the large segments of the population that do not participate in other forms of regular exercise. As previously described, some activity is clearly better than none.

Lifestyle physical activity has wellness benefits. Reduction in disease risk and early death are important. But equally important is quality of life. Many of the **wellness benefits** previously described result from moderate lifestyle physical activity. For example, people who do moderate exercise have been shown to take less time to go to sleep and sleep nearly an hour longer. One study showed that functional limitations are much lower in moderately active people than in those who are sedentary. Lifestyle activity is also associated with enhanced self-esteem and less incidence of depression and anxiety.

Table 3 ▶ The FIT Formula for Lifestyle Physical Activity

	Threshold of Training	Target Zone
Frequency	Most days of the week	All, or most, days of the week
Intensity [a]	• Equal to brisk walking[b] • Approximately 150 calories accumulated per day • 3 to 5 METs[b]	• Equal to brisk to fast walking[b] • Approximately 150–300 calories accumulated per day • 3.0 to 7 METs[b]
Time (duration)	30 minutes or three 10-minute sessions per day	30–60 minutes accumulated in sessions of at least 10 minutes

[a]Heart rate and relative perceived exertion can also be used to determine intensity (see Concept 7).

[b]Depends on fitness level (see Table 2).

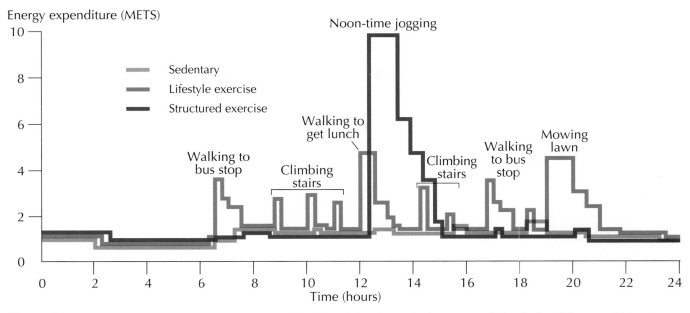

Figure 2 ▶ Comparison of structured exercise and lifestyle activity: theoretical patterns of physical activity over 24 hours.

Regular activity is important to achieving health, fitness, and wellness benefits. For the benefits of activity, especially lifestyle physical activity, to be optimal, it is important to exercise regularly. Daily, or nearly daily, lifestyle activity is recommended because each activity session has relatively short-term benefits that do not occur if the activity is not frequent enough. This is sometimes referred to as the **last bout effect.** Some aspects of metabolic fitness seem to be dependent on this last bout effect. For example, regular exercise provides an important stimulus that helps maintain insulin sensitivity and improves glucose regulation. Another example is the beneficial effect of exercise on stress management. In this case, the periodic stimulus from exercise helps directly counter the negative physical and physiological responses to stress. To maximize the benefits of physical activity, it is important to try to get some activity every day.

How Much Lifestyle Physical Activity Is Enough?

There is a FIT formula for lifestyle physical activity. The concept of a threshold of training is used in this book to describe the minimum activity needed for benefits. While there is no absolute threshold for lifestyle activity, public health guidelines endorsed by the ACSM and the CDC have recommended that adults try to accumulate at least 30 minutes of moderate-intensity activity each day. The recommendation of the surgeon general is similar but is expressed in terms of energy expenditure (about 1,000 kcal/day or about 150 kcal/day from moderate activity). The threshold levels for frequency, intensity, and time (duration) are summarized in Table 3. It is important to note that these are considered minimal, or threshold, levels. The target zone calls for the accumulation of up to 60 minutes or the expenditure of approximately 300 kcal/day.

Keeping track of accumulated minutes per day and per week is an easy way to monitor physical activity. Brisk walking is often used as an example of moderate intensity physical activity. Some people think that, because walking was used as an example, that is the only lifestyle activity that is recommended. Any activity equal in intensity to brisk walking can be used to meet the target of 30-60 minutes per day. Periodic monitoring of lifestyle activity can help ensure that you are obtaining a sufficient amount.

You can accumulate lifestyle physical activity to meet the recommendation. Previous recommendations suggested that physical activity had to be continuous to be effective. The evidence now indicates that all of the activity need not be done in one session to be effective. To achieve the health benefits, you can "accumulate activity" throughout the day. Figure 2 demonstrates the different

Performance Benefit An improved ability to score well on physical fitness tests or to perform well in athletic or work activities requiring high-level performance.

Cardiovascular Fitness Benefits Improvements in cardiovascular function that contribute to cardiovascular fitness.

Wellness Benefits Increases in quality of life and well-being.

Last Bout Effect Some of the benefits of physical activity are short-term.

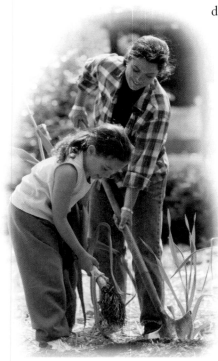

Gardening is a popular lifestyle activity among adults.

daily patterns of physical activity. The blue line reveals the pattern of a typical "exerciser" performing short bouts of vigorous activity, while the green line shows a lifestyle activity pattern. Note that both lines have a lot more daily activity than the low levels of activity for a sedentary individual. Although the bulk of the energy, or calories, expended should be in moderate activities, some light activity can also be beneficial. When some of the accumulated activity is in light activity, the duration of the activity should be increased to meet the guidelines for daily physical activity. Some lifestyle physical activities, such as shoveling snow or digging in the garden, may be considered vigorous. These activities can be counted in the accumulation of daily activities. Performing some of these activities can offset the performance of light activity and make it possible to expend adequate calories in a 30-minute period.

Tracking energy expenditure from physical activity can help in monitoring lifestyle physical activity. As shown in Table 3, an energy expenditure of between 150 and 300 kcal/day from physical activity is sufficient for meeting physical activity guidelines. While not as simple as tracking time, calories expended from physical activity can be estimated if the approximate MET value of the activity is known. The energy cost of resting energy expenditure (1 MET) is approximately 1 calorie per kilogram of body weight per hour (1 kcal/kg/hour). An activity such as walking (4 mph) requires an energy expenditure of about 4 METS, or 4 kcal/kg/hour. A 150 lb. person (~ 70 kg) walking for an hour would expend about 280 kcal (4 kcal/kg/hour × 70 kg × 1 hr.). Note that a 30-minute walk would burn approximately 150 calories and satisfy the guideline.

Energy expenditure estimates are often provided by many commercial pieces of fitness equipment. The work-load MET level is determined by the pace or heart rate and the time is usually tracked internally. If body weight is recorded by the device during the start-up process, it can estimate energy expenditure using the same algorithm. To assist in using energy expenditure estimates, a listing of calories expended in many activities is provided in Table 4. The table provides estimates for people of different weights performing exercise for an hour. Additional information about calculating energy expenditure from physical activity is available at Web05.

Many people use pedometers to monitor daily activity levels. Digital pedometers are a popular self-monitoring tool used to track physical activity patterns. They provide information about the number of steps a person takes. Stride length and weight can be entered into most pedometers to provide estimates of distance traveled and/or calories burned. Some newer pedometers include timers, which track the total amount of time spent moving; some allow step information to be stored over a series of days.

Pedometers provide a helpful reminder about the importance of being active during the day. They also are useful for tracking activity patterns over a series of days. The interest in and popularity of pedometers has resulted in media stories promoting the standard of 10,000 steps as the level of activity needed for good health. This standard was originally developed in Japan, where pedometers were popularized before gaining popularity elsewhere in the world. Experts have warned against using an absolute step count standard, such as 10,000 steps for all people. It will likely be too hard for some and not hard enough for others based on current activity patterns.

Studies on large numbers of people provide data to help classify people into activity categories based on step

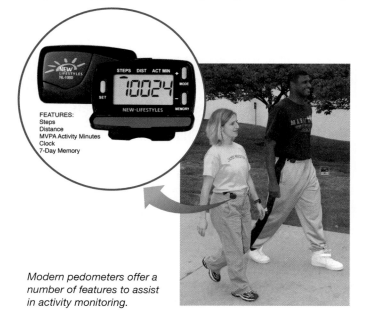

Modern pedometers offer a number of features to assist in activity monitoring.

Table 4 ► Calories Expended in Lifestyle Physical Activities

Activity Classification / Description	METs[a]	Calories Used per Hour for Different Body Weights					
		100 lb. (45 kg)	120 lb. (55 kg)	150 lb. (70 kg)	180 lb. (82 kg)	200 lb. (91 kg)	220 lb. (100 kg)
Gardening Activities							
Gardening (general)	5.0	227	273	341	409	455	502
Mowing lawn (hand mower)	6.0	273	327	409	491	545	599
Mowing lawn (power mower)	4.5	205	245	307	368	409	450
Raking leaves	4.0	182	218	273	327	364	401
Shoveling snow	6.0	273	327	409	491	545	599
Home Activities							
Child care	3.5	159	191	239	286	318	350
Cleaning, washing dishes	2.5	114	136	170	205	227	249
Cooking / food preparation	2.5	114	136	170	205	227	249
Home / auto repair	3.0	136	164	205	245	273	301
Painting	4.5	205	245	307	368	409	450
Strolling with child	2.5	114	136	170	205	227	249
Sweeping / vacuuming	2.5	114	136	170	205	227	249
Washing / waxing car	4.5	205	245	307	368	409	450
Leisure Activities							
Bocci ball / croquet	2.5	114	136	170	205	227	249
Bowling	3.0	136	164	205	245	273	301
Canoeing	5.0	227	273	341	409	455	501
Cross-country skiing (leisure)	7.0	318	382	477	573	636	699
Cycling (<10 mph)	4.0	182	218	273	327	364	401
Cycling (12–14 mph)	8.0	364	436	545	655	727	799
Dancing (social)	4.5	205	245	307	368	409	450
Fishing	4.0	182	218	273	327	364	401
Golf (riding)	3.5	159	191	239	286	318	350
Golf (walking)	5.5	250	300	375	450	500	550
Horseback riding	4.0	182	218	273	327	364	401
Swimming (leisure)	6.0	273	327	409	491	545	599
Table tennis	4.0	182	218	273	327	364	401
Walking (4 mph)	4.0	182	218	273	327	364	401
Walking (3 mph)	3.5	159	191	239	286	318	350
Occupational Activities							
Bricklaying / masonry	7.0	318	382	477	573	636	699
Carpentry	3.5	159	191	239	286	318	350
Construction	5.5	250	300	375	450	500	550
Electrical work / plumbing	3.5	159	191	239	286	318	350
Digging	7.0	318	382	477	573	636	699
Farming	5.5	250	300	375	450	500	550
Store clerk	3.5	159	191	239	286	318	350
Waiter / waitress	4.0	182	218	273	327	364	401

Note: MET values and caloric estimates are based on values listed in *The Compendium of Physical Activities* (see *Suggested Readings*).

[a]Based on values of those with "good fitness" ratings.

counts (see Table 5), but actual step goals should vary from individual to individual. The approach most frequently recommended is to first wear the pedometer for 1 week to establish a baseline step count (average steps per day). Once this has been done, setting a goal of increasing steps per day by 1,000 to 3,000 steps per day is recommended. Keeping records of daily step counts will help you determine if you are meeting your goal. Setting a goal that you are likely to meet will help you find success. As you meet your goal, you can increase your step counts gradually.

Pedometers do have some limitations as indicators of total physical activity. A person with longer legs will accumulate fewer steps over the same distance than someone with shorter strides (due to a longer stride length). A person running will also accumulate fewer steps over the same distance than a person who walks. There is considerable variability in the quality (and accuracy) of commercial pedometers, so it is important to consider this when purchasing one.

Lifestyle Activity and the Environment

The sedentary nature of our society is due in part to environmental factors. Many people would like to be more active but they may not live in an area conducive to activity. Studies have demonstrated that the extent of urban sprawl is associated with population levels of physical inactivity and obesity. Researchers have also determined that certain characteristics of an environment can make it more or less "walkable." Sidewalks, safe neighborhoods, aesthetic surroundings, and good lighting are considered to be among the key factors that define walkable areas. In Lab 6B you will evaluate the walkability of your community based on some of these characteristics.

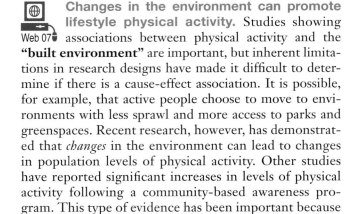

Changes in the environment can promote lifestyle physical activity. Studies showing associations between physical activity and the **"built environment"** are important, but inherent limitations in research designs have made it difficult to determine if there is a cause-effect association. It is possible, for example, that active people choose to move to environments with less sprawl and more access to parks and greenspaces. Recent research, however, has demonstrated that *changes* in the environment can lead to changes in population levels of physical activity. Other studies have reported significant increases in levels of physical activity following a community-based awareness program. This type of evidence has been important because it indicates that our environment does contribute to our physical activity patterns. The results also help justify expenses to make communities more walkable since, it has been shown to make a difference.

One organization called Active Living by Design (**www.activelivingbydesign.org**) is dedicated to promoting more active environments in society. The vision is for neighborhoods that allow physical activity to be built into a person's normal routine (going to the store, visiting friends) and communities with integrated biking paths and walking paths. These concepts are consistent with

Table 5 ▶ Activity Classification for Pedometer Step Counts in Healthy Adults		
Category		**Steps/Day**
Sedentary		< 5000
Low active		5,000–7,500
Somewhat active	Threshold	7,500–9,999
Active	Target Zone	10,000–12,500
Very active		> 12,500

Source: Based on values from Tudor-Locke.

Technology Update
Google Earth

Google Earth is an exciting new web technology that allows users to view real images from almost anywhere in the world simply by typing in an address or coordinates. The Google Earth Web site (**www.googleearth.com**) refers to it as a "3D interface to the planet." The system takes advantage of the network of satellites that orbit above earth to allow you to zoom in and out of different locations with the click of the mouse. Researchers have been using this type of technology for years, but the release of Google Earth has made it possible for anyone to access these images.

Researchers in the physical activity field use the somewhat related technologies of geodemographic information systems (GIS) and global positioning systems (GPS) to study physical activity. Researchers can accurately map cities and determine distances from residential areas to stores, parks, and greenspaces. Correlations are then made between these variables and measures of physical activity. New personal GPS monitors from Garmin, Inc. (**www.garmin.com**) directly interface with Google Earth, allowing you to see an image of your running route, bike trip, or other outdoor adventures. Visit **www.googleearth.com**.

other recommendations for urban planning (e.g., Smart Growth Movement). Additional information about environmental issues related to lifestyle activity can be found at Web07.

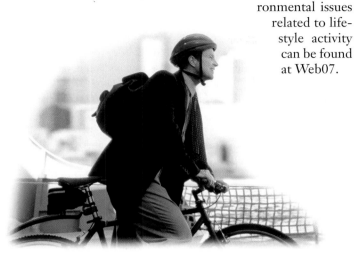

Bike commuting is an effective way to add physical activity to your day.

 Consider personal strategies for increasing lifestyle activity. While the environment has an impact on population levels of physical activity, it does not determine individual behavior. People are autonomous beings and can make decisions about where they go and what they do. The key is to take stock of your lifestyle and your environment and determine ways to integrate more activity into your daily routine. One activity that is often overlooked is commuting to work or school. In addition to providing beneficial amounts of physical activity, commuting can save time, gas, and money. The benefits to the individual, the environment and to society as a whole are significant. See Web08 for additional information about the benefits of active commuting.

Web 08

Built Environment A term used to describe aspects of our created physical environment (e.g., buildings, roads).

Strategies for Action

A regular plan of lifestyle physical activity is a good place to start. Lifestyle physical activity is something that virtually anyone can do. In Lab 6A, you can set lifestyle physical activity goals and plan a 1-week lifestyle physical activity program. In the plan, you can indicate the lifestyle activities you plan to do on all or most days of the week. For some, this plan may be the main component of a lifetime plan. For others, it may be only a beginning that leads to the selection of activities from other levels of the physical activity pyramid. Even the most active people should consider regular lifestyle physical activity because it is a type of activity that can be done throughout life.

Self-monitoring lifestyle physical activity can help you stick with it. Self-monitoring is a self-management skill that can be valuable in encouraging long-term activity adherence. A self-monitoring chart is provided in Lab 6A to help you keep a log of the lifestyle activities (or step counts) you perform during a 1-week time period. This is a short-term record sheet. However, charts such as this can be copied to make a log book to allow long-term activity self-monitoring.

Because environmental factors have an influence on our lifestyle physical activity patterns, it is important to become sensitive to different aspects of your environment. In Lab 6B, you will conduct an evaluation of the walkability of your community and an evaluation of community resources available for physical activity. The purpose of this lab is to increase your awareness of the importance of active environments for promoting physical activity. Becoming an advocate for physical activity in your community is a great way to help promote local change.

Online Learning Center

www.mhhe.com/corbin7e
The Online Learning Center contains a variety of Web-based resources that will help you get the most out of this book and your course. In addition to the On the Web pages, there are video activities, interactive quizzes, application assignments, and a variety of other useful study aids. Log on to the URL above to access these resources.

Web Resources

 America on the Move **www.americaonthemove.org**
American College of Sports Medicine **www.acsm.org**
Web 09 ACSM's Health and Fitness Journal
   www.acsm-healthfitness.org
Centers for Disease Control and Prevention **www.cdc.gov**
National Coalition for Promoting Physical Activity **www.ncppa.org**
National Sporting Good Manufacturers Association
   www.nsga.org

Suggested Readings

Web 10

Additional reference materials for Concept 6 are available on Web10.

Active Living Partners. 2006. *First Steps: Your Healthy Living Journal.* Champaign, IL: Human Kinetics.

Addy, C. L., et al. 2004. Associations of perceived social and physical environmental supports with physical activity and walking behavior. *American Journal of Public Health* 94(3):440–443.

Ainsworth, B. E. 2003. The compendium of physical activities. *President's Council on Physical Fitness and Sports Research Digest* 4(2):1–8.

American College of Sports Medicine. 2006. *ACSM's Guidelines for Exercise Testing and Prescription.* 7th ed. Philadelphia: Lippincott, Williams and Wilkins.

Brown, D. W., et al. 2004. Associations between physical activity dose and health-related quality of life. *Medicine and Science in Sports and Exercise* 36(5):890–896.

Brown, W. J., et al. 2006. 10,000 steps Rockhampton: Evaluation of whole community approach to improving population levels of physical activity. *Journal of Physical Activity and Health.* 3(1):1–14.

Dannenberg, A. C., et al. 2005. Assessing the walkability in the workplace: A new audit tool. *American Journal of Health Promotion* (5):39–44.

Ewing, R., et al. 2003. Relationship between urban sprawl and physical activity, obesity, and morbidity. *American Journal of Health Promotion* 18(1):47–57.

Eyler, A. A. 2004. The epidemiology of walking for physical activity in the United States. *Medicine and Science in Sports and Exercise* 35(9):1529–1536.

Frank, L. D., et al. 2005. Linking objectively measured physical activity with objectively measured urban form: Findings from SMARTRAQ. *American Journal of Preventive Medicine* 28(2 Suppl):117–125.

Hultquist, C. N. et al. 2005. Comparison of walking recommendations in previously inactive women. *Medicine and Science in Sport and Exercise* 37(4):676–683.

Humpel, N., et al., 2004. Changes in neighborhood walking are related to changes in perceptions of environmental attributes. *Annals of Behavioral Medicine* 27(1):60–67.

Le Masurier, G. C. 2004. Walk this way? *ACSM's Health and Fitness Journal* 8(1):7–10.

Moudon, A.V., et al. 2006. Operational definitions of walkable neighborhood: Theoretical and empirical insights. *Journal of Physical Activity and Health* 3(S1):S99–117.

Murtagh, E. M. et al., 2005. The effects of 60 minutes of brisk walking per week, accumulated in two different patterns, on cardiovascular risk. *Preventive Medicine* 41(1):92–97.

Peterson, J., et al. 2006. Differential effects of active living on quality of life at various levels of income. *Health Education Research* 21(1):146–56.

Sallis, J. F., et al. 2005. An ecological approach to creating active living communities. *Annual Review of Public Health.*

Tudor-Locke, C. 2002. Taking steps toward increased physical activity: Using the pedometer to measure and motivate. *President's Council on Physical Fitness and Sports Research Digest* 3(17):1–8.

Tudor-Locke, C. 2004. How many steps/day are enough? Preliminary pedometer indices for public health. *Sports Medicine* 34(1):1–8.

Tudor-Locke, C., et al. 2005. How many days of pedometer monitoring predict weekly physical activity in adults? *Preventive Medicine* 40(3):293–298.

Tullya, M. A., et al. 2005. Brisk walking, fitness, and cardiovascular risk: A randomized controlled trial in primary care. *Preventive Medicine* 41(2):622–628.

In the News

Large-Scale Physical Activity Promotions

A number of nonprofit agencies have taken major steps to help promote awareness of physical activity and good health. The America on the Move Foundation has received perhaps the biggest amount of national media coverage for its Web-based activity logging tool, which promotes self-monitoring of physical activity and diet (www.americaonthemove.org). The message of this promotion is simple: move more and eat less by making two small daily changes.

- Take 2000 more steps (about 1 mile).
- Eat 100 fewer calories (about a pat of butter).

Individuals can register online for free and track their activity on a Web-based interface.

Many communities across the United States have used the interface to create customized activity promotions for their local residents. One state-based program that has received a lot of recognition is the Lighten Up Iowa program (www.lightenupiowa.org). This promotion uses a team-based approach that allows individuals to work together to maintain active lifestyles for the 5 month promotion. These are just a few of the exciting community-based initiatives that are helping people lead more active lifestyles

Lab 6A   Planning and Self-Monitoring (Logging) Your Lifestyle Physical Activity

Name	Section	Date

Purpose: To self-monitor (log) physical activity and use it to plan a lifestyle physical activity program

Directions: Record the number of 5- or 10-minute activity blocks or steps taken each day (see back for procedures).

Chart 1 ▶ Lifestyle Activity Log

		5-Minute Blocks										10-Minute Blocks						Total Minutes or Steps
		1	2	3	4	5	6	7	8	9	10	1	2	3	4	5	6	
Day 1 Date:	Activity: Activity: Activity: Activity:																	Daily Total
Day 2 Date:	Activity: Activity: Activity: Activity:																	Daily Total
Day 3 Date:	Activity: Activity: Activity: Activity:																	Daily Total
Day 4 Date:	Activity: Activity: Activity: Activity:																	Daily Total
Day 5 Date:	Activity: Activity: Activity: Activity:																	Daily Total
Day 6 Date:	Activity: Activity: Activity: Activity:																	Daily Total
Day 7 Date:	Activity: Activity: Activity: Activity:																	Daily Total

Total Minutes or Steps for Week

Procedures

1. On Chart 1, record the time spent or steps taken per day in the various lifestyle activities.
2. If you record time spent in lifestyle activity, list all activities you perform each day. For each activity, record the number of minutes that you were active using combinations of 5- or 10-minute blocks. For example, if you perform 15 minutes of brisk walking, place an X over one 5- and one 10-minute block for that activity. If you cannot keep the log with you during the day, complete it at the end of the day. Total the minutes of activity accumulated during the day and record it in the Daily Total Box.
3. If you wear a pedometer to count daily activity, simply wear the pedometer from the time you get up in the morning until the time you go to bed. Record the number of steps taken in the Daily Total Box.
4. Sum the total for each day to determine the total minutes or steps taken for that week.
5. Use the weekly log to help you develop a weekly plan. In Chart 2, record the number of minutes you plan to perform each activity in the coming week, or record the number of steps you plan to take. If you use minutes in your plan, try to reach 30 per day. If you use step counts in your plan, try to achieve 2,000–3,000 steps above your daily count (if you averaged less than 10,000 steps a day in Chart 1), or at least 10,000 steps per day (if you averaged near or above 10,000 steps per day in Chart 1). Try to get your steps in blocks of time lasting at least 5 minutes.
6. Make a copy of Chart 1 and use it to self-monitor your activity for the week that you institute your plan.
7. Answer the questions in the Results and Conclusions and Interpretations sections.

Chart 2 ▶ Lifestyle Physical Activity Plan

Record the minutes or steps planned for each day. You may mix activities each day.

Activity	Day 1	Day 2	Day 3	Day 4	Day 5	Day 6	Day 7
Brisk walking							
Yard work/gardening							
Active housework							
Social dancing							
Occupational activity							
Wheeling self in wheelchair							
Bicycling							
Walking up and down stairs							
Other							
Other							
Other							
Daily Totals							

Results

Do you think you can consistently do 30 minutes of activity or meet your step goal each day?   (Yes)   (No)

Conclusions and Interpretations

1. Do you feel that you will use lifestyle physical activity as a regular part of your lifetime physical activity plan, either now or in the future? Use several sentences to explain your answer.
2. Did the logging of your activity make you more aware of your daily activity patterns? Explain why or why not.

Lab 6B   Evaluating Physical Activity Environments

Name	Section	Date

Purpose: To help you assess community factors that may influence your ability to perform lifestyle physical activity

Procedures

1. Use the community audit forms on the back page to conduct an evaluation of the walkability of your community and the availability of community resources for physical activity. The walkability audit requires that you take a brief walk in your neighborhood to note key features in the environment that may help or hinder walking. The community audit will require you to evaluate the quality of resources and programming available in your community. You can choose your campus community or your hometown.
2. For each question, first use the check boxes to note the presence or absence of key features in the environment. Then base your score for this question on the number of checks and your overall perception.
3. After you have completed both the Walkability Audit and the Community Resource Audit, total the scores for each tool and report the total scores in the bottom. Add up both scores to compute the Combined (physical activity) Environmental Audit.

Results: Record your rating for each of three healthy lifestyles in the following chart.

Environmental Activity Scoring Chart	Score	Rating
Walkability Audit		
Community Resource Audit		
Combined Environmental Audit		

Rating Chart for Environmental Audits	Good	Marginal	Poor
Walkability	16–20	12–15	<12
Community	16–20	12–15	<12
Combined	32–40	24–30	<24

Conclusions and Implications

Provide a brief summary of the physical activity environment in your community. Describe your experiences in evaluating the walkability of and resources in your community. If the environment is close to ideal, comment on how this may facilitate active lifestyles. If the environment is not ideal, comment on what needs to be done to improve it.

Comments on Walkability Audit

Comments on Community Resource Audit

Walkability and Community Resource Audits

Directions. Place a check by each box in each questionnaire. Based on the number of boxes checked for each question, place an X over the circle to rate each question (1=poor, 2=marginal, 3=good, 4=very good). Add rating numbers to get walkability scores and community resource scores. Total the two to get a combined environmental score.

Walkability Audit — Rating

1. Did you have room to walk? ① ② ③ ④
   - [ ] Sidewalks blocked or not continuous
   - [ ] Sidewalks were broken, cracked
   - [ ] No sidewalks, paths, or shoulders
   - [ ] Too much traffic on sidewalk
   - [ ] Other _____

2. Was it easy to cross streets? ① ② ③ ④
   - [ ] Road was too wide
   - [ ] Traffic signals were too short/too long
   - [ ] Parked cars blocked view of street
   - [ ] No striped or designated crosswalks
   - [ ] Other _____

3. Was it safe for walking? ① ② ③ ④
   - [ ] Too much traffic
   - [ ] Drivers too fast / too close
   - [ ] Inadequate lighting
   - [ ] Area of high crime
   - [ ] Other _____

4. Were there places to go? ① ② ③ ④
   - [ ] No stores in the area
   - [ ] No restaurants in the area
   - [ ] No friends nearby
   - [ ] Nothing interesting to see in area
   - [ ] Other _____

5. Was your walk pleasant? ① ② ③ ④
   - [ ] Not enough grass and trees
   - [ ] Scary dogs or people
   - [ ] Not well lighted
   - [ ] Too dirty
   - [ ] Other _____

Community Resource Audit — Rating

6. Are there walking/biking paths in the area? ① ② ③ ④
   - [ ] Paths are in unsafe areas
   - [ ] Paths need to be repaired
   - [ ] Paths are too crowded
   - [ ] Paths are too far away to be useful
   - [ ] Other _____

7. Is there a community fitness/rec center? ① ② ③ ④
   - [ ] Center is too expensive
   - [ ] Center is not clean or updated
   - [ ] Center is too far away
   - [ ] Center has old or limited equipment
   - [ ] Other _____

8. Are there bicycle lanes on streets? ① ② ③ ④
   - [ ] Lines not painted well
   - [ ] Lines not on all streets
   - [ ] Bike lanes not wide enough
   - [ ] Cars too close
   - [ ] Other _____

9. Are there parks, fields, and playgrounds? ① ② ③ ④
   - [ ] Parks in unsafe areas
   - [ ] Equipment/resources in poor repair
   - [ ] Too crowded
   - [ ] Too far away
   - [ ] Other _____

10. Are there community activity programs? ① ② ③ ④
    - [ ] Not enough programs
    - [ ] Not the right type of programs
    - [ ] Too expensive
    - [ ] Too far / inconvenient
    - [ ] Other _____

Total Score for Walkability Audit: [____] (Sum of Questions 1–5)

Total Score for Community Resources Audit: [____] (Sum of Questions 6–10)

Combined Environmental Audit: [____] (Sum of Questions 1–10)

Walkability checklist adapted from resources developed by the Partnership for a Walkable America. For information on this organization, visit this Web site: **www.walkableamerica.org**.

Cardiovascular Fitness

Health Goals for the year 2010

- Increase proportion of people who do vigorous physical activity that promotes cardiovascular fitness 3 or more days a week for 20 minutes per occasion.

- Decrease deaths from heart attack and stroke.

- Decrease incidence of heart attack, high blood pressure, stroke, and high blood lipids.

- Decrease heart disease among females.

- Increase public awareness of symptoms of heart disease.

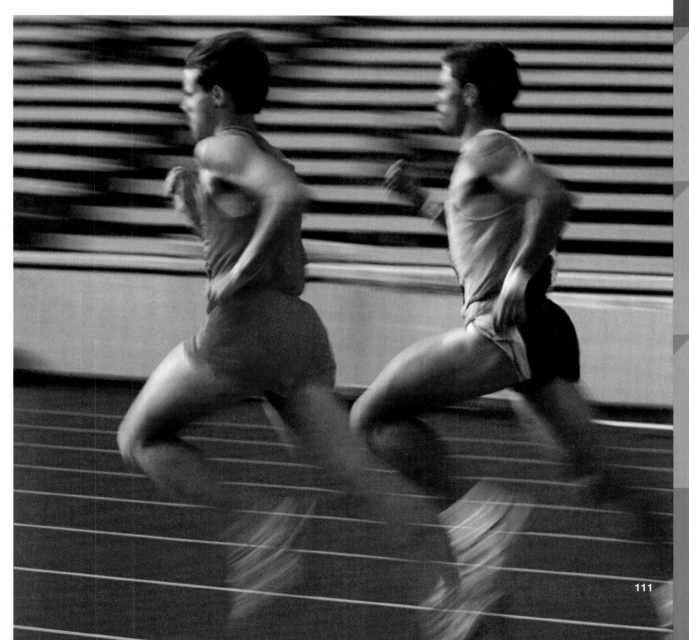

Cardiovascular fitness is probably the most important aspect of physical fitness because of its importance to good health and optimal physical performance.

Cardiovascular fitness is generally considered to be the most important aspect of physical fitness. Those who possess reasonable amounts of fitness have a decreased risk for heart disease, reduced risk for premature death, and improved quality of life. Regular cardiovascular exercise promotes fitness and provides additional health and wellness benefits that extend well beyond reducing risks for disease. This concept will describe the function of the cardiovascular system and explain how to determine the appropriate intensity of exercise needed to promote cardiovascular fitness.

Cardiovascular Fitness

Cardiovascular fitness is a term that has several synonyms. Cardiovascular fitness is sometimes referred to as *cardiovascular endurance* because a person who possesses this type of fitness can persist in physical activity for long periods of time without undue fatigue. It has been referred to as *cardiorespiratory fitness* because it requires delivery and utilization of oxygen, which is only possible if the circulatory and respiratory systems are capable of these functions.

The term *aerobic fitness* has also been used as a synonym for *cardiovascular fitness* because **aerobic capacity** is considered to be the best indicator of cardiovascular fitness, and aerobic physical activity is the preferred method for achieving it. Regardless of the words used to describe it, cardiovascular fitness is complex because it requires fitness of several body systems.

Good cardiovascular fitness requires a fit heart muscle. The heart is a powerful muscle that pumps blood through the body. The heart of a normal individual beats reflexively about 40 million times a year. In a single

day, the heart pumps over 4,000 gallons of blood through the body. To keep the cardiovascular system working effectively, it is crucial to have a strong and fit heart.

Like other muscles in the body, the heart becomes stronger if it is exercised. With regular exercise, the size and strength of the heart increase and it can pump more blood with each beat. This allows the heart to accomplish the same amount of work with fewer beats. Typical resting heart rate (RHR) values are around 70–80 beats per minute, but a highly trained endurance athlete may have a resting heart rate in the 40s or 50s. There is some individual variability in RHR, but a decrease in your RHR with training indicates clear improvements in cardiovascular fitness.

Good cardiovascular fitness requires a fit vascular system. The heart has four chambers, which pump and receive blood in a rhythmical fashion to maintain good circulation (see Figure 1). Blood containing a high concentration of oxygen is pumped by the left ventricle through the aorta (a major artery), where it is carried to the tissues. Blood flows through a sequence of arteries to capillaries and to veins. Veins carry the blood containing lesser amounts of oxygen back to the right side of the heart, first to the atrium and then to the ventricle. The right ventricle pumps the blood to the lungs. In the lungs, the blood picks up oxygen (O_2), and carbon dioxide (CO_2) is removed. From the lungs, the oxygenated blood travels back to the heart, first to the left atrium and then to the left ventricle. The process then repeats itself. A dense network of arteries distributes the oxygenated blood to the muscles, tissues, and organs (see Figure 2).

Healthy arteries are elastic, are free of obstruction, and expand to permit the flow of blood. Muscle layers line the arteries and control the size of the arterial opening upon the impulse from nerve fibers. Unfit arteries may have a reduced internal diameter (atherosclerosis) because of deposits on the interior of their walls, or they may have hardened, nonelastic walls (arteriosclerosis).

Fit coronary arteries are especially important to good health. The blood in the four chambers of the heart does not directly nourish the heart. Rather, numerous small arteries within the heart muscle provide for coronary circulation. Poor coronary circulation precipitated by unhealthy arteries can be the cause of a heart attack.

Deoxygenated blood flows back to the heart through a series of veins (see Figure 2d). The veins are intertwined

On the Web
www.mhhe.com/corbinweb

Web 01 Log on to this URL before reading this concept. See On the Web list of concepts. Click on the concept number you want to view. To access supplemental information, click on the number shown at each Web icon.

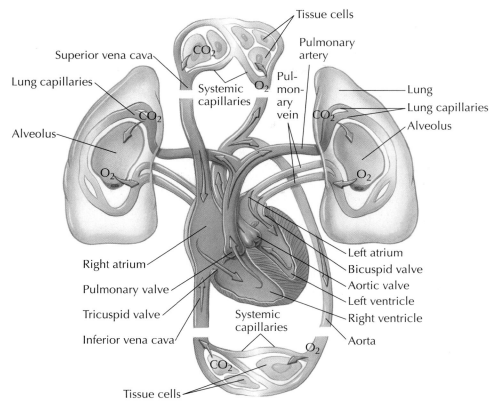

Figure 1 ▶ Cardiovascular system.

in the skeletal muscle and this allows normal muscle action to facilitate the return of blood to the heart. When a muscle is contracted, the vein is squeezed and this pushes the blood back to the heart. Small valves in the veins prevent the backward flow of the blood, but defects in the valves can lead to pooling of blood in the veins. A common condition, known as varicose veins, is associated with the pooling of blood in the leg. Regular physical activity helps reduce pooling of blood in the veins and helps keep the valves of the veins healthy.

Capillaries are the transfer stations where oxygen and fuel are released, and waste products, such as carbon dioxide, are removed from the tissues. The veins receive the blood from the capillaries for the return trip to the heart.

Good cardiovascular fitness requires a fit respiratory system and fit blood. The process of taking in oxygen (through the mouth and nose) and delivering it to the lungs, where it is picked up by the blood, is called external respiration (see Figure 2b). External respiration requires fit lungs as well as blood with adequate **hemoglobin** in the red blood cells (erythrocytes). Insufficient oxygen-carrying capacity of the blood is called **anemia,** a condition caused by lack of hemoglobin.

Delivering oxygen to the tissues from the blood is called internal respiration. Internal respiration requires

an adequate number of healthy capillaries. In addition to delivering oxygen to the tissues, these systems remove carbon dioxide. Good cardiovascular fitness requires fitness of both the external and internal respiratory systems.

Cardiovascular fitness requires fit muscle tissue capable of using oxygen. Once the oxygen is delivered, the muscle tissues must be able to use oxygen to sustain physical performance (see Figure 2e). Physical activity that promotes cardiovascular fitness stimulates changes in muscle fibers that make them more effective in using oxygen. Outstanding distance runners have high numbers of well-conditioned muscle fibers that can readily use oxygen to produce energy for sustained running. Training in other activities would elicit similar adaptations in the specific muscles used in those activities.

Aerobic Capacity A measure of aerobic or cardiovascular fitness.

Hemoglobin The oxygen-carrying pigment of red blood cells.

Anemia A condition in which hemoglobin and the blood's oxygen-carrying capacity is below normal.

Major Blood Vessels   Cardiovascular Fitness Characteristics

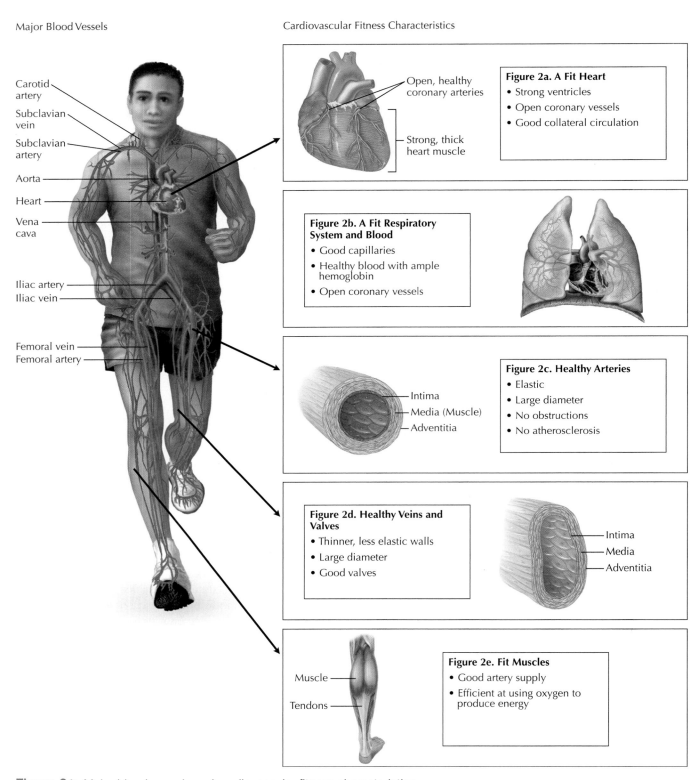

Carotid artery

Subclavian vein

Subclavian artery

Aorta

Heart

Vena cava

Iliac artery
Iliac vein

Femoral vein
Femoral artery

Open, healthy coronary arteries

Strong, thick heart muscle

Figure 2a. A Fit Heart
• Strong ventricles
• Open coronary vessels
• Good collateral circulation

Figure 2b. A Fit Respiratory System and Blood
• Good capillaries
• Healthy blood with ample hemoglobin
• Open coronary vessels

Intima
Media (Muscle)
Adventitia

Figure 2c. Healthy Arteries
• Elastic
• Large diameter
• No obstructions
• No atherosclerosis

Figure 2d. Healthy Veins and Valves
• Thinner, less elastic walls
• Large diameter
• Good valves

Intima
Media
Adventitia

Muscle

Tendons

Figure 2e. Fit Muscles
• Good artery supply
• Efficient at using oxygen to produce energy

Figure 2 ▶ Major blood vessels and cardiovascular fitness characteristics.

The performance and function of the cardiovascular system is maximized during exercise. During exercise, a number of changes occur to increase the availability of oxygen to the muscles (see Table 1). Breathing rate and heart rate increase allowing the body to take in more oxygen and distribute it more quickly. Activation of the sympathetic nervous system leads to a redistribution of the blood flow, so that more of it gets shunted to the working skeletal muscle. During rest, the muscles get about 20 percent of the available blood flow but this increases to about 70 percent during vigorous exercise. Within the muscles, a larger percentage of the available oxygen is also extracted from the muscles during exercise. Collectively, these changes help provide the muscles with the oxygen needed to maintain aerobic metabolism (see Web01 for more details).

Web 01

Cardiovascular fitness is typically evaluated using an indicator known as maximum oxygen uptake, or $\dot{V}O_2$ max. A person's **maximum oxygen uptake ($\dot{V}O_2$ max),** commonly referred to as aerobic capacity, is determined in a laboratory by measuring how much oxygen a person can use in maximal exercise. The test is usually done on a treadmill using specialized gas analyzers to measure oxygen use. The treadmill speed and grade are gradually increased and, when the exercise becomes very hard, oxygen use reaches

Web 02

its maximum. The test is a good indicator of overall cardiovascular fitness because you cannot take in and use a lot of oxygen if you do not have good fitness throughout the cardiovascular system (heart, blood vessels, blood, respiratory system, and muscles).

Elite endurance athletes can extract 5 or 6 liters of oxygen per minute from the environment, and this high aerobic capacity is what allows them to maintain high speeds in both training and competition without becoming excessively tired. In comparison, an average person typically extracts about 2 to 3 liters per minute. $\dot{V}O_2$ max is typically adjusted to account for a person's body size because bigger people may have higher scores due to their larger size. Scores are reported in milliliters (mL) of oxygen (O_2) per kilogram (kg) of body weight per minute (mL/kg/min.).

A number of field tests have been developed to provide good estimates of maximum aerobic capacity (see *Lab Resource Materials*). These tests are developed and validated based on comparisons with laboratory protocols that directly measure the amount of oxygen that is consumed. (for details, see Web02).

Cardiovascular Fitness and Health Benefits

Good cardiovascular fitness reduces risk for heart disease, other hypokinetic conditions, and early death. Numerous studies over the past 30–40 years have confirmed that good cardiovascular fitness is associated with a reduced risk for heart disease and a number of other chronic, hypokinetic conditions (see Figure 3). Recent studies employing better designs and improved measurement techniques have further strengthened the evidence—particularly with regard to effects of fitness on risks of diabetes. One recent report demonstrated that individuals classified in the least fit category were 3–6 times more likely to develop symptoms of metabolic syndrome or diabetes over a 15 year period than the most fit group. Clearly having at least a basic level of cardiovascular fitness (i.e., not being in the low fitness category) is important to disease prevention.

Web 03

In terms of longevity, one report indicated that moderately fit individuals live approximately 5–6 years longer than low-fit individuals. Moving from the moderate fit

Table 1 ▶ Changes in Cardiovascular Function between Rest and Exercise for a Person with Good Cardiovascular Fitness

		Rest	Maximal Exercise
Lungs	Breathing Rate (# / Minute)	12	30
Heart	Heart Rate (Beats / Minute)	70	190–200
	Stroke Volume (mL / Beat)	75	150
	Cardiac Output[a] (L / Minute)	5.2	28.5
Arteries	Blood Flow Distribution (%)	20%	70%
Muscle	Oxygen Extraction (%)	5%	20%
	VO₂ (mL/kg/min.)[b]	3.5	60

[a]Cardiac output (CO) = heart rate x stroke volume.
[b]$\dot{V}O_2$ = oxygen consumption = CO x avO2 difference.

Maximum Oxygen Uptake ($\dot{V}O_2$ max) A laboratory measure held to be the best measure of cardiovascular fitness. Commonly referred to as $\dot{V}O_2$ max or the volume ($\dot{V}$) of oxygen used when a person reaches his or her maximum (max) ability to supply it during exercise.

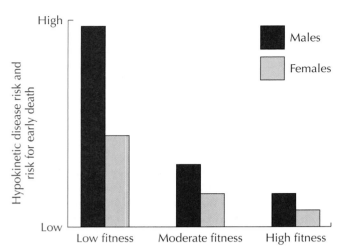

Figure 3 ▶ Risk reduction associated with cardiovascular fitness. Adapted from Blair et al.

to the high fit category provides additional benefits (and perhaps a few more years of life) but the key is to be out of the low fitness category. (See Web03 for more details on this type of research.)

The risk for low cardiovascular fitness is independent of other risk factors. Physical activity has been shown to have beneficial effects on some other established heart disease risk factors, such as cholesterol, blood pressure, and body fat. It is important to note that the beneficial effects of cardiovascular fitness on risk for heart disease and early death are considered to be independent of these other effects. This means that active/fit people would still have lower health risks even if their cholesterol, blood pressure, and body fat levels were identical to a matched set of inactive/unfit people. This evidence contributed to the labeling of physical inactivity as a major, independent risk factor for heart disease. The risk associated with physical inactivity is as large as (or larger than) risks associated with any of the other established risk factors.

Good fitness provides protection against the health risks associated with obesity. Some people think that they cannot be fit if they are overweight or overfat. It is now known that appropriate physical activity can build cardiovascular fitness in all types of people, including those with excess body fat. In fact, having good cardiovascular fitness greatly reduces risk for those who are overweight. Poor cardiovascular fitness, on the other hand, increases risk for both lean and overfat people. The greatest risk is among people who are unfit and overfat.

Recent studies have helped explain how physical activity protects against risks from overweight/obesity. Individuals with higher levels of activity (and/or higher

levels of fitness) have been shown to have lower levels of abdominal body fatness, even after correcting for differences in body mass index. In other words, individuals can be about the same size (i.e., similar weight for a given height) but active/fit individuals tend to have lower levels of abdominal body fat. The beneficial effects of physical activity are due, in part, to the ability of physical activity to help reduce levels of abdominal body fat. (See Web04 for more information.)

Good cardiovascular fitness enhances the ability to perform various tasks, improves the ability to function, and is associated with a feeling of well-being. Moving out of the low fitness zone is of obvious importance to disease risk reduction. Achieving the good zone on tests further reduces disease and early death risk and promotes optimal wellness benefits, and a position statement by the American College of Sports Medicine shows an improved ability to function among older adults. Other wellness benefits include the ability to enjoy leisure activities and meet emergency situations, as well as the health and wellness benefits described earlier in this book. Cardiovascular fitness in the high performance zone enhances the ability to perform in certain athletic events and in occupations that require high performance level (e.g., firefighters).

Heredity influences your cardiovascular fitness. It would be nice if all people who did appropriate physical activity achieved high levels of cardiovascular fitness. Genetic researchers have shown that the type of cardiovascular system you inherit has a good deal to do with your cardiovascular fitness. Research has also shown that heredity can influence the rate and extent of adaptations that occur from training.

You should not conclude from this information, however, that achieving good cardiovascular fitness is impossible for some people. Rather, you should understand that it is harder for some people to get fit than it is for others. With regular physical activity in the target zone virtually anyone can improve cardiovascular fitness.

Threshold and Target Zones for Improving Cardiovascular Fitness

Aerobic physical activity that is more vigorous than lifestyle physical activities is necessary to produce optimal gains in cardiovascular fitness. Activities at the second level of the physical activity pyramid, including active aerobics and active sports and recreation, are recommended for promoting good cardiovascular fitness (see Figure 4). The word *active* implies that these activities are more vigorous than lower-intensity activities from the lifestyle category. All physical activity can contribute to good health, but vigorous activity can also strengthen the cardiovascular system.

Cardiovascular fitness can be developed by exercising 3 to 6 days per week. Unlike less intense lifestyle physical activities, the types of activities that promote cardiovascular fitness may be done as few as 3 days a week. Additional benefits occur with added days of activity. However, because more vigorous physical activity has been shown to increase risk for orthopedic injury if done too frequently, most experts recommend at least 1 day a week off.

Various methods can be used to determine the appropriate intensity of aerobic activity. Like all dimensions of fitness, adaptations to cardiovascular fitness are based on the overload principle. When the body is regularly challenged, it essentially adapts to make the same amount of exercise easier on itself. Because individuals vary in their level of fitness, the appropriate intensity of exercise needed to maintain or improve fitness also varies. The relative intensity of a given bout of exercise can be directly determined if you have a measure of your **oxygen uptake reserve (VO₂R)** and the actual oxygen cost of a given activity. You would simply calculate what percentage of oxygen consumption the task requires, compared with your maximal capacity. Because these values cannot be calculated without special equipment, other indicators of relative intensity are more commonly used.

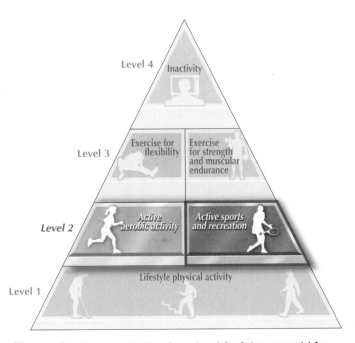

Figure 4 ▶ Select activities from level 2 of the pyramid for optimal cardiovascular fitness.

Heart rate provides a good indicator of the relative challenge presented by a given bout of exercise. Therefore, guidelines for the intensity of physical activity to build cardiovascular fitness are typically based on percentages of **heart rate reserve (HRR)** or maximal heart rate (max HR). Current guidelines from the ACSM indicate that exercise should be between 40 and 85 percent of your HRR or from 55 to 90 percent of your max HR to maintain or improve cardiovascular fitness. A fit individual will be able to work harder at a given heart rate, but the relative intensity of exercise will be equivalent for fit and unfit individuals using these types of ranges. Calculations of these ratings will be described in detail later.

Ratings of perceived exertion (RPE) have also been shown to be useful in assessing the intensity of aerobic physical activity. The RPE rating scale ranges from 6 (very very light) to 20 (very very hard), with 1 point increments in between. If the values are multiplied by 10, the RPE values loosely correspond to HR values (e.g., 60 = rest HR and 200 = max HR). The target zone for aerobic activity is from 12 to 16 (see Table 2).

The duration of physical activity for building cardiovascular fitness is 20 to 60 minutes. In the past, it was thought that the 20 to 60 minutes of active aerobic activity necessary to promote cardiovascular fitness should be done continuously in one session. Recent ACSM guidelines indicate that activity can be either intermittent or continuous if the total amount of exercise is the same and if the shorter sessions last at least 10 minutes. In other words, three 10-minute exercise sessions appear to give you the same benefit as one 30-minute session if the exercise is at the same intensity level.

There is a FIT formula for building cardiovascular fitness. Table 2 illustrates the threshold of training and target zones for performing physical activity designed to promote cardiovascular fitness.

Your current fitness level determines the appropriate type and amount of physical activity for your program. Adaptations to physical activity are based on

Oxygen Uptake Reserve (VO₂R) The difference between maximum oxygen uptake and resting oxygen uptake. A percentage of this value is often used to determine appropriate intensities for physical activities.

Heart Rate Reserve (HRR) The difference between maximum heart rate (highest heart rate in vigorous activity) and resting heart rate (lowest heart rate at rest).

Ratings of Perceived Exertion (RPE) The assessment of the intensity of exercise based on how the participant feels; a subjective assessment of effort.

Table 2 ▶ Threshold of Training and Target Zones for Activities Designed to Promote Cardiovascular Fitness[a]

	Threshold of Training	Target Zone
Frequency	3 days a week	At least 3 days and no more than 6 days a week
Intensity		
Heart rate reserve (HRR)	40%[a]	40–85%
Maximal heart rate (maxHR)	55%[a]	55–90%
Relative perceived exertion (RPE)	12[a]	12–16
Time	20 minutes	20–60 minutes

[a]These values are for beginners—the threshold for fit individuals reaches higher into the target zone.

ness improvements for fit and active people are best when activity is at least 50 percent HRR, 65 percent max HR, and 13 RPE. Your current fitness and activity status will affect how quickly you progress. The type of activity you choose should be appropriate for the intensity of activity at each stage of the progression.

Learning to count heart rate can help you monitor the intensity of your physical activity. To determine the intensity of physical activity for building cardiovascular fitness, it is important to know how to count your pulse. Each time the heart beats, it pumps blood into the arteries. The surge of blood causes a pulse, which can be felt by holding a finger against an artery. The major arteries that are easy to locate and are frequently used for pulse counts are the radial just below the base of the thumb on the wrist (see Figure 5) and the carotid on either side of the Adam's apple (see Figure 6). Counting the pulse at the carotid is the most popular procedure, probably because the carotid pulse is easy to locate. The radial pulse is a bit harder to find because of the many tendons near the wrist, but it works better for some people.

To count the pulse rate, simply place the fingertips (index and middle finger) over the artery at the wrist or neck location. Move the fingers around until a strong pulse can be felt. Press gently so as not to cut off the blood flow through the artery. Counting the pulse with the thumb is *not* recommended because the thumb has a relatively strong pulse of its own, and it could be confusing when counting another person's pulse.

the overload principle and the principle of progression. It is important to provide an appropriate challenge to your cardiovascular system (overload), but it is important to also progress gradually (progression). The amount of activity performed by a beginner differs from that performed by a person who is more advanced.

Beginners with low fitness may choose to start with lifestyle physical activity of relatively moderate intensity. Performing this type of activity at about 40 percent of HRR or an RPE of 12 (rated as somewhat hard) for several weeks will allow the beginner to adapt gradually. Initial bouts of activity may be less than the recommended 20 minutes, but as fitness increases, at least 20 minutes a day should be accumulated. As fitness improves from the low to marginal range, the frequency, intensity, and time of activity can be increased (see Table 3). Cardiovascular fit-

Counting heart rates during exercise presents some additional challenges. To obtain accurate exercise heart rate values, it is best to count heart beats or pulses while moving; however, this is difficult during most activities.

The most practical method is to count the pulse immediately after exercise. During physical activity, the heart rate increases, but immediately after exercise, it begins

Table 3 ▶ Progression of Activity Frequency, Intensity, and Time Based on Fitness Level

	Low Fitness	Marginal Fitness	Good Fitness
Frequency	3 days a week	3 to 5 days a week	3 to 6 days a week
Intensity			
Heart rate reserve (HRR)	40–50%	50–60%	60–85%
Maximum heart rate (maxHR)	55–65%	65–75%	75–90%
Relative perceived exertion (RPE)	12–13	13–14	14–16
Time	10–30 min	20–40 min	30–60 min

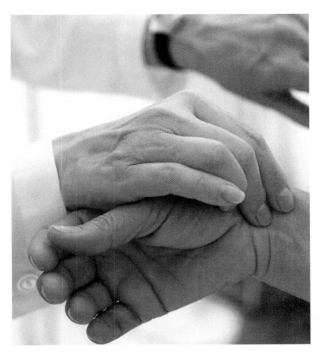

Figure 5 ► Counting your radial (wrist) pulse.

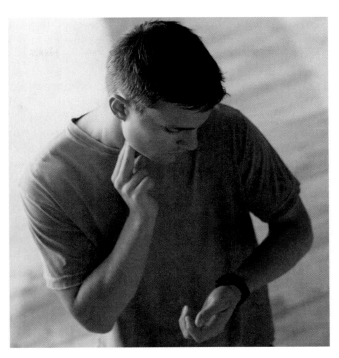

Figure 6 ► Counting your carotid (neck) pulse.

to slow and return to normal. In fact, the heart rate has already slowed considerably within 1 minute after activity ceases. Therefore, it is important to locate the pulse quickly and to count the rate for a short period of time in order to obtain accurate results. For best results, keep moving while quickly locating the pulse; then stop and take a 15-second count. Multiply the number of pulses by 4 to convert heart rate to beats per minute.

You can also count the pulse for 10 seconds and multiply by 6, or count the pulse for 6 seconds and multiply by 10 to estimate a 1-minute heart rate. The latter method allows you to calculate heart rates easily by adding 0 to the 6-second count. However, short-duration pulse counts increase the chance of error because a miscount of 1 beat is multiplied by 6 or 10 beats rather than by 4 beats.

The pulse rate should be counted after regular activity, not after a sudden burst. Some runners sprint the last few yards of their daily run and then count their pulse. Such a burst of exercise will elevate the heart rate considerably. This gives a false picture of the actual exercise heart rate. It would be wise for every person to learn to determine resting heart rate accurately and to estimate exercise heart rate by quickly and accurately making pulse counts after activity (see Lab 7A).

A person's maximal heart rate can be estimated reasonably with formulas. Calculations of threshold and target zone heart rates require an estimate of your maximal heart rate (maxHR). Your maxHR is the highest heart rate attained in maximal exercise. It could be determined using an electrocardiogram while exercising to exhaustion; however, for most people it is easier to estimate by using a formula. Until recently, a simple formula has been used ($220 - \text{age} = \text{maxHR}$). Although this formula gives a general estimate, recent research has found that it tends to overpredict for young people (20 to 40) and underpredict for those over 40. Based on the extensive research involving a review of hundreds of past studies and new laboratory research, a new formula is now recommended: $\text{maxHR} = 208 - (.7 \times \text{age})$. The formula has been shown to be useful for both sexes and for people of all activity levels. Table 4 illustrates the calculation of maxHR for a 22-year-old using the new formula. The 193 (rounded up from 192.6) heart rate for the 22-year-old example is five beats lower than if the old formula had been used.

The new formula is especially beneficial to older adults. Because the previous formula underpredicted

Table 4 ► Calculating Maximal Heart Rate (maxHR)

$$\text{age} = 22$$
$$\text{maxHR} = 208 - (.7 \times 22)$$
$$= 208 - 15.4$$
$$= 192.6 \approx 193$$

maxHR, it also underestimated the true level of physical stress during a treadmill test and underestimated target heart rate values for older adults.

Two methods can be used to determine threshold and target zone heart rates. The procedures used in determining target heart rates vary in complexity and accuracy. The preferred method, known as the percent of heart rate reserve method (often referred to as the Karvonnen method), involves calculating a percentage of your HRR. This method is considered more accurate because it takes into account your individual resting heart rate (an indicator of fitness) in making the calculations. A simpler procedure, known as the percent of maximal heart rate method, is easier to calculate but less personalized. The two methods of determining threshold and target zone heart rates are compared in Table 5 and are described in the following sections. You can also use Chart 8 in the *Lab*

Resource Materials to determine your threshold and target heart rates using your resting heart rate and your age.

Percent of Heart Rate Reserve (HRR) Method

To calculate your HRR, you must know your resting heart rate in addition to your maxHR. Resting heart rate is easily determined by counting the pulse for 1 minute while sitting or lying down. Ideally, this should be done early in the morning when you are rested, rather than late in the day when you have been involved in many activities.

HRR is determined by subtracting the resting heart rate from the maximal heart rate. The heart always works in the range between the resting (the lowest) and the maximal (the highest) rate of your pulse. The formula for calculating the working heart rate and an example for the 22-year-old with a resting heart rate of 68 beats per minute are shown in Table 5.

Table 5 ▶ Comparison of the Two Primary Methods for Calculating Target Heart Rate

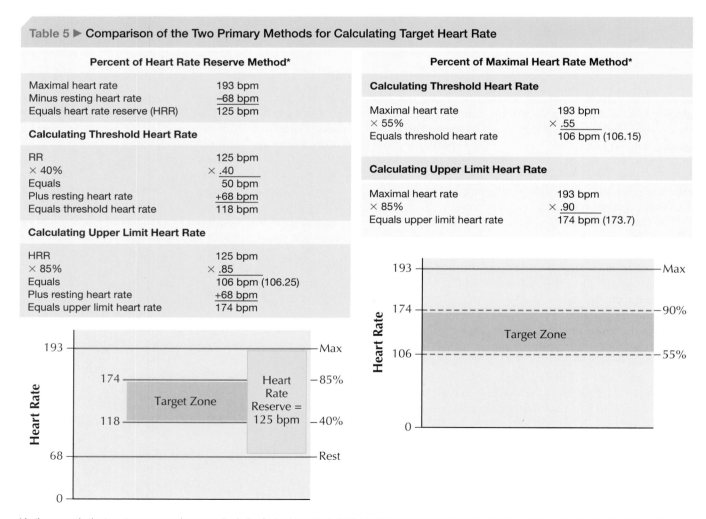

Percent of Heart Rate Reserve Method*

Maximal heart rate	193 bpm
Minus resting heart rate	−68 bpm
Equals heart rate reserve (HRR)	125 bpm

Calculating Threshold Heart Rate

RR	125 bpm
× 40%	× .40
Equals	50 bpm
Plus resting heart rate	+68 bpm
Equals threshold heart rate	118 bpm

Calculating Upper Limit Heart Rate

HRR	125 bpm
× 85%	× .85
Equals	106 bpm (106.25)
Plus resting heart rate	+68 bpm
Equals upper limit heart rate	174 bpm

Percent of Maximal Heart Rate Method*

Calculating Threshold Heart Rate

Maximal heart rate	193 bpm
× 55%	× .55
Equals threshold heart rate	106 bpm (106.15)

Calculating Upper Limit Heart Rate

Maximal heart rate	193 bpm
× 85%	× .90
Equals upper limit heart rate	174 bpm (173.7)

* In the example the target zone upper heart rate is similar for both methods (174) but the threshold heart rate is under predicted using the Maximal Heart Rate Method (106 as opposed to 118 for the HRR method). Example is of a 22-year-old person with a resting heart rate of 68 bpm.

The threshold of training, or minimum heart rate, for achieving health benefits is determined by calculating 40 percent of the working heart rate and then adding it to the resting heart rate. The upper limit of the target zone is 85 percent of the working heart rate. Because resting heart rate and max heart rate will vary, each person will have a unique threshold and target zone. Table 6 allows you to look up the appropriate target zone and threshold based on your resting heart rate and age. Locate your resting heart rate on the left-hand column and your age across the top. The values at the point where they intersect are your threshold and target heart zone values.

For best results, begin using heart rates at the lower part of the zone and gradually increase exercise intensity. Some athletes or advanced exercisers may occasionally exercise at heart rate values above 85 percent of heart rate reserve (i.e. above the target zone). This type of exercise may be necessary for high level training or performance but it is not necessary for improving cardiovascular fitness associated with good health and wellness.

Percent of Maximal Heart Rate Method

To use this method, first estimate your maximal heart rate, just as you did for the previous method; then determine the threshold heart rate by calculating 55 percent of the maximal heart rate. The upper limit of the target zone is determined by calculating 90 percent of the maximal heart rate. This procedure, using a percent of maximal heart rate, is deemed an acceptable alternative to the procedure using a percent of heart rate reserve because it provides target heart rates similar to those using 40–85 percent of the HRR method (see Table 5 for a worked example).

The ACSM recently increased the percentage of maxHR for calculating threshold heart rates because the percentage formerly used was underestimating these values. As the example in Table 5 indicate, the percent of maximal heart rate formula still underestimates threshold values but provides accurate values for the upper limit of the target zone.

Threshold and target zone heart rates should be used as general guidelines for cardiovascular exercise. You should learn to calculate your threshold and target

Table 6 ▶ Determining Threshold of Training* and Target Zone Heart Rates Using Resting Heart Rate and Age

Resting Heart Rate		Age									
		Less Than 25	25–29	30–34	35–39	40–44	45–49	50–54	55–59	60–64	Over 65
Below 50	Threshold	107	105	103	102	101	99	98	97	96	95
	target zone	107–170	105–167	103–164	102–161	101–159	99–155	98–151	97–148	96–146	95–139
50–54	Threshold	110	108	106	104	102	101	102	100	99	98
	target zone	110–170	108–167	106–164	104–162	102–160	101–156	102–153	100–150	99–147	98–140
55–59	Threshold	113	111	109	107	106	105	104	103	102	101
	target zone	113–171	111–168	109–163	107–162	106–160	105–157	104–154	103–150	102–146	101–140
60–64	Threshold	116	113	111	109	108	107	106	105	104	104
	target zone	116–171	113–169	111–166	109–163	108–161	107–159	106–155	105–151	104–147	104–141
65–69	Threshold	118	117	115	112	111	110	109	108	107	108
	target zone	118–172	117–170	115–166	112–163	111–161	110–159	109–155	108–152	107–148	108–142
70–74	Threshold	121	120	118	119	116	114	113	112	111	110
	target zone	121–173	120–171	118–167	119–164	116–162	114–160	113–156	112–153	111–149	110–143
75–79	Threshold	124	123	122	121	119	117	116	114	113	112
	target zone	124–173	123–172	122–168	121–164	119–163	117–160	116–157	114–155	113–151	112–143
80–85	Threshold	127	124	123	122	121	119	118	117	116	114
	target zone	127–174	124–172	123–169	122–165	121–164	119–161	118–158	117–156	116–152	114–144
86 and over	Threshold	130	125	126	125	124	123	121	119	117	117
	target zone	130–175	125–173	126–169	125–166	124–164	123–162	121–159	119–157	117–154	117–145

*Threshold for beginners. Mid target or above recommended after becoming a regular exerciser.

zone heart rate values using one of the two methods described. Regardless of which method you use, the key is to bring your heart rate above threshold and into the target zone to get the health benefits from cardiovascular fitness. The ranges that result from these methods should be used as general guidelines because there are several possible sources of error that can influence the values.

First, the method of calculating maximal heart rate is an estimate based on typical values for typical people. Second, errors in counting heart rate are possible. Finally, it is possible that the count you make *after* exercise may not actually reflect your heart rate *during* the activity. For this reason, it is important that you make several estimates of your threshold and target heart rates, especially when you are first starting a cardiovascular fitness program.

Heart rate monitors can help monitor the intensity and duration of cardiovascular exercise. Heart rate monitors have been used for years by competitive endurance athletes to monitor their training programs. Athletes learn what their heart rate is for certain paces and know how hard they can push to optimize their performance in a race. Technological advances have continued to enhance the utility of these devices, and the costs of the devices are now within the reach of many recreational exercisers.

A watch (receiver), typically worn on the wrist, receives a signal from a transmitter attached to a strap worn around the chest. Basic units display heart rate only, whereas more advanced models have alarms to indicate time spent in target zones and software that allows the heart rate signals to be downloaded and processed on a personal computer. The software can automatically track time spent in different target zones and allow users to see a graphical display of how hard they exercised. The immediate feedback on heart rate during exercise and the ability to log workouts over time may help some individuals maintain interest in their exercise program. Though these computerized monitors are helpful to some, they are not a requirement for accurate assessment of physical activity intensity.

Ratings of perceived exertion can be used to monitor the intensity of physical activity. The ACSM suggests that people experienced in physical activity can use RPE to determine if they are exercising in the target zone (see Table 7). Ratings of perceived exertion have been shown to correlate well with VO_2R and HRR. For this reason, RPE can be used to estimate exercise intensity among those who have learned to use the RPE rating categories. This avoids the need to stop and count heart rate during exercise. A rating of 12 is equal to threshold, and a rating of 16 is equal to the upper limit of the target zone. With practice, most people can recognize when they are in the target zone using ratings of perceived exertion.

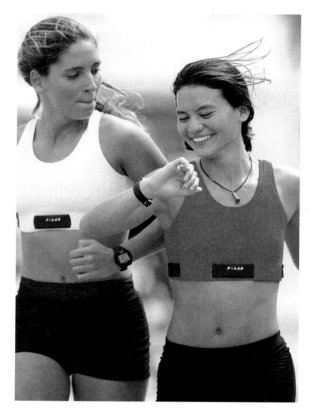

Heart rate monitors provide an effective way to track heart rate during exercise.

Table 7 ▶ Ratings of Perceived Exertion (RPE)

Rating	Description
6	
7	Very, very light
8	
9	Very light
10	
11	Fairly light
12	
13	Somewhat hard
14	
15	Hard
16	
17	Very hard
18	
19	Very, very hard
20	

Source: Data from Borg.

Strategies for Action

Web 05 ┃ An important step in taking action to develop and maintain cardiovascular fitness is assessing your current status. For an activity program to be most effective, it should be based on personal needs. Some type of testing is necessary to determine your personal need for cardiovascular fitness. As noted earlier, the best measure of cardiovascular fitness is a laboratory assessment of $\dot{V}O_2$ max, but this is not possible for most people. To provide alternatives, researchers have developed other tests that provide reasonable estimates. Commonly used tests are the step test, the swim test, the 12-minute run, the Astrand-Ryhming bicycle test, and the walking test. These tests are developed based on comparisons with measured $\dot{V}O_2$ max and are good general indicators of cardiovascular fitness.

In Lab 7B you will be able to compare estimates from several tests.

Web 06 ┃ The self-assessment you choose depends on your current fitness and activity levels, the availability of equipment, and other factors. The walking test is probably best for those at beginning levels because more vigorous forms of activity may cause discomfort and may discourage future participation. The step test is somewhat less vigorous than the running test and takes only a few minutes to complete. The bicycle test is also sub-maximal or relatively moderate in intensity. It is quite accurate but requires more equipment than the other tests and requires more expertise. You may need help from a fitness expert to do this test properly. The swim test is especially useful to those with musculoskeletal problems and other disabilities. The running test is the most vigorous and for this reason may not be best for beginners. On the other hand, more advanced exercisers with high levels of motivation may prefer this test.

Results on the walking, running, and swimming tests are greatly influenced by the motivation of the test taker. If the test taker does not try hard, fitness results are underestimated. The bicycle and step tests are influenced less by motivation because one must exercise at a specified workload and at a regular pace. Because heart rate can be influenced by emotional factors, exercise prior to the test, and other factors, tests using heart rate can sometimes give incorrect results. It is important to do your self-assessments when you are relatively free from stress and are rested.

Prior to performing any of these, be sure that you are physically and medically ready. Prepare yourself by doing some regular physical activity for 3 to 6 weeks before actually taking the tests. If possible, take more than one test and use the summary of your test results to make a final assessment of your cardiovascular fitness. In Lab 7B, you will have the opportunity to self-assess your cardiovascular fitness using one or more tests. A nonexercise estimate of cardiovascular fitness is also provided for comparison. While this self-report tool has limitations, it is increasingly being used as a screening tool in physicians' offices to determine if patients have risks associated with poor fitness. (See Jurca, 2005, in *Suggested Readings.*)

Online Learning Center

www.mhhe.com/corbin7e
The Online Learning Center contains a variety of Web-based resources that will help you get the most out of this book and your course. In addition to the On the Web pages, there are video activities, interactive quizzes, application assignments, and a variety of other useful study aids. Log on to the URL above to access these resources.

Web Resources

Web 07 ┃ American College of Sports Medicine **www.acsm.org**
American Heart Association **www.americanheart.org**
The Cooper Institute **www.cooperinst.org**

Suggested Readings

Web 08 ┃ Additional reference materials for Concept 7 are available at Web08.

American College of Sports Medicine. 2006. *ACSM's Guidelines for Exercise Testing and Prescription*. 7th ed. Philadelphia: Lippincott, Williams and Wilkins.

Bassuk, S. S., and J. E. Manson. 2004. Preventing cardiovascular disease in women: How much physical activity is good enough? *President's Council on Physical Fitness and Sports Research Digest* 5(3):1–8.

Blair, S. N., et al. 1996. Influence of cardiorespiratory fitness and other precursors on cardiovascular disease and all-cause mortality in men and women. *Journal of American Medical Association* 276(3):205–211.

Borg, G. 1982. Psychological bases of perceived exertion. *Medicine and Science in Sports and Exercise* 14:377.

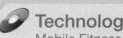

Technology Update
Mobile Fitness Testing for National Study

The importance of cardiovascular fitness for good health has led the public health service to incorporate objective measures of aerobic fitness into a large-scale surveillance study known as National Health and Nutrition Examination Survey (NHANES). In this fourth (IV) version of the study, data collection teams travel around the country in mobile examination centers and complete comprehensive health and fitness assessments on a representative sample of adults. The mobile trailers have the latest technology for fitness and health assessments and are designed to facilitate this type of distributed data collection. Visit the NHANES Web site at **www.cdc.gov/nchs/nhanes.htm** to take a virtual tour of the mobile testing center and to learn how this major public health study is being conducted. There have been many surveillance studies conducted using self-report measures of physical activity, but this is the first effort to systematically evaluate the fitness levels of the U.S. population using laboratory measures of physical fitness.

Bouchard, C. 1999. Heredity and health-related fitness. In C. B. Corbin and R. P. Pangrazi (eds.). *Toward a Better Understanding of Physical Fitness and Activity* Scottsdale, AZ: Holcomb-Hathaway.

Carnethon, M. R., et al. 2005. Prevalence and cardiovascular disease correlates of low cardiorespiratory fitness in adolescents and adults. *Journal of the American Medical Association* 294(23):2981–2988.

Centers for Disease Control and Prevention. 2005. Adult participation in recommended levels of physical activity—United States, 2001 and 2003. *MMWR Morbidity and Mortality Weekly Report* (54):208–1212.

Chenoweth, D., et al. 2006. The cost of sloth: Using a tool to measure the cost of physical inactivity. *ACSM's Health and Fitness Journal* 10(2):8–13.

Dziura, J., et al. 2004. Physical activity reduces Type 2 diabetes risk in aging independent of body weight change. *Journal of Physical Activity and Health* 1(1):19–28.

Franks, P. W., et al. 2004. Does the association of habitual physical activity with the metabolic syndrome differ by level of cardiorespiratory fitness? *Diabetes Care* 27(5):1187–1193.

Gulati, M., et al. 2005. The prognostic value of a nomogram for exercise capacity in women. *New England Journal of Medicine* 353(5):468–475.

Hills, A. P., et al. 2006. Validation of the intensity of walking for pleasure in obese adults. *Preventive Medicine* 42(1):47–50.

Jurca, R. 2005. Assessing cardiorespiratory fitness without performing exercise testing. *American Journal of Preventive Medicine* 29(3):185–193.

Lakka, T. A. 2004. Sedentary lifestyle, poor cardiorespiratory fitness, and the metabolic syndrome. *Medicine and Science in Sports and Exercise* 35(8):1279–1286.

Schnirring, L. 2001. New formula estimates maximal heart rate. *The Physician and Sportsmedicine* 29(7):13–14.

Tanaka H., K. D. Monahan, and D. R. Seals. 2001. Age-predicted maximal heart rate revisited. *Journal of the American College of Cardiology* 37(1):153–156.

U.S. Department of Health and Human Services. 1996. *Physical Activity and Health: A Report of the Surgeon General*. Atlanta: U.S. Department of Health and Human Services.

Williams, P. T. 2001. Physical fitness and activity as separate heart disease risk factors: A meta-analysis. *Medicine and Science in Sports and Exercise* 33(5):754–761.

Wong, S. L., et al. 2004. Cardiorespiratory fitness is associated with lower abdominal fat independent of body mass index. *Medicine and Science in Sports and Exercise* 36(2):286–291.

In the News

Curves

Curves Fitness Centers have had a profound effect on the fitness industry and on the physical fitness levels of women. There are an estimated 9,000 Curves locations that currently provide fitness opportunities to over 4 million women. In fact, there are about two Curves centers for every McDonald's restaurant in America, with worldwide exposure in 35 countries.

The success of Curves can be attributed, in part, to a simple fitness philosophy that resonates with many women. The Curves program provides a quick and efficient workout for women without a lot of extra hype. Women go into Curves, complete a circuit on the machines, and can be done in 30 minutes. The circuit consists of hydraulic resistance machines alternating with recovery pads, which allow the women to walk, dance, or jog in place. This allows participants to maintain an aerobic pace during the workout. The quick, structured workouts have made it easy for women to incorporate the program into their lives. Because members can go to any Curves location, it is easy for many to stick with their program. Check out Curves at **www.curves.com**.

Lab Resource Materials: Evaluating Cardiovascular Fitness

The Walking Test

- Warm up; then walk 1 mile as fast as you can without straining. Record your time to the nearest second.
- Immediately after the walk, count your heart rate for 15 seconds; then multiply by 4 to get a 1-minute heart rate. Record your heart rate.
- Use your walking time and your postexercise heart rate to determine your rating using Chart 1.

Chart 1 ▶ Walking Ratings for Males and Females

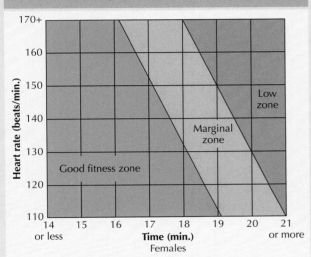

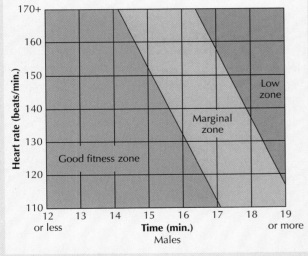

Source: James M. Rippe, M.D.

The ratings in Chart 1 are for ages 20 to 29. They provide reasonable ratings for people of all ages.

Note: The walking test is not a good indicator of high performance; the running and bicycle tests are recommended.

Step Test

- Step up and down on a 12-inch bench for 3 minutes at a rate of 24 steps per minute. One step consists of 4 beats—that is, "up with the left foot, up with the right foot, down with the left foot, down with the right foot."
- Immediately after the exercise, sit down on the bench and relax. Don't talk.
- Locate your pulse or have someone locate it for you.
- Five seconds after the exercise ends, begin counting your pulse. Count the pulse for 60 seconds.
- Your score is your 60-second heart rate. Locate your score and your rating on Chart 2.

Chart 2 ▶ Step Test Rating Chart

Classification	60-Second Heart Rate
High-performance zone	84 or less
Good fitness zone	85–95
Marginal zone	96–119
Low zone	120 and above

Source: Kasch and Boyer.

As you grow older, you will want to continue to score well on this rating chart. Because your maximal heart rate decreases as you age, you should be able to score well if you exercise regularly.

The Astrand-Ryhming Bicycle Test

- Ride a stationary bicycle ergometer for 6 minutes at a rate of 50 pedal cycles per minute (one push with each foot per cycle). Cool down after the test.
- Set the bicycle at a workload between 300 and 1,200 kpm. For less fit or smaller people, a setting in the range of 300 to 600 is appropriate. Larger or fitter people will need to use a setting of 750 to 1,200. The workload should be enough to elevate the heart rate to at least 125 bpm but no more than 170 bpm during the ride. The ideal range is 140–150 bpm.
- During the sixth minute of the ride (if the heart rate is in the correct range—see previous step), count the heart rate for the entire sixth minute. The carotid or radial pulse may be used.
- Use Chart 3 (males) or 4 (females) to determine your predicted oxygen uptake score in liters per minute. Locate your heart rate for the sixth minute of the ride in the left column and the work rate in kp·m/min. across the top. The number in the chart where the heart rate and work rate intersect represents your predicted O_2 uptake in liters per minute. The bicycle you use must allow you to easily and accurately determine the work rate in kp·m/min.

- Ratings are typically assigned based on milliliters per kilogram of body weight per minute. To convert your score to milliliters per kilogram per minute (mL/kg/min.) the first step is to multiply your score from Chart 3 or 4 by 1,000. This converts your score from liters to milliliters. Then divide your weight in pounds by 2.2. This converts your weight to kilograms. Then divide your score in milliliters by your weight in kilograms. This gives you your score in mL/kg/min.

- Example: An oxygen uptake score of 3.5 liters is equal to a 3,500-milliliter score (3.5 _ 1,000). If the person with this score weighed 150 pounds, his or her weight in kilograms would be 68.18 kilograms (150 divided by 2.2). The person's oxygen uptake would be 51.3 mL/kg/min. (3,500 divided by 68.18).
- Use your score in mL/kg/min. to determine your rating (Chart 5).

Chart 3 ▶ Determining Oxygen Uptake Using the Bicycle Test—Men (Liters O$_2$/min.)

Heart Rate	Work Rate (kp·m/min.)				Heart Rate	Work Rate (kp·m/min.)					Heart Rate	Work Rate (kp·m/min.)				
	450	600	900	1,200		450	600	900	1,200	1,500		450	600	900	1,200	1,500
123	3.3	3.4	4.6	6.0	139	2.5	2.6	3.6	4.8	6.0	155	2.0	2.2	3.0	4.0	5.0
124	3.3	3.3	4.5	6.0	140	2.5	2.6	3.6	4.8	6.0	156	1.9	2.2	2.9	4.0	5.0
125	3.2	3.2	4.4	5.9	141	2.4	2.6	3.5	4.7	5.9	157	1.9	2.1	2.9	3.9	4.9
126	3.1	3.2	4.4	5.8	142	2.4	2.5	3.5	4.6	5.8	158	1.8	2.1	2.9	3.9	4.9
127	3.0	3.1	4.3	5.7	143	2.4	2.5	3.4	4.6	5.7	159	1.8	2.1	2.8	3.8	4.8
128	3.0	3.1	4.2	5.6	144	2.3	2.5	3.4	4.5	5.7	160	1.8	2.1	2.8	3.8	4.8
129	2.9	3.0	4.2	5.6	145	2.3	2.4	3.4	4.5	5.6	161	1.7	2.0	2.8	3.7	4.7
130	2.9	3.0	4.1	5.5	146	2.3	2.4	3.3	4.4	5.6	162	1.7	2.0	2.8	3.7	4.6
131	2.8	2.9	4.0	5.4	147	2.3	2.4	3.3	4.4	5.5	163	1.7	2.0	2.8	3.7	4.6
132	2.8	2.9	4.0	5.3	148	2.2	2.4	3.2	4.3	5.4	164	1.6	2.0	2.7	3.6	4.5
133	2.7	2.8	3.9	5.3	149	2.2	2.3	3.2	4.3	5.4	165	1.6	1.9	2.7	3.6	4.5
134	2.7	2.8	3.9	5.2	150	2.2	2.3	3.2	4.2	5.3	166	1.6	1.9	2.7	3.6	4.5
135	2.7	2.8	3.8	5.1	151	2.2	2.3	3.1	4.2	5.2	167	1.5	1.9	2.6	3.5	4.4
136	2.6	2.7	3.8	5.0	152	2.1	2.3	3.1	4.1	5.2	168	1.5	1.9	2.6	3.5	4.4
137	2.6	2.7	3.7	5.0	153	2.1	2.2	3.0	4.1	5.1	169	1.5	1.9	2.6	3.5	4.3
138	2.5	2.7	3.7	4.9	154	2.0	2.2	3.0	4.0	5.1	170	1.4	1.8	2.6	3.4	4.3

Chart 4 ▶ Determining Oxygen Uptake Using the Bicycle Test—Women (Liters O$_2$/min.)

Heart Rate	Work Rate (kp·m/min.)					Heart Rate	Work Rate (kp·m/min.)					Heart Rate	Work Rate (kp·m/min.)			
	300	450	600	750	900		300	450	600	750	900		400	600	750	900
123	2.4	3.1	3.9	4.6	5.1	139	1.8	2.4	2.9	3.5	4.0	155	1.9	2.4	2.8	3.2
124	2.4	3.1	3.8	4.5	5.1	140	1.8	2.4	2.8	3.4	4.0	156	1.9	2.4	2.8	3.2
125	2.3	3.0	3.7	4.4	5.0	141	1.8	2.3	2.8	3.4	3.9	157	1.8	2.3	2.7	3.2
126	2.3	3.0	3.6	4.3	5.0	142	1.7	2.3	2.8	3.3	3.9	158	1.8	2.3	2.7	3.1
127	2.2	2.9	3.5	4.2	4.8	143	1.7	2.2	2.7	3.3	3.8	159	1.8	2.3	2.7	3.1
128	2.2	2.8	3.5	4.2	4.8	144	1.7	2.2	2.7	3.2	3.8	160	1.8	2.2	2.6	3.0
129	2.2	2.8	3.4	4.1	4.8	145	1.6	2.2	2.7	3.2	3.7	161	1.8	2.2	2.6	3.0
130	2.1	2.7	3.4	4.0	4.7	146	1.6	2.2	2.6	3.2	3.7	162	1.8	2.2	2.6	3.0
131	2.1	2.7	3.4	4.0	4.6	147	1.6	2.1	2.6	3.1	3.6	163	1.7	2.2	2.5	2.9
132	2.0	2.7	3.3	3.9	4.6	148	1.6	2.1	2.6	3.1	3.6	164	1.7	2.1	2.5	2.9
133	2.0	2.6	3.2	3.8	4.5	149	1.5	2.1	2.6	3.0	3.5	165	1.7	2.1	2.5	2.9
134	2.0	2.6	3.2	3.8	4.4	150	1.5	2.0	2.5	3.0	3.5	166	1.7	2.1	2.5	2.8
135	2.0	2.6	3.1	3.7	4.4	151	1.5	2.0	2.5	3.0	3.4	167	1.6	2.0	2.4	2.8
136	1.9	2.5	3.1	3.6	4.3	152	1.4	2.0	2.5	2.9	3.4	168	1.6	2.0	2.4	2.8
137	1.9	2.5	3.0	3.6	4.2	153	1.4	2.0	2.4	2.9	3.3	169	1.6	2.0	2.4	2.8
138	1.8	2.4	3.0	3.5	4.2	154	1.4	2.0	2.4	2.8	3.3	170	1.6	2.0	2.4	2.7

Chart 5 ▶ Bicycle Test Rating Scale (mL/O$_2$/kg/min.)

	Women				
Age	**17–26**	**27–39**	**40–49**	**50–59**	**60–69**
High-performance zone	46+	40+	38+	35+	32+
Good fitness zone	36–45	33–39	30–37	28–34	24–31
Marginal zone	30–35	28–32	24–29	21–27	18–23
Low zone	<30	<28	<24	<21	<18

	Men				
Age	**17–26**	**27–39**	**40–49**	**50–59**	**60–69**
High-performance zone	50+	46+	42+	39+	35+
Good fitness zone	43–49	35–45	32–41	29–38	26–34
Marginal zone	35–42	30–34	27–31	25–28	22–25
Low zone	<35	<30	<27	<25	<22

Source: Charts 4, 5, and 6 based on data from Astrand and Rodahl.

The 12-Minute Run Test

- Locate an area where a specific distance is already marked, such as a school track or football field, or measure a specific distance using a bicycle or automobile odometer.
- Use a stopwatch or wristwatch to accurately time a 12-minute period.
- For best results, warm up prior to the test; then run at a steady pace for the entire 12 minutes (cool down after the tests).
- Determine the distance you can run in 12 minutes in fractions of a mile. Depending upon your age, locate your score and rating in Chart 6.

Chart 6 ▶ Twelve-Minute Run Test Rating Chart (Score in Miles)

	Men (Age)			
Classification	**17–26**	**27–39**	**40–49**	**50+**
High-performance zone	1.80+	1.60+	1.50+	1.40+
Good fitness zone	1.55–1.79	1.45–1.59	1.40–1.49	1.25–1.39
Marginal zone	1.35–1.54	1.30–1.44	1.25–1.39	1.10–1.24
Low zone	<1.35	<1.30	<1.25	<1.10

	Women (Age)			
Classification	**17–26**	**27–39**	**40–49**	**50+**
High-performance zone	1.45+	1.35+	1.25+	39+
Good fitness zone	1.25–1.44	1.20–1.34	1.15–1.24	1.05–1.14
Marginal zone	1.15–1.24	1.05–1.19	1.00–1.14	.95–1.04
Low zone	<1.15	<1.05	<1.00	<.94

Source: Based on data from Cooper.

For a metric version of this chart, see Appendix A.

The 12-minute Swim Test

- Locate a swimming area with premeasured distances, preferably 20 yards or longer.
- After a warm-up, swim as far as possible in 12 minutes using the stroke of your choice.

- For best results, have a partner keep track of your time and distance. A degree of swimming competence is a prerequisite for this test.
- Determine your score and rating using Chart 7.

Chart 7 ▶ Twelve-Minute Swim Rating Chart (Score in Yards)

	Men (Age)			
Classification	17–26	27–39	40–49	50+
High-performance zone	700+	650+	600+	550+
Good fitness zone	600–699	550–649	500–599	450–549
Marginal zone	500–599	450–459	400–499	350–449
Low zone	Below 500	Below 450	Below 400	Below 350

	Women (Age)			
Classification	17–26	27–39	40–49	50+
High-performance zone	600+	550+	500+	450+
Good fitness zone	500–599	450–549	400–499	450–549
Marginal zone	400–499	350–359	300–399	250–349
Low zone	Below 400	Below 350	Below 300	Below 250

Source: Based on data from Cooper.

For a metric version of this chart, see Appendix A.

Chart 8 ▶ Non-Exercise Fitness Assessment Rating Chart

Rating	Score
Needs Improvement	1–4
Marginal	5–9
Good Conditioning	10–13
Highly Conditioned	13+

Lab 7A Counting Target Heart Rate and Ratings of Perceived Exertion

Name	Section	Date

Purpose: To learn to count heart rate accurately and to use heart rate and/or ratings of perceived exertion (RPE) to establish the threshold of training and target zones

Procedure

1. Practice counting the number of pulses felt for a given period of time at both the carotid and radial locations. Use a clock or watch to count for 15, 30, and 60 seconds. To establish your heart rate in beats per minute, multiply your 15-second pulse by 4, and your 30-second pulse by 2.
2. Practice locating your carotid and radial pulses quickly. This is important when trying to count your pulse after exercise.
3. Run a quarter-mile; then count your heart rate at the end of the run. Try to run at a rate you think will keep the rate of the heart above the threshold of training and in the target zone. Use 15-second pulse counts (choose either carotid or radial) and multiply by 4 to get heart rate in beats per minute (bpm). Record the bpm in the Results section.
4. Rate your perceived exertion (RPE) for the run (see RPE chart below). Record your results.
5. Repeat the run a second time. Try to run at a speed that gets you in the heart rate and RPE target zone. Record your heart rate and RPE results.

Results: Record your *resting* heart rates in the boxes below.

Carotid Pulse		Heart Rate per Minute	Radial Pulse		Heart Rate per Minute
	15 seconds × 4			15 seconds × 4	
	30 seconds × 2			30 seconds × 2	
	60 seconds × 1			60 seconds × 1	

Record your heart rate and rating of perceived exertion for run 1.

Pulse Count		Heart Rate per Minute
	15 seconds × 4	
Rating of Perceived Exertion		

Record your heart rate and rating of perceived exertion for run 2.

Pulse Count		Heart Rate per Minute
	15 seconds × 4	
Rating of Perceived Exertion		

Ratings of Perceived Exertion (RPE)

Rating	Description
6	
7	Very, very light
8	
9	Very light
10	
11	Fairly light
12	
13	Somewhat hard
14	
15	Hard
16	
17	Very hard
18	
19	Very, very hard
20	

Source: Data from Borg, G.

Answer the following questions:

Which pulse-counting technique did you use after the runs?   Carotid ◯   Radial ◯

What is your heart rate target zone (calculate, see pages 119 and 120, or see Table 6, page 121)? [＿＿＿＿＿] bpm

Was your heart rate for run 1 enough to get in the heart rate target zone?   Yes ◯   No ◯

Was your RPE for run 1 enough to get in the target zone (12–16)?   Yes ◯   No ◯

Was your heart rate for run 2 enough to get in the heart rate target zone?   Yes ◯   No ◯

Was your RPE for run 2 enough to get in the target zone (12–16)?   Yes ◯   No ◯

Conclusions and Implications: In several sentences, discuss your results, including which method you would use to count heart rate and why. Also discuss heart rate versus RPE (Rating of Perceived Exertion) for determining the target zone.

Lab Supplement*: You may want to keep track of your exercise heart rate over a week's time or longer to see if you are reaching the target zone in your workouts. Shade your target zone with a highlight pen and plot your exercise heart rate for each day of the week (see sample).

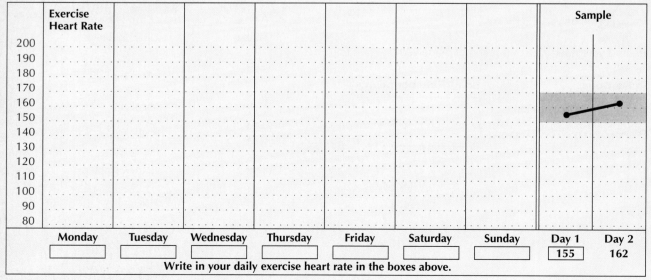

*Thanks to Ginnie Atkins for suggesting this lab supplement.

Lab 7B Evaluating Cardiovascular Fitness

Name	**Section**	**Date**

Purpose: To acquaint you with several methods for evaluating cardiovascular fitness and to help you evaluate and rate your own cardiovascular fitness

Procedure

1. Perform one or more of the four cardiovascular fitness tests and determine your ratings using the information in the Lab Resource Materials.
2. Perform each of the four steps for the Non-Exercise Estimate of Cardiovascular Fitness using the information on the back of this page. Learning this technique will allow you to estimate your fitness when you are injured or for some other reason cannot do a performance test.

Results

1. Record the information from your cardiovascular fitness test(s) in the spaces provided.
2. After you have completed the four steps for the Non-Exercise Estimate of Cardiovascular Fitness, use Chart 1 to determine your fitness rating.

Walking Test

Time		minutes
Heart rate		bpm
Rating		(see Chart 1, page 125)

Bicycle Test

Workload		kpm
Heart rate		bpm
Weight		pounds
Weight in kg*		
mL/O_2/kg		
Rating		(see Chart 5, page 127)

Non-Exercise Test

Score		
Rating		(see Chart 8, page 128)

*Weight in lb. ÷ 2.2.

Step Test

Heart rate		bpm
Rating		(see Chart 2, page 125)

12-Minute Run

Distance		miles
Rating		(see Chart 6, page 127)

12-Minute Swim Test

Distance		yards
Rating		(see Chart 7, page 128)

Non-Exercise Cardiovascular Fitness Rating

- Look up your activity score on Chart 1. Place activity estimate score here. _____ (A)

- Record your resting heart rate here (see Lab 7a). _____ × 0.30 = _____ (B)

- Record your BMI score here (see Lab 13b). _____ × 0.17 = _____ (C)

- Record gender here (female = 0/male = 1). _____ × 2.77 = _____ (D)

- Record your age in years here. _____ × 0.10 = _____ (E)

- Use the following formula to calculate your score and use Chart 9 to rate your fitness.

A – B – C + D – + 18.07 = Estimated Cardiovascular fitness (METS)

☐ – ☐ – ☐ + ☐ – + 18.07 = ☐

Chart 1 ▶ Self-Reported Activity Score (for Step Number 1 Above)

Activity Score	Choose the Score That Best Describes Your Physical Activity Level
0.00	I am inactive or do little activity other than usual daily activities.
0.32	I regularly (> 5 d/wk) participate in physical activities requiring low levels of exertion that result in slight increases in breathing and heart rate for at least **10 minutes** at a time.
1.06	I participate in aerobic exercises such as brisk walking, jogging, or running, cycling, swimming, or vigorous sports at a comfortable pace, or activities requiring similar levels of exertion for **20–60 minutes per week.**
1.76	I participate in aerobic exercises such as brisk walking, jogging, or running at a comfortable pace, or other activities requiring similar levels of exertion for **1–3 hours per week.**
3.03	I participate in aerobic exercises such as brisk walking, jogging, or running at a comfortable pace, or other activities requiring similar levels of exertion for **over 3 hours per week.**

Conclusions and Implications

1. In several sentences, explain why you selected the tests you selected. Discuss your current level of cardiovascular fitness and steps you will need to take to maintain or improve it. Comment on the effectiveness of the tests you selected.

2. In several sentences, explain your results from the non-exercise assessment by comparing the results with the other test(s). Did the self-report version classify you into the same fitness category? Try to explain any differences you noted.

Active Aerobics, Sports, and Recreational Activities

Health Goals for the year 2010

- Increase proportion of people who do vigorous physical activity that promotes cardiovascular fitness 3 or more days a week for 20 minutes per occasion.

- Increase adoption and maintenance of daily physical activity.

- Increase leisure-time physical activity.

- Decrease incidence of and deaths from heart diseases.

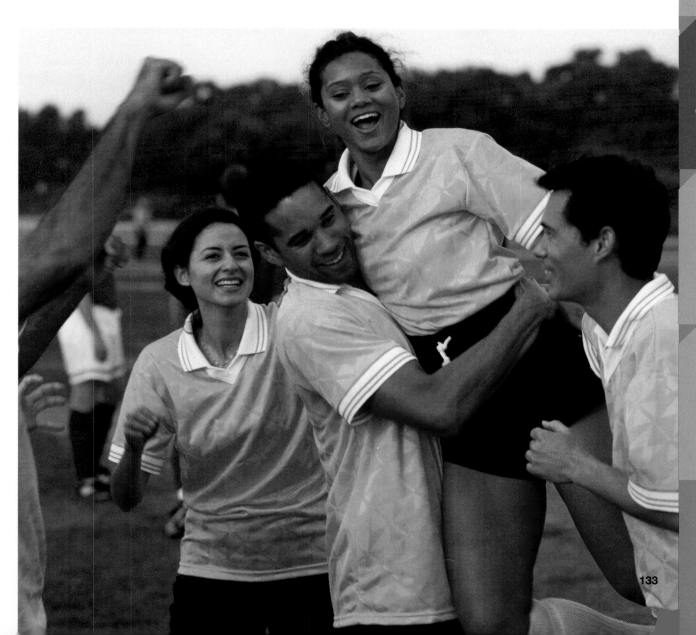

Active aerobics, sports, and recreational activities can promote health, develop fitness, and enhance performance.

Aerobic physical activity is the foundation for comprehensive fitness programs. Aerobic activity provides numerous health benefits, contributes to long-term weight control, and can be helpful in reducing stress. Improvements in cardiovascular fitness that result from aerobic activity also contribute to high quality of life and are essential for enhancing sports performance. Aerobic activity is generally defined as activity that is rhythmical, utilizes large muscle groups, and is performed in a continuous manner. However, aerobic activity does not have to be continuous to promote health or improve cardiovascular fitness.

The word *aerobic* literally means "with oxygen," but the reference to *aerobic activity* was popularized by Dr. Kenneth Cooper in his pioneering book *Aerobics*, published in 1968. Dr. Cooper was an early advocate of and a leader in the fitness movement, and his book helped increase awareness about the importance of regular physical activity. The Cooper Aerobic Points System emphasized that a variety of aerobic activities can contribute to cardiovascular health. Today, the concept of using various types of activities as part of an overall aerobic activity program is known as cross training.

This concept will review the diverse range of aerobic activities that are categorized at the second level of the activity pyramid (see Figure 1). These activities are more vigorous than the lifestyle activities at the first level of the pyramid. While it is beneficial to perform both types of activity, sufficient health benefits can be obtained with involvement in active aerobics and active sports and recreation. Because they are more vigorous, they do not need to be performed as frequently (see the FIT formula in Concept 7). Determining the types of aerobic activities that are most suited to you will help you establish and maintain a more active lifestyle.

Physical Activity Pyramid: Level 2

A variety of popular aerobic activities are included at level 2 of the pyramid. Swimming, exercising with machines, cycling, and jogging are among the most popular activities among adults. These activities, when done with enough intensity, are considered active aerobics and are included at level 2 of the pyramid.

An advantage of these **active aerobic activities** is that they provide a good cardiovascular workout in a short time and can often be done by oneself. A disadvantage (or barrier) for some people is that they are generally more vigorous and fast-paced than other forms of activity. The more vigorous nature is the most likely explanation for the age-related patterns that exist for participation in active aerobic activity. Young adults are far more likely to participate in active aerobic activity than are older adults. Most statistics report three- to five-fold differences in participation rates for young adults and older

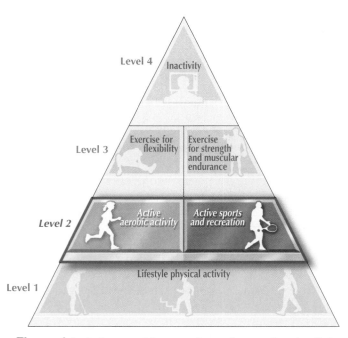

Figure 1 ► Active aerobics, sports, and recreational activities are included in the second level of the physical activity pyramid.

adults (40 to 60). The declining interest in vigorous activity for older adults is only a concern to public health officials if older adults fail to substitute moderate physical activity when they discontinue more vigorous activity.

Active recreation and sports are included at level 2 because they can provide the same benefits as structured aerobic activity. Activities such as hiking, boating, fishing, horseback riding, and other outdoor activities are generally classified as recreation. Because many of these activities can be performed at intensities suitable for building cardiovascular fitness, some can be categorized as **active recreational activities.** Hiking, skiing, kayaking, canoeing, hunting, and rock climbing are examples of active recreation activities that typically involve a considerable amount of activity. Recreation activities such as fishing and boating are typically done at lower intensities and can be considered as lifestyle activities.

Active sports can also be included in level 2 of the pyramid because they are vigorous. Examples of aerobic sports include basketball, racquetball, tennis, soccer, and hockey. These activities involve intermittent activity but typically are at an intensity that provides cardiovascular benefits. When performed regularly, they can provide benefits similar to those of active aerobics. Swimming and cycling are also popular activities that can be considered sports. However, most people do these activities noncompetitively, so they are considered as active aerobics in this book. Sports such as golf, bowling, and billiards/pool are aerobic but are light to moderate in intensity. For this reason, they are classified as lifestyle physical activities.

Physical activities at level 2 of the pyramid produce improvements in cardiovascular fitness and health in addition to those produced by lifestyle physical activities. Participation in lifestyle activity provides important health benefits, and additional vigorous aerobic activity results in additional health benefits. In fact, vigorous aerobic activity and active sports produce more benefits even if the total amount of activity (or energy expenditure) is the same. This difference can be seen in Figure 2. The green and blue bars show that a person's disease risk decreases as the amount of moderate activity increases. The black bar reveals the additional benefits provided by more vigorous activity. For each level of total activity, health risks are lower if a person performs more vigorous forms of physical activity. The surgeon general's report and other public health documents have encouraged Americans to meet at least the minimal activity threshold. The American College of Sports Medicine also emphasizes that "additional benefits can be gained through greater amounts of physical activity."

Not all activities at level 2 of the pyramid are equally safe. Sports medicine experts indicate that certain types of physical activities are more likely than others to result

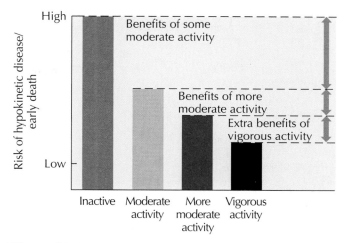

Figure 2 ▶ The extra benefits of vigorous physical activities.

in injury (see Table 1). Walking and low-impact dance aerobics are among the least risky activities. Skating, an aerobic activity, is the most risky, followed by basketball and competitive sports. Among the most popular aerobic activities, running has the greatest risk, with cycling, high-impact dance aerobics, and step aerobics having moderate risk for injury. Water activities were not considered in the study on which Table 1 was based, but other studies show that swimming and water aerobics are among those least likely to cause injuries because they do not involve impact, falling, or collision.

Injury rates vary among populations—for example, studies of high school and college athletes show that cheerleading and gymnastics are activities that result in the most injuries. A recent study of baby boomers, adults aged 35 to 54, showed that bicycling, basketball, baseball/softball, running/jogging, and aerobic dance exercise were among the activities most likely to result in emergency room treatment for that age group. No matter what the age group, activities that require high-volume training (aerobics and jogging), collision (football, basketball, and softball), falling (biking, skating, cheerleading, and

Active Aerobic Activities Physical activities of enough intensity to produce improvements in cardiovascular fitness. They are more intense than aerobic lifestyle physical activities.

Active Recreational Activities Activities done during leisure time that do not meet the characteristics of sports. Many types of active aerobics are recreational activities.

Active Sports Typically considered to be competitive physical activities that have an organized set of rules, along with winners and losers.

Table 1 ▶ Risk for Injury in Exercise

Activity	Injury per 1,000 Hours of Activity
Skating (including rollerblading)	20
Basketball	18
Average competitive sports	16
Running/jogging	16
Racquetball	14
Average aerobic activity	10
Tennis	8
Cycling	6
High-impact dance aerobics	6
Step aerobics	5
Aerobic exercise machines	3
Walking	2
Low-impact dance aerobics	2

Source: Data from the Center for Sports Medicine at St. Francis Hospital, San Francisco, CA.

gymnastics), the use of specialized equipment that can fail (biking), and repetitive movements that stress the joints (tennis and high-impact aerobics) increase risk for injury. These statistics point out the importance of using proper safety equipment, proper performance techniques, and proper training techniques.

Active Aerobic Activities

A variety of active aerobic activities are available for meeting individual needs and interests. Because there are so many choices, many beginning exercisers want to know which type of aerobic exercise is best. The best form of exercise is clearly whatever one you enjoy and will do regularly. Some people tend to be very consistent in performing their favorite form of activity, while others stay active by participating in a variety of activities. Seasonal differences are also common with physical activity participation. Many people choose to remain indoors during very hot or very cold weather and perform outdoor activities when temperatures are more moderate.

The charts in Figure 3 show the frequency of participation in a variety of active aerobic activities. These data were compiled from the recent Sporting Goods Manufacturers

Web 01

Association (SGMA) Survey, a nationally representative survey designed to track trends in the fitness and sports industry. While the survey is designed primarily for marketing purposes, it provides valuable information about activity interests in the United States. The results revealed a 7.8 percent increase in people who reported frequent exercise, the first increase in the past 10 years. According to the survey, approximately 54.9 million Americans aged 6 and older (21.1 percent) are considered "regular" exercisers—defined as participating in exercise at least 100 days a year.

Active aerobic activities are generally rhythmical and typically involve the large muscle groups of the legs. The rhythmical nature of aerobic activity allows it to be performed continuously and in a controlled manner. The activation of a large muscle mass is important in providing an appropriate challenge to the cardiovascular system. Descriptions of the most common individual forms of aerobic activity are provided below in order of their popularity (see Figure 3A). Additional information is available in the On the Web features.

Walking

Web 02

Walking is generally considered as a lifestyle physical activity and is effective in promoting metabolic fitness and overall health. If cardiovascular fitness is desired, walking must be done intensely enough to elevate the heart rate to target zone levels. For elderly and unfit individuals, walking often provides an intensity sufficient to maintain or improve cardiovascular fitness. For younger and more fit individuals, walking needs to be quite brisk to enhance cardiovascular fitness.

As shown in Figure 3, a large segment of the population has embraced fitness walking as their predominant conditioning activity. Over 10 million women and 6 million men report walking for exercise more than 100 days a year.

Jogging/Running

Web 03

A consistently popular form of active aerobics among both adult men and women is jogging or running. Though no official distinction exists between jogging and running, those who run more than a few miles per day, who participate in races, and who are concerned about improving the time in which they run a certain distance often prefer to be called "runners" rather than "joggers."

The popularity of jogging and running declined during the 1990s, but trends show progressive increases in participation rates since 2000. Over 25 million Americans report jogging/running for exercise; approximately 10 million (about 6 million males and 4 million females) report running regularly. A major advantage of running is that it requires little equipment and can be done almost anywhere.

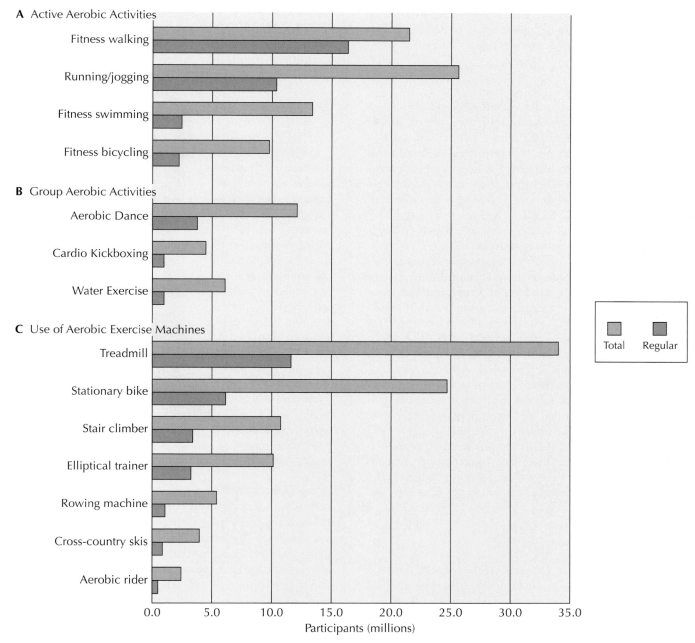

Figure 3 ▶ Participation rates for various active aerobic activities in the United States. *Total* refers to the total number of participants that report doing the activity (including occasional participants). *Regular* refers to participants who are active 100 or more days per year.

Swimming

Swimming is a popular recreational activity, but a relatively small percentage of Americans are considered to be regular fitness swimmers. According to the SGMA survey, nearly 100 million people report participating in "recreational swimming." The number of people that report regular fitness swimming is only about 2.5 million, but this figure is increasing. A 7 percent increase in swimming among women occurred over the past 5 years.

Because it requires considerable skill to move efficiently through the water, many individuals are not able to swim long enough to benefit. Even highly trained athletes can be exhausted after a few hundred yards if they do not have good skills. For those who do swim, it can be an excellent form of physical activity to promote cardiovascular fitness. Because of the water environment and the non-weight-bearing status, the heart rate response to swimming is typically lower for the same intensity of exercise.

The heart rate does not increase as rapidly in response to swimming, so target heart rates should be set about 5 to 10 beats lower than for other aerobic activities.

Bicycling

Bicycling can be an excellent active aerobic activity, but it requires a properly fitted bike, as well as safety equipment, such as a helmet and light if done after dark. There are different types of bikes to fit the needs and interests of the rider. Road bikes are most common but mountain bikes are becoming increasingly popular. Many people appreciate having a versatile bike suitable for different conditions and select a "city bike," which has upright handlebars but more durable wheels and tires for more rugged conditions.

Cycling is more efficient than running and some other aerobic activities because of the mechanical efficiency of the bicycle. Cycling on the level at 5 mph is about three times less intense than running the same speed. It would take a pace of 13 mph to expend a similar number of calories, compared with running at 5 mph. The speed of cycling will give you an indicator of intensity, but this can be influenced by hills and wind. A better indicator of intensity is heart rate or a rating of perceived exertion (RPE). Because biking may involve periods of coasting, it may need to be performed for longer periods of time than jogging to get the same benefit.

According to the SGMA survey, an estimated 50 million Americans report riding their bike for recreation. A smaller number (15 million) report frequent recreational bike riding, and a still smaller segment of the population (about 2 million) can be classified as a regular fitness bicyclist.

Cross-Country Skiing

In most colder climates, cross-country skiing is one of the more popular forms of aerobic activity. Of course, this activity requires snow and specialized equipment. Because it involves both the arms and legs in a coordinated movement, cross-country skiing is one of the most effective types of cardiovascular fitness exercises. The downside is that it requires some degree of skill to be able to perform the movements correctly. There are two main types of cross-country skiing: classic, or diagonal stride, and skating. Each requires a different type of ski and technique.

Inline Skating

Because of the speed and freedom of movement, inline skating has become a popular aerobic activity. Technological advances in equipment have made it much safer, though injury rates are still high,

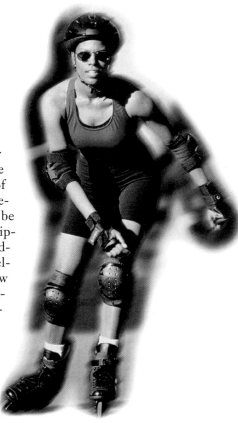

Inline skating is an effective, enjoyable type of aerobic exercise.

compared with other aerobic activities (see Table 1). Because of the injury risk, precautions should be taken. Special equipment is recommended, including a helmet, knee and elbow pads, wrist supporters, and hand protectors. Some degree of skill is necessary to perform skating safely and effectively, so it is wise to practice a bit in a controlled environment before taking to the streets.

Many types of active aerobics can be done in group settings. Although most aerobic activities can be done individually, many people prefer the social interactions and challenge of group exercise classes (see Figure 3B). Group exercise classes are offered at many fitness centers and community recreation centers.

An advantage of group exercise classes is that there is a social component, which helps to increase motivation and promote consistency. A disadvantage is that all participants are generally guided through the same exercise. A vigorous routine can cause unfit people to overextend themselves, while an easy routine may not be intense enough for experienced exercisers. A well-trained group exercise leader is able to help participants adjust the exercise to their own level and ability. Check the qualifications of the exercise leader to be sure that he or she is certified to lead group exercise. Descriptions of the most common group aerobic activities follow.

Dance and Step Aerobics

Dance aerobics is a choreographed series of dance steps and exercises done to music. A variety of forms of dance aerobics are available for different interests and abilities. "Low-impact" aerobics were developed to reduce the risk for injury or soreness. In this form, one foot stays on the floor at all times. Low-impact is an especially wise choice for beginners or older exercisers. Traditional "high-impact" is still common in many settings. In this form, both feet leave the ground simultaneously for a good part of the routine. It is recommended only for advanced exercisers. Even for these people high-impact aerobics can increase risk for injuries. A hybrid aerobic dance format known as "hi-lo" is gaining in popularity. This form integrates the two types of impact to provide a more balanced routine. The use of alternating sequences moderates the risks associated with both types and is considered to reflect movements more typical of the activities of daily living. Step aerobics, also known as bench stepping and step training, is an adaptation of dance aerobics. In this activity, the performer steps up and down on a bench when performing various dance steps. In most cases, step aerobics is considered to be low-impact, but higher in intensity than many forms of dance aerobics.

Martial Arts Exercise

A variety of martial arts have become popular active aerobic activities. In addition to traditional martial arts, such as karate and tae kwon do, a number of other alternative formats have been developed, including kickboxing, aerobic boxing, cardio-karate, box-fitness, and tae-bo. These activities involve intermittent bouts of high-intensity movements and lower-intensity recovery phases. Because martial arts involve a lot of arm work, they can be effective in promoting good overall fitness. Some activities are more intense than others, so consider the alternatives to find the best fit for you. Good instruction is critical for this form of activity, so look for appropriate certifications and credentials before choosing a facility or setting. Many of the disciplines involve a number of contraindicated movements that may increase risk for injury, so it is important to be aware of the risks and minimize your use of bad movements (see Concept 11). If contact is involved, it is important to be matched with a person of similar size and ability.

Spinning

Spinning is a type of stationary cycling typically performed in a group. A group leader typically instructs participants on what pace, gear, and/or cadence to use. In most cases, the routines involve intermittent bursts of high-intensity intervals followed by spinning at lower resistance to recover. The instructor may help riders simulate hill climbing or extended sprints to simulate competitive biking conditions. Although the class relates most directly to cy-

cling, the format has appealed to a broader set of fitness enthusiasts who just enjoy the challenge it provides.

Water Exercise

Swimming is not the only activity done in the water. Water walking and water exercise are two popular alternatives to swimming. Although these activities can be done alone, they are typically conducted in group settings to provide access to pools and certified instructors trained in water safety. Water aerobics are especially good for people with arthritis or other musculoskeletal problems and for people relatively high in body fat. The body's buoyancy in water assists the participant and reduces injury risk. The resistance of the water provides an overload that helps the activity promote health and cardiovascular benefits. Exercises done in shallow water are low in impact, and deeper-water exercises are considered to be higher-impact activities. An advantage of water walking and water exercise is that neither requires the ability to swim. Many classes include activities designed to promote flexibility and muscle fitness development, as well as cardiovascular benefits. Many injured athletes use water activity as a way to rehabilitate from injuries without losing too much fitness.

There has been an increasing trend in the use of cardiovascular exercise machines. Since 1990, the number of fitness walkers and joggers has remained fairly consistent, but the use of cardiovascular machines has increased by over 40 percent. The increased availability of this equipment at commercial fitness centers and the convenience of being able to exercise indoors at any time of day are the main reasons for the popularity of cardiovascular machines (see Figure 3C). Treadmills are the most commonly used exercise machine, followed by stationary bikes and stair climbers. However, trends within the fitness industry change quickly. Elliptical trainers have increased in popularity, and this has led to corresponding reductions in the use of other equipment, such as rowing machines and ski machines. Use of these machines can be fun and interesting initially, but that interest may decrease with repeated use. Many people enjoy using different machines to provide some degree of cross training and to have more variety in their program.

Many new features have been developed to enhance interest and ease of use. Most newer machines feature feedback systems, which provide continuous readouts of total exercise time, distance traveled, target and goal intensity, and estimates of calories burned. Most models also include modes that provide built-in warm-up and cool-down phases or a series of predetermined intervals with varying intensities. Some devices have built in heart rate monitors to allow more precise monitoring of exercise intensity.

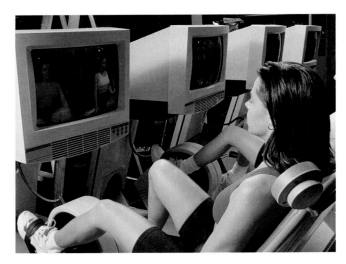

Interactive technology has made machine exercise more appealing for some people.

There is considerable competition within fitness clubs to offer the latest technology in exercise machines. Some clubs have personalized key systems, which automatically track personal preferences and settings and record time spent on each machine. This information can then be downloaded onto computers for automatic logging. Other fitness clubs have installed video monitors for individual pieces of equipment to allow users to select TV programs or to view interactive displays that allow you to compete against a virtual or real opponent. These features provide additional feedback that may enhance motivation or provide for a customized experience. See Web08 for comparisons of new aerobic exercise machines.

Active aerobics can be done either continuously or intermittently. We generally think of active aerobics as being continuous. Jogging, swimming, and cycling at a steady pace for long periods are classic examples. Experts have shown that aerobic exercise can be done intermittently as well as continuously. Both **continuous** and **intermittent aerobic activities** can build cardiovascular fitness. For example, studies have shown that three 10-minute exercise sessions in the target zone are as effective as one 30-minute exercise session. Still, experts recommend bouts of 20 to 60 minutes in length, with several 10- to 15-minute bouts being an acceptable alternative when longer sessions are not possible.

Active Recreation Activities

Active recreation can provide important health benefits and contribute to high quality of life. Activities that you do in your free time for personal enjoyment or to "re-create" yourself are considered to be recreation activities. Recreation activities that exceed threshold

intensity for cardiovascular fitness are considered to be "active." They are more vigorous than recreation activities such as fishing, bowling and golf, which are typically classified as lifestyle or moderate-level activities (level 1 in the pyramid).

Many of the active aerobic activities, such as cycling, jogging, and skiing, could easily be classified in the active recreation as well as in the active aerobics section. Also, many of the sports that are described in a later section of this concept can be considered as active recreation activities. The distinction somewhat depends on how the activities are viewed by the individual. Some people may view recreation as what they do for fun, but it can also contribute to a healthy lifestyle.

Active recreation is popular, but participation rates in the population generally vary over time. Active recreation provides ways to experience new things, to socialize, and to obtain important health benefits. Participation rates for some common recreation activities are highlighted in Table 2, along with 5-year trends. As indicated in the table, some activities seem to gain participants, while others lose them.

Outdoor recreation activities (e.g., hiking, fishing, camping, and mountain biking) typically have a strong core of dedicated participants who have been participating for a long time. There are fewer new participants but the changes over time are generally pretty small. Other recreation activities vary widely in participation rates over time due to changing interests and demographics.

Extreme sports have become popularized through the X Games and other media outlets, and there have been corresponding trends for participation in these activities in recent years. As shown in Table 2, activities such as surfing, snowboarding, and skateboarding have had some of the highest increases in reported participation. Other activities highlighted in the SGMA survey with strong growth over the past 10–15 years are mountain biking (68 percent growth rate), kayaking (80 percent growth rate) and wakeboarding (50 percent growth rate).

Active Sport Activities

Some sports are more active than others. Some sports require more activity than others. Activities that involve muscles from different parts of the body are more active than those that involve fewer muscles. Some are of high intensity and others are less intense. When done vigorously, tennis and basketball involve many different muscle groups and are high in intensity. Soccer involves many muscle groups and is high in intensity but does not emphasize the use of the arms. Golf, on the other hand, is less intense and relies more on skill and technique. The action in basketball, tennis, and soccer involves bursts of

Table 2 ▶ Participation Rates for Common Recreational Activities

Activity	Participants (Millions)	Participants (% of Population)	Five-Year Trend (% Change)
Recreation—Outdoor			
Fishing—nonfly	43.8	16.8	-4.4
Camping—tent	41.9	16.1	-1.9
Hiking—day	39.1	15.0	1.3
Camping—RV	19.0	7.3	4.4
Horseback riding	16.0	6.1	-3.0
Wall climbing	8.6	3.3	83.0
Mountain biking	6.9	2.6	-19.8
Hiking—backpack	6.2	2.4	-8.8
Trail running	6.1	2.3	17.3
Fishing—fly	6.0	2.3	-17.8
Rock climbing	2.2	0.8	10.0
Recreation—Indoor			
Exercise to music	14.3	5.5	3.6
Martial arts	6.9	2.6	27.8
Recreation—Skating			
Inline skating	19.2	7.4	-40.0
Ice skating	17.0	6.5	-9.1
Roller skating	11.7	4.5	-20.4
Skateboarding	11.1	4.3	54.2
Roller hockey	2.7	1.0	-30.8
Recreation—Snow			
Skiing	13.6	5.2	-8.1
Snowboarding	7.8	3.0	41.8
Snowmobiling	5.5	2.1	-15.4
XC skiing	4.2	1.6	-10.6
Snowshoeing	2.5	1.0	47.1
Recreation—Water			
Canoeing	11.6	4.5	-14.7
Jet skiing	10.6	4.1	-5.4
Snorkeling	10.2	3.9	-3.8
Water skiing	8.4	3.2	-17.6
Kayaking	6.3	2.4	80.0
Sailing	5.2	2.0	-11.9
Rafting	4.5	1.7	-19.6
Wakeboarding	3.3	1.3	50.0
Scuba diving	3.2	1.2	-5.9
Surfing	2.1	0.8	50.0
Boardsailing	0.8	0.3	-27.3
Recreation—Shooting			
Hunting—gun	15.2	5.8	-9.0
Target shooting	13.8	5.3	14.0
Paintball	9.8	3.8	66.1
Archery	7.1	2.7	0.0
Trap / skeet	4.5	1.7	66.7
Hunting—bow	4.1	1.6	-12.8

Data from the Sporting Goods Manufacturers Association Survey (see Web Resources).

activity followed by rest but requires persistent, vigorous activity over a relatively long period of time. Golf requires little vigorous activity. Sports that have characteristics similar to those of basketball, tennis, and soccer have benefits like those of active aerobic activities. Of course, any sport can be more or less active, depending on how you perform it. Shooting baskets or even playing half-court basketball is not as vigorous as playing a full-court game.

The most popular sports share characteristics that contribute to their popularity. The most popular sports are often considered to be lifetime sports because they can be done at any age. The characteristics that make these sports appropriate for lifelong participation probably contribute significantly to their popularity. Often, the popular sports are adapted so people without exceptional skill can play them. For example, bowling uses a handicap system to allow people with a wide range of abilities to compete. Slow-pitch softball is much more popular than fast-pitch softball or baseball because it allows people of all abilities to play successfully.

One of the primary reasons sports participation is so popular is that sports provide a challenge. For the greatest enjoyment, the challenge of the activity should be balanced by the person's skill in the sport. If you choose to play against a person with lesser skill, you will not be challenged. On the other hand, if you lack skill or your opponent has considerably more skill, the activity will be frustrating. For optimal challenge and enjoyment, the skills of a given sport should be learned before competing. Likewise, choose an opponent who has a similar skill level.

Participation rates for some common recreation activities are highlighted in Table 3. These figures reflect total participation and not those that regularly participate. Because the survey also collects data on adolescents, the figures for some of the team sports are not accurate indicators of adult involvement. While adults still enjoy these activities as spectators there are fewer opportunities to regularly participate in them. The figures are intended primarily to show overall patterns and shouldn't be interpreted as being indicative of actual participation rates among adults.

Continuous Aerobic Activities Aerobic activities that are slow enough to be sustained for relatively long periods without frequent rest periods.

Intermittent Aerobic Activities Aerobic activities, relatively high in intensity, alternated with frequent rest periods.

Table 3 ▶ Participation Rates for Common Sports*

Activity	Participants (Millions)	Participants (% of Population)	Five-Year Trend (% Change)
Sports—Team			
Basketball	35.4	13.6	−16.5
Softball	16.0	6.1	−24.9
Football	17.9	6.9	−5.8
Soccer	17.7	6.8	−2.7
Baseball	10.9	4.2	−11.4
Cheerleading	3.6	1.4	9.1
Ice hockey	2.8	1.1	−3.4
Sports—Racquet			
Tennis	17.8	6.8	5.3
Table tennis	13.5	5.2	−10.0
Badminton	5.9	2.3	−40.4
Racquetball	4.9	1.9	−15.5
Squash	0.5	0.2	62.1
Sports—Other			
Golf	27.3	10.5	−9.0
Bowling	55.0	21.1	8.7

Data from the Sporting Goods Manufacturers Association.

*Results are based on responses from adolescents and adults.

Becoming skillful will help you enjoy sports. Improving your skill can increase the probability that you will do sports for a lifetime. The following self-management guidelines can help you improve your sport performance:

- *When learning a new activity, concentrate on the general idea of the skill first; worry about details later.* For example, a diver who concentrates on pointing the toes and keeping the legs straight at the end of a flip may land flat on his or her back. To make it all the way over, the diver should concentrate on merely doing the flip. When the general idea is mastered, then concentrate on details.

- *The beginner should be careful not to emphasize too many details at one time.* After the general idea of the skill is acquired, the learner can begin to focus on the details, one or two at a time. Concentration on too many details at one time may result in **paralysis by analysis.** For example, a golfer who is told to keep the head

down, the left arm straight, and the knees bent cannot possibly concentrate on all of these details at once. As a result, neither the details nor the general idea of the golf swing is performed properly.

- *Once the general idea of a skill is learned, a skill analysis of the performance may be helpful.* Be careful not to overanalyze; it may be helpful to have a knowledgeable person help you locate strengths and weaknesses. Movies and videotapes of skilled performances can be helpful to learners.

- *In the early stages of learning a lifetime sport or physical activity, it is not wise to engage in competition.* Beginners who compete are likely to concentrate on beating their opponent rather than on learning a skill properly. For example, in bowling, the beginner may abandon the newly learned hook ball in favor of the sure thing straight ball. This may make the person more successful immediately, but is not likely to improve the person's bowling skills for the future.

- *To be performed well, sports skills must be overlearned.* Often, when you learn a new activity, you begin to play the game immediately. The best way to learn a skill is to overlearn it, or practice it until it becomes habit. Frequently, games do not allow you to overlearn skills. For example, during a tennis match is not a good time to learn how to serve because there may be only a few opportunities to do so. For the beginner, it is much more productive to hit many serves (overlearn) with a friend until the general idea of the serve is well learned. Further, the beginner *should not* sacrifice speed to concentrate on serving for accuracy. Accuracy will come with practice of a properly performed skill.

- *When unlearning an old (incorrect) skill and learning a new (correct) skill, a person's performance may get worse before it gets better.* For example, a golfer with a baseball swing may want to learn the correct golf swing. It is important for the learner to understand that the score may worsen during the relearning stage. As the new skill is overlearned, skill will improve, as will the golf score.

- *Mental practice may aid skill learning.* Mental practice (imagining the performance of a skill) may benefit performance, especially if the performer has had previous experience in the skill. Mental practice can be especially useful in sports when the performer cannot participate regularly because of weather, business, or lack of time.

- *For beginners, practicing in front of other people may be detrimental to learning a skill.* An audience may inhibit the beginner's learning of a new sports skill. This is especially true if the learner feels that his or her performance is being evaluated by someone in the audience.

- *There is no substitute for good instruction.* Getting good instruction, especially at the beginning level, will help you learn skills faster and better. Instruction will help you apply these rules and use practice more effectively.

Strategies for Action

You can take steps to become successful in physical activity. You can use self-management skills to enjoy activities at the second level of the pyramid:

- *Select self-promoting activities.* **Self-promoting activities** require relatively little skill and can be done in a way that avoids comparison with other people. They allow you to set your own standards of success and can be done individually or in small groups that are suited to your personal needs. Examples include wheelchair distance events, jogging, resistance training, swimming, bicycling, and dance exercise.
- *Find activities that you enjoy.* There is no best form of activity! The key for long-term exercise adherence is to find exercises that you enjoy and that fit into your lifestyle. Sports are a common form of activity for younger people, but other aerobic and recreational activities have become more common among adults. This is partially because of changing interests, but also because of changing opportunities and lifestyles.

In Lab 8A, you will evaluate predisposing, enabling, and reinforcing factors that may help you identify the types of activity that are best suited to you.

- *Self-monitor your activity to help you stick with your plan.* Self-monitoring is a self-management skill that can be valuable in encouraging long-term activity adherence. A self-monitoring chart is provided in Lab 8B to help you plan and log the activities you perform in a 1-week period. This is a short-term record sheet. However, it can be copied to make a log book to allow long-term self-monitoring.
- *Improve your performance skills and technique.* Consider taking lessons and practice the skills you want to learn. Also, work to try to improve your technique. Better skills and better technique can make exercise more enjoyable (and safer). Guidelines for evaluating running technique are included in a supplemental lab found in the Online Learning Center.

Online Learning Center

www.mhhe.com/corbin7e
The Online Learning Center contains a variety of Web-based resources that will help you get the most out of this book and your course. In addition to the On the Web pages, there are video activities, interactive quizzes, application assignments, and a variety of other useful study aids. Log on to the URL above to access these resources.

Web Resources

American Council on Exercise **www.acefitness.org**
American Running Association **www.americanrunning.org**
Disabled Sports USA **www.dsusa.org**
National Association for Sports and Physical Education **www.aahperd.org/naspe/**
President's Council on Physical Fitness and Sports **www.fitness.gov**
Special Olympics International **www.specialolympics.org**
Sport Quest **www.sportQuest.com**
Sporting Goods Manufacturers Association **www.sgma.com**
X Sports **www.expn.com**

Technology Update
Dance Dance Revolution

An interactive computer game called Dance Dance Revolution (DDR) has become a popular fitness option for adolescents. The game is played on a dance pad with four arrow panels activated by the feet. The arrows are synchronized to the rhythm and beat of a chosen song, and the computer tracks the number of correct steps made on the pad. The game has multiple levels for different abilities and allows multiple people to play at one time. The game has become so popular among youth that many schools have purchased the technology for school-based physical education programs. A number of other games have developed based on this type of interaction. As game and computer technology continue to evolve, it is likely that these applications will become even more common. There are a number of Web sites devoted to DDR fans. The following site—**www.ddrfreak.com**—is just one of many.

Paralysis by Analysis An overanalysis of skill behavior. This occurs when more information is supplied than a performer can use or when concentration on too many details results in interference with performance.

Self-Promoting Activities Activities that do not require a high level of skill to be successful.

Suggested Readings

Additional reference materials for Concept 8 are available at Web10.

Web 10

Angus, R. 2006. *Competitive Judo.* Champaign, IL: Human Kinetics.

Barry, D. D., et al. 2006. *Fitness Cycling.* Champaign, IL: Human Kinetics.

Beck, K. M. 2005. *Running Strong.* Champaign, IL: Human Kinetics.

Bishop, J. G. 2005. *Fitness Through Aerobics.* San Francisco: Benjamin Cummings.

Brownson, R. C., et al. 2005. Declining rates of physical activity in the United States: What are the contributors? *Annual Review of Public Health.* 26: 421–443.

Clarke, B. 2006. *5 and 10K Training.* Champaign. IL: Human Kinetics.

Cooper, K. H. 1982. *The Aerobics Program for Total Well-Being.* New York: M. Evans.

Iknoian, T. 2005. *Fitness Walking.* 2nd ed. Champaign, IL: Human Kinetics.

Jensen, C. R. 2006. *Outdoor Recreation in America.* 6th ed. Champaign, IL: Human Kinetics.

Kil, Y. S. 2006. *Competitive Taekwondo.* Champaign, IL: Human Kinetics.

Magill, R. A. 2007. *Motor Learning and Control: Concepts and Applications.* 8th ed. New York: McGraw-Hill.

Maglischo, E. 2003. *Swimming Fastest.* Champaign, IL: Human Kinetics.

Matsuzaki, C. 2004. *Tennis Fundamentals.* Champaign, IL: Human Kinetics.

Miller, L. 2003. *Get Rolling: A Beginners Guide to In-Line Skating.* Camden, ME: Ragged Mountain Press.

Mood, D. P., et al. 2007. *Sports and Recreational Activities.* 14th ed. New York: McGraw-Hill.

Schmidt, R., & T. Lee. 2005. *Motor Control and Learning.* 4th ed. Champaign, IL: Human Kinetics.

Thomas, D. 2005. *Swimming.* 3rd ed. Champaign. IL: Human Kinetics.

U.S. Consumer Product Safety Commission. 2000. Baby boomer sports injuries. www.cpsc.gov.

In the News

Ecotourism

The popularity of physical activity for recreation and the relative ease of international travel have led to increases in the popularity of Ecotourism and adventure travel. You can book trips to go kayaking in Baja or trekking in Nepal. Others prefer bike tours through the French wine country or hiking expeditions through Mayan ruins. The common feature of these trips is that they involve active forms of recreation and exploration in distant locales. Touring companies are available to handle many of the logistical challenges—leaving vacationers with time to enjoy the scenery and the adventure.

The World Tourism Organization (WTO) cites adventure travel as one of fastest-growing segments of the tourism industry. In 2004, there were a record 763 million international tourists (an 11 percent increase over 2003 figures), and a sizable percentage of these involved planned forms of active recreation and physical activity. To ensure that resources and the environment are not damaged through their increasing use, the WTO has established clear guidelines for sustainable ecotourism. See the WTO Web site for details (**www.world-tourism.org**). The globalization of our society will likely help maintain trends for ecotourism and active travel vacations in the future.

Lab 8A The Physical Activity Adherence Questionnaire

Name		Section	Date

Purpose: To help you understand the factors that influence physical activity adherence and to see which factors you might change to improve your chances of achieving the action or maintenance level for physical activity

Procedures

1. The factors that predispose, enable, and reinforce adherence to physically active living are listed below. Read each statement. Place an X in the circle under the most appropriate response for you: very true, somewhat true, or not true.
2. When you have answered all of the items, determine a score by summing the four numbers for each type of factor. Then sum the three scores (predisposing, enabling, reinforcing) to get your total score.
3. Record your scores in the Results section and answer the questions in the Conclusions and Implications section.

	Very True	Somewhat True	Not True	
Predisposing Factors				
1. I am very knowledgeable about physical activity.	3	2	1	
2. I have a strong belief that physical activity is good for me.	3	2	1	
3. I enjoy doing regular exercise and physical activity.	3	2	1	
4. I am confident of my abilities in sports, exercise, and other physical activities.	3	2	1	
		Predisposing Score	**=**	
Enabling Factors				
5. I possess good sports skills.	3	2	1	
6. I know how to plan my own physical activity program.	3	2	1	
7. I have a place to do physical activity near my home or work.	3	2	1	
8. I have the equipment I need to do physical activities I enjoy.	3	2	1	
		Enabling Score	**=**	
Reinforcing Factors				
9. I have the support of my family for doing my regular physical activity.	3	2	1	
10. I have many friends who enjoy the same kinds of physical activities that I do.	3	2	1	
11. I have the support of my boss and my colleagues for participation in activity.	3	2	1	
12. I have a doctor and/or an employer who encourages me to exercise.	3	2	1	
		Reinforcing Score	**=**	
		Total Score (Sum 3 Scores)	**=**	

Results: Record your scores in the "score" column. Use your score and the Physical Activity Adherence Rating Chart to determine your ratings. Record your ratings in the "rating" column below.

Physical Activity Adherence Ratings

Adherence Category	Score	Rating
Predisposing		
Enabling		
Reinforcing		
Total		

Physical Activity Adherence Ratings Chart

Classification	Predisposing Score	Enabling Score	Reinforcing Score	Total Score
Adherence likely	11–12	11–12	11–12	33–36
Adherence possible	9–10	9–10	9–10	25–32
Adherence unlikely	<9	<9	<9	<25

Conclusions and Implications: In several sentences, discuss your ratings from this questionnaire. Also discuss the predisposing, enabling, and reinforcing factors that you may need to alter or increase your prospects for lifetime activity.

In several sentences, discuss what type of activiy you find most enjoyable (active aerobics, active recreation, or active sports). Comment on *why* you enjoy the acivities that you have selected.

Lab 8B Planning and Logging Participation in Active Aerobics, Sports, and Recreation

Name		Section	Date

Purpose: To set 1-week lifestyle physical activity goals, to prepare a plan, and to self-monitor progress in your 1-week active aerobics, active sports, and active recreation plan

Procedures

1. Use the planning calendar (Chart 1) to schedule several physical activity sessions for the week. Plan at least three sessions, but be realistic in your plan. Schedule activities that you enjoy and that you can perform conveniently. You may mix different activities each day for variety. Indicate the days you expect to do them and the length of time you expect to do the activity.
2. Keep a 1-week log of your actual participation using Chart 2. If possible, keep the log with you during the day. Anytime you perform an activity for 10 minutes, check one of the boxes. If you perform more than 10 minutes of activity in one session, check additional 10-minute blocks. If you cannot keep the log with you, fill in the log at the end of the day. If you choose to keep a log for more than 1 week, make copies of the extra log sheet.
3. Log only those activities for which you meet the target zone for cardiovascular fitness. Remember that 5 or 6, rather than 7, days a week of more vigorous activity is recommended. You can create a log book using several log sheets.
4. Sum the total number of minutes for each day by tallying the number of activity blocks.
5. Answer the questions in the Results section.

Results

	Yes	No
Did you do 20 or more minutes at each session?	◯	◯
Did you do 20 or more minutes of activity on at least 3 days?	◯	◯

Conclusions and Implications

1. Do you feel that you will use active aerobics, active sports, or active recreation as a regular part of your lifetime physical activity plan, either now or in the future? Use several sentences to explain your answer.

2. Did the logging of your activity make you more aware of your daily activity patterns? In several sentences, explain why or why not.

Write the number of minutes you plan to do each activity each day. You may use a mix of activities each day.

Chart 1 ▶ Planning Calendar

Activity	Monday	Tuesday	Wednesday	Thursday	Friday	Saturday	Sunday
Active Aerobics (name)							
1.							
2.							
3.							
4.							
Active Recreation (name)							
1.							
2.							
3.							
4.							
Active Sports (name)							
1.							
2.							
3.							
4.							
Total Minutes Per Day							

Chart 2 ▶ Activity Log

Record the length of each activity session you actually performed.
Make a check in the appropriate box for each 10-minute time block under the day that you did the activity.

Activity	Monday	Tuesday	Wednesday	Thursday	Friday	Saturday	Sunday
Active Aerobics (name)							
1.							
2.							
3.							
4.							
Active Recreation (name)							
1.							
2.							
3.							
4.							
Active Sports (name)							
1.							
2.							
3.							
4.							
Total Minutes Per Day							

You may wish to make a copy of this page to use for future planning.

Lab 8B

Planning and Logging Participation in Active Aerobics, Sports, and Recreation

Flexibility

Health Goals for the year 2010

- Increase proportion of people who regularly perform exercises for flexibility.

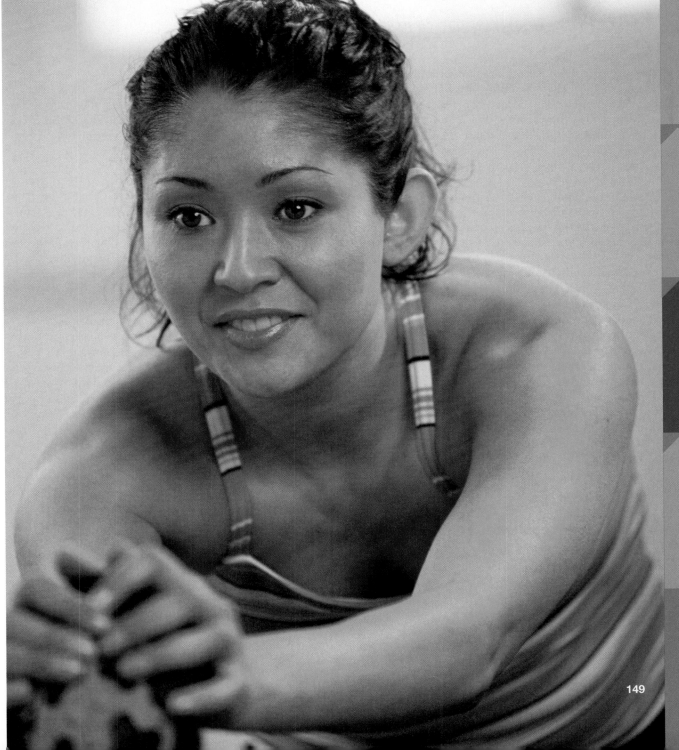

149

*Regular stretching exercises promote flexibility—
a component of fitness—that permits freedom of
movement, contributes to ease and economy of muscular
effort, allows for successful performance in certain
activities, and provides less susceptibility to some types of
injuries or musculoskeletal problems.*

Flexibility refers to the amount of motion that is possible at a given joint or series of joints. A joint with limited ability to bend or straighten is said to be tight or stiff, while joints with a high degree of flexibility are referred to as loose-jointed, or hypermobile. A reasonable amount of flexibility is needed to perform efficiently and effectively in daily life, but excessive flexibility is not desirable.

Flexibility is highly specific. An individual may demonstrate optimal flexibility in one region of the body while having stiffness in other joints. For example, a person may have good flexibility of the spine, hips, and legs in order to reach down and touch the toes but be unable to clasp both hands behind the back due to stiffness of the shoulder joints. The optimal amount of flexibility for a given joint is dependent on the specific needs of the individual. For instance, a figure skater requires a greater degree of trunk and hip flexibility for skill performance than does a hockey player. An electrician doing overhead work requires a greater degree of shoulder flexibility than does a receptionist.

This concept will explain how flexibility is assessed and will describe how much flexibility is needed for good health. Guidelines are also provided on proper stretching techniques to help you establish a program that will build good flexibility.

On the Web

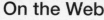

www.mhhe.com/corbinweb
Log on to this URL before reading this concept. See On the Web list of concepts. Click on the concept number you want to view. To access supplemental information, click on the number shown at each Web icon.

Flexibility Fundamentals

Flexibility is not the same thing as stretching. Flexibility is a component of health-related physical fitness. It is a state of being. Stretching is the primary technique used to improve the state of one's flexibility.

The range of motion in a joint or joints is a reflection of the flexibility at that joint. Clinically, the **range of motion (ROM)** of a joint is the extent *and* direction of movement that is possible. The extent of movement is described by the arc through which a joint moves and is typically measured in degrees using a tool called a goniometer. The direction of movement at a specific joint is determined by the shapes of the boney surfaces that are in contact. Certain types of joints allow for a greater degree of movement than others.

Doctors and physical therapists use a specific vocabulary to describe the movement of joints. Figure 1 illustrates the use of some of these movement terms as they relate to hip, knee, or ankle motion. Similar terms are applied in describing movement of the spine and upper body. Note that the same terms (such as *flexion/extension*) can be applied to different joints of the body, while other terms (such as *dorsiflexion/plantar flexion*) are unique to a specific joint such as the ankle.

The shape, size, and orientation of a joint greatly influence the amount of motion available. The circular surface of the ball-and-socket joint of the hip, for example, allows for considerable mobility including movement to the side (adduction and abduction), forward and backward (flexion and extension), and in and out (internal and external rotation). The hinge joint of the knee is more restrictive and limits movement to primarily forward and backward (flexion and extension). Motion at other joints, such as the ankle, involve the combined movements of numerous bony surfaces. A hinge-type portion permits the up and down motion of the foot (dorsiflexion and plantar

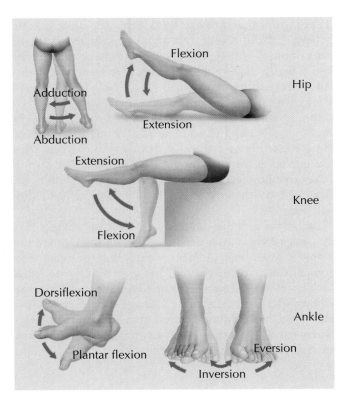

Figure 1 ▶ Ranges of joint motion.

flexion), while a separate planar-type joint allows the side to side motion (inversion and eversion) of the foot. A basic understanding of this terminology is important in understanding principles of flexibility and stretching.

Factors Influencing Flexibility

Long muscle-tendon units (MTUs) are important to flexibility. The extent of movement available at a specific joint is determined by the shape of the joint, as well as by the tautness of the ligaments and the action of the muscles and tendons that cross the joint. **Ligaments** are bands of connective tissue that connect bones together at a joint. They provide rigidity and stability to the joint capsule and restrict excessive motion at the joint. Damage to ligaments from repeated sprains can lead to excessive joint **laxity** and increase risk for injuries. **Tendons** are also made of connective tissue, but they attach muscles to bone. Having long muscles and tendons allows for greater range of motion and better flexibility. Together, the muscles and tendons are referred to as a **muscle-tendon unit (MTU)**. Muscle fibers are more extensible and elastic than tendons but both are stretched together. However, for ease of understanding, the phrase "muscle

stretching" rather than MTU stretching will be used in this concept.

The properties of connective tissue and muscle impact flexibility. Nearly one-fourth of the body's protein is collagen, a connective tissue making up the ligaments, tendons, and noncontractile elements of muscle. Collagen has both viscous and elastic properties. Viscous tissue will lengthen permanently when a force is applied to it, much like a piece of taffy being pulled and stretched. Elastic tissue, on the other hand, returns to its original length, much like the recoil of a rubber band or spring after being stretched. Stretching must be performed for an adequate time to allow the viscous tissues to stretch and lengthen. Stretching must also be done frequently to keep elastic tissues from returning to their normal length.

Static flexibility is different from dynamic flexibility. A joint's flexibility can be described differently depending on how it is assessed. Static flexibility is the maximum range a joint can achieve under stationary conditions. An example is the hip ROM achieved during a hamstring stretch. Static flexibility is limited by passive viscous and elastic properties of the MTU. Dynamic flexibility is the maximum range a joint can achieve under active conditions. An example is the maximum height and position of a hurdler's lead leg. While it may seem logical that dynamic flexibility would be greater than static, the opposite is true. Dynamic flexibility is affected by both passive and active elements of the MTU. The hurdler's performance depends on passive MTU extensibility as well as the ability to move against gravity, at fast speeds, and without elicitation of a stretch reflex. While good static flexibility is necessary for good dynamic flexibility, it does not ensure it. Athletes must train both static and dynamic flexibility for optimal performance.

Flexibility varies considerably across the life span. Flexibility is generally high in children but declines during adolescence because of the rapid changes

---

Range of Motion (ROM) The full motion possible in a joint or series of joints.

Ligaments Bands of tissue that connect bones. Unlike muscles and tendons, overstretching ligaments is not desirable.

Laxity Motion in a joint outside the normal plane for that joint, due to loose ligaments.

Tendons Fibrous bands of tissue that connect muscles to bones and facilitate movement of a joint.

Muscle-Tendon Unit (MTU) The skeletal muscles and the tendons that connect them to bones. Stretching to improve flexibility is associated with increased length of the MTU.

in growth—essentially, the bones grow faster than the MTU. In early adulthood, the MTU catches up to the skeletal system, causing flexibility to peak in the mid- to late twenties. With increasing age, range of motion tends to decline again. The reduced flexibility is due to a loss of elasticity in the MTU and cross-linkages within the collagen fibers of the tendons, ligaments, and joint capsules. Over the span of their working lives, adults typically lose 3 to 4 inches of lower back flexibility as measured by the common "sit-and-reach" test. Research studies have confirmed that the declines in flexibility are not as evident in individuals who maintain regular patterns of physical activity. The use of planned stretching programs has also been shown to help maintain flexibility with age.

Gender differences exist in flexibility. Girls tend to be more flexible than boys at young ages, but the gender difference becomes smaller for adults. The greater flexibility of females is generally attributed to anatomical differences (e.g., wider hips) and hormonal influences. Preferred activity patterns may also explain some of the difference, as females tend to be involved in sports and activities that require good flexibility and involve regular stretching (e.g., dance, gymnastics, swimming).

Genetic factors can explain some individual variability in flexibility. In some families, the trait for loose joints is passed from generation to generation. This **hypermobility** is sometimes referred to as joint looseness. Studies show that people with this trait may be more prone to joint dislocation.

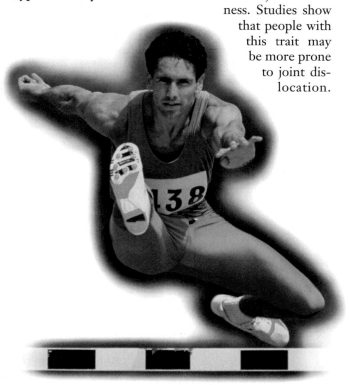

Dynamic flexibility is important in many sports.

There is not much research evidence, but some experts believe that those with hypermobility may also be more susceptible to athletic or dance injuries, especially to the knee, ankle, and shoulder, and may be more apt to develop premature osteoarthritis.

Lack of use or misuse can cause reductions in flexibility. Lack of physical activity is one of the major factors contributing to poor flexibility. When muscles are moved as part of normal daily activities or during structured physical activity, the muscles and tendons get stretched. Without this regular stimulation, flexibility will decrease.

Improper exercise can lead to muscle imbalances that may negatively impact flexibility. The most common example is when body builders overdevelop their biceps in comparison to their triceps. This leads to a *muscle-bound* look characterized by a restricted range of motion in the elbow joint. To avoid this, it is important to exercise muscles through the full range of motion and to provide sufficient exercise for the **antagonist muscles** involved in a specific movement.

Health Benefits of Flexibility and Stretching

No ideal standard for flexibility exists. It is not known how much flexibility any one person should have in a joint. Norms are available that list how hundreds of subjects of various ages, of both sexes, and in many walks of life have performed on different tests. But there is little scientific evidence to indicate that a person who can reach 2 inches past his or her toes on a sit-and-reach test is less fit than a person who can reach 8 inches past the toes. Too much flexibility could be as detrimental as too little. The standards presented in the *Lab Resource Materials* are based on the best available evidence.

Adequate flexibility is necessary for achieving and maintaining optimal posture. Short and tight muscles in certain body regions can result in poor posture. Shortness of muscles of the chest and back of the neck can result in "rounded shoulders" and a "forward head" position. Tightness of the hip flexor muscles can result in excessive lordosis, or arching, of the low back.

Extremes of inflexibility and hyperflexibility increase the likelihood of injury. Research linking stretching to the prevention of injury has been equivocal, with some studies showing benefits but others not. A number of recent articles have systematically reviewed the literature on stretching to try to explain the different findings. The general consensus is that the problems lie in the extremes. Short, tight muscles and tendons are more likely to be

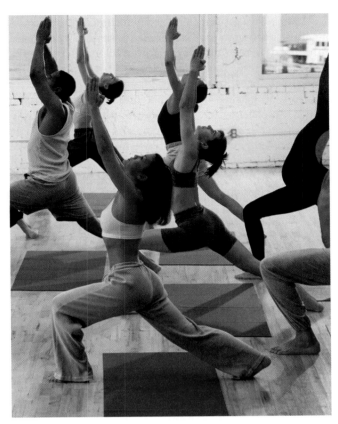

Yoga and other movement classes involving stretching are becoming increasingly popular.

While good flexibility is beneficial, the most recent evidence indicates that warm-up stretching prior to competition can actually impair performance in some activities. For example, warm-up stretching has been shown to reduce strength performance jumping height, and running economy. Because of this, experts suggest that flexibility training (different from a stretching warm-up) should not be done on the day of a performance. A stretching warm-up is still recommended after a general warm-up, but the warm-up period is not the time to conduct an extensive flexibility program—especially for those preparing for high-level performance. Stretching to improve flexibility should be conducted at the end of training, when the muscles are warm and performance is not imminent.

Stretching may help to relieve muscle cramps, stiffness, and some local or referred pain. A muscle spasm or cramp may result for various reasons, including overexertion, dehydration, and heat stress. Stretching a cramped (but not a strained) muscle will help relieve the cramp. When body parts are held in static positions for long periods, or when muscles are chronically overloaded, fatigued, or chilled, **trigger points** may cause stiffness and local or referred pain. Often, the trigger point can be deactivated and the pain relieved by gentle but persistent stretching of the muscle, especially if heat or cold packs are applied.

Stretching is probably *ineffective* in preventing muscle soreness. In the past, it was suggested that stretching during a cool-down will *prevent* muscular soreness. In a controlled study, however, muscle soreness was deliberately induced in a group of subjects. When half of the group stretched immediately afterward and at intervals for 48 hours, they had as much soreness as the group who did not stretch.

Overstretching may make a person susceptible to injury or hamper performance. Muscles and tendons can lengthen (extensibility) and return to their normal

involuntarily overstretched (strained) than are long ones. However, excess flexibility can compromise the integrity of the joint capsule and increase tissue compliance to an extent that injuries are more likely. An appropriate amount of flexibility provides benefits without the risks. For individual bouts of activity, a good cardiovascular warm-up is definitely more important than a preexercise bout of stretching.

Adequate flexibility may help prevent muscle strain and such orthopedic problems as backache. Back pain is a leading medical complaint in Western culture. One common cause of backache is shortened lower back muscles and hip flexor muscles. Short hamstrings (muscles in the back of the leg) are also associated with lower back problems. Improving flexibility can decrease risk for back problems.

There are questions about the value of stretching prior to competition. The longer length and reduced **stiffness** in muscles in people with good flexibility allows greater **stretch tolerance** that lead to improved performance. For example, a diver must have flexibility to perform a pike dive, and a hurdler must have good flexibility in the back, hip, and leg to perform well.

Hypermobility Looseness or slackness in the joint and of the muscles and ligaments (soft tissue) surrounding the joint.

Antagonist Muscles In this concept, *antagonist* refers to the muscle group on the opposite side of the limb from the muscle group being stretched (e.g., biceps is the antagonist of triceps).

Stiffness Elasticity in the MTU; measured by force needed to stretch.

Stretch Tolerance Greater stretch for the same pain level.

Trigger Points Especially irritable spots, usually tight bands or knots in a muscle or fascia (a sheath of connective tissue that binds muscles and other tissues together). Trigger points often refer pain to another area of the body.

length after stretching (elasticity). Ligaments and the joint capsule are extensible but lack elasticity. When stretched, they remain in the lengthened state. If this occurs, the joint may lack stability and is susceptible to chronic dislocation or movement in an undesirable plane. This is particularly true of weight-bearing joints, such as the hip, knee, and ankle. Loose ligaments may allow the joint to twist abnormally, tearing the cartilage and other soft tissue.

Stretching Methods

To develop flexibility, do exercises from the flexibility exercise section of the physical activity pyramid. The activities in the first two levels of the physical activity pyramid (see Figure 2) do little to develop flexibility. To build this important part of fitness, stretching exercises from the third level of the pyramid are essential. Three commonly used types of stretching exercises are **static stretch, proprioceptive neuromuscular facilitation (PNF),** and **ballistic stretch.**

Static stretching is widely recommended because most experts believe it is less likely to cause injury. Static stretching is done slowly and held for a period of several seconds. With this type of stretch, the probability of tearing the soft tissue is low if performed properly. Static stretches can be performed with **active assistance** or with **passive assistance.**

When active assistance is used, you contract the opposing muscle group to produce a reflex relaxation (**reciprocal inhibition**) in the muscles you are stretching. This enables you to stretch the muscle more easily. For example, when doing a calf stretch exercise (see Figure 3A), the muscles on the front of the shin are contracted to assist in the stretch of the muscles of the calf. However, active assistance to static stretching has one problem. It is almost impossible to produce adequate overload by simply contracting the opposing muscles.

When passive assistance (see Figure 3B, C) is used, an outside force, such as a partner, aids you in stretching. For example, in the calf stretch, passive assistance can be provided by another person (Figure 3B), another body part (Figure 3B), or gravity (Figure 3C). This type of stretch does not create the relaxation in the muscle associated with active assisted stretch. An unrelaxed muscle cannot be stretched as far, and injury may happen. Therefore, it is best to combine the active assistance with a passive assistance when performing a static stretch. This gives the advantage of a relaxed muscle and a sufficient force to provide an overload to stretch it.

A good way to begin static stretching exercises is to stretch until you begin to feel tension, back off slightly and hold the position several seconds, and then gradually stretch a little farther, back off, and hold. Decrease the stretch slowly after the hold.

Ballistic stretching is not recommended for most people. A ballistic stretch uses momentum to produce the stretch. Momentum is produced by vigorous motion, such as flinging a body part (bobbing) or rocking it back and forth to create a bouncing movement. As with static stretching, the ballistic movement can be provided either actively or passively. For example, in the calf stretch shown

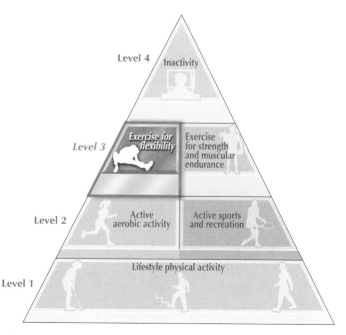

Figure 2 ▶ Flexibility or stretching exercises should be selected from level 3 of the physical acivity pyramid.

Static Stretch A muscle is slowly stretched, then held in that stretched position for several seconds.

Proprioceptive Neuromuscular Facilitation (PNF) A type of static stretch most commonly characterized by a precontraction of the muscle to be stretched and a contraction of the antagonist muscle during the stretch.

Ballistic Stretch Muscles are stretched by the force of momentum of a body part that is bounced, swung, or jerked.

Active Assistance An assist to stretch from an active contraction of the opposing (antagonist) muscle.

Passive Assistance Stretch imposed on a muscle with the assistance of a force other than the opposing muscle.

Reciprocal Inhibition Reflex relaxation in stretched muscle during contraction of the antagonist.

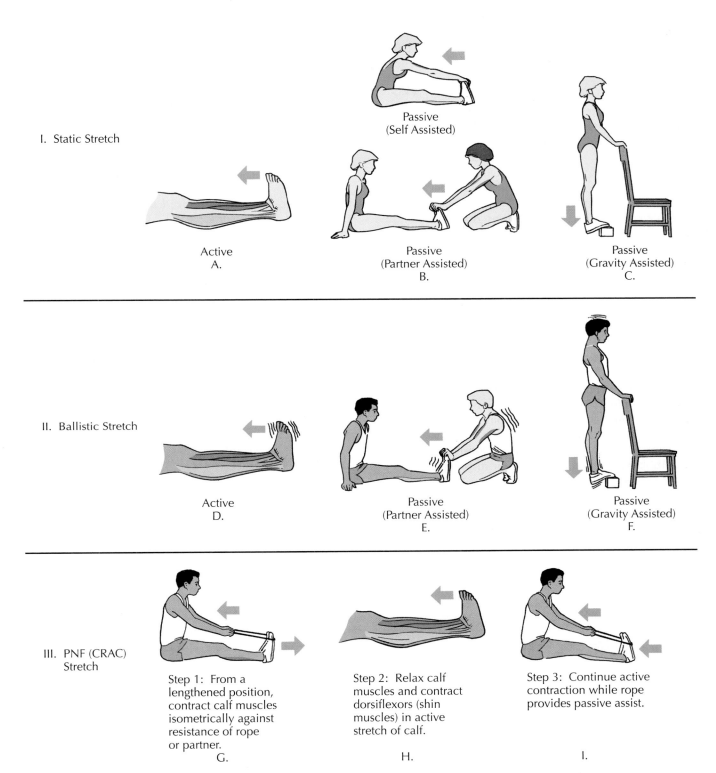

Figure 3 ▶ Examples of static, ballistic, PNF, active, and passive stretches of the calf muscles (gastronemius and soleus). Muscles shown in dark pink are the muscles being contracted. Muscles shown in light pink are those being stretched.

I. Static Stretch

Passive
(Self Assisted)

Active
A.

Passive
(Partner Assisted)
B.

Passive
(Gravity Assisted)
C.

II. Ballistic Stretch

Active
D.

Passive
(Partner Assisted)
E.

Passive
(Gravity Assisted)
F.

III. PNF (CRAC)
Stretch

Step 1: From a lengthened position, contract calf muscles isometrically against resistance of rope or partner.
G.

Step 2: Relax calf muscles and contract dorsiflexors (shin muscles) in active stretch of calf.
H.

Step 3: Continue active contraction while rope provides passive assist.
I.

in Figure 3D, E, and F, the foot is actively bounced forward by the antagonist muscle force or passively by an assist from another person or gravity. The forceful movement in ballistic stretching may increase risks for injury. Therefore, this form of stretching is not recommended for most people.

The inherent problem with most ballistic stretching is the lack of control over the force and range of movement. Experts have begun to characterize *dynamic stretching* as a safe derivative of ballistic stretching. This form of stretching uses gradual and controlled movement of body parts up to the limit of a joint's range of motion. Stretches may involve arm or leg swings of increasing reach or increasing speed. The key is to perform the movement in a controlled manner through the normal range of motion. This approach allows dynamic stretching to be a safe and efficient means of using active stretching techniques.

PNF techniques have proven to be most effective at improving flexibility. PNF has been popular for rehabilitation since the 1960s. It consists of dozens of techniques to stimulate muscles to contract more strongly or to relax more fully, so that they can be stretched. Several PNF techniques have become popular in fitness programs to improve the flexibility of healthy people. The contract-relax-antagonist-contract (CRAC) technique is the most popular. CRAC PNF involves three steps: (1) Move the limb so the muscle to be stretched is elongated initially; then contract it **(agonist muscle)** isometrically for several seconds (against an immovable object or the resistance of a partner); (2) relax

the muscle; and (3) immediately statically stretch the muscle with the active assistance of the antagonist muscle and an assist from a partner, gravity, or another body part. Figure 3G, H, and I provide a detailed illustration of how this technique is applied to the calf stretch. Research shows that this and other types of PNF stretch are more effective than a simple static stretch.

How Much Stretch Is Enough

Stretching exercises should be done regularly to achieve optimal benefits. Threshold and target zones for each type of stretching to improve and maintain flexibility are presented in Table 1. The values in this table illustrate how the principles of overload and progression are best applied to promote and maintain flexibility through regular stretching.

Note that stretching should be done at least three times a week and that daily stretching is preferable. Evidence suggests that even 1 week without stretching can lead to decreases in muscle length and increases in stiffness, so it is important to develop a regular routine of stretching. However, like other forms of activity, 1 day is clearly better than none.

To increase the length of a muscle, you must stretch it more than its normal length (overload) but not overstretch it. The best evidence suggests that muscles should be stretched to about 10

Table 1 ▶ Flexibility Threshold of Training and Target Zones

	Threshold of Training			Target Zones		
	Static	**Ballistic**	**PNF (CRAC)**	**Static**	**Ballistic**	**PNF (CRAC)**
Frequency	• 3 days per week for all methods			• 3 to 7 days per week for all methods		
Intensity	• Stretch as far as you can without pain; with slow movement, hold at the end of the range of motion.	• Stretch muscle beyond normal length with gentle bounce or swing, but do not exceed 10 percent of active-static range of motion.	• Same as static, except use a maximum isometric contraction of muscle prior to stretch	• Add assist. • Avoid over-stretch and pain for all methods.	• Same as threshold	• Same as static • Add assist.
Time	• Hold 15 seconds. • 3 reps • Rest 30 seconds between reps.	• Continuous reps for 30 seconds (this is 1 set)	• Hold isometric contraction 3 seconds. • Hold stretch 15 seconds. • 3 reps • Rest 30 seconds between reps.	• Hold 15–60 seconds. • 3–5 reps • Rest 30 seconds between reps. • Rest 1 minute between sets.	• 1–3 sets • Rest 1 minute between sets.	• 3–5 reps of 3- second con-traction and 15- to 60-second hold • Rest 30 seconds between reps. • 1–3 sets • Rest 1 minute between sets.

percent beyond their normal length to bring about an improvement in flexibility. More practical indicators of the intensity of stretching are to stretch just to the point of tension or just before discomfort. Exercises that do not cause an overload will not increase flexibility. Once adequate flexibility has been achieved, **range of motion (ROM) exercises** that do not require stretch greater than normal can be performed to maintain flexibility and joint range of motion.

For flexibility to be increased, you must stretch and hold muscles beyond normal length for an adequate amount of time. When a muscle is stretched (lengthened), the stretch reflex acts to resist the stretch (see Figure 4). Sensory receptors (A) in the muscle tendon unit (MTU), send a signal to the sensory neurons (B), and these neurons signal the motor neurons (C) to contract (shorten) the muscles (D). This reflex restricts initial efforts at stretching; however, if the stretch is held and maintained over time, the stretch reflex subsides and allows the muscle to lengthen (this phase is called the development phase because it is at this time that improvements occur). This reflex is important to understand because it explains why it is important to hold a stretch for an extended period of time. Attempts to stretch for shorter durations are limited by the opposing action of the stretch reflex (see Figure 4). In the past, stretches of 10 to 30 seconds were recommended. New studies, however, suggest that, to get the most benefit for the least effort, stretching for at least 15 seconds and up to 30 to 60 seconds for each repetition is recommended (see Figure 5).

For flexibility to be increased, you must repeat stretching exercises an adequate number of times. Figure 5 shows the typical responses to a stretched muscle during a series of stretches. Tension in a muscle decreases as the stretch is held. Most of the decrease occurs in the first 15 seconds. The tension curves are lower with each successive repetition of stretching, which is why multiple sets of stretching are recommended. The ACSM recommends three or four repetitions because this number seems to give the most benefits for the amount of time spent in exercise. Recent evidence suggests that one or two repetitions are adequate for most healthy people not interested in high-level performance.

Performing warm-up exercises is not the same as doing a stretching workout for flexibility development. The warm-up typically includes stretching exercises to prepare you for the workout and to reduce the risk for injury. Modest static stretching exercises done after a general warm-up are recommended by most experts (see Concept 3). Stretching exercises are typically done later in the workout to promote flexibility.

The best time for stretching is when the muscles are warm. Some studies have shown that increasing the temperature of the muscle through warm-up exercises or heat packs has resulted in improved ability to stretch muscle.

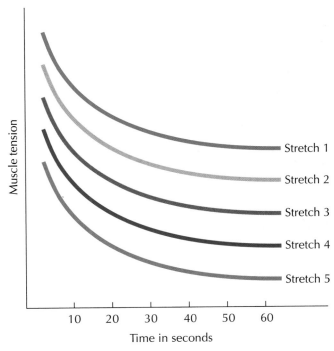

Figure 5 ► Typical responses to a stretched muscle during a series of stretches.

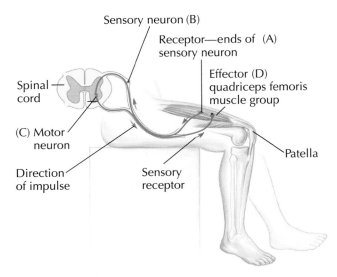

Figure 4 ► The stretch reflex.
Source: Shier, Butler, and Lewis.

Agonist Muscles Muscle group being stretched.

Range of Motion (ROM) Exercises Exercises used to maintain existing joint mobility (to prevent loss of ROM).

Other studies have failed to find a difference between the flexibility of subjects who warmed up and those who did not warm up. Some experts believe that cooling the muscle with ice packs in the final phases of stretching aids in lengthening the muscle, but one study failed to confirm this. Until scientists reach a consensus, it seems wise to perform the stretching phase of your workout when the muscles are warm. This means that stretching can be done in the middle or near the end of the workout. Since some people do not want to interrupt their workout in the middle, they prefer to stretch at the end. Stretching at the end of the workout serves a dual purpose—building flexibility and cooling down. It is, however, appropriate to stretch at any time in the workout after the muscles have been active and are warm.

Flexibility-Based Activities and Training Aids

Web 04

The popularity of flexibility-based activity has increased in recent years. Movement disciplines such as yoga, Tai Chi, and Pilates, have been around for many years, but they have only recently become popular among fitness enthusiasts. While popularity of these activities is high, the health benefits of some of them have not been well established. The positions and movements recommended in some of the activity sessions may be contraindicated exercises that could increase risk for injuries. If you choose to participate in these activities, make sure that you find qualified instructors and that you progress very gradually. See Concept 11 for more information about safe and contraindicated exercise.

Tai Chi is one of the safest and more established movement disciplines. Tai Chi (often translated as Chinese shadow boxing) is considered a martial art but involves the execution of slow, flowing movements called forms. Recent studies have confirmed that regular participation in Tai Chi may provide health benefits. One study demonstrated that Tai Chi instruction improved balance and strength in people age 70 and older and reduced the risk of falling in this group. It has also been associated with reduced anxiety and stress.

Yoga is a diverse and controversial movement discipline. *Yoga* is an umbrella term that refers to a number of yoga traditions. The foundation for most yoga traditions is Hatha Yoga, which incorporates a variety of asanas (postures). Iyengar yoga is another popular variation. It uses similar asanas as Hatha Yoga but uses props and cushions to enhance the movements. Emphasis is placed on balance through coordinated breathing and precise body alignment. Most forms of yoga are considered to be safe but positions in some of the extreme yoga disciplines have been criticized by movement specialists and physical therapists as causing

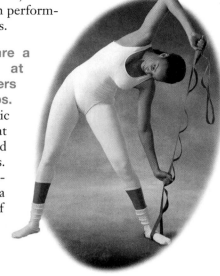

more harm than good, so care should be used when performing some movements.

Pilates classes are a popular offering at many fitness centers and health clubs. Pilates is a therapeutic exercise regimen that combines strength and flexibility movements. It was originally developed as more of a therapeutic form of exercise, but it is increasingly being promoted as an overall form of conditioning. Emphasis in Pilates exercise is on core

Stretching ropes can enhance stretching exercise.

stabilization movements and enhanced body awareness, but classes typically include some stretching activities as well.

Specialized equipment may help improve the effectiveness and ease of stretching exercise. One advance in equipment technology for flexibility training is the development of "stretching ropes." These ropes have multiple loops, which enable individuals to change the length of the rope and perform a variety of different exercises. This feature provides an easy way to put muscles on stretch and to vary the degree of stretch. Because you can apply resistance through the elastic straps, it is even possible to perform PNF stretching without the assistance of a partner. A variety of stretching ropes are available on the market, and they all provide similar functionality. Foam rollers are another stretching aid that may facilitate flexibility exercise (see Technology Update).

Technology Update
Foam Rollers

Web 05

Foam rollers are cylindrical pieces of exercise equipment being widely used in rehabilitation clinics and fitness centers. In conjunction with specific exercises, they are used to improve strength, balance, and flexibility by challenging movement in two planes. The rollers come in a variety of sizes and densities. A typical roller is 6 inches in diameter by 3 feet long. Half rollers possess a flat side, which provides greater stability and increased ease of exercise in a supine position. Rollers can be used to stretch a variety of muscles. Examples of their use are provided in the On the Web feature.

Guidelines for Safe and Effective Stretching Exercise

There is a correct way to perform flexibility exercises. Remember that stretching can *cause* muscle soreness, so "easy does it." Start at your threshold if you are unaccustomed to stretching a given muscle group; then increase within the target zone. The list in Table 2 will help you gain the most benefit from your exercises.

Stretching is specific to each muscle or muscle group. No single exercise can produce total flexibility. For example, stretching tight hamstrings can increase the length of these muscles but will not lengthen the muscles in other areas of the body. For total flexibility, it is important to stretch each of the major muscle groups and to use the major joints of the body through full range of normal motion.

Table 2 ▶ Do and Don't List for Stretching	
Do	**Don't**
Do warm muscles before you attempt to stretch them.	Don't stretch to the point of pain. Remember, you want to stretch muscles, not joints.
Do stretch with care if you have osteoporosis or arthritis.	Don't use ballistic stretches if you have osteoporosis or arthritis.
Do use static or PNF stretching rather than ballistic stretching if you are a beginner.	Don't perform ballistic stretches with passive assistance unless you are under the supervision of an expert.
Do stretch weak or recently injured muscles with care.	Don't ballistically stretch weak or recently injured muscles.
Do use great care in applying passive assistance to a partner; go slowly and ask for feedback.	Don't overstretch a muscle after it has been immobilized (such as in a sling or cast) for a long period.
Do perform stretching exercises for each muscle group and at each joint where flexibility is desired.	Don't bounce a muscle through excessive range of motion. Ballistic stretches should be gentle and should not involve excessive range of motion.
Do make certain the body is in good alignment when stretching.	Don't stretch swollen joints without professional supervision.
Do stretch muscles of small joints in the extremities first; then progress toward the trunk with muscles of larger joints.	Don't stretch several muscles at one time until you have stretched individual muscles. For example, stretch muscles at the ankle, then the knee, then the ankle and knee simultaneously.
Do precede sport-specific ballistic stretch with static or PNF stretching.	

Strategies for Action

Web 06

An important step for developing and maintaining flexibility is assessing your current status. An important early step in taking action to improve fitness is self-assessment. There are dozens of tests of flexibility. Four tests that assess range of motion in the major joints of the body, that require little equipment, and that can be easily administered are presented in the *Lab Resources Materials* at the end of this concept. In Lab 9A, you will get an opportunity to try these self-assessments. It is recommended that you perform these assessments before you begin your regular stretching program and use these assessments to reevaluate your flexibility periodically.

Scores on flexibility tests may be influenced by several factors. Your range of motion at any one time may be influenced by your motivation to exert maximum effort, warm-up preparation, muscular soreness, tolerance for pain, room temperature, and ability to relax. Recent studies have found a relationship between leg or trunk length and the scores made on the sit-and-reach test. The sit-and-reach test used in this book is adapted to allow for differences in body build.

Select exercises that promote flexibility in all areas of the body. The ACSM recommends that adults regularly perform 8 to 10 stretching exercises for the major muscle groups of the body. Table 3 describes some of the most effective exercises for a basic flexibility routine. Individual stretching needs may vary, but the most common areas to target are the trunk, the legs, and the arms. A variety of stretches for these areas are described in Tables

3, 4, and 5. Most are designed for static stretching, but the pectoral stretch and back-saver hamstring stretch use PNF techniques. Ballistic stretching exercises are discussed in more detail in Concept 14.

Keeping records of progress is important to adhering to a stretching program. An activity logging sheet is provided in Lab 9B to help you keep records of your progress as you regularly perform stretching exercises to build and maintain good flexibility.

Online Learning Center

www.mhhe.com/corbin7e
The Online Learning Center contains a variety of Web-based resources that will help you get the most out of this book and your course. In addition to the On the Web pages, there are video activities, interactive quizzes, application assignments, and a variety of other useful study aids. Log on to the URL above to access these resources.

Web Resources

Orthopedic Physical Therapy Products (source for stretching ropes) **www.optp.com**
Web 07 ▮ The Physician and Sportsmedicine
www.physsportsmed.com

Suggested Readings

Additional reference materials for Concept 9 are available at Web08.

Web 08 ▮

Alter, M. J. 1996. *Science of Flexibility*. Champaign, IL: Human Kinetics.

Bracko, M. R. 2002. Can stretching prior to exercise and sports improve performance and prevent injury? *ACSM's Health and Fitness Journal* 6(5):17–22.

Chewning, B., T. M. A. Yu, and J. Johnson. 2000. Tai chi: Effects on health. *ACSM's Health and Fitness Journal* 4(3):17–19.

Choi, J. H. 2005. Effects of Sun-style Tai Chi exercise on physical fitness and fall prevention in fall-prone older adults. *Journal of Advanced Nursing* 51:150–157.

Clay, C. C., et al. 2005. The metabolic cost of Hatha Yoga. *Journal of Strength and Conditioning Research* 19:604–610.

DiBrezzo, R., et al. 2005. Exercise intervention designed to improve strength and dynamic balance among community-dwelling older adults. *Journal of Aging and Physical Activity* 13:198–209.

Greiner, S. G., C. Russell, and S. M. McGill. 2003. Relationships between lumbar flexibility, sit-and-reach test, and a previous history of low back pain in industrial workers. *Canadian Journal of Applied Physiology* 28(2):165–171.

Hootman, J. M., et al. 2002. Epidemiology of musculoskeletal injuries among sedentary and physically active adults. *Medicine and Science in Sports and Exercise* 34(5):838–844.

Knudsen, D. V. 2000. Stretching during warm-up: Do we have enough evidence? *Journal of Physical Education, Recreation and Dance* 70(2):271–277.

Knudsen, D. V., et al. 2000. Current issues in flexibility fitness. *President's Council on Physical Fitness and Sports Research Digest* 2(10):1–8.

Lemmink, K. A., et al. 2003. The validity of the sit-and-reach test and the modified sit-and-reach test in middle-aged to older men and women. *Research Quarterly for Exercise and Sport* 74(3):331–336.

Li, J. X., et al. 2001. Tai chi: Physiological characteristics and beneficial effects on health. *British Journal of Sports Medicine* 35(3):148–156.

McAtee, R. 1993. *Facilitated Stretching*. Champaign, IL: Human Kinetics.

Parks, K. A., et al. 2003. A comparison of lumbar range of motion and functional ability scores in patients with low back pain: Assessment for range of motion validity. *Spine* 28(4): 380–384.

Sherman, K.J., et al., 2005. Comparing yoga, exercise, and a self-care book for chronic low back pain: A randomized, controlled trial. *Annals of Internal Medicine* 143(12):849–56.

Shier, D., J. Butler, and R. Lewis. 2007. *Hole's Essentials of Anatomy and Physiology*. 11th ed. New York: McGraw-Hill.

Shrier, I. 2004. Does stretching improve performance?: A systematic and critical review of the literature. *Clinical Journal of Sport Medicine* Volume 14(5):267–273.

Shrier, I. 2005. When and how to stretch. *The Physician and Sports Medicine* 33(3):22–26.

Shrier, I., and K. Gossal. 2000. Myths and truths of stretching. *The Physician and Sportsmedicine* 28(8):57–63.

Thacker, S. B., et al. 2004. The impact of stretching on sports injury risk: A systematic review of the literature. *Medicine and Science in Sports and Exercise* 36(3):371–378.

In the News

Increasing Popularity of Tai Chi, Yoga, and Pilates

In recent years, there has been increasing interest in movement disciplines related to flexibility and stretching. Data from the recent Superstudy of Sports Participation conducted by the Sporting Goods Manufacturers Association (SGMA) indicated that yoga and Tai Chi were among the fastest-growing activities with 15.6 percent increases in participation rates from the previous survey. Increases in Pilates classes have been even more pronounced, with rates of irregular participants doubling in the past years. The popularity of these activities suggests that people may be more interested in flexibility-related activity when it is presented in a more engaging and interactive format.

An increasing array of classes, videos, and resources are now available for these programs. When reviewing these programs, it is important to consider that there is no strong scientific basis for yoga and Pilates programming. When performed safely with a qualified instructor, they probably can be beneficial. It is also not necessary to participate in these type of programs to improve flexibility. In fact, a recent study demonstrated that yoga was not as good as a basic stretching program for flexibility benefits.

Table 3 The Basic Eight for Trunk Stretching Exercises

Table 3

1. Upper Trapezius/Neck Stretch

This exercise stretches the muscles on the back and sides of the neck. To stretch the right trapezius, place hand on top of your head. Gently look down towards your left underarm, tucking your chin towards your chest. Let the weight of your arm gently draw your head forward. Hold. Repeat to the opposite side.

Scalenes: The stretch above may be modified to stretch the muscles on the front and sides of the neck. Start from the stretch position described above. Keep your left ear near your left shoulder. Turn your head slightly and look up toward the ceiling, lifting your chin 2–3″. Hold.

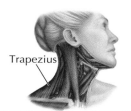

Trapezius

2. Chin Tuck

This exercise stretches the muscles at the base of the skull and reduces headache symptoms. Sit up straight, with chest lifted and shoulders back. Gently tuck in the chin by making a slight motion of nodding "yes." Imagine a string attached to the back of your head, which is pulling your head upward, like a puppet. As your chin draws inward, attempt to lengthen the back of your neck. Hold.

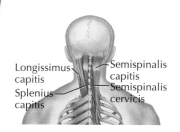

Longissimus capitis
Splenius capitis
Semispinalis capitis
Semispinalis cervicis

3. Pectoral Stretch

This exercise stretches the chest muscles (pectorals).
1. Stand erect in doorway, with arms raised 45 degrees, elbows bent, hands grasping the door-jamb and feet in front-stride position. Press out on door frame, contracting your arms maximally for 6 seconds. Relax and shift weight forward on legs. Lean into doorway, so that the muscles on the front of your shoulder joint and chest are stretched. Hold.
2. Repeat with your arms raised 90 degrees.
3. Repeat with your arms raised 135 degrees. This exercise is useful to prevent or correct round shoulders and sunken chest.

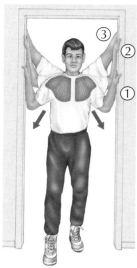

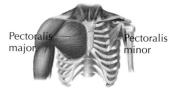

Pectoralis major
Pectoralis minor

4. Lateral Trunk Stretch

This exercise stretches the trunk muscles. Sit on the floor. Stretch the left arm over your head, to the right. Bend to the right at the waist, reaching as far to the right as possible with your left arm and as far as possible to the left with your right arm; hold. Do not let your trunk rotate. Repeat on the opposite side. For less stretch, your overhead arm may be bent at the elbow. This exercise can be done in the standing position, but is less effective.

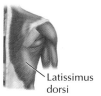

Latissimus dorsi

Table 3

The Basic Eight for Trunk Stretching Exercises Table 3

5. Leg Hug

This exercise stretches the hip and back extensor muscles. Lie on your back. Bend one leg and grasp your thigh under the knee. Hug it to your chest. Keep the other leg straight and on the floor. Hold. Repeat with the opposite leg.

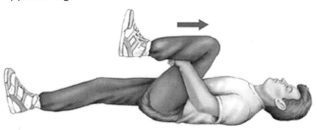

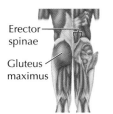

Erector spinae

Gluteus maximus

7. Trunk Twist

This exercise stretches the trunk muscles and the muscles on the outside of the hip. Sit with your right leg extended, left leg bent and crossed over the right knee. Place your right arm on the left side of the left leg and push against that leg while turning the trunk as far as possible to the left. Place the left hand on the floor behind the buttocks. Stretch and hold. Reverse position and repeat on the opposite side.

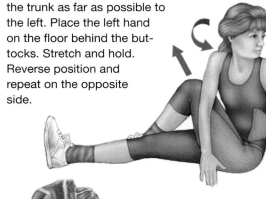

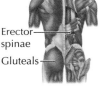

Erector spinae

Gluteals

6. Heel Sit

This exercise stretches the muscles of the lower back. Begin on hands and knees with eyes looking down toward the floor. Keep your hands on the floor directly below your shoulders. Rock backwards, bringing your buttocks toward your heels. Gently round the lower back outward. Hold.

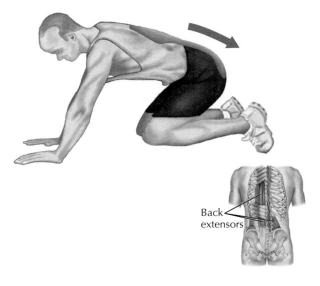

Back extensors

8. Spine Twist

This exercise stretches the trunk rotators and lateral rotators of the thighs. Start in hook-lying position, arms extended at shoulder level. Cross your left knee over the right. Push the right knee to the floor, using the pressure of the left knee and leg. Keep your arms and shoulders on the floor while touching your knees to the floor on the left. Stretch and hold. Reverse leg position and lower your knees to right.

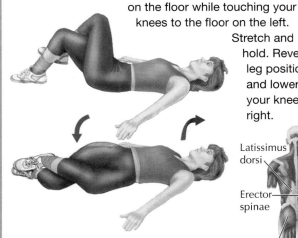

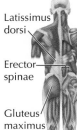

Latissimus dorsi

Erector spinae

Gluteus maximus

Table 4 The Basic Eight for Leg Stretching Exercises

Table 4

1. Calf Stretch

This exercise stretches the calf muscles and Achilles tendon. Face a wall with your feet 2' or 3' away. Step forward on your left foot to allow both hands to touch the wall. Keep the heel of your right foot on the ground, toe turned in slightly, knee straight, and buttocks tucked in. Lean forward by bending your front knee and arms and allowing your head to move nearer the wall. Hold. Bend your right knee, keeping your heel on floor. Stretch and hold. Repeat with the other leg.

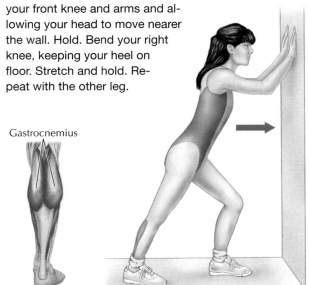

Gastrocnemius

2. Shin Stretch

This exercise relieves shin muscle soreness by stretching the muscles on the front of the shin. Kneel on your knees, turn to the right, and press down and stretch your right ankle with your right hand. Move your pelvis forward. Hold. Repeat on the opposite side. Except when they are sore, most people need to strengthen rather than stretch these muscles.

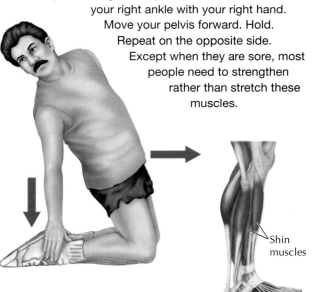

Shin muscles

3. Back-Saver Hamstring Stretch

This exercise stretches the hamstrings and calf muscles and helps prevent or correct backache caused in part by short hamstrings. Sit on the floor with the feet against the wall or an immovable object. Bend left knee and bring foot close to buttocks. Clasp hands behind back. Contract the muscles on the back of the upper leg (hamstrings) by pressing the heel downward toward the floor; hold; relax. Bend forward from hips, keeping lower back as straight as possible. Let bent knee rotate outward so trunk can move forward. Lean forward keeping back flat; hold and repeat on each leg.

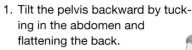

Hamstrings

4. Hip and Thigh Stretch

This exercise stretches the hip (iliopsoas) and thigh muscles (quadriceps) and is useful for people with lordosis and back problems. Place your right knee directly above your right ankle and stretch your left leg backward so your knee touches the floor. If necessary, place your hands on floor for balance.

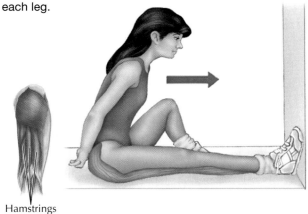

Iliopsoas

Quadriceps

1. Tilt the pelvis backward by tucking in the abdomen and flattening the back.
2. Then shift the weight forward until a stretch is felt on the front of the thigh; hold. Repeat on the opposite side. Caution: Do not bend your front knee more than 90 degrees.

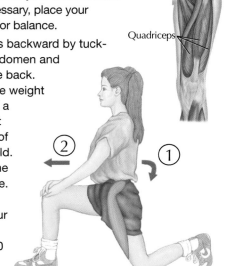

5. Sitting Stretch

This exercise stretches the muscles on the inside of the thighs. Sit with the soles of your feet together; place your hands on your knees or ankles and lean your forearms against your knees; resist (contract) by attempting to raise your knees. Hold. Relax and press the knees toward the floor as far as possible; hold. This exercise is useful for pregnant women and anyone whose thighs tend to rotate inward, causing backache, knock-knees, and flat feet.

Adductors

7. Inner Thigh Stretch

This exercise stretches the muscles of the inner thigh. Stand with feet spread wider than shoulder-width apart. Shift weight onto the right foot and bend the right knee slightly. Straighten left knee and raise toes of left foot off the floor. Lean forwards slightly from the waist keeping back straight/shoulders back. Shift weight back over the right foot by moving hips diagonally away from the left foot. Hold. Repeat in the opposite direction.

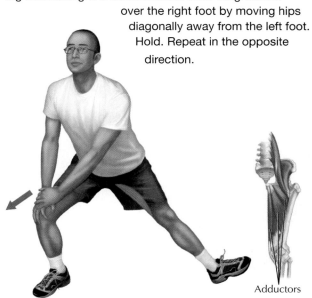

Adductors

6. Lateral Thigh and Hip Stretch

This exercise stretches the muscles and connective tissue on the outside of the legs (iliotibial band and tensor fascia lata). Stand with your left side to the wall, left arm extended and palm of your hand flat on the wall for support. Cross the left leg behind the right leg and turn the toes of both feet out slightly. Bend your left knee slightly and shift your pelvis toward the wall (left) as your trunk bends toward the right. Adjust until tension is felt down the outside of the left hip and thigh. Stretch and hold. Repeat on the other side.

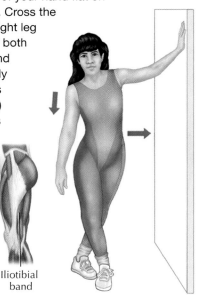

Iliotibial band

8. Deep Buttock Stretch

This exercise stretches the deep buttock muscles, such as the piriformis. Lie on your back with knees bent and one ankle crossed over opposite knee. Hold thigh of bottom leg and pull gently toward your chest. Hold. Repeat on the other side.

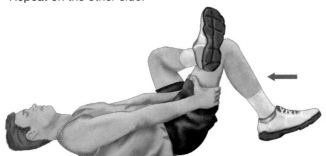

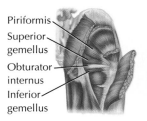

Piriformis
Superior gemellus
Obturator internus
Inferior gemellus

Table 5 The Basic Four for Arm Stretching Exercises

Table 5

1. Forearm Stretch

This exercise stretches the muscles on the front and back sides of the lower arm. It is particularly useful in relieving stress from excessive keyboarding activity. Hold your right arm straight out in front, with your palm facing down. Use your left hand to gently stretch the fingertips of your right hand toward the floor. Hold. Turn your right arm over with your palm facing up. Use your left hand to gently stretch the fingertips of your right hand toward the floor. Hold. Repeat on the opposite side.

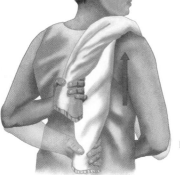
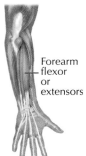

Forearm flexor or extensors

2. Back Scratcher

Stand straight with back of left hand held flat against back. With right hand, throw one end of a towel over right shoulder from front to back. Grab end of towel with left hand. Pull down gently on the towel with right hand, raising arm in back as high as is comfortable. Hold. Repeat to opposite side.

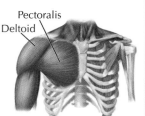

Pectoralis
Deltoid

3. Overhead Arm Stretch

This exercise stretches the triceps and latissimus dorsi muscles. Stretch your arms up overhead. Grasp your right elbow with your left hand. Pull your right elbow back behind your head. Hold. Repeat on opposite side.

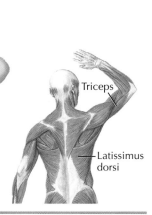

Triceps

Latissimus dorsi

4. Arm Pretzel

This exercise stretches the shoulder muscles (lateral rotators). Stand or sit with your elbows flexed at right angles, palms up. Cross your right arm over your left; grasp your right thumb with your left hand and pull gently downward, causing your right arm to rotate laterally. Stretch and hold. Reverse arm position and repeat on your left arm.

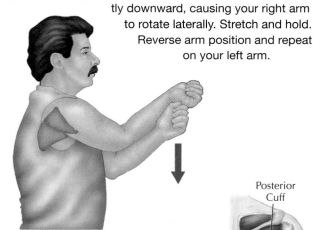
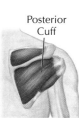

Posterior Cuff

Lab Resource Materials: Flexibility Tests

Directions: To test the flexibility of all joints is impractical. These tests are for joints used frequently. Follow the instructions carefully. Determine your flexibility using Chart 1.

Test

1. *Modified Sit-and-Reach* (Flexibility Test of Hamstrings)

   a. Remove shoes and sit on the floor. Place the sole of the foot of the extended leg flat against a box or bench, and place the head, back, and hips against a wall with a 90-degree angle at the hips.

   b. Place one hand over the other and slowly reach forward as far as you can with arms fully extended. Keep head and back in contact with the wall. A partner will slide the measuring stick on the bench until it touches the fingertips.

   c. With the measuring stick fixed in the new position, reach forward as far as possible, three times, holding the position on the third reach for at least 2 seconds while the partner reads the distance on the ruler. Keep the knee of the extended leg straight (see illustration).

   d. Repeat the test a second time and average the scores of the two trials.

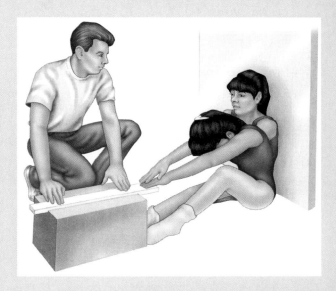

Test

2. *Shoulder Flexibility* ("Zipper" Test)

   a. Raise your arm, bend your elbow, and reach down across your back as far as possible.

   b. At the same time, extend your left arm down and behind your back, bend your elbow up across your back, and try to cross your fingers over those of your right hand as shown in the accompanying illustration.

   c. Measure the distance to the nearest half-inch. If your fingers overlap, score as a plus. If they fail to meet, score as a minus; use a zero if your fingertips just touch.

   d. Repeat with your arms crossed in the opposite direction (left arm up). Most people will find that they are more flexible on one side than the other.

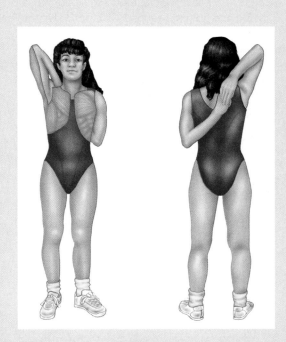

Test

3. *Hamstring and Hip Flexor Flexibility*

   a. Lie on your back on the floor beside a wall.

   b. Slowly lift one leg off the floor. Keep the other leg flat on the floor.

   c. Keep both legs straight.

   d. Continue to lift the leg until either leg begins to bend or the lower leg begins to lift off the floor.

   e. Place a yardstick against the wall and underneath the lifted leg.

   f. Hold the yardstick against the wall after the leg is lowered.

   g. Using a protractor, measure the angle created by the floor and the yardstick. The greater the angle, the better your score.

   h. Repeat with the other leg.*

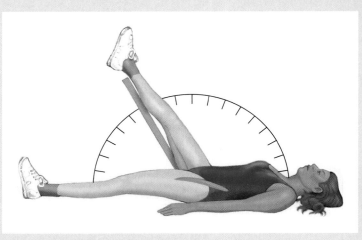

*Note: For ease of testing, you may want to draw angles on a piece of posterboard, as illustrated. If you have goniometers, you may be taught to use them instead.

Test

4. *Trunk Rotation*

   a. Tape two yardsticks to the wall at shoulder height, one right side up and the other upside down.

   b. Stand with your left shoulder an arm's length (fist closed) from the wall. Toes should be on the line, which is perpendicular to the wall and even with the 15-inch mark on the yardstick.

   c. Drop the left arm and raise the right arm to the side, palm down, fist closed.

   d. Without moving your feet, rotate the trunk to the right as far as possible, reaching along the yardstick, and hold it 2 seconds. Do not move the feet or bend the trunk. Your knees may bend slightly.

   e. A partner will read the distance reached to the nearest half-inch. Record your score. Repeat two times and average your two scores.

   f. Next, perform the test facing the opposite direction. Rotate to the left. For this test, you will use the second yardstick (upside down) so that, the greater the rotation, the higher the score. If you have only one yardstick, turn it right side up for the first test and upside down for the second test.

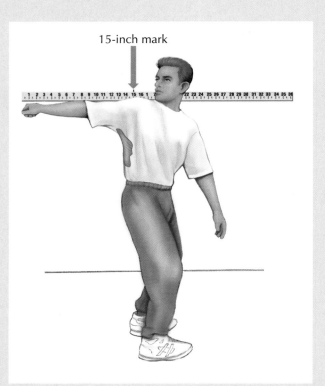

15-inch mark

Chart 1 ▶ Flexibility Rating Scale for Tests 1–4

Classification	Men					Women				
	Test 1	Test 2		Test 3	Test 4	Test 1	Test 2		Test 3	Test 4
		Right Up	Left Up				Right Up	Left Up		
High performance*	16+	5+	4+	111+	20+	17+	6+	5+	111+	20.5 or >
Good fitness zone	13–15	1–4	1–3	80–110	16–19.5	14–16	2–5	2–4	80–110	17–20
Marginal zone	10–12	0	0	60–79	13.5–15.5	11–13	1	1	60–79	14.5–16.5
Low zone	<9	<0	<0	<60	<13.5	<10	<1	<1	<60	<14.5

*Though performers need good flexibility, hypermobility may increase injury risk.

Lab 9A Evaluating Flexibility

Name	Section	Date

Purpose: To evaluate your flexibility in several joints

Procedures

1. Take the flexibility tests outlined in *Lab Resource Materials.*
2. Record your scores in the Results section.
3. Use Chart 1 in *Lab Resource Materials* to determine your ratings on the self-assessments; then place an X over the circle for the appropriate rating.

Results

Flexibility Scores and Ratings

Record Scores

Record Ratings

			High Performance	Good Fitness	Marginal	Poor
Modified sit-and-reach						
Test 1	Left		○	○	○	○
	Right		○	○	○	○
Zipper						
Test 2	Left		○	○	○	○
	Right		○	○	○	○
Hamstring/hip flexor						
Test 3	Left		○	○	○	○
	Right		○	○	○	○
Trunk rotation						
Test 4	Left		○	○	○	○
	Right		○	○	○	○

Do any of these muscle groups need stretching? Check one circle for each muscle group.

	Yes	No
Back of the thighs and knees (hamstrings)	○	○
Calf muscles	○	○
Lower back (lumbar region)	○	○
Front of right shoulder	○	○
Back of right shoulder	○	○
Front of left shoulder	○	○
Back of left shoulder	○	○
Most of the body	○	○
Trunk muscles	○	○

Conclusions and Implications: In several sentences, discuss your current flexibility and your flexibility needs for the future. Include comments about your current state of flexibility, need for improvement in specific areas, and special flexibility needs for sports or other special activities.

Lab 9B Planning and Logging Stretching Exercises

Name	**Section**	**Date**

Purpose: To set 1-week lifestyle goals for stretching exercises, to prepare a stretching for flexibility plan, and to self-monitor progress in your 1-week plan

Procedures

1. Using Chart 1, provide some background information about your experience with stretching exercise, your goals, and your plans for incorporating these exercises into your normal exercise routine.
2. In Chart 2, keep a log of your actual participation in stretching exercise. You can choose from any of the stretching exercises described in Table 3, 4, or 5. Try to pick at least eight exercises and try to perform them at least 3 days in the week (ideally every day).
3. Describe your experiences with your stretching exercise program. Be sure to comment on your plans for future stretching exercise.

Chart 1 ▶ Stretching Exercise Survey

1. What is your level of experience with stretching exercise (check the circle)
   ◯ Beginner
   ◯ Intermediate
   ◯ Advanced

2. What are your primary goals for resistance exercise
   ◯ General conditioning
   ◯ Sports improvement (specify sport:_____)
   ◯ Health benefits

3. Are you currently involved in a regular stretching program. If yes, describe your program. If no, describe barriers that have prevented you from stretching.
   ◯ Yes
   ◯ No

Results

	Yes	No
Did you do eight exercises at least 3 days in the week?	◯	◯
Did you do eight exercises more than 3 days in the week?	◯	◯

Chart 2 ▶ Stretching Exercise Log

Check the stretching exercises you actually performed and the days on which you performed them.	Day 1 Date:	Day 2 Date:	Day 3 Date:	Day 4 Date:	Day 5 Date:	Day 6 Date:	Day 7 Date:
1.							
2.							
3.							
4.							
5.							
6.							
7.							
8.							

Conclusions and Interpretations

1. Do you feel that you will use stretching exercises as part of your regular lifetime physical activity plan, either now or in the future? Use several sentences to explain your answer.

2. Discuss the exercises you feel benefited you and the ones that did not. What exercises would you continue to do and which ones would you change? Use several sentences to explain your answer.

Muscle Fitness and Resistance Exercise

Health Goals for the year 2010

- Increase proportion of people who regularly perform exercises for strength and muscular endurance.

- Reduce steroid use, especially among youth.

- Increase screening and reduce incidence of osteoporosis.

- Reduce activity limitations due to chronic back pain.

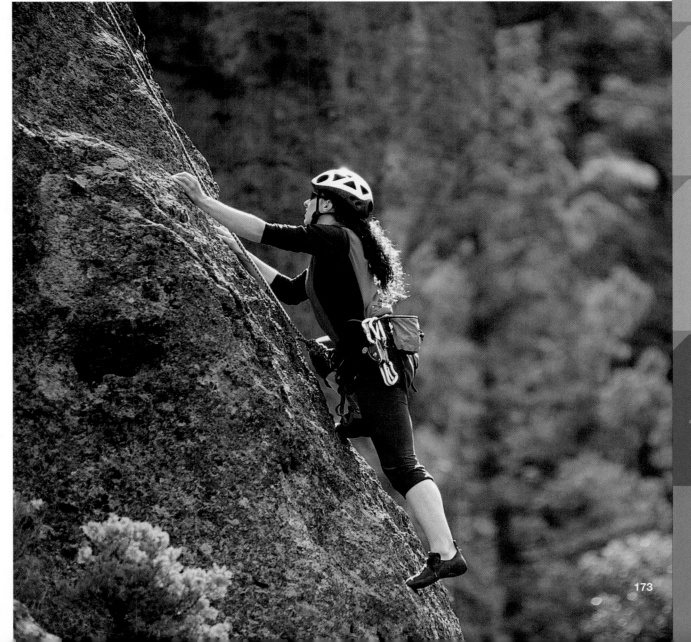

Progressive resistance exercise promotes muscle fitness that permits efficient and effective movement, contributes to ease and economy of muscular effort, promotes successful performance, and lowers susceptibility to some types of injuries, musculoskeletal problems, and some illnesses.

There are two components of muscle fitness: strength and muscular endurance. Strength is the amount of force you can produce with a single maximal effort of a muscle group. Muscular endurance is the capacity of the skeletal muscles or group of muscles to continue contracting over a long period of time. You need both strength and muscular endurance to increase work capacity; to decrease the chance of injury; to prevent low back pain, poor posture, and other hypokinetic conditions; to improve athletic performance; and perhaps to save a life or property in an emergency. Muscle fitness training increases the fitness of the bones, tendons, and ligaments, as well as the muscles. It has been found to be therapeutic for patients with chronic pain.

Progressive resistance exercise (PRE) is the type of physical activity done with the intent of improving muscle fitness. *Weight training* is frequently used as a synonym for *PRE* but it should not be confused with the various competitive events related to resistance exercise. Weight lifting is a competitive sport that involves two lifts: the snatch and the clean and jerk. Powerlifting, also a competitive sport, includes three lifts: the bench press, the squat, and the dead lift. Bodybuilding is a competition in which participants are judged on the size and **definition** of their muscles. Participants in these competitive events rely on highly specialized forms of PRE to optimize their training. Individuals interested in general muscular fitness also rely on PRE but do not need to follow the same routines or regimens to achieve good results. This concept will cover the scientific basis of muscular fitness and will provide guidelines and principles that can be used to establish an appropriate PRE program.

Factors Influencing Strength and Muscular Endurance

There are three types of muscle tissue. The three types of muscle tissue—smooth, cardiac, and skeletal—have different structures and functions. Smooth muscle tissue consists of long, spindle-shaped fibers, with each fiber containing only one nucleus. The fibers are involuntary and are located in the walls of the esophagus, stomach, and intestines, where they move food and waste products through the digestive tract. Cardiac muscle tissue is also involuntary and, as its name implies, is found only in the heart. These fibers contract in response to demands on the cardiovascular system. The heart muscle contracts at a slow, steady rate at rest but contracts more frequently and forcefully during physical activity. Skeletal muscle tissues consist of long, cylindrical, multinucleated fibers. They provide the force needed to move the skeletal system and can be controlled voluntarily.

Leverage is an important mechanical principle that influences strength. The body uses a system of levers to produce movement. Muscles are connected to bones via tendons, and some muscles (referred to as "primary movers") cross over a particular joint to produce movement. The movement occurs because when a muscle contracts it physically shortens and pulls the two bones connected by the joint together. Figure 1 shows the two heads of the biceps muscle inserting on the forearm. When the muscle contracts, the forearm is pulled up toward the upper arm (elbow flexion). A person with long arms and legs has a mechanical advantage in most movements, since the force

On the Web
www.mhhe.com/corbinweb

Web 01 Log on to this URL before reading this concept. See On the Web list of concepts. Click on the concept number you want to view. To access supplemental information, click on the number shown at each Web icon.

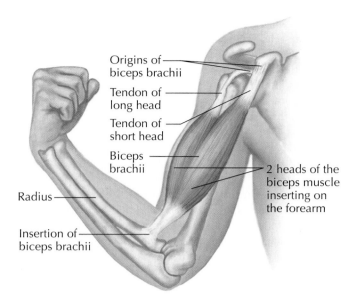

Origins of
biceps brachii

Tendon of
long head

Tendon of
short head

Biceps
brachii

2 heads of the
biceps muscle
inserting on
the forearm

Radius

Insertion of
biceps brachii

Figure 1 ▶ Muscle action on body levers.

that is exerted can act over a longer distance. Although it is not possible to change the length of your limbs, it is possible to learn to use your muscles more effectively. The ability of Tiger Woods to hit golf balls 350 yards is due to his ability to generate torque and power rather than to his actual strength.

Skeletal muscle tissue consists of different types of fibers that respond and adapt differently to training. There are three distinct types of muscle fibers, slow-twitch (Type I), fast-twitch (Type IIb), and intermediate (Type IIa). The slow-twitch fibers are generally red in color and are well suited to produce energy with aerobic metabolism. Slow-twitch fibers generate less tension but are more resistant to fatigue. Endurance training leads to adaptations in the slow-twitch fibers that allow them to produce energy more efficiently and to better resist fatigue. Fast-twitch fibers are generally white in color and are well suited to produce energy with anaerobic processes. They generate greater tension than slow-twitch fibers, but they fatigue more quickly. These fibers are particularly well suited to fast, high-force activities, such as explosive weight-lifting movements, sprinting, and jumping. Resistance exercise enhances strength primarily by increasing the size (muscle **hypertrophy**) of fast-twitch fibers, but cellular adaptations also take place to enhance various metabolic properties. Intermediate fibers have biochemical and physiological properties that are between those of the slow-twitch and fast-twitch fibers. A distinct property of these intermediate fibers is that they are highly adaptable, depending on the type of training that is performed.

An example of fast-twitch muscle fiber in animals is the white meat in the flying muscles of a chicken. The chicken is heavy and must exert a powerful force to fly a few feet up to a perch. A wild duck that flies for hundreds of miles has dark meat (slow-twitch fibers) in the flying muscles for better endurance.

People who want large muscles will use PRE designed to build strength (fast-twitch fibers). People who want to be able to persist in activities for a long period of time without fatigue will want to use PRE programs designed to build muscular endurance (slow-twitch fibers).

Muscular endurance and strength are part of the same continuum. Though strength and muscular endurance are developed in different ways, they are part of the same continuum. **Absolute strength** is the maximal force that can be exerted at one time, while **absolute endurance** reflects the ability to sustain a submaximal force over an extended period of time. Most activities rely on various combinations of strength and endurance. For this reason, it is important to have sufficient amounts of strength and endurance. Studies show that a person who is strength-trained will fatigue as much as four times faster than a person who is endurance-trained. However, there is a modest correlation between strength and endurance. A person who trains for strength will develop some endurance, and a person who trains for endurance will develop some strength.

Genetics, gender, and age affect muscle fitness performance. Each person inherits a certain percentage of fast-twitch and slow-twitch muscle fibers. This allocation influences the potential a person has for muscle fitness activities. Individuals with a larger percentage of fast-twitch fibers will generally increase

Web 02

Web 03

Progressive Resistance Exercise (PRE) The type of physical activity done with the intent of improving muscle fitness.

Definition The detailed external appearance of a muscle.

Hypertrophy Increase in the size of muscles as a result of strength training; increase in bulk.

Absolute Strength The maximum amount of force one can exert—e.g., the maximum number of pounds or kilograms that can be lifted on one attempt.

Absolute Endurance Muscular endurance measured by the maximum number of repetitions one can perform against a given resistance—e.g., the number of times you can bench press 50 pounds.

muscle size and strength more readily than individuals endowed with a larger percentage of slow-twitch fibers. People with a larger percentage of slow-twitch fibers have greater potential for muscular endurance performance. Regardless of genetics, all people can improve their strength and muscular endurance with proper training.

Women have smaller amounts of the anabolic hormone testosterone and, therefore, have less muscle mass than men. Because of this, women typically have 60 to 85 percent of the absolute strength of men. When expressed relative to lean body weight, women have **relative strength** similar to that of men. For example, a 150-pound female who lifts 150 pounds has relative strength equivalent to that of a 250-pound male who lifts 250 pounds, even though she has less absolute strength. Absolute muscular endurance is also greater for males, but the difference again is negated if **relative muscular endurance** is considered. Relative strength and endurance are better indicators of muscle fitness, since they take into account differences in size and muscle mass, but, for some activities, absolute strength and endurance are more important.

Maximum strength is usually reached in the twenties and typically declines with age. Though muscular endurance declines with age, it is not as dramatic as decreases in strength. As people grow older, regardless of gender, strength and muscular endurance are better among people who train than people who do not. This suggests that PRE is one antidote to premature aging.

Muscular endurance is related to cardiovascular endurance, but it is not the same thing. Cardiovascular endurance depends on the efficiency of the heart muscle, circulatory system, and respiratory system. It is developed with activities that stress these systems, such as running, cycling, and swimming. Muscular endurance depends on the efficiency of the local skeletal muscles and the nerves that control them. Most forms of cardiovascular exercise, such as running, require good cardiovascular and muscular endurance. For example, if your legs lack the muscular endurance to continue contracting for a sustained period of time, it will be difficult to perform well in running and other aerobic activities.

Health Benefits of Muscle Fitness and Resistance Exercise

Good muscle fitness is associated with reduced risk for injury. People with good muscle fitness are less likely to suffer joint injuries (e.g., neck, knee, ankle) than those with poor muscle fitness. Weak muscles are more likely to be involuntarily overstretched than are strong muscles.

Muscle balance is important in reducing the risk for injury. Resistance training should build both agonist and antag-

onist muscles. For example, if you do resistance exercise to build the quadriceps muscles (front of the thigh), you should also exercise the hamstring muscles (back of the thigh). In this instance, the quadriceps are the agonist (muscle being used), and the hamstrings are the antagonist. If the quadriceps become too strong relative to the antagonist hamstring muscles, the risk for injury increases (see Figure 2).

Good muscle fitness is associated with good posture and reduced risk for back problems. When muscles in specific body regions are weak or overdeveloped, poor posture can result. Lack of fitness of the abdominal and low back muscles is particularly related to poor posture and potential back problems. Excessively strong hip flexor muscles can lead to swayback. Poor balance in muscular development can also result in postural problems. For example, the muscles on the sides of the body must be balanced to maintain an erect posture.

Good muscle fitness can bring about improved athletic performance. Many sports depend on strength and muscular endurance. A football player must have good muscle strength to block and tackle effectively. A swimmer or a wrestler requires good muscular endurance to perform optimally. Also, people in jobs requiring high-level performance, such as law enforcement and fire safety, are likely to benefit from good muscle fitness.

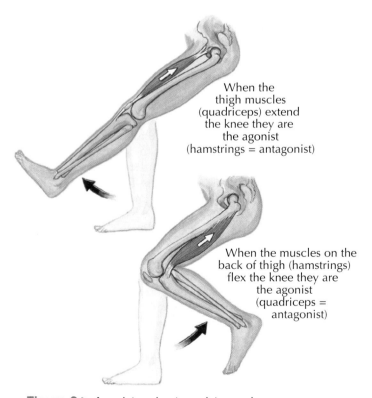

When the thigh muscles (quadriceps) extend the knee they are the agonist (hamstrings = antagonist)

When the muscles on the back of thigh (hamstrings) flex the knee they are the agonist (quadriceps = antagonist)

Figure 2 ▶ Agonist and antagonist muscles.

Good muscle fitness is associated with wellness and quality of life. Wellness is reflected in quality of life and well-being. A person with muscle fitness is able to perform for long periods of time without undue fatigue. As a result, the person has energy to perform daily work efficiently and effectively and has reserve energy to enjoy leisure time. Among older people, maintenance of strength is associated with increased balance, less risk for falling, and greater ability to perform the tasks of daily living independently. Muscle fitness also contributes to looking one's best.

Resistance exercise is associated with reduced risk for osteoporosis. Resistance exercises provide a positive stress on the bones. Together with good diet, including adequate calcium intake, this stress on the bones reduces the risk for osteoporosis. Evidence suggests that young people who do PRE develop a high bone density. As we grow older, bone mass decreases, so people who have a high bone density when they are young have a "bank account" from which to draw as they grow older. These people have bones that are less likely to fracture or be injured. Injuries to the bones, particularly the hip and back, are common among older adults. Regular PRE can reduce the risk for these conditions. Post-menopausal women are especially at risk for osteoporosis (see Concept 4).

PRE contributes to weight control. Regular PRE results in muscle mass increases. Muscle or lean body mass takes up less space than fat, contributing to attractive appearance. Further, muscle burns calories at rest, so extra muscle built through PRE can contribute to increased resting and basal metabolism. For each pound of muscle gained, a person can burn approximately 35 to 50 calories more per day. A typical strength training program performed at least three times a week can lead to 2 additional pounds of muscle after 8 weeks, so this can amount to an expenditure of an additional 100 calories a day, or 700 a week. Conversely, muscle mass tends to decrease with age, and this can slow metabolism by a similar amount and contribute to gradual increases in body fatness. PRE can help people retain muscle mass as they grow older.

Core strength is an important health parameter. Core strength refers to strength of the abdominal, paraspinal (back), and gluteal muscles. In the past core muscle training has not been emphasized in PRE programs. However, there is a new emphasis on core muscle exercises because of their importance to daily life. Good core strength can help reduce back pain, prevent injuries, and improve performance in many applied tasks and sport movements. Many athletes view core strength training as an important part of their conditioning. Core strength is also important as you grow older. It promotes functional balance and may help prevent falls.

Types of PRE

There are different types of PRE, and each has its advantages and disadvantages. The main types of PRE are isotonic, isometric, and isokinetic. These terms refer to the way in which a load or stimulus is provided to the muscles. The differences among these types of exercise are described below and are also illustrated in Figure 3. The advantages of each type are summarized in Table 1 (see Web04 for details).

Web 04

- **Isotonic** exercises are the most common type of PRE. When isotonic exercises are performed the muscles shorten and lengthen to cause movement. The most common types of isotonic exercises are calisthenics, resistance machine exercises, free weight exercises, and exercises using other types of resistance such as exercise bands. Isotonic exercise allows for the use of resistance through a full range of joint motion and provides an effective stimulus for muscle development.

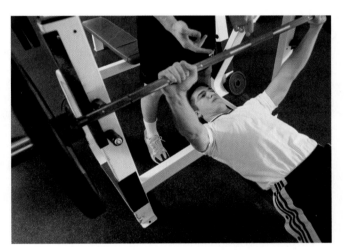

Progressive resistance exercises are methods of training designed to build muscle fitness.

Relative Strength Amount of force that one can exert in relation to one's body weight or per unit of muscle cross section.

Relative Muscular Endurance Endurance measured by the maximum number of repetitions one can perform using a given percent of absolute strength—e.g., the number of times you can lift 50 percent of your absolute strength.

Isotonic Type of muscle contraction in which the muscle changes length, either shortening (concentrically) or lengthening (eccentrically).

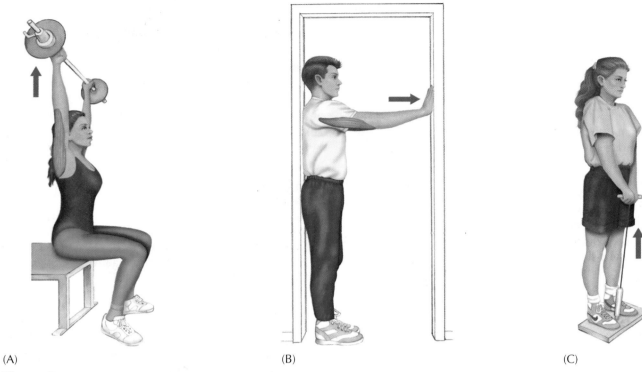

(A)   (B)   (C)

Figure 3 ▶ Examples of three types of muscle fitness exercises: (A) isotonic, (B) isometric, and (C) isokinetic.

Table 1 ▶ Advantages and Disadvantages of Isotonic, Isometric, and Isokinetic Exercises

	Advantages	Disadvantages
Isotonic	• Can effectively mimic movements used in sport skills • Enhance dynamic coordination • Promote gains in strength	• Do not challenge muscles through the full range of motion • Require equipment or machines • May lead to soreness
Isometric	• Can be done anywhere • Require only low cost/little equipment • Can rehabilitate an immobilized joint	• Build strength at only one position • Cause less muscle hypertrophy • Are a poor link or transfer to sport skills
Isokinetic	• Build strength through a full range of motion • Are beneficial for rehabilitation and evaluation • Are safe and less likely to promote soreness	• Require specialized equipment • Cannot replicate natural acceleration found in sports • Are more complicated to use and cannot work all muscle groups

When performing isotonic exercise, both **concentric** (shortening) and **eccentric** (lengthening) contractions should be used. For example in the overhead press exercise, the muscles on the back of the arms (triceps) shorten (contract concentrically) to overcome resistance or lift a weight. When the same muscles contract eccentrically, lengthening occurs allowing a slow and controlled return of the muscle to its normal length (see Figure 3A). Because isotonic exercises involves movement against a resistance such as a resistance machine or lifting of a weight when using free weights, it is helpful for building both **dynamic strength** and **dynamic muscular endurance.** Dynamic refers to movement, so strength and muscular endurance that causes movement are referred to as dynamic.

- **Isometric** exercises are those in which no movement takes place while a force is exerted against an immovable object (see Figure 3B). When properly done, they are effective for developing strength and endurance but it is important to recognize that they promote **static strength** and **static endurance** since they work the muscle only at the angle of the joint used in the exercise and is therefore not emphasized in most exercise programs.

- **Isokinetic** exercises are isotonic-concentric muscle contractions performed on machines that keep the velocity of the movement constant through the full range of motion. Isokinetic devices essentially match the resistance to the effort of the performer, permitting maximal tension to be exerted throughout the range of motion (see Figure 3C). Isokinetic exercises are effective, but they are typically only found in sport training or rehabilitation settings.

Plyometrics is a form of isotonic exercise that promotes athletic performance. Plyo-

Web 05

metrics is a form of isotonic exercise that is especially useful for athletes training for power development. High jumpers, long jumpers, and volleyball and basketball players often use this technique, which includes jumping from boxes, hopping on one foot, and engaging in similar types of activities. For most people interested primarily in the health benefits of physical activity, plyometrics are not a preferred type of exercise. In fact, they can increase risk for injury, especially among beginners. For more information on plyometrics, refer to Concept 12.

Functional balance training is a specialized form of training aimed at improving core strength and balance. Balance tends to deteri-

Web 06

orate with age, and this is partly due to corresponding declines in muscle strength, range of motion, and a lower ability to coordinate muscle movements. Functional balance training has been shown to help improve balance and mobility in the elderly. It is also used in rehabilitation and in specialized training regimens for sports. This type of training is typically conducted with specialized devices, such as exercise balls (Swiss balls), BOSU platforms, and balance boards. Because these devices challenge you to remain balanced, they recruit muscles that are not typically worked in most strength training regimens. They can be used to perform a variety of movements and to work a variety of muscles (see the Technology Update and Web06 for details).

Resistance Training Equipment

Free weights are the most commonly used equipment for resistance exercise. Free weight equipment consists of weights that are typically loaded onto a barbell or a dumbbell. They have often been considered to be the domain of serious weight lifters, but recent statistics indicate that they are more widely used than previously thought. According to the Sporting Goods Manufacturers Association (SGMA), over 50 million Americans use free weights with approximately 10 million classified as regular users. Factors that contribute to their popularity

are their versatility, the ability to change weight in gradual increments, and the ability to modify exercises for specific muscles or movements (see Table 2 on page 180). Because free weights require balance and technique, they may be more difficult for beginners to use.

Resistance training machines offer many advantages for overall conditioning. Resis-

Web 07

tance training machines can be effective in developing strength and muscular endurance if used properly. They can save time because, unlike free weights, the resistance can be changed easily and quickly. They may be safer because you are less likely to drop weights. A disadvantage is that the kinds of exercises that can be done on these machines are more limited than free weight exercises. They also may not promote optimal balance in muscular development, since a stronger muscle can often make up for a weaker muscle in the completion

Concentric Contractions Isotonic muscle contractions in which the muscle gets shorter as it contracts, such as when a joint is bent and two body parts move closer together.

Eccentric Contractions Isotonic muscle contractions in which the muscle gets longer as it contracts—that is, when a weight is gradually lowered and the contracting muscle gets longer as it gives up tension. Eccentric contractions are also called negative exercise.

Dynamic Strength A muscle's ability to exert force that results in movement. It is typically measured isotonically.

Dynamic Muscular Endurance A muscle's ability to contract and relax repeatedly. This is usually measured by the number of times (repetitions) you can perform a body movement in a given time period. It is also called isotonic endurance.

Isometric Type of muscle contraction in which the muscle remains the same length. Also known as static contraction.

Static Strength A muscle's ability to exert a force without changing length; also called isometric strength.

Static Muscular Endurance A muscle's ability to remain contracted for a long period. This is usually measured by the length of time you can hold a body position.

Isokinetic Isotonic-concentric exercises done with a machine that regulates movement velocity and resistance.

Plyometrics A training technique used to develop explosive power. It consists of isotonic-concentric muscle contractions performed after a prestretch or an eccentric contraction of a muscle.

of a lift. Some machines have mechanisms that provide variable, or accommodating, resistance. These features allow the machine to provide a more appropriate resistance across the full range of motion. More recent developments have allowed machines to allow movement to take place in multiple dimensions. This allows for independent arm/leg movements to provide a more realistic training stimulus and reduce the likelihood of creating muscle imbalances. See the *On the Web* feature for additional details about strength training machines.

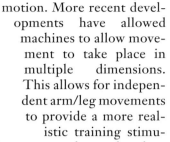

Elastic bands can provide resistance to build muscle fitness.

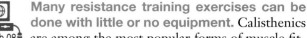
Many resistance training exercises can be done with little or no equipment. Calisthenics are among the most popular forms of muscle fitness exercise among adults. Calisthenics, such as curl-ups and push-ups, are suitable for people of different ability levels and can be used to improve both strength and muscular endurance. Many variations can be added to increase the difficulty of various calisthenic exercises. For example, push-ups can be made more challenging by elevating your feet. Performing regular calisthenics can help build and maintain good muscular fitness.

Other alternatives to expensive resistance training machines or commercially made free weights are homemade weights and elastic exercise bands. Homemade weights can be constructed from pieces of pipe or broom sticks and plastic milk jugs filled with water. Elastic tubes or bands available in varying strengths may be substituted for the weights and for the pulley device used in many resistance training machines to impart resistance.

Progressive Resistance Exercise: How Much Is Enough?

PRE is the best type of training for muscle fitness. PRE is the most common type of training for building muscle fitness and it is the most effective. It is sometimes referred to as progressive resistive training (PRT). The word *progressive* is used in both instances because the frequency, intensity, and length of time of muscle overload are gradually, or progressively, increased as muscle

Table 2 ▶ Advantages (+) and Disadvantages (−) of Free Weights and Machine Weights

		Free Weights		**Machine Weights**
Isolation of Major Muscle Groups	−/+	Movements require balance and coordination; more muscles are used for stabilization.	+/−	Other body parts are stabilized during lift, allowing isolation, but muscle imbalances can develop.
Applications to Real-Life Situations	+	Movements can be developed to be truer to real life.	−	Movements are determined by the paths allowed on the machine.
Risk for Injury	−	There is more possibility for injury because weights can fall or drop on toes.	+	They are safer because weights cannot fall on participants.
Needs for Assistance	−	Spotters are needed for safety with some lifts.	+	No spotters are required.
Time Requirement	−	More time is needed to change weights.	+	It is easy and quick to change weights or resistance.
Number of Available Exercises	+	Unlimited number of exercises is possible.	−	Exercise options are determined by the machine.
Cost	+	They are less expensive but good (durable) weights are still somewhat expensive.	−	They are expensive; access to a club is usually needed, since multiple machines are usually needed.
Space Requirement	+/−	Equipment can be moved but loose weights may clutter areas.	−/+	Machines are stationary but take up large spaces.

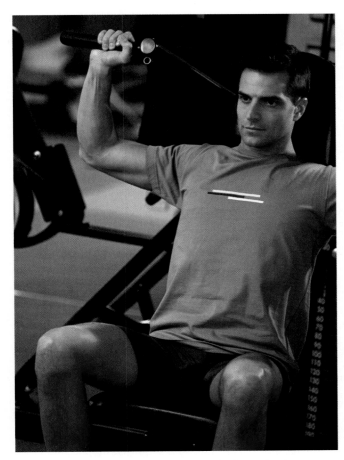

Well-planned resistance training helps you look your best.

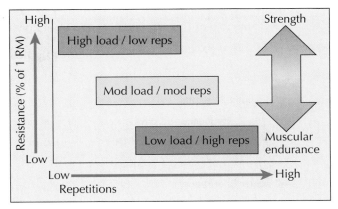

Figure 4 ▶ Comparison of muscular endurance with muscle strength by different repetitions and resistance.

fitness increases. PREs are typically done in one to three sets, though more are used in some instances, such as for high-performance benefits. A set is a group of repetitions (reps) done in succession, followed by a rest period. For most people, a set consists of 3 to 25 reps.

The stimulus for strength is different than for muscular endurance. The stimulus for strength is maximal exertion. Strength training should, therefore, use high resistance overload with low repetitions. The stimulus for muscular endurance is repeated contractions with short rests. Muscular endurance exercises should be performed with a relatively high number of repetitions and lower resistance.

The graph in Figure 4 illustrates the relationship between strength and muscular endurance. Training that requires high resistance and low repetitions (top bar) results in the least gain in endurance but the greatest gain in strength. Training with moderate resistance and moderate repetitions (second bar) results in moderate gains in both strength and endurance. Training that requires a high number of repetitions and a relatively low resistance

(third bar) results in small gains in strength but large increases in muscular endurance.

There are different thresholds and target zones for muscle fitness development. The amount of resistance used in a PRE program is based on a percentage of your **1 repetition maximum (1RM)**—the maximum amount of resistance you can move (or weight you can lift) one time. The 1RM value provides an indicator of your maximum strength, but desired levels of resistance are determined using percentages of the 1RM value. The specific prescription depends on the program goals. For strength, the percentages typically vary 60 to 80 percent of the 1RM value, whereas for endurance the percentages vary from 20 to 40 percent. Evidence suggests that very strong people interested in high-level performance can train at 80 percent and above. Individuals interested in a combination of strength and endurance should use values ranging from 40 to 60 percent. A summary of the FIT formulas for muscular strength and muscular endurance are included in Table 3 (see p. 182), along with guidelines for general muscle fitness.

A combined strength/muscle endurance program is the best choice for most individuals. Research has shown that for healthy adults most health benefits can be achieved using a combined strength/muscular endurance program. The American College of Sports Medicine guidelines indicate that young adults can achieve significant

1 Repetition Maximum (1RM) The maximum amount of resistance you can move a given number of times—for example, 1RM = maximum weight lifted one time; 6RM = maximum weight lifted six times.

Table 3 ▶ Threshold of Training and Fitness Target Zones for Muscular Fitness

	Threshold of Training	Fitness Target Zones
Isotonic Exercise		
Muscular Strength		
Frequency	2 days a week for each muscle group	2–3 days per week for each muscle group
Intensity	60% of 1RM for every repetition	60–80% of 1RM for number of reps on every set
Time	1 set of 3–8 reps	1–3 sets of 3–8 reps
Muscular Endurance		
Frequency	2 days per week	Every other day
Intensity	Move 20% of 1RM	Move 20%–60% of 1RM
Time	One set of 9 repetitions of each exercise	2–5 sets of 9–25 repetitions of each exercise
General Muscular Fitness		
Frequency	2–3 days a week	3 days a week
Intensity	40% of 1RM for young adults	40–60% of 1RM for young adults
	30% for adults >50 years old	30–50% for adults >50 years old
Time	1 set of 8–12 reps for young adults	1–3 sets of 8–12 reps for young adults
	1 set of 10–15 reps for adults >50 years old	1–3 sets of 10–15 reps for adults >50
Isometric Exercise		
Static Muscular Fitness		
Frequency	3 days per week	Every other day
Intensity	Hold a resistance 50% of the weight you ultimately need to hold in your work or leisure activity.	Hold a resistance 50–150% of the weight you ultimately need to hold in your work or leisure activity.
Time	Hold for lengths of time that are 50% of the time for the actual work or leisure task; repeat 10–20 times and rest 30 seconds between repetitions.	Hold for lengths of time that are 50–120% of the time for the actual work or leisure task (for longer times use fewer repetitions); rest 30–60 seconds between repetitions⁴

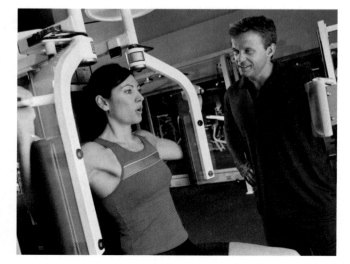

Resistance machines provide a safe and efficient way to exercise.

health benefits by performing one set of 8 to 12 repetitions at least 2 days a week. For older adults (50 and older), less intense exercises performed 10 to 15 times appears to be sufficient. For both age groups, 8 to 10 basic exercises are recommended to promote good muscle fitness for the whole body. Individuals who want pure strength or high-level endurance for performance will benefit from extra sets and from more specific training protocols.

Circuit resistance training (CRT) is an effective way to build muscular endurance and cardiovascular endurance. CRT consists of the performance of high repetitions of an exercise with low to moderate resistance, progressing from one station to another, performing a different exercise at each station. The stations are usually placed in a circle to facilitate movement. CRT typically uses about 20 to 25 reps against a resistance that is 30 to 40 percent of 1RM for 45 seconds. Fifteen seconds of rest is provided while changing stations. Approximately 10 exercise stations are used, and the participant repeats the circuit two to three times (sets). Because of the short rest periods, significant cardiovascular benefits have been reported in addition to muscular endurance gains.

Programs intended to slim the figure/physique should be of the muscular endurance type. Many men and women are interested in exercises designed to decrease girth measurements. High-repetition, low-resistance exercise is suitable for this because it usually brings about some strengthening and may decrease body fatness, which in turn changes body contour. Exercises do not spot-reduce fat, but they do speed up metabolism, so more calories are burned. However, if weight or fat reduction is desired, aerobic (cardiovascular) exercises are best. To increase girth, use strength exercises.

Endurance training may have a negative effect on strength and power. Some studies have shown that, for athletes who rely primarily on strength and power in their sport, too much endurance training can cause a loss of strength and power because of the modification of different muscle fibers. Strength and power athletes need some endurance training, but not too much, just as endurance athletes need some strength and power training, but not too much.

Training Principles for PRE

The overload principle provides the basis for PRE. For the body to adapt and improve, the muscles and systems of the body must be challenged. As noted earlier, the concept behind PRE is that the frequency, intensity, and duration of lifts are progressively increased to maintain an effective stimulus as the muscle fitness improves. It was in the area of muscle fitness development that the overload principle was first clearly outlined. Legend holds that centuries ago a Greek named Milo of Crotona became progressively stronger by repeatedly lifting his calf. As the calf grew into a bull, its weight increased, and Milo's strength increased as well. We know now that for most people, PREs are necessary if muscle fitness is to be developed and maintained. Activities from other levels of the physical activity pyramid do not provide an adequate stimulus, so specific resistance exercise is needed to improve this dimension of fitness (see Figure 5).

The muscle fitness workout should be based on the principle of progression. Many beginning resistance trainers experience soreness after the first few days of training. The reason for the soreness is that the principle of progression has been vio-

Web 09

lated. Soreness can occur with even modest amounts of training if the volume of training is considerably more than normal. In the first few days or weeks of training, the primary adaptations in the muscle are due to motor learning factors rather than to muscle growth. Because these adaptations occur no matter how much weight is used, it is prudent to start your program slowly with light weights. After these adaptations occur and the rate of improvement slows down, it is necessary to follow the appropriate target zone to achieve proper overload.

The most common progression used in resistance training is the double progressive system, so-called because this system periodically adjusts both the resistance and the number of repetitions of the exercise performed. For example, if you are training for strength, you may begin with three repetitions in one set. As the repetitions become easy, additional repetitions are added. When you have progressed to eight repetitions, increase the resistance and decrease the repetitions in each set back to three and begin the progression again. Additional details on progression of resistance exercise are provided at the *On the Web* feature.

The principle of specificity applies to PRE. Depending on the specific muscles you want to develop, you will use different types of resistance training programs. Factors that can be varied in your program are the type of muscle contraction (isometric or isotonic), the speed or cadence of the movement, and the amount of resistance being moved. For example, if you want strength in

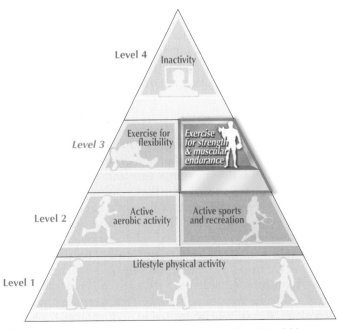

Figure 5 ▶ To build muscle fitness, activities should be selected from level 3 of the physical activity pyramid.

the elbow extensor muscles (e.g., triceps) so that you can more easily lift heavy boxes onto a shelf, you can train using isotonic contractions, at a relatively slow speed, with a relatively high resistance. If you want muscle fitness of the fingers to grip a heavy bowling ball, much of your training should be done isometrically using the fingers the same way you normally hold the ball. If you are training for a skill that requires explosive power, such as in throwing, striking, kicking, or jumping, your strength exercises should be done with less resistance and greater speed. If you are training for a skill that uses both concentric and eccentric contractions, you should perform exercises using these characteristics (e.g., plyometrics).

If you are not training for a specific task, but merely wish to develop muscle fitness for daily living, consider the advantages and disadvantages of isotonics, isometrics, and isokinetics, listed in Table 1. You may wish to use a variety of methods.

The principle of diminishing returns applies to resistance training. To get optimal strength gains from progressive resistance training, one or more sets of exercise repetitions are performed. Some high-level performers use as many as five sets of a particular exercise. Research indicates that most of the fitness and health benefits, however, are achieved in one set. Considerably more than 50 percent of the benefits may result in the first set, with each additional set producing less benefit. Because compliance with resistance training programs is less likely as the time needed to complete the program increases, the American College of Sports Medicine (ACSM) recommends single-set programs for most adults. It acknowledges that additional benefits are likely with more multiset routines, but the ACSM believes that adults are more likely to participate if they can get most of the benefits in a relatively short amount of time. In sports or competition where small performance differences make a big difference, doing multiple sets is important.

The principle of rest and recovery especially applies to strength development. Progressive resistance training for strength development done every day of the week does not allow enough rest and time for recovery. Studies have shown that the greatest proportion of strength is accomplished in 2 days of training per week. Exercise done on a third day does result in additional increases, but the amount of gain is relatively small, compared with gains resulting from 2 days of training per week. For people interested in health benefits rather than performance benefits, 2 days a week saves time and may result in greater adherence to a strength-training program. For people interested in performance benefits, more frequent training may be warranted. Rotating exercises so that certain muscles are exercised on one day

and other muscles are exercised the next allows for more frequent training.

The amount of exercise necessary to maintain strength is less than the amount needed to build it. Recent evidence suggests that, once strength is developed, it can be maintained by performing fewer sets or exercising fewer days per week. For example, if you have performed three sets of an exercise 3 days a week to build strength, you may be able to maintain current levels of strength with one set a week. Also, you may be able to maintain strength by exercising 1 or 2 rather than 3 days per week. If schedules of fewer sets or days per week result in strength loss, frequency must be increased. Smaller muscles seem to need more frequent exercise than larger muscles.

Is There Strength in a Bottle?

Anabolic steroids are used by some athletes and a significant number of nonathletes to enhance performance and build muscular bodies. **Anabolic steroids** are a synthetic reproduction of the male hormone testosterone. They have important clinical roles for treating various medical conditions but are known primarily for their illegal use by athletes. Strength athletes use steroids for their documented effects on increasing muscle mass and strength. Endurance athletes have also been known to take steroids to help prevent overtraining or to improve recovery. In recent years, the issues associated with steroid use have become widely publicized. The congressional hearings on steroids in 2005, the Balco steroid trial, and the candid commentary from former baseball player Jose Canseco (on TV and in books) are just a few examples of the media coverage of steroids. The problems associated with steroid abuse have garnered such visibility that it was directly discussed in the president's State of the Union address in 2006.

Most of the focus on steroids has been on their use by elite athletes but exercise science and public health researchers have determined that there is a growing problem of steroid abuse in nonathletes as well. While elite athletes typically obtain pharmaceutical drugs, nonathletes get steroids primarily from the black market. In addition to the existing risks from steroids, there are risks associated with the ingestion of contaminated drugs and of products that are not what they are purported to be.

Taking anabolic steroids is a dangerous way to build muscle fitness and is illegal. Steroids, Web 10 like other illegal drugs, are dangerous. Research has identified numerous side effects associated with steroid use—many irreversible (see Figure 6). Because steroids are addictive, it is hard for users to stop and the continued (or extended) use of steroids contributes to

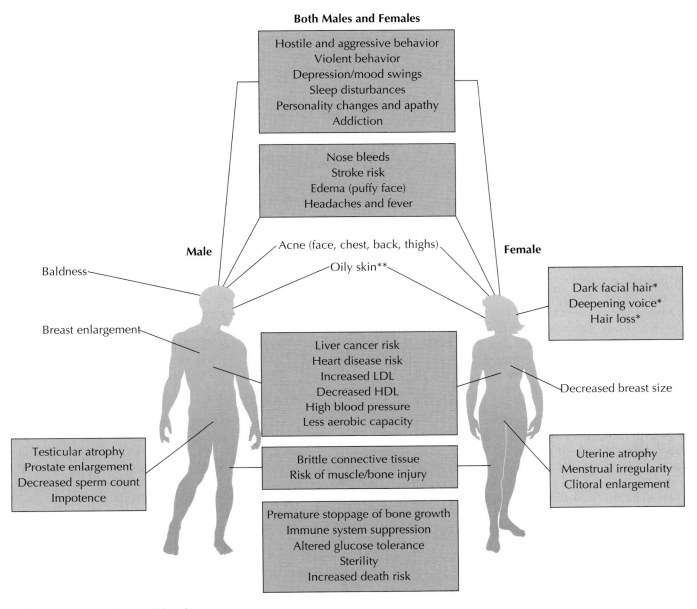

Both Males and Females

Hostile and aggressive behavior
Violent behavior
Depression/mood swings
Sleep disturbances
Personality changes and apathy
Addiction

Nose bleeds
Stroke risk
Edema (puffy face)
Headaches and fever

Male

Baldness

Breast enlargement

Acne (face, chest, back, thighs)
Oily skin**

Female

Dark facial hair*
Deepening voice*
Hair loss*

Liver cancer risk
Heart disease risk
Increased LDL
Decreased HDL
High blood pressure
Less aerobic capacity

Decreased breast size

Testicular atrophy
Prostate enlargement
Decreased sperm count
Impotence

Brittle connective tissue
Risk of muscle/bone injury

Uterine atrophy
Menstrual irregularity
Clitoral enlargement

Premature stoppage of bone growth
Immune system suppression
Altered glucose tolerance
Sterility
Increased death risk

*Among women, irreversible when use stops.
**Among women, partially reversible when use stops.

Figure 6 ▶ Adverse effects of anabolic steroids.

even greater risk. The most severe risk is that of early death. While cause and effect cannot always be proven, steroids have been implicated in a number of cases.

Former major league baseball player Ken Caminiti admitted that he had used steroids and suggested that many other athletes also used them. His death at a very young age was directly attributed to a drug overdose; however, many have speculated that steroid use contributed to his early death. Studies show that most athletes who use steroids are familiar with the adverse effects but use them anyway. Most later say they regret this choice.

Injuries are more likely and some may last longer in people who use steroids. Although the use of steroids allows more frequent training and can lead to stronger muscles, steroid use does not lead to stronger tendons

Anabolic Steroids Synthetic hormones similar to the male sex hormone testosterone. They function androgenically to stimulate male characteristics and anabolically to increase muscle mass, weight, bone maturation, and virility.

and ligaments. In fact, steroid use may make connective tissue more brittle, leading to connective tissue injury. Connective tissue injuries take longer to heal than muscle injuries. There is some evidence that the high levels of strength resulting from use of steroids and very heavy training may be involved in bone injuries.

Androstenedione and THG are *not* safe alternatives to steroids. Androstenedione (andro) is a precursor of naturally occurring testosterone and estrogen. Early studies suggested that andro use did not lead to increases in testosterone levels, but more recent evidence suggests that andro would probably have anabolic effects at the high doses most likely used by athletes. The side effects of andro use are similar to those of anabolic steroids, including disruption of normal sexual development, infertility, and increased risk for some forms of cancer. Use in children can lead to premature puberty and premature closure of the growth plates in bones. Andro has been banned by the International Olympic Committee, the NCAA, the NFL, and most recently major league baseball. The clear documentation of risks has also caused the FDA to require manufacturers to stop distributing products with androstenedione.

Tetrahydrogestrinone (THG) is a chemically engineered steroid that, until recently, has been undetectable by standard drug tests. Many well-known athletes have tested positive for THG, and ongoing drug investigations will likely identify other THG users. The American College of Sports Medicine condemned THG as a threat to the health of athletes and the integrity of sports. The FDA declared that THG is a drug and not a "dietary supplement," as some purveyors and users of the product maintain. It is a purely synthetic steroid, which exhibits the same properties (and risks) of other anabolic steroids.

The sale of steroid precursors is prohibited by law. Eighteen substances, including andro and THG, are classified as illegal steroids and steroid alternatives.

Human growth hormone (HGH), taken to increase strength, may be even more dangerous than anabolic steroids. HGH is produced by the pituitary gland but is also made synthetically. Some athletes are taking it in addition to anabolic steroids or in place of anabolic steroids because it is difficult to detect in urine tests. HGH primarily increases bone size, not muscle size. Athletes often use growth hormone in combination with anabolic steroids so they can gain muscle mass along with bone-strength. Athletes assume that this will protect them from some of the bone injuries that occur among steroid users. However, these athletes are further risking their health, as the health risks of steroid use are compounded further with HGH use. Risks of HGH use include irreversible acromegaly (giantism) and growth

deformities, cardiovascular disease, goiter, menstrual disorder, excessive sweating, lax muscles and ligaments, premature bone closure, decreased sexual desire, and impotence. In addition, the life span can be shortened by as much as 20 years. Like steroids, there are some medical uses for HGH, but HGH should be used only with physician recommendations and prescriptions.

Creatine is used by some people hoping to build muscle fitness. Creatine is a nutrient involved in the production of energy during short-term, high-intensity exercise, such as resistance exercise. The body produces creatine naturally from foods containing protein, but some athletes take creatine supplements (usually a powder dissolved into a liquid) to increase the amounts available in the muscle. The concept behind supplementation is that additional creatine intake enhances energy production and therefore increases the body's ability to maintain force and delay fatigue. Some studies have shown improvements in athletic performance with creatine, but reviews indicate that the supplement may be effective only for athletes who are already well trained. Studies have been more consistent with regard to the performance enhancing effects of creatine on muscle strength. It is important to recognize, though, that the benefits are due to the ability to work the muscles harder during an exercise session, not to the supplement itself. Increases in body weight may result, but this is likely due to water retention. At present, creatine usage hasn't been linked to any major health problems but the long-term effects are unknown.

The safety and efficacy of many strength-related dietary supplements are not established. Performance-related supplements have continued to grow in popularity, despite clear evidence that the overwhelming majority of the supplements are not effective. There are over 29,000 dietary supplements available to American consumers, and over 1,000 new products are released each year. Sales data demonstrate that consumers seem willing to try almost any new product that hits the shelves and presumably believe that commercially available products are either reasonably or completely safe. Under current guidelines from the Dietary Supplement Health and Education Act (DSHEA), manufacturers are not required to provide safety data on their products as drug companies are. Instead, dietary supplements are regulated as foods, meaning that they are considered safe unless proved otherwise. The Food and Drug Administration (FDA) is responsible for determining whether a substance is harmful but, with so many products, it is impossible for the FDA to keep up.

Concerns about the largely unregulated food supplement industry have led the Institute of Medicine (IOM) to recommend alternative procedures to help ensure the safety and efficacy of dietary supplements. The goal is to develop a system to identify supplement ingredients that may pose risks, prioritize them based on their level of potential risk, and then evaluate them for safety. To facilitate this process, the IOM wants to require manufacturers and distributors to report adverse events to the FDA in a timely fashion. According to recent estimates, the FDA receives reports on less than 0.5% of all adverse events associated with supplement use. A requirement to report health problems would allow better detection of potentially harmful supplements. Additional information on supplements and quackery in the fitness field is found in Concept 23.

Guidelines for Safe and Effective Resistance Training

There are many fallacies, superstitions, and myths associated with resistance training. Web 12 Some common misconceptions about resistance training are described in Table 4.

There is a proper way to perform. Although PRE offers considerable health benefits, there are also some risks if the exercises are not performed correctly or if safety procedures are not followed. Before using unfamiliar equipment get instruction in proper use.

Beginners should emphasize lighter weights and progress their program gradually. When beginning a resistance training program, start with light weights so that you can learn proper technique and avoid soreness and injury. Most of the adaptations that occur in the first few months of a program are due to improvements in the body's ability to recruit muscle fibers to contract effectively and efficiently. These neural adaptations occur in response to the movement itself and not the weight that is used. Therefore, beginning lifters can achieve significant benefits from lighter weights.

As experience and fitness levels improve, it is necessary to use heavier loads and more challenging sets to continually challenge the muscles. Information on how to determine appropriate workloads and how to balance more complex training programs is available in several articles by Kraemer and Ratamess (see *Suggested Readings*).

Table 4 ▶ Fallacies and Facts about Resistance Training

Fallacies	Facts
Resistance training will make you muscle-bound and cause you to lose flexibility.	Normal resistance training will not reduce flexibility if exercises are done through the full range of motion and with proper technique. Powerlifters who do highly specific movements have been shown to have poorer flexibility than other weight lifters.
Women will become masculine-looking if they gain strength.	Women will not become masculine-looking from resistance exercise. Women have less testosterone and do not bulk up from resistance training to the same extent as men. Women and men can make similar relative gains in strength and hypertrophy from a resistance training program, however. The greater percentage of fat in most women prevents the muscle definition possible in men and camouflages the increase in bulk.
Strength training makes you move more slowly and look uncoordinated.	Strength training, if done properly, can enhance sport-specific strength and increase power. There are no effects on coordination from having high levels of muscular fitness.
No pain, no gain.	It is not true that you have to get to the point of soreness to benefit from resistance exercise. It may be helpful to strive until you can't do a final repetition but you should definitely stop before it is painful. Slight tightness in the muscles is common 1 to 2 days following exercise but is not necessary for adaptations.
Soreness occurs because lactic acid builds up in the muscles.	Lactic acid is produced during muscular work but is converted back into other substrates within 30 minutes after exercising. Soreness is due to microscopic tears or damage in the muscle fibers, but this damage is repaired as the body builds the muscle. Excessive soreness occurs if you violate the law of progression and do too much too soon.
Strength training can build cardiovascular fitness and flexibility.	Resistance exercise can increase heart rate, but this is due primarily to a pressure overload rather than a volume overload on the heart that occurs from endurance (aerobic) exercise. Gains in muscle mass do cause an increase in resting metabolism that can aid in controlling body fatness.
Strength training is beneficial only for young adults.	Studies have shown that people in their eighties and nineties can benefit from resistance exercise and improve their strength and endurance. Most experts would agree that resistance exercise increases in importance with age rather than decreases.

Table 5 ▶ How to Prevent Injury
• Warm up 10 minutes before the workout and stay warm.
• Do not hold your breath while lifting. This may cause blackout or hernia.
• Avoid hyperventilation before lifting a weight.
• Avoid dangerous or high-risk exercises.
• Progress slowly.
• Use good shoes with good traction.
• Avoid arching the back. Keep the pelvis in normal alignment.
• Keep the weight close to the body.
• Do not lift from a stoop (bent over with back rounded).
• When lifting from the floor, do not let the hips come up before the upper body.
• For bent-over rowing, lay your head on a table and bend the knees, or use one-arm rowing and support the trunk with your free hand.
• Stay in a squat as short a time as possible and do not do a full squat.
• Be sure collars on free weights are tight.
• Use a moderately slow, continuous, controlled movement and hold the final position a few seconds.
• Overload but don't overwhelm! A program that is too intense can cause injuries.
• Do not allow the weights to drop or bang.
• Do not train without medical supervision if you have a hernia, high blood pressure, a fever, an infection, recent surgery, heart disease, or back problems.
• Use chalk or a towel to keep your hands dry when handling weights.

maintain good flexibility. Some safety tips are presented in Table 5.

Perform lifts in a slow, controlled manner to enhance both effectiveness and safety. Lifting at a slow cadence will provide a greater stimulus to the muscles and increase strength gains. A good recommendation is to take 2 seconds on the lifting phase (concentric) and 4 seconds on the lowering (eccentric) phase.

Provide sufficient time to rest during and between workouts. The body needs time to rest in order to allow beneficial adaptations to occur. Choose an exercise sequence that alternates muscle groups so muscles have a chance to rest before another set. Lifting every other day or alternating muscle groups (if lifting more than 3 or 4 days per week) is also important in providing rest for the muscles.

Include all body parts and balance the strength of antagonistic muscle groups. A common mistake made by many beginning lifters is to perform only a few different exercises or to emphasize a few body parts. Training the biceps without working the triceps, for example, can lead to muscle imbalances that can compromise flexibility and increase risks for injury. In some cases, training must be increased in certain areas to compensate for stronger antagonist muscle groups. Many sprinters, for example, pull their hamstrings because the quadriceps are so overdeveloped that they overpower the hamstrings. The recommended ratio of quadriceps to hamstring strength is 60:40.

Customize your training program to fit your specific needs. Athletes should train muscles the way that they will be used in their skill, using similar patterns, range of motion, and speed (the principle of specificity). If you wish to develop a particular group of muscles, remember that the muscle group can be worked harder when isolated than when worked in combination with other muscle groups.

Use good technique to reduce the risks for injury and to isolate the intended muscles. An important consideration in resistance exercise is to complete all lifts through the full range of motion using only the intended muscle groups. A common cause of poor technique is using too heavy of a weight. If you have to jerk the weight up or use momentum to lift the weight, it is too heavy. Using heavier weights will only provide a greater stimulus to your muscles if your muscles are actually doing the work. Therefore, it is best to use a weight that you can control safely. By lifting through the full range of motion, you will increase the effectiveness of the exercise and

Choose exercises that build muscle fitness in the major muscle groups of the body. The ACSM recommends 8 to 10 basic exercises for muscle fitness. Table 6 (page 192) provides eight basic exercises for free weights. Table 7 (page 194) presents eight basic exercises for resistance machines. For additional options in resistance training, see the eight calisthenic exercises in Table 8 (page 196) and the eight core strength exercises in Table 9 (page 198). Since good muscular fitness in the abdominals is important, it is recommended that some abdominal or core training be performed as part of any program. Isometric exercises are available at Web04.

Strategies for Action

An important step in taking action for developing and maintaining muscle fitness is assessing your current status. An important early step in taking action to improve fitness is self-assessment. A 1RM test of isotonic strength is described in *Lab Resource Materials*. This test allows you to determine absolute and relative strength for the arms and legs. In addition, the 1RM values can be used to help you select the appropriate resistance for your muscle fitness training program. A grip strength test of isometric strength is also provided in *Lab Resource Materials* for Lab 10A. In addition to descriptions of the 1RM test, a body weight test for isotonic strength is provided in the *On the Web* feature for people who do not have the equipment to perform the 1RM assessment.

Three tests of muscular endurance are described in the *Lab Resource Materials* for Lab 10B. It is recommended that you perform the assessments for both strength and muscular endurance before you begin your progressive resistance training program. Periodically reevaluate your muscle fitness using these assessments.

Many factors other than your own basic abilities affect muscle fitness test scores. If muscles are warmed up before lifting, more force can be exerted and heavier loads can be lifted. Muscle endurance performance may also be enhanced by a warm-up. Do not perform your self-assessments after vigorous exercise because that exercise can cause fatigue and result in sub-optimal test results. It is appropriate to practice the techniques in the various tests on days preceding the actual testing. People who have good technique achieve better scores and are less likely to be injured when performing tests than those without good technique. It is best to perform the strength and muscular endurance tests on different days.

Keeping records of progress is important to adhering to a PRE program. Activity logging sheets are provided in Labs 10C and 10D to help you keep records of your progress as you regularly perform PRE to build and maintain good muscle fitness. A guide to the different muscles of the body is presented in Figure 7.

Online Learning Center

Web Resources

American College of Sports Medicine **www.acsm.org**
National Athletic Trainers Association **www.nata.org**
National Strength and Conditioning Association
www.nsca-cc.org
The Physician and Sportsmedicine Online
www.physsportsmed.com

Web 14

Suggested Readings

Additional reference materials for Concept 10 are available at Web15.

Web 15

American College of Sports Medicine. 2006. *ACSM's Guidelines for Exercise Testing and Prescription.* 7th ed. Philadelphia: Lippincott, Williams and Wilkins.

Technology Update
BOSU® Balance Trainers

BOSU® Balance Trainers (made by Fitness Quest Inc.) have become a popular piece of exercise equipment in many fitness centers. The unique features of the Bosu® are the domed shape and the firm resistance provided by the air-filled bladder. The Bosu® evolved in some ways from the large, inflatable balls (Swiss balls) that are frequently used in gyms and physical therapy clinics. While the Swiss balls have proven to be highly effective, their unstable nature has made some movements complicated and difficult to perform. The Bosu® Balance Trainer provides a stable surface while maintaining some of the same benefits of the stability balls. They can be used for a wide array of movements and have been found useful for rehabilitation purposes, sport enhancement, and general core strength training. Visit **www.bosu.com** for details.

BOSU is a registered trademark of BOSU Fitness LLC. Used with permission

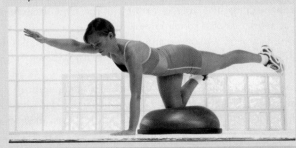

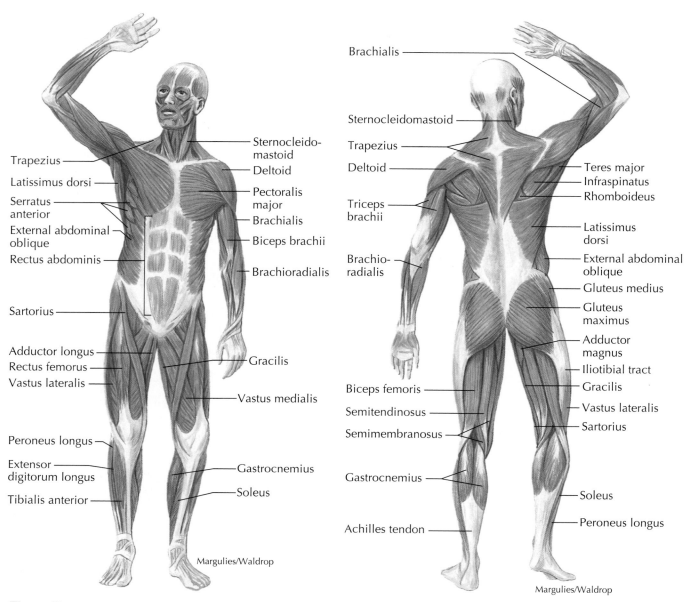

Trapezius
Latissimus dorsi
Serratus anterior
External abdominal oblique
Rectus abdominis
Sartorius
Adductor longus
Rectus femorus
Vastus lateralis
Peroneus longus
Extensor digitorum longus
Tibialis anterior

Sternocleido-mastoid
Deltoid
Pectoralis major
Brachialis
Biceps brachii
Brachioradialis
Gracilis
Vastus medialis
Gastrocnemius
Soleus

Margulies/Waldrop

Brachialis
Sternocleidomastoid
Trapezius
Deltoid
Triceps brachii
Brachio-radialis
Biceps femoris
Semitendinosus
Semimembranosus
Gastrocnemius
Achilles tendon

Teres major
Infraspinatus
Rhomboideus
Latissimus dorsi
External abdominal oblique
Gluteus medius
Gluteus maximus
Adductor magnus
Iliotibial tract
Gracilis
Vastus lateralis
Sartorius
Soleus
Peroneus longus

Margulies/Waldrop

Figure 7 ▶ Muscles in the body.

American College of Sports Medicine. "Creatine Supplementation: Current Content." (www.acsm.org).

Baechle, T. R. and R. W. Earle. 2006. *Weight Training*. 3rd ed. Champaign, IL: Human Kinetics.

Bird, S. P. 2005. Designing resistance training programmes to enhance muscular fitness: A review of the acute programme variables. *Sports Medicine* 35:841–851.

Brown, G. A., M. Vukovich, and D. S. King. 2006. Testosterone prohormone supplements. *Medicine and Science in Sports and Exercise* 38(8):1451–1461.

Cauza, E., et al. 2005. The relative benefits of endurance and strength training on the metabolic factors and muscle function of people with type 2 diabetes mellitus. *Archives of Physical Medicine and Rehabilitation* 86:1527–1533.

Delavier, F. 2006. *Strength Training Anatomy*. 2nd ed. Champaign, IL: Human Kinetics

Downing, J. H., and J. E. Lander. 2002. Performance errors in weight training and their correction. *Journal of Physical Education, Recreation and Dance* 73(9):44–52.

Fahey, T. D. 2007. *Basic Weight Training for Men and Women*. 6th ed. New York: McGraw-Hill.

Holt, S. 2001. Mechanics of machines: Selecting the right piece of equipment. *Fitness Management* (July):56+.

Jones, C. S., C. Christenson, and M. Young. 2000. Weight training injury trends: A 20-year survey. *The Physician and Sportsmedicine* 28(7):61–72.

Jurca, R., et al. 2005. Association of muscular strength with incidence of metabolic syndrome in men. *Medicine and Science in Sports and Exercise* 37:1849–1855.

Kraemer, W. 2005. Progression and resistance training. *President's Council on Physical Fitness and Sports Research Digest* 6(3):1–8.

Kraemer, W. J., and N. A. Ratamess. 2004. Fundamentals of resistance training: Progression and exercise prescription. *Medicine and Science in Sports and Exercise* 36(4):674–688.

Kristal, A. R., A. J. Littman, D. Benitez, and E. White. 2005. Yoga practice is associated with attenuated weight gain in healthy, middle-aged men and women. *Alternative Therapy in Medicine and Health* 11:28–33.

Manini, T. M., et al. 2005. Misconceptions about strength exercise among older adults. *Journal of Aging and Physical Activity* 13:422–433.

Misic, M., and G. A. Kelley. 2002. The impact of creatine supplementation on anaerobic performance: A meta-analysis. *American Journal of Sportsmedicine* 4:116–124.

Nissen, S. L., and B. R. Sharp. 2003. Effects of dietary supplements on lean mass and strength gains with resistance exercise: A meta analysis. *Journal of Applied Physiology* 94(2):651–659.

Ohira, T., et al. 2006. Effects of weight training on quality of life in recent breast cancer survivors: The Weight Training for Breast Cancer Survivors (WTBS) study. *Cancer* 106(9):2076–2083.

Peterson, M. D., M. R. Rhea, and B. A. Alvar. 2005. Applications of the dose-response for muscular strength development: A review of meta-analytic efficacy and reliability for designing training prescription. *Journal of Strength and Conditioning Research* 19(4):950–958.

Rhea, M. R., et al. 2002. A comparison of linear and daily undulating periodized programs with equated volume and intensity for strength. *Journal of Strength and Conditioning Research* 16(2):250–255.

Rhea, M. R., et al. 2003. A meta analysis to determine the dose response for strength development. *Medicine and Science in Sports and Exercise* 35(3): 456–464.

Shiner, J., et al. 2005. Integrating low-intensity plyometrics into strength and conditioning programs. *Strength and Conditioning Journal* 27(6):10–20.

Urhausen, A., et al. 2004. Are the cardiac effects of anabolic steroids abuse in strength athletes reversible? *Heart* 90:496–501.

Volek, J. S. 2004. Influence of nutrition on responses to resistance training. *Medicine and Science in Sports and Exercise* 36(4):689–696.

Yesalis, C. E., and M. S. Bahrke. 2005. Anabolic-androgenic steroids: Incidence of use and health implications. *President's Council on Physical Fitness and Sports Research Digest* 6(1):1–8.

Westcott, W. 2003. *Building Strength and Stamina.* 2nd ed. Champaign, IL: Human Kinetics.

Zatsiorsky, V. M., and W. J. Kraemer. 2006. *Science and Practice of Strength Training.* 2nd ed. Champaign, IL: Human Kinetics.

 In the News

Prohormone Nutritional Supplements Shown to Be Ineffective and Potentially Harmful

A variety of nutritional supplements are marketed as alternatives to steroids. Most of these products are referred to as testosterone prohormones because they are thought to lead to the production of testosterone and testosterone analogs. Many companies marketed these products as having anabolic and ergogenic effects based on the notion that increases in testosterone could enhance adaptations to resistance training. Examples of common ingredients in these products are dehydroepiandrosterone (DHEA), andostenedione, and androstenediol. Because the safety of these products had not been established, the U.S. Food and Drug Association passed the Anabolic Steroid Control Act of 2004, which labeled these products as controlled substances that cannot be purchased or used without a prescription. A recent study (Brown et al., 2006) provides convincing evidence that this decision was well founded. The study reviewed the safety and efficacy of the most common testosterone prohormones and found that they did not produce anabolic or ergogenic effects. More importantly, the supplements were found to increase the risks of negative health consequences.

Table 6 The Basic Eight for Free Weights

Table 6

1. Bench Press

This exercise develops the chest (pectoral) and triceps muscles. Lie supine on bench with knees bent and feet flat on bench or flat on floor in stride position. Grasp bar at shoulder level. Push bar up until arms are straight. Return and repeat. Do not arch lower back. Note: Feet may be placed on floor if lower back can be kept flattened. Do not put feet on the bench if it is unstable.

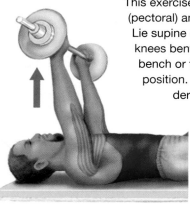

Pectoralis major

Triceps

2. Overhead (Military Press)

This exercise develops the muscles of the shoulders and arms. Sit erect, bend elbows, palms facing forward at chest level with hands spread (slightly more than shoulder width). Have bar touching chest; spread feet (comfortable distance). Tighten your abdominal and back muscles. Move bar to overhead position (arms straight). Lower bar to chest position. Repeat. Caution: Keep arms perpendicular and do not allow weight to move backward or wrists to bend backward. Spotters are needed.

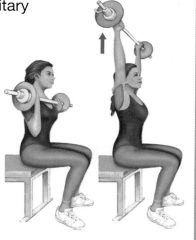

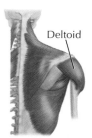

Deltoid

3. Biceps Curl

This exercise develops the muscles of the upper front part of the arms (biceps). Stand erect with back against a wall, palms forward, bar touching thighs. Spread feet in comfortable position. Tighten abdominals and back muscles. Do not lock knees. Move bar to chin, keeping body straight and elbows near the sides. Lower bar to original position. Do not allow back to arch. Repeat. Spotters are usually not needed. Variations: Use dumbbell and sit on end of bench with feet in stride position; work one arm at a time. Or use dumbbell with the palm down or thumb up to emphasize other muscles.

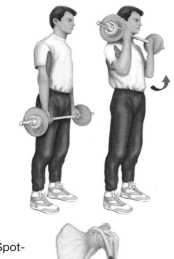

Biceps

4. Triceps Curl

This exercise develops the muscles on the back of the upper arms (triceps). Sit erect, elbows and palms facing up, bar resting behind neck on shoulders, hands near center of bar, feet spread. Tighten abdominal and back muscles. Keep upper arms stationary. Raise weight overhead, return bar to original position. Repeat. Spotters are needed. Variation: Substitute dumbbells (one in each hand, or one held in both hands, or one in one hand at a time).

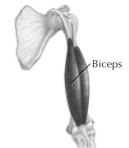

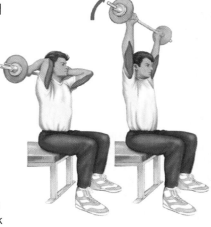

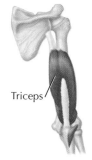

Triceps

5. Wrist Curl

This exercise develops the muscles of the fingers, wrist, and forearms. Sit astride a bench with the back of one forearm on the bench, wrist and hand hanging over the edge. Hold a dumbbell in the fingers of that hand with the palm facing forward. To develop the flexors, lift the weight by curling the fingers then the wrist through a full range of motion. Slowly lower and repeat. To strengthen the extensors, start with the palm down. Lift the weight by extending the wrist through a full range of motion. Slowly lower and repeat. Note: Both wrists may be exercised at the same time by substituting a barbell in place of the dumbbell.

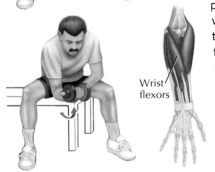

Wrist flexors

7. Half-Squat

This exercise develops the muscles of the thighs and buttocks. Stand erect, feet shoulder-width apart and turned out 45 degrees. Rest bar behind neck on shoulders. Spread hands in a comfortable position. Begin squat by first moving hips backwards, keeping back straight, eyes ahead. By moving first at the hips and then bending knees, shins will remain vertical. Bend knees to approximately 90 degrees. Pause; then stand. Repeat. Spotters are needed. Variations: Substitute dumbbell in each hand at sides.

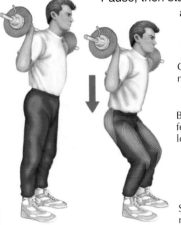
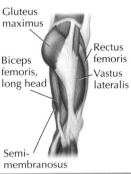

Gluteus maximus

Biceps femoris, long head

Rectus femoris

Vastus lateralis

Semi-membranosus

6. Dumbbell Rowing

This exercise develops the muscles of the upper back. It is best performed with the aid of a bench or chair for support. Grab a dumbbell with one hand and place opposite hand on the bench to support the trunk. Slowly lift the weight up until the elbow is parallel with the back. Lower the weight and repeat to complete the set. Switch hands and repeat with the opposite arm. The exercise can also be performed with one leg kneeling on the bench.

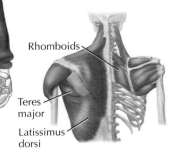

Rhomboids

Teres major

Latissimus dorsi

8. Lunge

This exercise develops the thigh and gluteal muscles. Place a barbell (with or without weight) behind your head and support with hands placed slightly wider than shoulder-width apart. In a slow and controlled motion, take a step forward and allow the leading leg to drop so that it is nearly parallel with the ground. The lower part of the leg should be nearly vertical and the back should be maintained in an upright posture. Take stride with opposite leg to return to standing posture. Repeat with other leg, remaining stationary or moving slowly in a straight line with alternating steps.

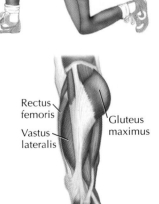

Rectus femoris

Vastus lateralis

Gluteus maximus

Table 7

Table 7 The Basic Eight for Resistance Machine Exercises

1. Chest Press

This exercise develops the chest (pectoral) and tricep muscles. Position seat height so that arm handles are directly in front of chest. Position backrest so that hands are at a comfortable distance away from the chest. Push handles forward to full extension and return to starting position in a slow and controlled manner. Repeat. Note: Machine may have a foot lever to help position, raise, and lower the weight.

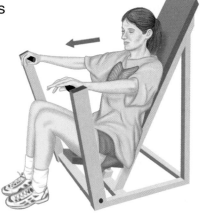

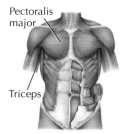

Pectoralis major

Triceps

2. Overhead Press

This exercise develops the muscles of the shoulders and arms. Position seat so that arm handles are slightly above shoulder height. Grasp handles with palms facing away and push lever up until arms are fully extended. Return to starting position and repeat. Note: Some machines may have an incline press.

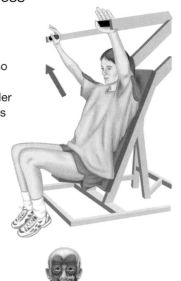

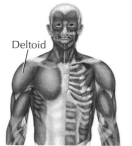

Deltoid

3. Bicep Curl

This exercise develops the elbow flexor muscles on the front of the arm, primarily the biceps. Adjust seat height so that arms are fully supported by pad when extended. Grasp handles palms up. While keeping the back straight, flex the elbow through the full range of motion.

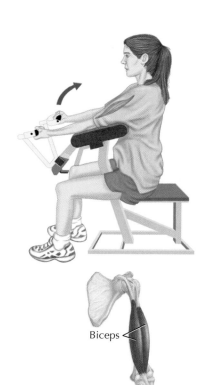

Biceps

4. Tricep Press

This exercise develops the extensor muscles on the back of the arm, primarily the triceps. Adjust seat height so that arm handles are slightly above shoulder height. Grasp handles with thumbs toward body. While keeping the back straight, extend arms fully until wrist contacts the support pad (arms straight). Return to starting position and repeat.

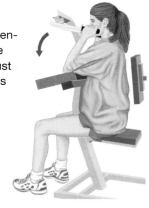

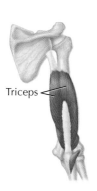

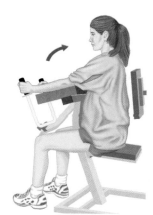

Triceps

The Basic Eight for Resistance Machine Exercises Table 7

Table 7

5. Lat Pull Down

This exercise primarily develops the latiss-mus dorsi, but the biceps, chest, and other back muscles may also be developed. Sit on the floor. Adjust seat height so that hands can just grasp bar when arms are fully extended. Grasp bar with palms facing away from you and hands shoulder-width (or wider) apart. Pull bar down to chest and return. Repeat.

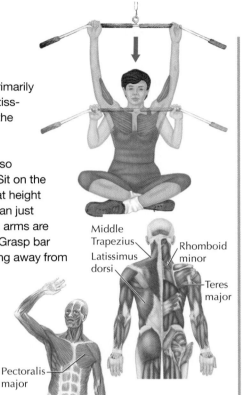

Middle Trapezius
Latissimus dorsi
Rhomboid minor
Teres major
Pectoralis major

7. Knee Extension

This exercise develops the thigh (quadriceps) muscles. Sit on end of bench with ankles hooked under padded bar. Grasp edge of table. Extend knees. Return and repeat. Alternative: Leg press (similar to half-squat). Note: The knee extension exercise iso-lates the quadriceps but places greater stress on the structures of the knee than the leg press or half-squat.

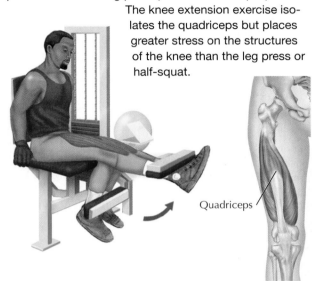

Quadriceps

6. Seated Rowing

This exercise develops the muscles of the back and shoulder. Adjust the machine so that arms are almost fully extended and parallel to the ground. Grasp handgrip with palms turned down and hands shoulder-width apart. While keeping the back straight, pull levers straight back to chest. Slowly return to starting posi-tion and repeat.

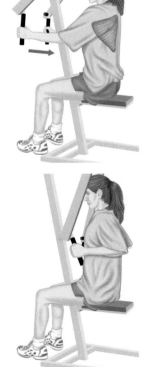

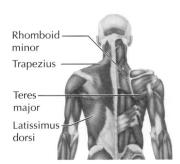

Rhomboid minor
Trapezius
Teres major
Latissimus dorsi

8. Hamstring Curl

This exercise develops the hamstrings (muscles on back of thigh) and other knee flexors. Lie prone on bench with ankles hooked under padded bar. Rest chin on hands or grasp bench. Flex knees as far as possible without allowing hips to raise. Return and repeat. Caution: Do not hyperextend the knees while assuming the starting position. If necessary, ask a partner to raise the pads while you place the heels under the bar.

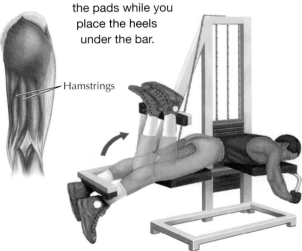

Hamstrings

Table 8

Table 8 The Basic Eight for Calisthenics

1. Bent Knee Push-Ups and Let-Down

This exercise develops the muscles of the arms, shoulders, and chest. Lie on the floor, face down with the hands under your shoulders. Keep your body straight from the knees to the top of the head. Push up until the arms are straight. Slowly lower chest (let-down) to floor. Repeat. Variation: full push-up and let-down performed the same way except body is straight from the toes to the top of head.

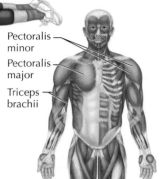

Pectoralis minor
Pectoralis major
Triceps brachii

Variation: Start from the up position and lower until the arm is bent at 90 degrees; then push up until arms are extended. Caution: Do not arch back.

2. Modified Pull-Ups

This exercise develops the muscles of the arms and shoulders. Hang (palms forward and shoulder-width apart) from a low bar (may be placed across two chairs), heels on floor, with the body straight from feet to head. Bracing the feet against a partner or fixed object is helpful. Pull up, keeping the body straight; touch the chest to the bar; then lower to the starting position. Repeat. Note: This exercise becomes more difficult as the angle of the body approaches horizontal and easier as it approaches the vertical. Variation: Perform so that the feet do not touch the floor (full pull-up). Variation: Perform with palms turned up. When palms are turned away from the face, pull-ups tend to use all the elbow flexors. With palms facing the body, the biceps are emphasized more.

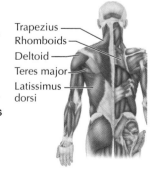

Trapezius
Rhomboids
Deltoid
Teres major
Latissimus dorsi

3. Dips

This exercise develops the latissimus dorsi, deltoid, rhomboid, and tricep. Start in a fully extended position with hands grasping the bar (palms facing in). Slowly drop down until the upper part of the arm is horizontal or parallel with the floor. Extend the arms back up to the starting position and repeat. Note: Many gyms have a dip/pull-up machine with accommodating resistance that provides a variable amount of assistance to help you complete the exercise.

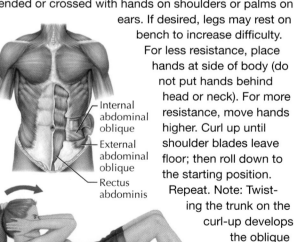

Rhomboid major
Deltoid
Triceps
Latissimus dorsi

4. Crunch (Curl-Up)

This exercise develops the upper abdominal muscles. Lie on the floor with the knees bent and the arms extended or crossed with hands on shoulders or palms on ears. If desired, legs may rest on bench to increase difficulty. For less resistance, place hands at side of body (do not put hands behind head or neck). For more resistance, move hands higher. Curl up until shoulder blades leave floor; then roll down to the starting position. Repeat. Note: Twisting the trunk on the curl-up develops the oblique abdominals.

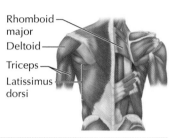

Internal abdominal oblique
External abdominal oblique
Rectus abdominis

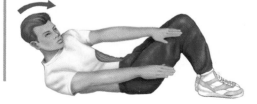

Table 8

5. (Trunk) Lift

This exercise develops the muscles of the upper back and corrects round shoulders. Lie face down with hands clasped behind the neck. Pull the shoulder blades together, raising the elbows off the floor. Slowly raise the head and chest off the floor by arching the upper back. Return to the starting position; repeat. For less resistance, hands may be placed under thighs. Caution: Do not arch the lower back. Lift only until the sternum (breastbone) clears the floor. Variations: arms down at sides (easiest), hands by head, arms extended (hardest).

Back extensors

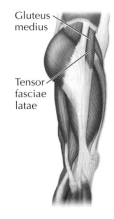

6. Side Leg Raises

This exercise develops the muscles on the outside of thighs. Lie on your side. Point knees forward. Raise the top leg 45 degrees; then return. Do the same number of repetitions with each leg. Caution: Keep knees and toes pointing forward. Variation: Ankle weights may be added for greater resistance.

Gluteus medius

Tensor fasciae latae

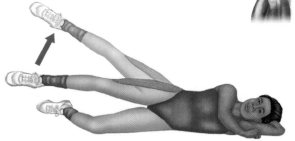

7. Lower Leg Lift

This exercise develops the muscles on the inside of thighs. Lie on the side with the upper leg (foot) supported on a bench. Note: If no bench is available, bend top leg and cross it in front of bottom leg for support. Raise the lower leg toward the ceiling. Repeat. Roll to opposite side and repeat. Keep knees pointed forward. Variation: An ankle weight may be added for greater resistance.

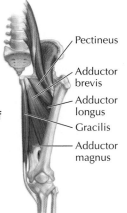

Pectineus

Adductor brevis

Adductor longus

Gracilis

Adductor magnus

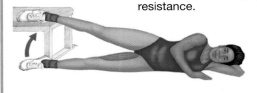

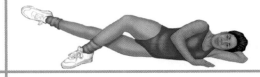

8. Alternate Leg Kneel

This exercise develops the muscles of the legs and hips. Stand tall, feet together. Take a step forward with the right foot, touching the left knee to the floor. The knees should be bent only to a 90-degree angle. Return to the starting position and step

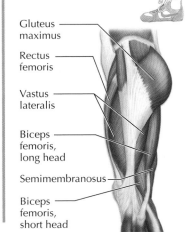

Gluteus maximus

Rectus femoris

Vastus lateralis

Biceps femoris, long head

Semimembranosus

Biceps femoris, short head

out with the other foot. Repeat, alternating right and left. Variation: Dumbbells may be held in the hands for greater resistance.

Table 9

Table 9 Exercises for Core Strength

1. Crunch (Curl-Up)

This exercise develops the upper abdominal muscles. Lie on the floor with the knees bent and the arms extended or crossed with hands on shoulders or palms on ears. If desired, legs may rest on bench to increase difficulty. For less resistance, place hands at side of body (do not put hands behind neck). For more resistance, move hands higher. Curl up until shoulder blades leave floor; then roll down to the starting position. Repeat. Note: Twisting the trunk on the curl-up develops the oblique abdominals.

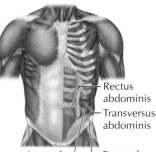

2. Reverse Curl

This exercise develops the lower abdominal muscles. Lie on the floor. Bend the knees, place the feet flat on the floor, and place arms at sides. Lift the knees to the chest, raising the hips off the floor. Do not let the knees go past the shoulders. Return to the starting position. Repeat.

3. Crunch with Twist (on Bench)

This exercise strengthens the oblique abdominals and helps prevent or correct lumbar lordosis, abdominal ptosis, and backache. Lie on your back with your feet on a bench, knees bent at 90 degrees. Arms may be extended or on shoulders or hand on ears (the most difficult). Same as crunch except twist the upper trunk so the right shoulder is higher than the left. Reach toward the left knee with the right elbow. Hold. Return and repeat to the opposite side.

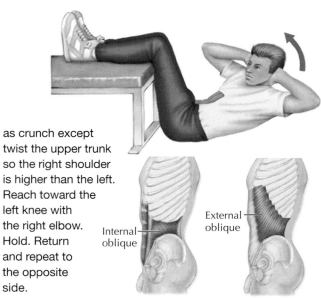

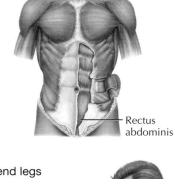

4. Sitting Tucks

This exercise strengthens the lower abdominals, increases their endurance, improves posture, and prevents backache. (This is an advanced exercise and is not recommended for people who have back pain.) Sit on floor with feet raised, arms extended for balance. Alternately bend and extend legs without letting back or feet touch floor.

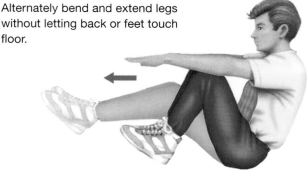

Table 9

5. Hands and Knees Balance

Begin with both hands and knees placed on Bosu®. Place hands directly below shoulders and knees directly below hips. Look straight down at floor. Draw in lower abdomen. Extend one leg and raise opposite arm to a horizontal position. Keep spine in neutral position. Hold. Relax. Repeat with opposite arm and leg. Do 10 or more repetitions on each side.

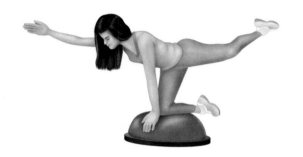

7. Side Step

Begin standing on the floor with Bosu® on your left. Step up onto the center of Bosu® with left foot. Tap right foot on top; then step back to the floor with first the right foot and then the left. Repeat for 60 seconds. Switch to the opposite side.

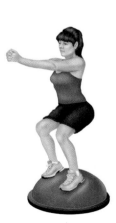

6. Marching

Stand in the middle of the Bosu® with shoulders back and lower abdomen drawn in. March in place, swinging arms in opposite directions—forward and backward—while maintaining spine in neutral position. Progress to jogging in place. Continue for 1 to 2 minutes or longer.

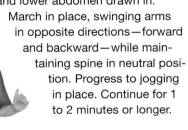

8. Squatting

Stand with feet apart on Bosu®. With knees angled outward slightly, draw abdomen in. Reach forward with hands clasped. Draw shoulder blades down and back. Squat up and down by moving hips backward and then bending knees. (Imagine the movement pattern involved in sitting back on a stool.) Repeat for 1 to 2 minutes.

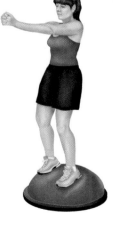

Table 10

Table 10 Strength and Muscular Endurance Self-Assessments

1. Seated Press (Chest Press)

This test can be performed using a seated press (see below) or using a bench press machine. When using the seated press, position the seat height so that arm handles are directly in front of the chest. Position backrest so that hands are at comfortable distance away from the chest. Push handles forward to full extension and return to starting position in a slow and controlled manner. Repeat. Note: Machine may have a foot lever to help position, raise, and lower the weight.

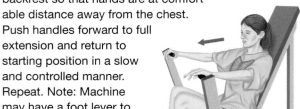

2. Leg Press

To perform this test, use a leg press machine. Typically, the beginning position is with the knees bent at right angles with the feet placed on the press machine pedals or a foot platform. Extend the legs and return to beginning position. Do not lock the knees when the legs are straightened. Typically, handles are provided. Grasp the handles with the hands when performing this test.

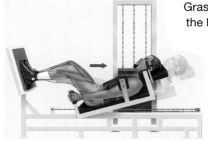

Lab Resource Materials: Muscle Fitness Tests

Evaluating Isotonic Strength: 1RM

1. Use a weight machine for the leg press and seated arm press (or bench press) for the evaluation.
2. Estimate how much weight you can lift two or three times. Be conservative; it is better to start with too little weight than too much. If you lift the weight more than 10 times, the procedure should be done again on another day when you are rested.
3. Using correct form, perform a leg press with the weight you have chosen. Perform as many times as you can up to 10.
4. Use Chart 1 to determine your 1RM for the leg press. Find the weight used in the left-hand column and then find the number of repetitions you performed across the top of the chart.
5. Your 1RM score is the value where the weight row and the repetitions column intersect.
6. Repeat this procedure for the seated arm press.
7. Record your 1RM scores for the leg press and seated arm press in the Results section.
8. Next, divide your 1RM scores by your body weight in pounds to get a "strength per pound of body weight" (str/lb./body wt.) score for each of the two exercises.
9. Finally, determine your strength rating for your upper body strength (arm press) and lower body (leg press) using Chart 2 (page 205).

Chart 1 ▶ Predicted 1RM Based on Reps-to-Fatigue

Wt.	1	2	3	4	5	6	7	8	9	10	Wt.	1	2	3	4	5	6	7	8	9	10
30	30	31	32	33	34	35	36	37	38	39	170	170	175	180	185	191	197	204	211	219	227
35	35	37	38	39	40	41	42	43	44	45	175	175	180	185	191	197	203	210	217	225	233
40	40	41	42	44	46	47	49	50	51	53	180	180	185	191	196	202	209	216	223	231	240
45	45	46	48	49	51	52	54	56	58	60	185	185	190	196	202	208	215	222	230	238	247
50	50	51	53	55	56	58	60	62	64	67	190	190	195	201	207	214	221	228	236	244	253
55	55	57	58	60	62	64	66	68	71	73	195	195	201	206	213	219	226	234	242	251	260
60	60	62	64	65	67	70	72	74	77	80	200	200	206	212	218	225	232	240	248	257	267
65	65	67	69	71	73	75	78	81	84	87	205	205	211	217	224	231	238	246	254	264	273
70	70	72	74	76	79	81	84	87	90	93	210	210	216	222	229	236	244	252	261	270	280
75	75	77	79	82	84	87	90	93	96	100	215	215	221	228	235	242	250	258	267	276	287
80	80	82	85	87	90	93	96	99	103	107	220	220	226	233	240	247	255	264	273	283	293
85	85	87	90	93	96	99	102	106	109	113	225	225	231	238	245	253	261	270	279	289	300
90	90	93	95	98	101	105	108	112	116	120	230	230	237	244	251	259	267	276	286	296	307
95	95	98	101	104	107	110	114	118	122	127	235	235	242	249	256	264	273	282	292	302	313
100	100	103	106	109	112	116	120	124	129	133	240	240	247	254	262	270	279	288	298	309	320
105	105	108	111	115	118	122	126	130	135	140	245	245	252	259	267	276	285	294	304	315	327
110	110	113	116	120	124	128	132	137	141	147	250	250	257	265	273	281	290	300	310	321	333
115	115	118	122	125	129	134	138	143	148	153	255	256	262	270	278	287	296	306	317	328	340
120	120	123	127	131	135	139	144	149	154	160	260	260	267	275	284	292	302	312	323	334	347
125	125	129	132	136	141	145	150	155	161	167	265	265	273	281	289	298	308	318	329	341	353
130	130	134	138	142	146	151	156	161	167	173	270	270	278	286	295	304	314	324	335	347	360
135	135	139	143	147	152	157	162	168	174	180	275	275	283	291	300	309	319	330	341	354	367
140	140	144	148	153	157	163	168	174	180	187	280	280	288	296	305	315	325	336	348	360	373
145	145	149	154	158	163	168	174	180	186	193	285	285	293	302	311	321	331	342	354	366	380
150	150	154	159	164	169	174	180	186	193	200	290	290	298	307	316	326	337	348	360	373	387
155	155	159	164	169	174	180	186	192	199	207	295	295	303	312	322	332	343	354	366	379	393
160	160	165	169	175	180	186	192	199	206	213	300	300	309	318	327	337	348	360	372	386	400
165	165	170	175	180	186	192	198	205	212	220	305	305	314	323	333	343	354	366	379	392	407

Source: JOPERD.

Evaluating Isometric Strength

Test: Grip Strength

Adjust a hand dynamometer to fit your hand size. Squeeze it as hard as possible. You may bend or straighten the arm, but do not touch the body with your hand, elbow, or arm. Perform with both right and left hands. *Note:* When not being tested, perform the basic eight isometric strength exercises, or squeeze and indent a new tennis ball (*after* completing the dynamometer test).

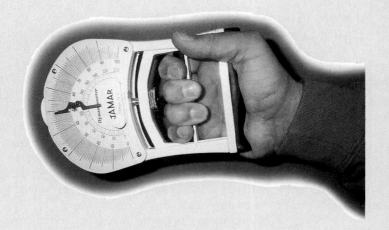

Evaluating Muscular Endurance

1. Curl-Up (Dynamic)

Sit on a mat or carpet with your legs bent more than 90 degrees so your feet remain flat on the floor (about halfway between 90 degrees and straight). Make two tape marks 4½ inches apart or lay a 4½-inch strip of paper or cardboard on the floor. Lie with your arms extended at your sides, palms down and the fingers extended so that your fingertips touch one tape mark (or one side of the paper or cardboard strip). Keeping your heels in contact with the floor, curl the head and shoulders forward until your fingers reach 4½ inches (second piece of tape or other side of strip). Lower slowly to beginning position. Repeat one curl-up every 3 seconds. Continue until you are unable to keep the pace of one curl-up every 3 seconds.

Two partners may be helpful. One stands on the cardboard strip (to prevent movement) if one is used. The second assures that the head returns to the floor after each repetition.

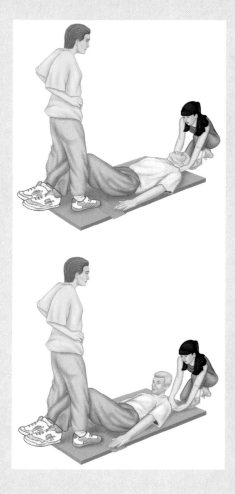

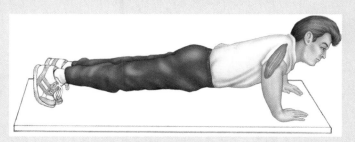

2. Ninety-Degree Push-Up (Dynamic)
Support the body in a push-up position from the toes. The hands should be just outside the shoulders, the back and legs straight, and toes tucked under. Lower the body until the upper arm is parallel to the floor or the elbow is bent at 90 degrees. The rhythm should be approximately 1 push-up every 3 seconds. Repeat as many times as possible up to 35.

3. Flexed-Arm Support (Static)
Women: Support the body in a push-up position from the knees. The hands should be outside the shoulders, the back and legs straight. Lower the body until the upper arm is parallel to the floor or the elbow is flexed at 90 degrees.
Men: Use the same procedure as for women except support the push-up position from the toes instead of the knees. (Same position as for 90-degree push-up.) Hold the 90-degree position as long as possible, up to 35 seconds.

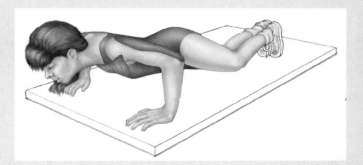

Chart 2 ▶ Fitness Classification for Relative Strength in Men and Women (1RM/Body Weight)

	Leg Press			Arm Press		
Age:	30 or Less	31–50	51+	30 or Less	31–50	51+
Ratings for Men						
High-performance zone	2.06+	1.81+	1.61+	1.26+	1.01+	.86+
Good fitness zone	1.96–2.05	1.66–1.80	1.51–1.60	1.11–1.25	.91–1.00	.76–.85
Marginal zone	1.76–1.95	1.51–1.65	1.41–1.50	.96–1.10	.86–.90	.66–.75
Low fitness zone	1.75 or less	1.50 or less	1.40 or less	.96 or less	.80 or less	.65 or less
Ratings for Women						
High-performance zone	1.61+	1.36+	1.16+	.75+	.61+	.51+
Good fitness zone	1.46–1.60	1.21–1.35	1.06–1.15	.65–.75	.56–.60	.46–.50
Marginal zone	1.31–1.45	1.11–1.20	.96–1.05	.56–.65	.51–.55	.41–.45
Low fitness zone	1.30 or less	1.10 or less	.95 or less	.55 or less	.50 or less	.40 or less

Chart 3 ▶ Isometric Strength Rating Scale (Pounds)

Classification	Left Grip	Right Grip	Total Score
Ratings for Men			
High-performance zone	125+	135+	260+
Good fitness zone	100–124	110–134	210–259
Marginal zone	90–99	95–109	185–209
Low fitness zone	<90	<95	<185
Ratings for Women			
High-performance zone	75+	85+	160+
Good fitness zone	60–74	70–84	130–159
Marginal zone	45–59	50–69	95–129
Low fitness zone	<45	<50	<95

Suitable for use by young adults between 18 and 30 years of age. After 30, an adjustment of 0.5 of 1 percent per year is appropriate because some loss of muscle tissue typically occurs as you grow older.

See Appendix A.

Chart 4 ▶ Rating Scale for Dynamic Muscular Endurance

Age:	17–26		27–39		40–49		50–59		60+	
Classification	Curl-Ups	Push-Ups	Curl-Ups	Push-Ups	Curl-Ups	Push-Ups	Curl-Ups	Push-Ups	Curl-Ups	Push-Ups
Ratings for Men										
High-performance zone	35+	29+	34+	27+	33+	26+	32+	24+	31+	22+
Good fitness zone	24–34	20–28	23–33	18–26	22–32	17–25	21–31	15–23	20–30	13–21
Marginal zone	15–23	16–19	14–22	15–17	13–21	14–16	12–20	12–14	11–19	10–12
Low fitness zone	<15	<16	<14	<15	<13	<14	<12	<12	<11	<10
Ratings for Women										
High-performance zone	25+	17+	24+	16+	23+	15+	22+	14+	21+	13+
Good fitness zone	18–24	12–16	17–23	11–15	16–22	10–14	15–21	9–13	14–20	8–12
Marginal zone	10–17	8–11	9–16	7–10	8–15	6–9	7–14	5–8	6–13	4–7
Low fitness zone	<10	<8	<9	<7	<8	<6	<7	<5	<6	<4

Chart 5 ▶ Rating Scale for Static Endurance (Flexed-Arm Support)

Classification	Score in Seconds
High-performance zone	30+
Good fitness zone	20–29
Marginal zone	10–19
Low fitness zone	10

Lab 10A Evaluating Muscle Strength: 1RM and Grip Strength

Name		Section	Date

Purpose: To evaluate your muscle strength using 1RM and to determine the best amount of resistance to use for various strength exercises

Procedures: 1RM is the maximum amount of resistance you can lift for a specific exercise. Testing yourself to determine how much you can lift only one time using traditional methods can be fatiguing and even dangerous. The procedure you will perform here allows you to estimate 1RM based on the number of times you can lift a weight that is less than 1RM.

Evaluating Strength Using Estimated 1RM

1. Use a resistance machine for the leg press and arm or bench press for the evaluation part of this lab.
2. Estimate how much weight you can lift two or three times. Be conservative; it is better to start with too little weight than too much. If you lift a weight more than 10 times, the procedure should be done again on another day when you are rested.
3. Using correct form, perform a leg press with the weight you have chosen. Perform as many times as you can up to 10.
4. Use Chart 1 in *Lab Resource Materials* to determine your 1RM for the leg press. Find the weight used in the left-hand column and then find the number of repetitions you performed across the top of the chart.
5. Your 1RM score is the value where the weight row and the repetitions column intersect.
6. Repeat this procedure for the arm or bench press using the same technique.
7. Record your 1RM scores for the leg press and bench press in the Results section.
8. Next divide your 1RM scores by your body weight in pounds to get a "strength per pound of body weight" (1RM/body weight) score for each of the two exercises.
9. Determine your strength rating for your upper body strength (arm press) and lower body (leg press) using Chart 2 in *Lab Resource Materials.* Record in the Results section. If time allows, assess 1RM for other exercises you choose to perform (see Lab 10C).
10. If a grip dynamometer is available, determine your right-hand and left-hand grip strength using the procedures in *Lab Resource Materials.* Use Chart 3 in *Lab Resource Materials* to rate your grip (isometric) strength.

Results

Arm press (or bench press):	Wt. selected ___	Reps ___	Estimated 1RM ___ (Chart 1, *Lab Resource Materials*)
	Strength per lb. body weight ___ (1RM ÷ body weight)		Rating ___ (Chart 2, *Lab Resource Materials*)
Leg press:	Wt. selected ___	Reps ___	Estimated 1RM ___ (Chart 1, *Lab Resource Materials*)
	Strength per lb. body weight ___ (1RM ÷ body weight)		Rating ___ (Chart 2, *Lab Resource Materials*)
Grip strength:	Right grip score ___		Right grip rating ___
	Left grip score ___		Left grip rating ___
	Total score ___		Total rating ___

Seated Press (Chest Press)

This test can be performed using a seated press (see below) or using a bench press machine. When using the seated press, position the seat height so that arm handles are directly in front of the chest. Position backrest so that hands are at comfortable distance away from the chest. Push handles forward to full extension and return to starting position in a slow and controlled manner. Repeat. Note: Machine may have a foot lever to help position, raise, and lower the weight.

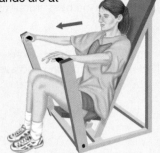

Leg Press

To perform this test, use a leg press machine. Typically, the beginning position is with the knees bent at right angles with the feet placed on the press machine pedals or a foot platform. Extend the legs and return to beginning position. Do not lock the knees when the legs are straightened. Typically, handles are provided. Grasp the handles with the hands when performing this test.

Conclusions and Implications: In several sentences, discuss your current strength, whether you believe it is adequate for good health, and whether you think that your "strength per pound of body weight" scores are representative of your true strength.

Lab 10B Evaluating Muscular Endurance

Name		Section	Date

Purpose: To evaluate the dynamic muscular endurance of two muscle groups and the static endurance of the arms and trunk muscles

Procedures

1. Perform the curl-up, push-up, and flexed-arm support tests described in *Lab Resource Materials* (pp. 204–205).
2. In Chart 1, record your test scores in the Results section. Determine and record your rating from Charts 4 and 5 in *Lab Resource Materials.*

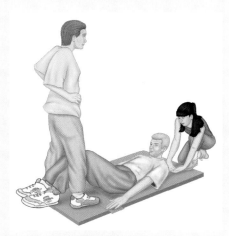

1. Curl-up (dynamic)

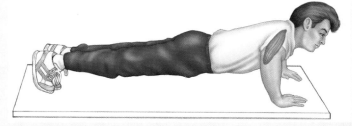

2. Ninety-degree push-up (dynamic)

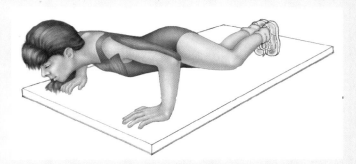

3. Flexed-arm support (static): women in knee position and men in full support position

Results

Record your scores below.

Curl-up [   ]   Push-up [   ]   Flexed-arm support (seconds) [   ]

Check your ratings in Chart 1.

Chart 1 ▶ Rating Scale for Static Endurance (Flexed-Arm Support)

	Curl-Up	Push-Up	Flexed-Arm Support
High	◯	◯	◯
Good	◯	◯	◯
Marginal	◯	◯	◯
Poor	◯	◯	◯

On which of the tests of muscular endurance did you score the lowest?

Curl-up ◯ Push-up ◯ Flexed-arm support ◯

On which of the tests of muscular endurance did you score the best?

Curl-up ◯ Push-up ◯ Flexed-arm support ◯

Conclusions and Implications: In several sentences, discuss your current level of muscular endurance and whether this level is enough to meet your health, work, and leisure-time needs in the future.

Lab 10C Planning and Logging Muscle Fitness Exercises: Free Weights or Resistance Machines

Name	**Section**	**Date**

Purpose: To set lifestyle goals for muscle fitness exercise, to prepare a muscle fitness exercise plan, and to self-monitor progress for the 1-week plan

Procedures

1. Using Chart 1, provide some background information about your experience with resistance exercise, your goals, and your plans for incorporating these exercises into your normal exercise routine.
2. In Chart 2, keep a log of your actual participation in resistance exercise. You can choose free weights, machines, or some of both. Try to do at least eight exercises on at least 2 different days and be sure to work different body parts. Also, be sure that you plan your exercise program so it fits with the goals you described in Chart 1. If you are just starting out, it is best to start with light weights and more repetitions 12–15. For best results, take the log with you during your workout, so you can remember the weights, reps, and sets you performed.
3. Describe your experiences with your resistance exercise program. Be sure to comment on your plans for future resistance exercise.

Chart 1 ▶ Muscle Fitness Survey

1. What is your level of experience with resistance training (check the box)?

   ◯ Beginner   ◯ Intermediate   ◯ Advanced

2. What are your primary goals for resistance exercise?

   ◯ General conditioning   ◯ Improved appearance   ◯ Other_____

   ◯ Sports training   ◯ Avoidance of back pain

3. Are you currently involved in a regular resistance exercise program?

   ◯ Yes   ◯ No

4. Describe your current program or your future goals.
   - What days and times do you lift weights (or when can you lift)?
   - Where do you lift (or where can you lift)?
   - Describe your goals (or plans for resistance exercise):

Chart 2 ▶ Muscle Fitness Exercise Log

Check the exercises you performed and the days you performed them. You can do all free weights, all machines, or some of both. List others that you added.

Exercises	Day 1 (date)			Day 2 (date)			Day 3 (date)		
	Wt.	Reps	Sets	Wt.	Reps	Sets	Wt.	Reps	Sets
Free Weight Exercises									
1 Bench press									
2 Overhead press									
3 Bicep curl									
4 Tricep curl									
5 Wrist curl									
6 Dumbbell rowing									
7 Half squat									
8 Lunge									
9									
10									
Machine Exercises									
11 Chest press									
12 Overhead press									
13 Bicep curl									
14 Tricep press									
15 Lat pull-down									
16 Seated rowing									
17 Knee extension									
18 Hamstring curl									
19									
20									

Results

Were you able to do your basic eight exercises at least 2 days in the week?   Yes ◯   No ◯

Conclusions and Implications: Do you feel that you will use muscle fitness exercises as part of your regular lifetime physical activity plan, either now or in the future? Comment on what modifications you would make in your program in the future. Use several sentences to answer.

Lab 10D Planning and Logging Muscle Fitness Exercises: Calisthenics or Core Exercises

Name **Section** **Date**

Purpose: To set lifestyle goals for muscle fitness exercises that can easily be performed at home, to prepare a muscle fitness exercise plan, and to self-monitor progress for a 1-week plan

Procedures

1. Using Chart 1, provide some background information about your experience with calisthenic or core exercise, your goals, and your plans for incorporating these exercises into your normal exercise routine.
2. In Chart 2, keep a log of your actual participation in these exercises. You can choose all calisthenic exercises, all core exercises, or some of both. Some of the core exercises require the use of a Bosu® balance trainer or a similar device. If you don't have access to this, you can substitute other exercises. Try to do at least eight exercises on at least 2 different days and be sure to work different body parts.
3. Describe your experiences with your resistance exercise program. Be sure to comment on your plans for future resistance exercise.

Chart 1 ▶ Muscle Fitness Survey

1. What is your level of experience with calisthenic exercises (refer to Table 8)? Check the box that best describes you.

   ◯ I have done calisthenic exercise during PE class but not on my own.

   ◯ I have done calisthenic exercise before and still do some on a periodic basis.

   ◯ I have done calisthenic exercise a lot and still use it in my regular exercise program.

2. What is your level of experience with core exercises (refer to Table 9)? Check the box that best describes you.

   ◯ I have done abdominal exercises but have never done the other core exercises.

   ◯ I have done abdominal exercises and have tried core exercises with the Bosu® or similar devices.

   ◯ I regularly perform core exercises and am very experienced with the Bosu® or similar devices.

3. What are your primary reasons for doing calisthenic or core exercise?

   ◯ General conditioning

   ◯ Sports training

   ◯ Improved appearance

   ◯ Avoidance of back pain

4. Describe your current program or your present or future goals.
   - What days and times do you exercise (or when can you exercise)?
   - Where do you perform these exercises (or where can you exercise)?
   - Describe your goals/plans:

Chart 2 ▶ Muscle Fitness Exercise Log

Check the exercises you performed and the days you performed them. List others that you added.

Exercises	Day 1 (date)		Day 2 (date)		Day 3 (date)	
	Reps	Sets	Reps	Sets	Reps	Sets
Calisthenic Exercises						
1 Bent knee push-ups						
2 Modified Pull-ups						
3 Dips						
4 Crunch (curl-up)						
5 Trunk lift						
6 Side leg raise						
7 Lower leg lift						
8 Alternate leg kneel						
9						
10						
Core Exercises						
11 Crunch						
12 Reverse curl						
13 Crunch with twist						
14 Sitting tucks						
15 Hands and knees balance						
16 Marching						
17 Side step						
18 Squatting						
19						
20						

Results

Were you able to do your planned exercises at least 2 days in the week?   Yes ◯   No ◯

Conclusions and Implications: Do you feel that you will use these muscle fitness exercises as part of your regular lifetime physical activity plan, either now or in the future? Discuss the exercises you feel benefited you and the ones that did not. What modifications would you make in your program for it to work better for you?

Body Mechanics: Posture, Questionable Exercises, and Care of the Back and Neck

Concept 11

Health Goals for the year 2010

- Increase healthy and active days.
- Reduce days with pain and activity limitations.
- Increase assistance to those with pain and activity limitations.
- Increase proportion of people who regularly perform exercises for strength and muscular endurance.
- Increase proportion of people who regularly perform exercises for flexibility.

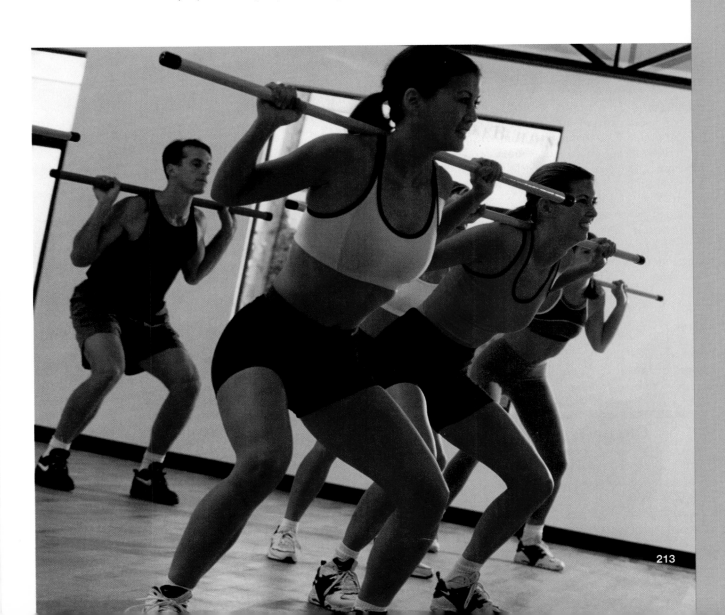

The health, integrity, and function of the neck and back are influenced by modifiable as well as nonmodifiable factors. Maintaining a healthy neck and back can be attained by using good posture, good body mechanics, and safe exercise technique.

The neck and back serve vital roles in supporting the weight of the head and body, producing movement, carrying loads, and protecting the spinal cord and nerves. These roles are facilitated by optimal alignment of the vertebrae and a balance between muscular strength and flexibility. Impairment of one or more of these functions can lead to injuries to the muscles, vertebrae, discs, ligaments, or nerves of the spine. Neck and back pain are common in today's society, with nearly 80 percent of the population experiencing an episode of low back pain sometime in their lives. A likely factor predisposing this region to injury is the spinal column's coupled role in producing large arrays of movement along with demands in bearing significant loads. The potential consequences of chronic neck and back pain are far-reaching and include emotional and economic costs to individuals and society.

In this concept, information about good posture, body mechanics, and safe exercise performance is provided to help you adopt preventive measures that may reduce your risk for back and neck problems. This information is intended to provide a basic foundation of knowledge. Those interested in more detailed information are encouraged to read further in textbooks of anatomy, physiology, or kinesiology. Persons with neck or back pain should always seek direction from their own medical provider.

Anatomy and Function of the Spine

The spinal column is arranged for movement. The bones that make up the spine are called vertebrae. There are 33 vertebrae in the spine, and most are separated from

one another by an **intervertebral disc** (see Figure 1). The vertebrae are divided into a number of types commonly referred to as cervical (neck), thoracic (upper back), and lumbar (low back). The fused vertebrae that comprise the tailbone are called the sacrum and coccyx. The vertebrae of the cervical, thoracic, and lumbar spine provide the

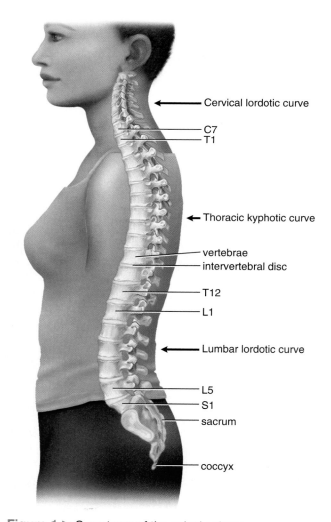

Figure 1 ▶ Curvatures of the spinal column.

Labels on figure:
Cervical lordotic curve
C7
T1
Thoracic kyphotic curve
vertebrae
intervertebral disc
T12
L1
Lumbar lordotic curve
L5
S1
sacrum
coccyx

On the Web

www.mhhe.com/corbinweb

Web 01 Log on to this URL before reading this concept. See On the Web list of concepts. Click on the concept number you want to view. To access supplemental information, click on the number shown at each Web icon.

large array of motion available to the trunk. The spine is capable of the motions of flexion (forward bending), extension (backward bending), sidebending, and rotation. Functionally, these movements often occur in combination with one another. For example, in executing a tennis serve, a player will both extend and rotate the spine. When you perform active movements repetitively, when you perform movements that cause the joints to move beyond a healthy range of motion, or when you perform activities that require heavy or inefficient lifting, the spine is at risk of injury.

The spinal column has an important role in bearing loads and protecting the neck and back from injury. The widest portion of each vertebra articulates with the intervertebral disc to form a strong pillar of support extending from the skull to the pelvis. While the vertebrae are capable of significant load bearing, it is the unique structure of the intervertebral discs that is critical in distributing force and absorbing shock. Another major function of the spinal column is to protect the nervous system from injury. The spinal cord and nerves are surrounded and protected by the bony armor of the vertebrae.

Good Posture Is Important for Neck and Back Health

Good posture has aesthetic benefits. Posture is an important part of nonverbal communication. The first impression a person makes is usually a visual one, and good posture can help convey an impression of alertness, confidence, and attractiveness.

Proper posture allows the body segments to be balanced. The body is made in segments, which are balanced in a vertical column by muscles and ligaments. Proper posture helps maintain an even distribution of force across the body, helps improve shock absorption, and helps minimize the degree of active muscle tension required to maintain the posture. When viewed from the side, three normal curvatures of the spine are present, causing the vertebral column to appear S-shaped. These curvatures are created by the **lordotic** (inward) **curve** of the cervical and lumbar spines and the **kyphotic** (outward) **curve** of the thoracic spine (see Figure 1). The curves help balance forces on the body and minimize muscle tension. They are also responsible for humans' unique ability to walk upright on two legs while maintaining a forward gaze.

The degree of curvature is influenced by the tilt of the pelvis. A forward pelvic tilt increases curvature in the neck and lower back, whereas a backward pelvic tilt flattens the lower back. The most desirable position is a **neutral spine** in which the spine has neither too much nor too little lordotic curve. The forces across the spine are balanced and muscular tension is at a minimum.

Awareness of good standing posture is important to a healthy spine. In the standing position, the head should be centered over the trunk; the shoulders should be down and back but relaxed, with the chest high and the abdomen flat. The spine should have gentle curves when viewed from the side but should be straight when seen from the back. When the pelvis is tilted properly, the pubis falls directly underneath the lower tip of the sternum. The knees should be relaxed, with the kneecaps pointed straight ahead. The feet should point straight ahead, and the weight should be borne over the heel, on the outside border of the sole, and across the ball of the foot and toes (see Figure 2, page 216).

Awareness of good seated posture is important to a healthy spine. A large percentage of our days are spent sitting as we attend class, commute to work, sit at a computer, dine out, or relax in front of the television. Good seated posture decreases pressure within the discs of the lower back and reduces fatigue of lower back muscles. In sitting, the head should be centered over the trunk, the shoulders down and back. If one is using a computer, the monitor should be at eye level with the screen 18–24 inches from the eyes. The seat of the chair should be at an angle that allows the knees to be positioned slightly lower than the hips. The back should firmly rest against the chair, with support to the lumbar spine. Feet should be supported on the floor and arms supported on armrests for ideal unloading of the spine (see Figure 3).

Intervertebral Discs Spinal discs; cushions of cartilage between the bodies of the vertebrae. Each disc consists of a fibrous outer ring (annulus fibrosus) and a pulpy center (nucleus pulposus).

Posture The relationship among body parts, whether standing, lying, sitting, or moving. Good posture is the relationship among body parts that allows you to function most effectively, with the least expenditure of energy and with a minimal amount of stress and strain on the body.

Lordotic Curve The normal inward curvature of the cervical and lumbar spine that is necessary for good posture and body mechanics.

Kyphotic Curve The normal outward curvature of the thoracic spine that is necessary for good posture and body mechanics.

Neutral Spine Proper position of the spine to maintain a normal lordotic curve. The spine has neither too much nor too little lordotic curve.

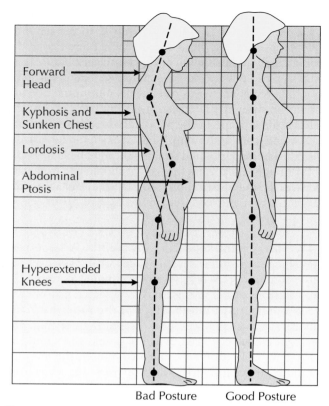

Forward
Head

Kyphosis and
Sunken Chest

Lordosis

Abdominal
Ptosis

Hyperextended
Knees

Bad Posture   Good Posture

Figure 2 ▶ Comparison of bad and good posture.

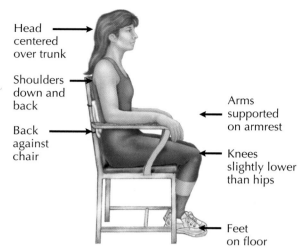

Head
centered
over trunk

Shoulders
down and
back

Back
against
chair

Arms
supported
on armrest

Knees
slightly lower
than hips

Feet
on floor

Figure 3 ▶ Good sitting posture.

Poor posture contributes to a variety of health problems. When posture deviates from neutral, weight distribution becomes uneven and tissues are at risk for injury. Examples of common postural deviations are described in Table 1, along with associated health problems. Two of those highlighted are that of lumbar lordosis (excessive curvature of the lower back) and flat back (reduced curvature of the lower back).

Lumbar lordosis posture occurs when the pelvis is tipped forward from a position of neutral tilt. With this posture, the hip muscles become shortened and tight, while the abdominal muscles become weak and long (with a reduced ability to "hold" within inner range). This muscle imbalance shifts body segment alignment toward a position of uneven loading, increasing pressure on the facet joints of the vertebrae. Over time, degenerative changes may occur, including a narrowing of the openings where spinal nerves exit, thus increasing risk for pain.

Flat back posture, on the other hand, occurs when the pelvis is tipped backward from a position of neutral tilt. With this posture, the lumbar spine is flexed, the lower back muscles are in a lengthened (weak) position, and the hamstring muscles are shortened and tight. A reduced lumbar curvature increases pressure on the intervertebral bodies and decreases shock absorption capabilities. Relative differences in flexibility between tight hamstring and long trunk muscles may also lead to a lack of accurate

segmental control. Laws of physics demonstrate that the body takes the path of least resistance during a chain of movement (e.g., forward bending), with the most flexible segment (i.e., the back) providing a greater contribution to the total range of movement. It follows that regions of greater movement will experience greater tissue strain. In the case of flat back posture, tight hamstrings may limit the contribution of hip motion during forward bending tasks, thus predisposing the lower back to become the fulcrum for movement and the site of injury.

Correcting postural deviations begins with restoring adequate muscle fitness and muscle length. Many postural problems are caused by a combination of weak and inflexible muscles. It is important to strengthen weak muscles in a shortened position and stretch tight muscles to help correct postural imbalance. For example, lumbar lordosis posture may be corrected by strengthening the abdominal muscles that pull the bottom of the pelvis upward and the hamstring muscles that keep the top of the pelvis tipped backward (see Figure 4). Postural correction is further enhanced by stretching tight hip flexor muscles.

In addition to body alignment problems, hereditary, congenital, and disease conditions, as well as certain environmental factors, can cause poor posture. Some environmental factors that contribute to poor posture include ill-fitting clothing and shoes, chronic fatigue, improperly fitting furniture (including poor chairs, beds, and mattresses), emotional and personality problems, poor work habits, poor physical fitness due to inactivity, and lack of knowledge relating to good posture. Some posture problems, such as **scoliosis,** may be congenital, hereditary, or acquired but can be improved with exercise, braces, and/or other medical procedures. Early detection is critical in treating scoliosis.

Table 1 ▶ Health Problems Associated with Poor Posture

Posture Problem	Definition	Health Problem
Forward head	The head aligned in front of the center of gravity	Headache, dizziness, and pain in the neck, shoulders, or arms
Kyphosis	Excessive curvature (flexion) in the upper back; also called humpback	Impaired respiration as a result of sunken chest and pain in the neck, shoulders, and arms
Lumbar lordosis	Excessive curvature (hyperextension) in the lower back (sway back), with a forward pelvic tilt	Back pain and/or injury, protruding abdomen, low back syndrome, and painful menstruation
Flat back	Reduced curvature in the lower back	Back pain, increased risk for injury due to reduced shock absorption
Abdominal ptosis	Excessive protrusion of abdomen, also called protruding abdomen	Back pain and/or injury, lordosis, low back syndrome, and painful menstruation
Hyperextended knees	The knees bent backward excessively	Greater risk for knee injury and excessive pelvic tilt (lordosis)
Pronated feet	The longitudinal arch of the foot flattened with increased pressure on inner aspect of foot	Decreased shock absorption, leading to foot, knee, and lower back pain

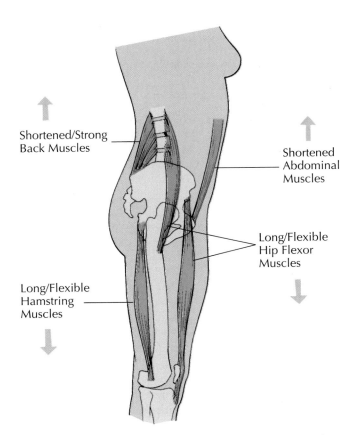

Shortened/Strong Back Muscles

Shortened Abdominal Muscles

Long/Flexible Hip Flexor Muscles

Long/Flexible Hamstring Muscles

Figure 4 ▶ Balanced muscle strength and length permit good postural alignment.

Good Body Mechanics Is Important for Neck and Back Health

Proper body mechanics can help prevent back and neck injury. Body mechanics is a discipline that applies mechanical laws and principles to the study of how the body can perform more efficiently and with less energy. Good body mechanics, as applied to back care, implies maintaining a neutral spine during activities of daily living. A neutral spine maintains the normal curvature of the spine, thus allowing an optimal balance of forces across the spine, reducing compressive forces and minimizing muscle tension. Table 2 (page 218) provides specific recommendations for and examples of good body mechanics in a variety of settings and positions.

Ergonomics is a discipline that uses biomechanical principles to develop tools and workplace settings that put the least amount of strain on the body. The modification of tools and occupational work stations can improve body mechanics and improve job efficiency. Many employers

Web 03

Scoliosis A lateral curvature with some rotation of the spine; the most serious and deforming of all postural deviations.

Table 2 ▶ Body Mechanics Guidelines for Posture and Back/Neck Care	
Sitting	• Use a hard chair with a straight back and armrests, placing the spine against the back of the chair. A footrest reduces fatigue (see Figure 3). • Keep one or both knees lower than the hips and feet supported on the floor. • If your back flattens when you sit, place a lumbar roll behind your lower back. • When sitting at a table, keep the back and neck in good alignment. • Do not sit in front-row theater seats, which forces you to tip your head back. • When driving a car, pull the seat forward, so the legs are bent when operating the pedals. If your back flattens when you drive, use a lumbar support pillow. • Whenever possible, sit while working but stand occasionally.
Standing	• When standing for long periods of time, keep the lower back flat by propping a foot on a stool; alternate feet. • Avoid tilting the head backward (when shaving or washing your hair).
Lying	• Avoid lying on the abdomen. • When lying on the back, a pillow or lift should be placed under the knees. Do not use a thick head pillow. • When lying on your side, keep your knees and hips bent; place a pillow between the knees.
Lifting and Carrying	• When lifting, avoid bending at the waist. Keep the back straight, bend the knees, and lift with the legs. Assume a side-stride position with the object between the feet to allow you to get low and near the object. • Perform one-hand lifting the same way as two-hand lifting; use the nonlifting hand for support. • When lifting, do not twist the spine. This can be more damaging from a sitting position than from a standing position. • When lifting, keep the object close to the body; do not reach to lift. Tighten the abdominal muscles before lifting. • If possible, avoid carrying objects above waist level. • When objects must be carried above the waist, carry them in the midline of the body, preferably on the back (use a backpack). Keep backpack weight low and use both straps for support. • Push or pull heavy objects, rather than lifting them. It takes 34 times more force to lift than to slide an object across the floor. Pushing is preferred over pulling. • Do not lift or carry loads too heavy for you. The most economical load for the average adult is about 35 percent of the body weight. Obviously, with strength training, you can lift a greater load, but heavy loads are a backache risk factor. • Divide the load if possible, carrying half in each hand/arm. If the load cannot be divided, alternate it from one side of the body to the other. • When lifting and lowering an object from overhead, avoid hyperextending the neck and the back. Any lift above waist level is inefficient. • When objects must be carried in front of the body above the level of the waist, lean backward to balance the load, and avoid arching the back.
Working	• When working above head level, get on a stool or ladder to avoid tipping the head backward. • Work at eye level; for example, computer monitors should not be too high or low. • To avoid back and neck strain, climb a ladder or stand on a stool so you don't have to raise your arms over your head. • When working with the hands, the workbench or kitchen cabinet should be about 2 to 4 inches below the waist. The office desk should be about 29 to 30 inches high for the average man and about 27 to 29 inches high for the average woman. • Tools most often used should be the closest to reach. • Avoid constant arm extension, whether forward or sideward. • The arms should move either together or in opposite directions. When the conditions allow, use both hands in opposite and symmetrical motions while working. • Organize work to save energy. Vary the working position by changing from one task to another before feeling fatigued. When working at a desk, get up and stretch occasionally to relieve tension. • Use proper tools and equipment to reduce neck strain; for example, use a paint roller with an extension to reach overhead, thus reducing the need to hold the arms overhead and to hyperextend the neck. • Avoid stooping or unnatural positions that cause strain.

take an active interest in ergonomic principles, since repetitive motion injuries and other musculoskeletal conditions are the leading cause of work-related ill health. One application of ergonomics is the design of effective workstations for computer users. Properly fitting desks and chairs and the effective positioning of computer screens and keyboards have been shown to minimize problems such as carpal tunnel syndrome (CTS), a painful and debilitating injury of the median nerve at the wrist. (More information on ergonomics, also known as human factors engineering, can be found at Web03.)

Good lifting technique focuses on using the legs. Keep in mind that the muscles of the legs are relatively large and strong, compared with the back muscles. Likewise, the hip joint is well designed for motion. It is less likely to suffer the same amount of wear and tear as the smaller joints of the spine. When lifting an object from the floor, an individual should do the following: straddle the object with a wide stance; squat down by hinging through the hips and bending the knees; maintain a slight arch to the lower back by sticking out the buttocks; test the load and get help if it is too heavy or awkward; rise by tightening the leg muscles, not the back; keep the load close to the waist; don't pivot or twist (see Figure 5).

Poor body mechanics can increase risks for back pain. A common cause of backache is muscle strain, frequently precipitated by poor body mechanics in daily activities, such as lifting or exercising. If lifting is done improperly, great pressure is exerted on the lumbar discs, and excessive stress and strain are placed on the lumbar muscles and ligaments. Many popular exercises also place too much strain on the back and should be avoided. Poor postures can also cause back strain. An example is sleeping flat on the back or abdomen on a soft mattress. By avoiding bad body mechanics, you can reduce your risk for back pain.

Causes and Consequences of Back and Neck Pain

Most people (more than half) will see a physician about a backache during their lifetime. Back pain is second only to headache as a common medical complaint. An estimated 30 to 70 percent of Americans have recurring back problems, and 2 million of these people cannot hold jobs as a result. Back problems most often affect people between the ages of 25 and 60, but one study indicated that up to 26 percent of teenagers report backaches. Athletes also have back problems, but the condition is more common in people who are not highly fit. Unfortu-

nately, studies also indicate that back pain is the leading cause of inactivity among individuals under the age of 45. Therefore, taking preventive measures to reduce the risk for back pain is important.

The prevention of back problems is an important goal in worksite health promotion Web 04 **programs.** Back pain is the most common reason for workers' compensations claims and for lost workdays among employed individuals. Statistics indicate that 27 percent of all workers' compensation claims result from musculoskeletal disorders of the neck and back. These disorders account for nearly 46 percent of the total workers' compensation costs. Given these statistics, it should come as no surprise that worksite health promotion programs place strong emphasis on measures to prevent or reduce back injury. These programs include structured exercise programs, the use of ergonomically designed workstations and equipment, and awareness education about proper lifting and carrying techniques.

Most back and neck pain stems from lifestyle choices or life experiences. The original cause (or causes) of back and neck pain are typically hard to identify. Although back and neck problems can result from an acute injury (e.g., a diving accident or car accident), most are caused by accumulated stresses over a lifetime. These factors include the avoidable effects of poor posture and body mechanics as well as from performing questionable exercises that put the back at risk (exercises to avoid are discussed later in the concept). Musculoskeletal injuries and degenerative changes to the discs, spinal joints, facets, ligaments, or vertebral canals protecting the spinal cord can predispose you to back and neck problems. Depression,

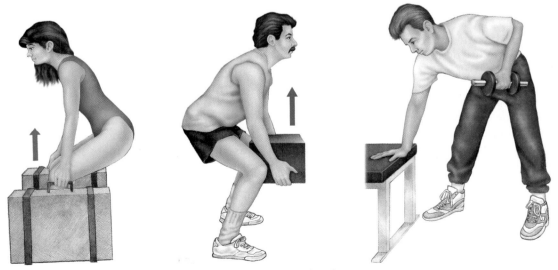

Figure 5 ► Good body mechanics can help prevent back and neck pain.

cancer, infections, and some visceral diseases (kidney, pelvic organs) can also contribute to back problems. While people have some control over these causes, some back pain stems directly from structural or functional disorders that a person is born with. Inherited causes include anomalies of the spine, such as scoliosis.

To reduce risk for back pain, it is important to try to reduce the risk factors that you have control over. Modifiable risk factors (factors for which you have the power to change) include regular heavy labor, the use of vibrational tools, routines of prolonged sitting, smoking, a hypokinetic lifestyle, coronary artery disease, and obesity. Nonmodifiable risk factors include a family history of joint disease, age, direct trauma (e.g., as a fall or rough athletic activity when young). A questionnaire is provided in Lab 11A for assessing your potential risk for back and neck pain.

The nervous system and various pain-sensitive structures contribute to back pain. Back pain can result from direct or indirect causes. Direct causes are typically the result of tissue trauma to areas in or around the spinal column. The most common sources of pain are ligaments, intervertebral discs, nerve roots, spinal joints and deep muscles. Indirect causes stem from the release of pain-causing chemicals from injured tissues. These chemicals cause nerves in the area to remain irritated and sensitive. Processes within the brainstem, spinal cord and peripheral nerves can also modulate the sensation of pain, either increasing or decreasing it. For example, some back pain can be caused by abnormal feedback loops that act to enhance or maintain the perception of pain—even when the original cause or problem is corrected.

The integrity of the neck and back are jeopardized by excessive stress and strain. Forces are constantly at work to bend, twist, shear, compress, or lengthen tissues of the body. Stress on these tissues may eventually create strain, a change in the tissue's size or dimension. Healthy tissues typically return to their normal state once the force is removed. Injury occurs when excessive stress and strains prevent the tissue from returning to its normal state.

Poor posture can cause body segments to experience stress and strain. For example, sitting with a slouched posture causes the upper back to round forward excessively. The cervical spine arches backward to compensate in order to maintain a normal forward gaze. Excessive stress and strain are then placed on the muscles of the posterior neck. Over time, chronic stress from poor alignment can lead to other postural deviations and degenerative changes to the neck. The postural fault of forward head also places a chronic strain on the posterior neck muscles. Tension in these muscles can lead to **myofascial trigger points,** causing headache or **referred pain** in the face, scalp, shoulder, arm, and chest. Stress and strain can also occur from bad body mechanics and improper lifting techniques. The lumbar vertebrae and the sacrum are most vulnerable to this type of injury due to the significant weight they support and the thinner ligamentous support at this level.

Web 05 **Some exercises and movements can produce microtrauma, which can lead to back and neck pain.** Most people are familiar with acute injuries, such as ankle sprains. These injuries are associated with immediate onset of pain and swelling. **Microtrauma** is "a silent injury"—that is, an injury that results from repetitive motions, such as those used in calisthenics or sports. These injuries also occur in occupations. Other terms that frequently appear in the scientific literature include *repetitive motion syndrome, repetitive strain injury (RSI), cumulative trauma disorder (CTD),* and *overuse syndrome.* They all refer to injury caused by repetitive movement. We may violate the integrity of our joints by performing, for example, 40 backward arm circles with the palms down 3 days per week for 10 or 20 years. We don't usually notice the wear and tear until the friction over time causes microscopic changes in the joint, such as fibrosis of the synovial lining, abnormal thickening of the surrounding joint capsule, thinning and roughening of the articular cartilage cushioning joint surfaces, and calcifications in the rotator cuff tendon. Because these changes are unseen and often unfelt, we view the exercise as harmless. Later in life, microtrauma becomes apparent, resulting in tendonitis, bursitis, arthritis, or nerve compression. Chances are, when the injury reaches an acute stage, the cause of the injury is not identified and is typically attributed to old age.

Web 06 **The lumbar region of the spine is a frequent site of injury and back pain.** The lumbar vertebrae are particularly vulnerable to injury due to the significant weight they support and their thinner ligamentous support. The intervertebral discs in the lumbar region are also susceptible to a type of injury known as a **herniated disc** (this injury has often been called a slipped disc but this is an outdated and technically incorrect term).

The primary function of the intervertebral discs is shock absorption. They are composed of a tirelike outer ring (annulus fibrosus) surrounding a gel-like center (nucleus pulposus). The greatest risk for injury to the discs occurs during excessive loading and twisting motions of the spine. Small tears begin to occur in the inner fibers of the annulus. The nucleus begins to move outward, much like toothpaste moving within a squeezed tube. Disc herniation is termed *incomplete* or *contained* as long as the migrating edge of the nucleus remains within the fibers of annulus. As damage continues (often the result of years of cumulative microtrauma) the annular fibers may reach a point of rupture at their periphery (see Figure 6). At this point, the nucleus pulposus moves into the space around the spinal cord and the herniation is termed *complete* or *non-contained*. Like the proverbial "straw that broke the camel's back," it may take just one incident to progress a damaged disc to a herniated disc.

Disc herniation is a frequently cited cause of back pain, but studies have shown that only 5 to 10 percent of persons with herniated discs experience pain. The reason for this is that pain is often not experienced until complete herniation occurs. The pain is experienced as the nuclear material begins to press on pain-sensitive structures in its path (additional information on the four stages of disc herniation is available at Web06). Interestingly, the risk for disc herniation is greatest for individuals in their thirties and forties. Risk decreases with increasing years as the disc degenerates and becomes less soft and pliable.

Degenerative disc disease is a common part of aging. Many elderly people appear to get shorter as they age, often due to degenerative changes within the discs. One notable change is flattening of the discs as a result of lost water content. This in turn causes the vertebrae to sit closer together, increasing compressive forces on both the small facet joints and vertebral bodies, decreasing the size of the canal where the spinal nerves exit and increasing the likelihood of nerve impingement, bone spur formation, and arthritis. (See Figure 7.)

Medical intervention is sometimes needed for neck or back pain. Most cases of back pain resolve spontaneously, with 70 percent having no symptoms at the end of 3 weeks and 90 percent recovered after 2 months, yet some cases of neck or back pain benefit from medical intervention in order to hasten recovery in acute cases or improve pain level/function in chronic cases. Conservative treatment typically involves the use of anti-inflammatory medications, muscle relaxants, therapeutic exercise, massage, heat, cryotherapy, traction, or electrical stimulation. When conservative care is unsuccessful, referral may occur to an alternative therapy, such as acupuncture, or to a pain clinic for steroidal anti-inflammatory injections. As a last measure, surgery may be needed for removal of a disc or for fusion.

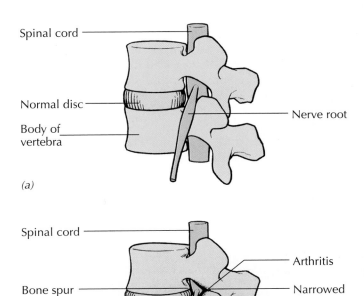

Figure 7 ► Normal disc (*a*) and degenerated disc with nerve impingement and arthritic changes (*b*).

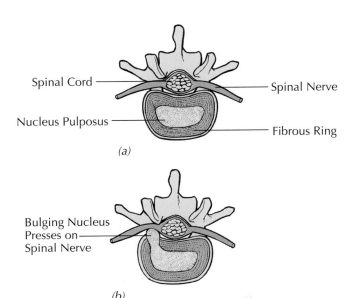

Figure 6 ► Normal disc (*a*) and herniated disc (*b*).

Myofascial Trigger Points Tender spots in the muscle or muscle fascia that refer pain to a location distant to the point.

Referred Pain Pain that appears to be located in one area, though it actually originates in another area.

Microtrauma Injury so small it is not detected at the time it occurs.

Herniated Disc The soft nucleus of the spinal disc that protrudes through a small tear in the surrounding tissue; also called prolapse.

Guidelines for Safe Physical Activity

Some exercises and movements may put the back and neck at risk. The human body is designed for motion. Nevertheless, certain movements can put the joints and musculoskeletal system at risk and should therefore be avoided. With respect to care of the spine, many **contraindicated** movements involve the extremes of hyperflexion and hyperextension. Hyperflexion causes increased pressure in the discs, potentially leading to disc herniation. Hyperextension causes compressive wear and tear on the facet joints that join vertebral segments (see Figure 8). Hyperextension of the spine also causes narrowing of the intervertebral canal, potentially causing nerve impingement. With respect to the knee, hyperextension places excessive stress on the ligaments and joint capsule at the back of the knee, whereas hyperflexion increases compressive forces under the kneecap (patello-femoral joint).

Following established exercise guidelines is important for safe exercise. "Safe" exercises are defined as those performed with normal body posture, mechanics, and movement in mind. They don't compromise the integrity or stability of one body part to the detriment of another. "Questionable" exercises, on the other hand, are exercises that may violate normal body mechanics and place the joints, ligaments, or muscles at risk for injury. No harm may occur from doing the exercise once, but repeated use over time can lead to injury. A number of commonly used exercises are regarded as poor choices (contraindicated) for nearly everyone in the general population due to the reasonable risk for injury over time. A separate category of questionable exercises are regarded as poor choices for only certain segments of the population because of a specific health issues or known physical problem.

Differentiating exercises as "safe" or "questionable" can be difficult—even experts in the field have different opinions on the subject. These views are known to change over time as new knowledge and research findings reshape our understanding of the effect of exercise on the human body.

Safe exercise includes performing activities of daily living properly.

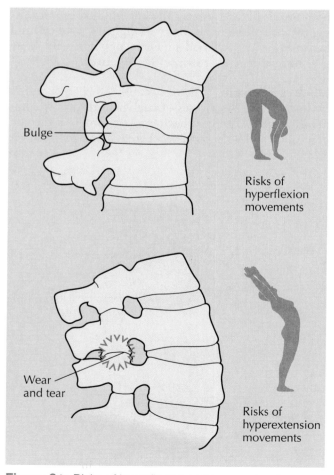

Figure 8 ▶ Risks of hyperflexion and hyperextension.

When considering the merits and risks of different exercises, it may be necessary to consult with an expert. Professionals such as athletic trainers, biomechanists, physical educators, physical therapists, and certified strength and conditioning specialists are appropriate people to consult. These individuals typically have college degrees and four to eight years of study in such courses as anatomy, physiology, kinesiology, preventive and therapeutic exercise, and physiology of exercise. On-the-job training, a good physique or figure, and good athletic or dancing ability are not sufficient qualifications for teaching or advising about exercise. Most fitness centers prefer to hire instructors and personal trainers with appropriate certifications. Unfortunately, certification is not a requirement. When searching for advice on training or exercise, it is certainly appropriate to inquire about an individual's qualifications.

Exercises that are prescribed for a particular individual differ from those that are good for everyone (mass prescription). In a clinical setting, a therapist works with one patient. A case history is taken and tests made to determine which muscles are weak or strong, short or long. Exercises are then prescribed for that person. For example, a tennis player with a recent history of shoulder dislocation would probably be prescribed specific shoulder-strengthening exercises to regain stability in the joint. Common shoulder stretching exercises would likely be contraindicated for this individual. In this case, the muscles and joint capsule on the front of the shoulder are already quite lax to have allowed dislocation to occur in the first place.

Exercises that are prescribed or performed as a group cannot typically take individual needs into account. For example, when a physical educator, an aerobics instructor, or a coach leads a group of people in exercise, there is little (if any) consideration for individual differences, except for some allowance made in the number of repetitions or in the amount of weight or resistance used. Some of the exercises performed in this type of group setting may not be appropriate for all individuals. Similarly, an exercise that is appropriate for a certain individual may not be appropriate for all members of a group. Since it is not always practical to prescribe individual exercise routines for everyone, it is often necessary to provide general recommendations that are appropriate for most individuals. The classification of exercises in this concept should be viewed in this context.

The risks associated with physical activity can be reduced by modifying the variables or conditions under which the activity is performed. While some exercises are contraindicated, it is almost always possible to find safer alternatives. Modifications in the way the exercise is performed can also reduce risks. The variables that are typically under the direct control of the participant include exercise frequency (the number of repetitions performed in a given time span), duration (the length of time activity is sustained), intensity (the amount of resistance), speed (the velocity of activity, or rate, at which resistance is applied), and quality (the posture and mechanics of the body parts involved in the movement). Table 3 (page 224) highlights these five activity variables, illustrates how each might be involved in potential injury, and provides suggestions for modifying the variable to reduce the risk for injury. In some cases, changing a single variable may significantly reduce risk but, in other cases, multiple factors may need to be changed. In many cases, the best strategy is to look for a safer exercise. A variety of contraindicated exercises and safer alternatives are presented in Table 4 (pages 228–234) at the end of the concept.

Risks from exercise can't be completely avoided. Variables that are not always under the direct control of the participant include environmental conditions, such as temperature, humidity, or exercise surface. Likewise, the demands of sport and certain occupations may require individuals to train or work to the maximal limit of these variables (up to or just short of injury). Circumstances may not always permit every variable to be modified to suit an individual. However, making an active effort to adjust variables that are modifiable will make a difference in reducing injury risk.

Prevention of and Rehabilitation from Back and Neck Problems

Exercise is a frequently prescribed treatment for back or neck pain. Exercise has been found to be helpful in treating many types of chronic pain. (Resistance exercises and aerobic exercise are frequently used in pain clinics.) Exercises that are selected to specifically help correct pain-related problems are classified as therapeutic. These exercises are aimed at correcting the underlying cause of neck or back pain by strengthening weak muscles, stretching short ones, and improving circulation to and nourishment of tissues of the body. Both therapeutic and health-related fitness exercises may be considered preventive. Done faithfully, and with the appropriate FIT formula, they improve the health of the musculoskeletal system, allowing greater efficiency of function and reduced incidence of injury.

Contraindicated Not recommended because of the potential for harm.

Table 3 ▶ Controllable Variables in Reducing Risk for Injury

Variables	Activity Examples	Potential Injury	Modifications to Reduce Risk
Frequency	• Repeated back hyperextension in a gymnast • Repeated wrist movement in an assembly-line worker	Microtrauma to the joints undergoing repeated motions	• Maintain a balance of flexibility and strength in the vulnerable regions of the body. • Provide rest/rotate work stations within the shift. • Use ergonomic modifications to the worksite.
Duration	• Sustained position of a deep squat in a baseball catcher • Forward head posture of an office worker	Stress and strain to the muscles and ligaments used to hold the posture	• Strengthen the muscles of the knees and maintain leg muscle flexibility in the catcher. • Take regular posture breaks in the office worker and modify computer station for good seated posture.
Intensity	Excessive loads and reaction forces experienced by a • Power lifter • Runner • Construction worker	Stress and strain to the musculoskeletal system, especially the weaker portions of the back and shoulders	• Do a proper warm-up and correct training progression. • Wear supportive shoes and clothing. • Be aware of personal limits, seeking help or a spot when needed.
Speed	High-velocity movement of • A 50-yd sprinter • The rapid fingering of a concert pianist	• Motions applied over a short duration of time under conditions of high tension predispose the muscles and tendons to injury. • With fast-paced motions, precision is often sacrificed (particularly with fatigue), possibly leading to faulty movement patterns.	• Follow activity-specific training protocols to optimize recruitment of appropriate muscle fiber types. • Maintain balance of flexibility and strength. • Use deep muscles for stability and superficial muscles for mobility.
Movement quality	• Extended range of motion during ballistic shoulder stretching of swimmers • Poor body mechanics when shoveling snow	• Movement through extreme ranges or at the limit of normal motion can lead to instability or wear/tear of joints. • Poor balance of forces throughout the body increases risk for stress and strain.	• Balance flexibility with strength and respect pain, the body's signal of injury. • Use good posture and body mechanics in recreational and lifestyle activities to balance forces.

Strengthening muscles involved in providing core stability can reduce the risk for back problems. As described in Concept 10, building core strength is important for overall muscular fitness. However, to reduce the risks for back and neck problems, it is also important to train the muscles involved in core stabilization. The main difference between core stability and core strengthening programs are the muscles trained. **Core stability** refers to strength of the muscles providing segmental stabilization of the spine, whereas **core strength** refers to strength of the muscles that bend, extend, and rotate the spine.

The primary core stabilizer muscles of the trunk are the transverse abdominus, multifidus, and deep neck flexors. They stabilize the small spinal joints and pelvis during active movements (such as stabilizing the trunk during a tennis serve or golf swing). They are deeply located muscles (slow-twitch) that are active during endurance activities and at low resistance, are poorly recruited, and often sag/lengthen due to weakness. Interestingly, neck and back pain often inhibit these muscles—in essence, "turning them off." Atrophy (muscle wasting) of these muscles occurs in 80 percent of patients with neck or back pain. Specific training of the multifidus, transverse abdominus, and deep neck flexors is thus critical for a full recovery. Exercises for improving core stability are described and illustrated in the exercise section at the end of the concept. Training requires that the muscles be activated at low levels of resistance and with slow movements in order to avoid substitution by the stronger mobilizer muscles. Their function as slow-twitch endurance muscles also necessitates that they be trained as such (low resistance, long duration holds, many repetitions).

The primary muscles of core strength are the rectus abdominus, the lateral fibers of the external obliques, and the erector spinae (back extensors). These muscles function as the prime movers of the trunk. They are characterized as superficial muscles, fast-twitch in nature, activated at higher resistance levels, and recruited preferentially over the stabilizers; they are often in a shortened (tight) position. Traditional abdominal and trunk extensor strengthening exercises are included in the exercise section at the end of the concept. These exercises can be performed at higher speeds and with greater resistance than core stabilization exercises.

Resistance exercise can often correct muscle imbalance, the underlying cause of many postural and back problems. If the muscles on one side of a joint are stronger than the muscles on the opposite side, the body part is pulled in the direction of the stronger muscles. Corrective exercises are usually designed to strengthen the long, weak muscles and to stretch the short, strong ones in order to have equal pull in both directions. For example, people with lumbar lordosis may need to strengthen the abdominals and hamstrings and stretch the lower back and hip flexor muscles.

Although general resistance training may help improve the strength and endurance of the back muscles, the exercises may not be specific enough to target the areas that may contribute to risk for low back pain. Because of this, there has been increased attention given to the development of back exercise machines that can more effectively rehabilitate and/or strengthen back musculature. The machines help isolate the muscles by restraining or preventing other muscles from assisting. For example, pelvic muscles are restrained in a back extension machine to help isolate the lumbar muscles. This isolation helps strengthen the lumbar muscles, an important target for reducing risks for back problems. Additional detail is provided at Web08.

Some additional general guidelines will help prevent postural, back, and neck problems. In addition to the suggestions for improving body mechanics noted in the previous sections, the following guidelines should be helpful:

- Do exercises to strengthen abdominal and hip extensors and to stretch the hip flexors and lumbar muscles if they are tight (see Tables 4–10).
- Avoid hazardous exercises.
- Do regular physical activity for the entire body, such as walking, jogging, swimming, and bicycling.
- Warm up before engaging in strenuous activity.
- Sleep on a moderately firm mattress or place a 3/4-inch-thick plywood board under the mattress.
- Avoid sudden, jerky back movements, especially twisting.
- Avoid obesity. The smaller the waistline, the less the strain on the lower back.
- Use appropriate back and seat supports when sitting for long periods.
- Maintain good posture when carrying heavy loads; do not lean forward, sideways, or backward.
- Adjust sports equipment to permit good posture; for example, adjust a bicycle seat and handle bars to permit good body alignment.
- Avoid long periods of sitting at a desk or driving; take frequent breaks and adjust the car seat and headrest for maximum support.

Specialized types of resistance exercise equipment are available to strengthen the back musculature.

Core Stability Strength of muscles which demonstrate optimal firing patterns and tension-generating capabilities to "brace" the trunk in anticipation of, and during movement of the head, arms, or legs.

Core Strength Strength of muscles which demonstrate optimal firing patterns and tension-generating capabilities to create movement of the trunk.

Strategies for Action

An important step in taking action is assessing your current status. An important early step in taking action is self-assessment. The Healthy Back Tests consist of eight pass or fail items that will give you an idea of the areas in which you might need improvement. The Healthy Back Tests are described in *Lab Resource Materials*. You will take these tests in Lab 11A. Experts have identified behaviors associated with potential future back and neck problems. A questionnaire is also provided for assessing these risk factors.

Web 09

Learning to adopt and maintain good posture is an important and effective way to promote good back health. A posture test is included in Lab 11B to help you evaluate your posture. Identifying possible postural problems can help you take appropriate corrective action that can reduce stress and strain on your back and neck.

Specific exercises are sometimes needed to prevent or help rehabilitate postural, neck, and back problems. Exercises included in previous concepts were presented with health-related fitness in mind. The exercises included in this concept are not so different. They are either flexibility or strength/muscle endurance exercises for specific muscle groups;

Web 10

however, each is selected specifically to help correct a postural problem or to remove the cause of neck and back pain. To that extent, these exercises may be classified as therapeutic. The same exercises may be called preventive because they can be used to prevent postural or spine problems. People who have back and neck pain should seek the advice of a physician to make certain that it is safe for them to perform the exercises.

The exercises in Tables 5–11 are not necessarily intended for all people. Rather, you should choose exercises based on your own individual needs. Use your results on the Healthy Back Tests and the posture test to determine the exercises that are most appropriate for you. Table 4 (pages 228–234) provides information on "Questionable Exercises and Safe Alternatives."

To facilitate the use of these exercises for back or postural problems, the most effective exercises for various maladies are organized in Tables 5–11. Lab 11C is designed to help you choose specific exercises related to test items in Lab 11A.

Keeping records of progress is important to adhering to a back care program. An activity logging sheet is provided in Lab 11C to help you keep records of your progress as you regularly perform exercises to build and maintain good back and neck fitness.

Online Learning Center

www.mhhe.com/corbin7e
The Online Learning Center contains a variety of Web-based resources that will help you get the most out of this book and your course. In addition to the On the Web pages, there are video activities, interactive quizzes, application assignments, and a variety of other useful study aids. Log on to the URL above to access these resources.

Web Resources

American Back Care Company
    www.americanback.com

Web 11   Back and Body Care **www.backandbodycare.com**
Guide to Clinical Preventive Services
    http://odphp.osophs.dhhs.gov/pubs/guidecps
MedX **www.medxonline.com**
National Osteoporosis Foundation **www.nof.org**
National Safety Council **www.nsc.org**

Technology Update
Core Stabilization Training Aids

The muscles that work to stabilize the core tend to be shorter and deeper than the muscles involved in large movement. Inadequate development of these muscles has been shown to be a risk factor for back pain, but it is difficult to develop effective training programs for these muscles. In most movements, the stronger, more superficial muscles tend to do most of the work. Physical therapists have used a variety of biofeedback devices to help patients learn how to control and activate different muscles more effectively. A new, pressure-based biofeedback device has been developed to facilitate training of the stabilizer muscles. Visit the following Web site for additional information: **http://backtrainer.com/The-Stabilizer.html.**

Suggested Readings

Web 12

Additional reference materials for Concept 11 are available at Web12.

Bracko, M. R. 2004. Can we prevent back injuries? *ACSM's Health and Fitness Journal* 8(4):5–11.

Frontera, W. R., et al. 2006. *Exercise in Rehabilitation Medicine.* 2nd ed. Champaign, IL: Human Kinetics.

Golderberg, L., and P. Twist. 2001. *Strength Ball Training: 69 Exercises Using Swiss Balls and Medicine Balls.* Champaign, IL: Human Kinetics.

Katzmarzyk, P. T., and L. C. Cora. 2002. Musculoskeletal fitness and risk of mortality. *Medicine and Science in Sports and Exercise* 34(5):740–744.

Kendall, F. P. (ed.) 2005. *Muscles: Testing and Function, with posture and pain.* Philadelphia: Lippencott, Williams & Wilkins.

Liemohn, W., and G. Pariser. 2002. Core strength: Implications for fitness and low back pain. *ACSM's Health and Fitness Journal* 6(5):10–16.

McGill, S. M. 2001. Low back stability. *Exercise and Sport Science Reviews* 29(1):26–31.

Norris, C. M. 2001. Functional load abdominal training: Part 2. *Physical Therapy in Sport* 2:149–156.

Plowman, S. A. 1999. Physical fitness and healthy low back function. In C. B. Corbin and R. P. Pangrazi (eds.). *Towards a Better Understanding of Physical Fitness and Activity.* Scottsdale, AZ: Holcomb-Hathaway.

Rainville, J., et al. 2004. Exercise as a treatment for chronic low back pain. *Spine* 4(1):106–115.

Richardson, C. A., et al. 2002. The relation between the transverse abdominis muscles, sacroiliac joint mechanics, and low back pain. *Spine* 27(4):399–405.

Sherman, K. J., et al. 2005. Comparing yoga, exercise, and a self-care book for chronic low back pain: A randomized, controlled trial. *Annals of Internal Medicine* 143(12):849–856.

Walters, P. H. 2000. Back to the basics: Strengthening the neglected lower back. *ACSM's Health and Fitness Journal* 4(4):19–25.

Worobey, S., et al. 2002. Strength training for posture. *Fitness Management* 6:46–49.

In the News

Worksite Health Promotion Programs

Worksite health promotion programs are widely used by companies to help control rising health care costs. Most programs emphasize the promotion of overall wellness and fitness but reducing risk of injury and promoting back health are often targeted as key focus areas. The reason for this is that back pain is one of the top reasons that employees seek medical care and it is also one of the primary causes of long term disability as well as absenteeism. Most employers today cover the majority of health care costs for their employees. Employers also lose productivity in their staff if employees are absent or on disability. By reducing medical claims/disability related to back problems and absenteeism related to back pain companies save money. Therefore, there are major economic incentives for companies to work to promote back health among employees. A summary in the *Guide to Clinical Preventive Services* summarized the effectiveness of different counseling and prevention strategies for back pain prevention (see Web Resources). The review concluded that "There is limited evidence that educational sessions in occupational settings (e.g., back schools) produce modest short-term benefits in adults with recurrent or chronic low back pain, but no evidence that such education prevents back pain in healthy individuals or those at risk for back pain."

Table 4

Table 4 Questionable Exercises and Safer Alternatives

1. Questionable Exercise: The Swan

This exercise hyperextends the lower back and stretches the abdominals. The abdominals are too long and weak in most people and should not be lengthened further. Extension can be harmful to the back, potentially causing nerve impingement, and facet joint compression. Other exercises in which this occurs include: cobras, backbends, straight-leg lifts, straight-leg sit-ups, prone-back lifts, donkey kicks, fire hydrants, backward trunk circling, weight lifting with the back arched, and landing from a jump with the back arched.

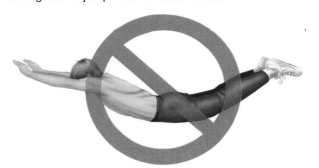

Safer Alternative Exercise: Back Extension

Lie prone over a roll of blankets or pillows and extend the back to a neutral or horizontal position.

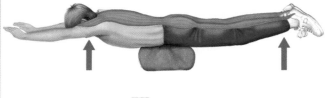

Deltoid

Erector spinae

Gluteus maximus

Hamstring

2. Questionable Exercise: Back-Arching Abdominal Stretch

This exercise can stretch the hip flexors, quadriceps, and shoulder flexors (such as the pectorals), but it also stretches the abdominals, which is not desired. Because of the armpull, it can potentially hyperflex the knee joint, and strain neck musculature.

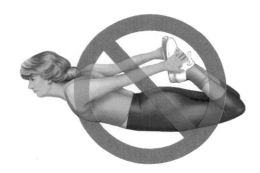

Note: All safer alternative exercises should be held 15 to 30 seconds unless otherwise indicated.

Safer Alternative Exercise: Wand Exercise

This exercise stretches the front of the shoulders and chest. Sit with wand grasped at ends. Raise wand overhead. Be certain that the head does not slide forward. Keep the chin tucked and neck straight. Bring wand down behind shoulder blades. Keep spine erect. Hold. Press forward on the wand simultaneously by pushing with the hands. Relax; then try to move the hands lower, sliding the wand down the back. Hold again. Hands may be moved closer together to increase stretch

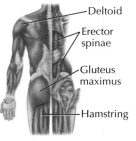

on chest muscles. If this is an easy exercise for you, try straightening the elbows and bringing the wand to waist level in back of you.

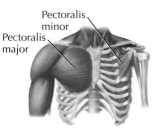

Pectoralis minor

Pectoralis major

3. Questionable Exercise: Seated Forward Arm Circles with Palms Down

This exercise (arms straight out to the sides) may cause pinching of the rotator cuff and biceps tendons between the bony structures of the shoulder joint and/or irritate the bursa in the shoulder. The tendency is to emphasize the use of the stronger chest muscles (pectorals) to perform the motion rather than emphasizing the weaker upper back muscles.

Safer Alternative Exercise: Seated Backward Arm Circles with Palms Up

Sit, turn palms up, pull in chin, and contract abdominals. Circle arms backward.

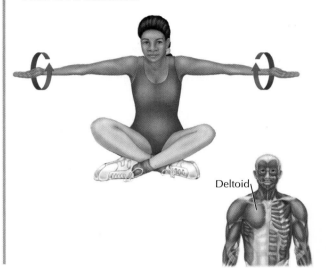

Deltoid

4. Questionable Exercise: Double-Leg Lift

This exercise is usually used with the intent of strengthening the abdominals, when in fact it is primarily a hip flexor (iliopsoas) strengthening exercise. Most people have overdeveloped the hip flexors and do not need to further strengthen those muscles because this may cause forward pelvic tilt. Even if the abdominals are strong enough to contract isometrically to prevent hyperextension of the lower back, the exercise produces excess stress on the discs.

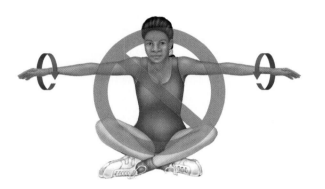

Safer Alternative Exercise: Reverse Curl

This exercise strengthens the lower abdominals. Lie on your back on the floor and bring your knees in toward the chest. Place the arms at the sides for support. For movement, pull the knees toward the head, raising the hips off the floor. Do not let knees go past the shoulders. Return to starting position and repeat.

Rectus abdominis

Table 4

Table 4 Questionable Exercises and Safer Alternatives

5. Questionable Exercise: The Windmill

This exercise involves simultaneous rotation and flexion (or extension) of the lower back, which is contraindicated. Because of the orientation of the facet joints in the lumbar spine, these movements violate normal joint mechanics, placing tremendous torsional stress on the joint capsule and discs.

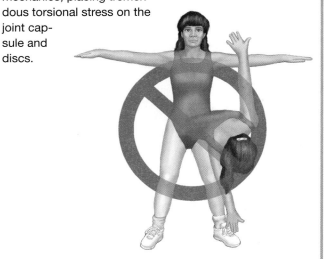

Safer Alternative Exercise: Back-Saver Toe Touch

Sit on the floor. Extend leg and bend the other knee, placing the foot flat on the floor. Bend at the hips and reach forward with both hands. Grasp one foot, ankle, or calf depending upon the distance you can reach. Pull forward with your arms and bend forward. Slight bend in the knee is acceptable. Hold. Repeat with the opposite leg.

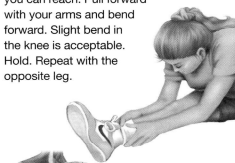

Erector spinae
Gluteals
Adductors

6. Questionable Exercise: Neck Circling

This exercise and other exercises that require neck hyperextension (e.g., neck bridging) can pinch arteries and nerves in the neck and at the base of the skull, cause wear and tear to small joints of the spine, and produce dizziness or myofascial trigger points. In people with degenerated discs, it can cause dizziness, numbness, or even precipitate strokes. It also aggravates arthritis and degenerated discs.

Safer Alternative Exercise: Head Clock

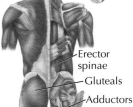

This exercise relaxes the muscle of the neck. Assume a good posture (seated with legs crossed or in a chair), and imagine that your neck is a clock face with the chin at the center. Flex the neck and point the chin at 6:00, hold, lift the chin; repeat pointing chin to 4:00, to 8:00, to 3:00 and finally to 9:00. Return to center position with chin up after each movement.

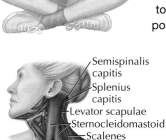

Semispinalis capitis
Splenius capitis
Levator scapulae
Sternocleidomastoid
Scalenes
Trapezius

7. Questionable Exercise: Shoulder Stand Bicycle

This exercise and the yoga positions called the plough and the plough shear (not shown) force the neck and upper back to hyperflex. It has been estimated that 80 percent of the population has forward head and kyphosis (humpback) with accompanying weak muscles. This exercise is especially dangerous for these people. Neck hyperflexion results in excessive stretch on the ligaments and nerves. It can also aggravate preexisting arthritic conditions. If the purpose for these exercises is to reduce gravitational effects on the circulatory system or internal organs, lie on a tilt board with the feet elevated. If the purpose is to warm up the muscles in the legs, slow jog in place. If the purpose is to stretch the lower back, try the leg hug exercise.

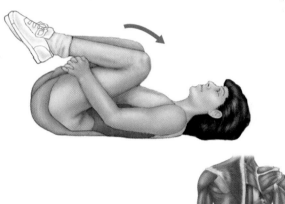

Safer Alternative Exercise: Leg Hug

Lie on your back with the knees bent at about 90 degrees. Bring your knees to the chest and wrap the arms around the back of the thighs. Pull knees to chest and hold.

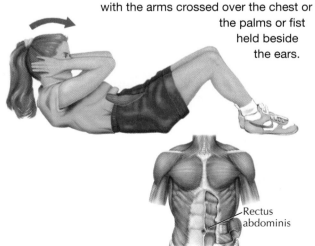

Erector spinae

Gluteals

8. Questionable Exercise: Straight-Leg and Bent-Knee Sit-Ups

There are several valid criticisms of the sit-up exercise. Straight-leg sit-ups can displace the fifth lumbar vertebra causing back problems. A bent-knee sit-up creates less shearing force on the spine, but some recent studies have shown it produces greater compression on the lumbar discs than the straight-leg sit-up. Placing the hands behind the neck or head during the sit-up or during a crunch results in hyperflexion of the neck.

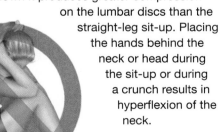

Safer Alternative Exercise: Crunch

Lie on your back with the knees bent more than 90 degrees. Curl up until the shoulder blades lift off the floor, then roll down to starting position and repeat. There are several safe arm positions. The easiest is with the arms extended straight in front of the body. Alternatives are with the arms crossed over the chest or the palms or fist held beside the ears.

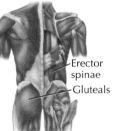

Rectus abdominis

Table 4 Questionable Exercises and Safer Alternatives

9. Questionable Exercise: Standing Toe Touches or Double-Leg Toe Touches

These exercises—especially when done ballistically—can produce degenerative changes at the vertebrae of the lower back. They also stretch the ligaments and joint capsule of the knee. Bending the back while the legs are straight may cause back strain, particularly if the movement is done ballistically. If performed only on rare occasions as a test, the chance of injury is less than if incorporated into a regular exercise program. Safer stretches of the lower back include the leg hug, the single knee-to-chest, the hamstring stretcher, and the back-saver toe touch.

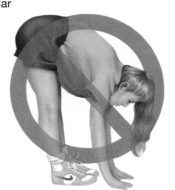

Safer Alternative Exercise: Back-Saver Hamstring Stretch

This exercise stretches the hamstring and lower back muscles. Sit with one leg extended and one knee bent, foot turned outward and close to the buttocks. Clasp hands behind back. Bend forward from the hips, keeping the low back as straight as possible. Allow bent knee to move laterally so trunk can move forward. Stretch and hold. Repeat with the other leg.

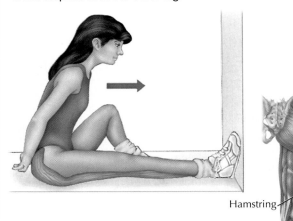

Hamstring

10. Questionable Exercise: Bar Stretch

This type of stretch may be harmful. Some experts have found that when the extended leg is raised 90 degrees or more and the trunk is bent over the leg, it may lead to **sciatica** and **piriformis syndrome,** especially in the person who has limited flexibility.

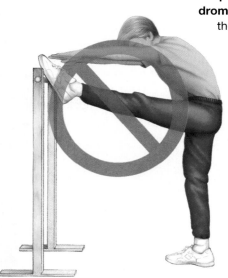

Safer Alternative Exercise: One-Leg Stretch

This exercise stretches the hamstring muscles. Stand with one foot on a bench, keeping both legs straight. Hinge forward from the hips keeping shoulders back and chest up. Bend forward until a pull is felt on the back side of the thigh. Hold. Repeat.

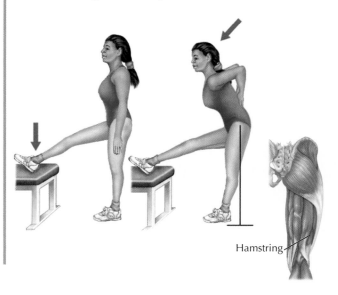

Hamstring

Table 4

11. Questionable Exercise: Shin and Quadriceps Stretch

This exercise causes hyperflexion of the knee. When the knee is hyperflexed more than 120 degrees and/or rotated outward by an external **torque,** the ligaments and joint capsule are stretched and damage to the cartilage may occur. Note: One of the quadriceps, the rectus femoris, is not stretched if the trunk is allowed to bend forward because it crosses the hip as well as the knee joint. If the exercise is used to stretch the quadriceps, substitute the hip and thigh stretch. For most people it is not necessary to stretch the shin muscles, since they are often elongated and weak; however, if you need to stretch the shin muscles to relieve muscle soreness, try the shin stretch.

Safer Alternative Exercise: Hip and Thigh Stretch

Kneel so that the front leg is bent at 90 degrees (front knee directly above the front ankle). The knee of the back leg should touch the floor well behind the front foot. Press the pelvis forward and downward. Hold. Repeat with the opposite leg forward. Do not bend the front knee more than 90 degrees.

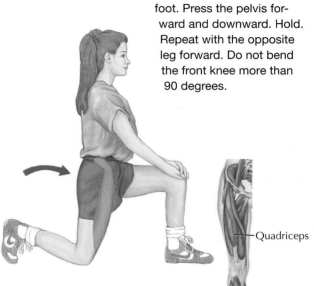

Quadriceps

12. Questionable Exercise: The Hero

Like the shin and quadriceps stretch this exercise causes hyperflexion of the knee. It also causes torque on the hyperflexed knee. For these reasons the ligaments and joint capsule are stretched and the cartilage may be damaged. For most people it is not necessary to stretch the shin muscles since they are often elongated and weak; however, if you need to stretch the shin muscles use the shin stretch. If this exercise is used to stretch the quadriceps substitute the hip and thigh stretch.

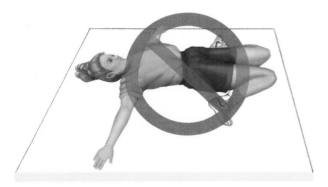

Safer Alternative Exercise: Shin Stretch

Kneel on your knees, turn to right and press down on right ankle with right hand. Hold. Keep hips thrust forward to avoid hyperflexing the knees. Do not sit on the heels. Repeat on the left side.

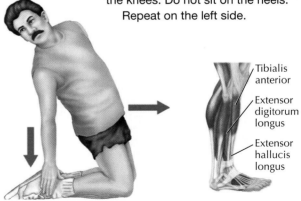

Tibialis anterior

Extensor digitorum longus

Extensor hallucis longus

Sciatica Pain along the sciatic nerve in the buttock and leg.

Piriformis Syndrome Muscle spasm and nerve entrapment in the pyriformis muscle of the buttocks region, causing pain in the buttock and referred pain down the leg (sciatica).

Torque A twisting or rotating force.

Table 4

Table 4 Questionable Exercises and Safer Alternatives

13. Questionable Exercise: Deep Squatting Exercises

This exercise, with or without weights, places the knee joint in hyperflexion, tends to "wedge it open," stretching the ligaments, irritating the synovial membrane, and possibly damaging the cartilage. The joint has even greater stress when the lower leg and foot are not in straight alignment with the knee. If you are performing squats to strengthen the knee and hip extensors, then try substituting the alternate leg kneel or half-squat with free weight or leg presses on a resistance machine.

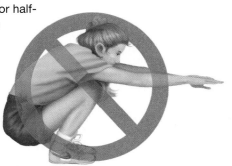

Safer Alternative Exercise: Half Squat

This exercise develops the muscles of the thighs and buttocks. Stand upright with feet shoulder width apart. Squat slowly by moving hips backwards, then bending knees. Keep shins vertical. Bend knees 45–90 degrees. Repeat.

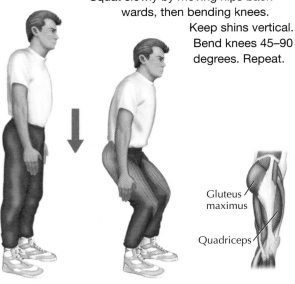

Gluteus maximus

Quadriceps

14. Questionable Exercise: Knee Pull-Down

This exercise can result in hyperflexion of the knee. The arms or hands placed on top of the shin places undue stress on the knee joint.

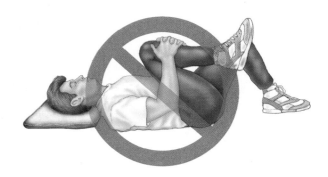

Safer Alternative Exercise: Single Knee-to-Chest

Lie down with both knees bent, draw one knee to the chest by pulling on the thigh with the hands, then extend the knee and point the foot toward the ceiling. Hold. Pull to chest again and return to starting position. Repeat with other leg.

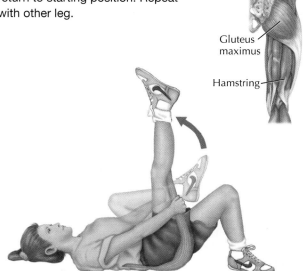

Gluteus maximus

Hamstring

Stretching Exercises for the Hip Flexors and Hamstrings and for Pelvic Stabilization

Table 5

Table 5

When performed on a regular basis, these exercises will help maintain neutral spine posture and improve the flexibility of the hip flexor and hip extensor musculature. (Tightness of these muscles can, respectively, contribute to a forward or backward pelvic tilt due to their attachments to the pelvis.) Hold stretches for 15 to 30 seconds.

1. Back-Saver Hamstring Stretch

This exercise stretches the hamstrings and calf muscles. Sit on the floor with the feet against the wall or an immovable object. Bend left knee and bring foot close to buttocks. Clasp hands behind back. Bend forward from hips, keeping lower back as straight as possible. Let bent knee rotate outward so trunk can move forward keeping back flat. Hold and repeat on each leg.

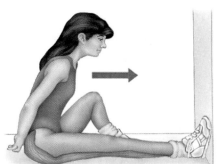

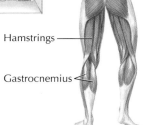

Hamstrings

Gastrocnemius

3. Hip and Low Back Stretch

This exercise stretches the hip flexors of one leg and the gluteals and lumbar muscles of the opposite leg. Lie on your back. Draw one knee up to the chest and pull thigh down tightly with the hands; then slowly return to the original position. Repeat with other knee. Do not grasp knee—grasp thigh. If a partner or a weight stabilizes the extended leg, the hip flexor muscles on that leg will be stretched.

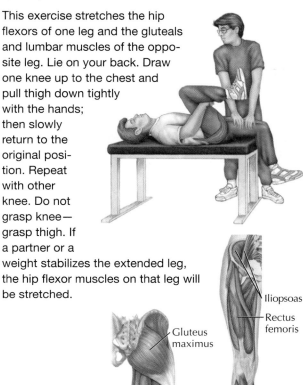

Iliopsoas

Rectus femoris

Gluteus maximus

2. Single Knee-to-Chest

This exercise stretches the lower back, gluteals, and hamstring muscles. Lie on your back with knees bent. Use hands on back of thigh to draw one knee to the chest. Hold. Then extend the knee and point the foot toward the ceiling. Hold. Return to the starting position without arching your back. Repeat with other leg.

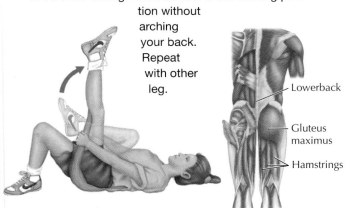

Lowerback

Gluteus maximus

Hamstrings

4. Hip and Thigh Stretch

This exercise stretches the hip flexor muscles and helps prevent or correct forward pelvic tilt, lumbar lordosis, and backache. Place right knee directly above right ankle and stretch left leg backward so knee touches floor. If necessary, place hands on floor for balance. Press pelvis forward and downward. Hold. Repeat on opposite side. Caution: Do not bend front knee more than 90 degrees.

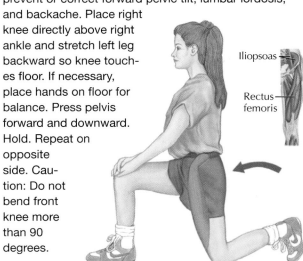

Iliopsoas

Rectus femoris

Table 6 Core Stabilization Exercises

Table 6

These exercises help train the abdominal and buttock muscles to provide postural stability by maintaining the pelvis in a neutral position during activity. They help prevent or correct lumbar lordosis, abdominal ptosis (see Table 1), and backache. Hold stretches for 15 to 30 seconds.

1. Abdominal Hollowing on Hands and Knees

Begin on hands and knees with lower back in a neutral position, stomach muscles relaxed and sagging and eyes looking at the floor. Hands should be aligned directly below shoulders and knees directly below hips. The action is to pull the belly button "in and up," drawing it toward the spine. If performed correctly, the muscles below the umbilicus will flatten, rather than bulge. Recruitment of the transverse abdominus may be facilitated by coughing and then holding the muscle contraction. The exercise is held for 10–30 seconds. Breathe normally throughout the contraction. Repeat 10 times.

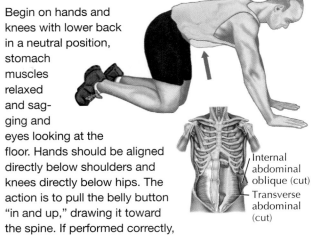

Internal abdominal oblique (cut)

Transverse abdominal (cut)

2. Abdominal Hollowing in Wall Support

Begin standing with feet 6 inches from the wall and back gently resting against the surface. Maintain a neutral spine. Contract the muscles below the belly button by pulling the abdominal wall "in and up." The pelvic floor may be contracted at the same time by pulling it "up and in" in a gripping motion. Breathe throughout the contraction. Hold 10–30 seconds. Repeat 10 times.

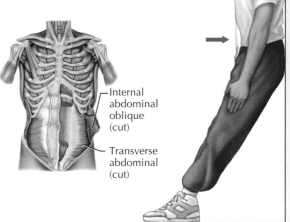

Internal abdominal oblique (cut)

Transverse abdominal (cut)

3. Horizontal Side Support

Begin in side lying position with the body resting on the forearm. Slowly lift the pelvis until the body forms a straight line from foot to shoulder. Hold 10 seconds. Repeat 8–12 times.

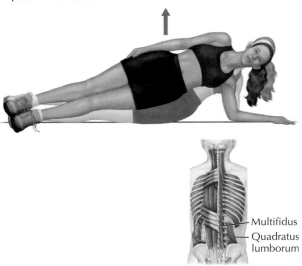

Multifidus
Quadratus lumborum

4. Head Nod

Lie flat on the back without a pillow. Gently nod the head in a "yes" motion. Motion should result in the tightening of muscles deep in the front of the neck. Place two fingers over the sides of the neck to monitor for the undesirable substitution of stronger muscles in this region. Hold 10–30 seconds (or as long as can be maintained without substitution). Repeat 10 times. Progress this exercise by first nodding "yes" and then lifting the head ¼ inch to ½ inch off the surface.

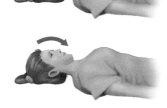

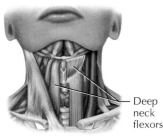

Deep neck flexors

Table 7

Exercises for Muscle Fitness of the Abdominals Table 7

These exercises are designed to increase the strength of the abdominal muscles. Strong abdominal muscles are important for maintaining a neutral pelvis, maintaining good posture, and preventing backache associated with lordosis. Hold stretches for 15 to 30 seconds.

1. Reverse Curl

Lie on your back. Bend the knees and bring knees in toward the chest. Place arms at sides for balance and support. Pull the knees toward the chest, raising the hips off the floor. Do not let the knees go past the shoulders. Return to the starting position. Repeat.

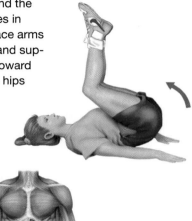

Rectus abdominis

3. Crunch with Twist (on Bench)

Lie on your back with your feet on a bench, knees bent at 90 degrees. Arms may be extended or on shoulders or hands on ears (the most difficult). Same as crunch except twist the upper trunk so the right shoulder is higher than the left. Reach toward the left knee with the right elbow. Hold. Return and repeat to the opposite side. (This exercise is not recommended for people with lower back pain due to the combined motions of flexion and rotation.)

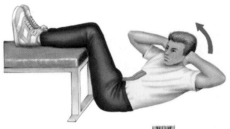

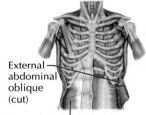

External abdominal oblique (cut)

Internal abdominal oblique

2. Crunch (Curl-Up)

Lie on your back with your knees bent and palms on ears. If desired, legs may rest on bench to increase difficulty. For less resistance, place hands at side of body. For more resistance, move hands higher. Curl up until shoulder blades leave floor, then roll down to the starting position. Repeat. Variation: extend the arms or cross the arms over your chest.

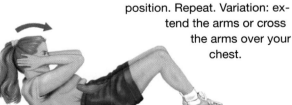

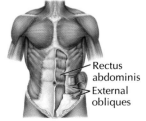

Rectus abdominis
External obliques

4. Sitting Tucks

Sit on floor with feet raised, arms extended for balance. Alternately bend and extend legs without letting your back or feet touch floor. (This is an advanced exercise and is not recommended for people who have back pain.)

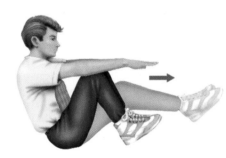

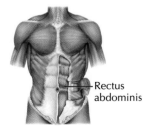

Rectus abdominis

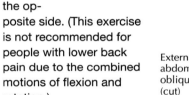

Table 8

Table 8 Stretching and Strengthening Exercises for the Muscles of the Neck

These exercises are designed to increase strength in the neck muscles and to improve neck range of motion. They are helpful in preventing and resolving symptoms of neck pain and for relieving trigger points. Hold stretches for 15 to 30 seconds.

1. Neck Rotation Exercise

This PNF exercise strengthens and stretches the neck rotators. It should always be done with the head and neck in axial extension (good alignment). It is particularly useful for relieving trigger point pain and stiffness. Place palm of left hand against left cheek. Point fingers toward ear and point elbow forward. Turn head and neck to the left; contract while gently resisting with left hand. Contract neck muscle for 6 seconds. Relax and turn head to right as far as possible; hold stretch. Repeat four times; repeat on opposite side.

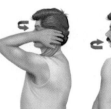
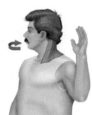

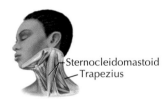

Sternocleidomastoid
Trapezius

3. Chin Tuck

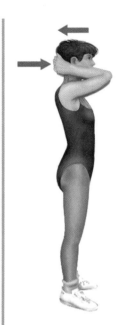

This exercise stretches the muscles at the base of the skull and reduces headache symptoms. Place hands together at the base of the head. Tuck in the chin and gently press head backward into your hands, while looking straight ahead. Hold.

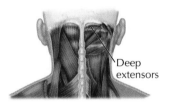

Deep extensors

2. Isometric Neck Exercises

This exercise strengthens the neck muscles. Sit and place one or both hands on the head as shown. Assume good head and neck posture by tucking the chin, flattening the neck, and pushing the crown of the head up (axial extension). Apply resistance (a) sideward, (b) backward, and (c) forward. Contract the neck muscles to prevent the head and neck from moving. Hold contraction for 6 seconds. Repeat each exercise up to six times. Note: For neck muscles, it is probably best to use a little less than a maximal contraction, especially in the presence of arthritis, degenerated discs, or injury.

Neck flexors

Neck rotator and extensors

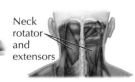

4. Upper Trapezius Stretch

This exercise stretches the upper trapezius muscle and relieves neck pain and headache. To stretch the right upper trapezius, place hand on top of head. Gently turn head toward left underarm and tilt chin toward chest. Increase stretch by gently drawing head forward with left hand. Hold. Repeat to opposite side.

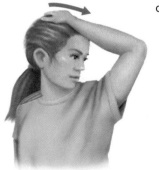

Trapezius

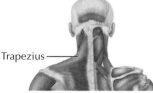

Exercises for the Trunk and Mobility Table 9

Table 9

These exercises are designed to increase the strength and mobility of the muscles that move the trunk. They are especially helpful for people with chronic back pain. Hold stretches for 15 to 30 seconds.

1. Upper Trunk Lift

Lie on a table, bench, or special-purpose bench designed for trunk lifts with the upper half of the body hanging over the edge. Have a partner stabilize the feet and legs while the trunk is raised parallel to the floor; then lower the trunk to the starting position. Lift smoothly, one segment of the back at a time. Place hands behind neck or on ears. Do not raise past the horizontal or arch the back or neck.

Back extensors

3. Side Bend

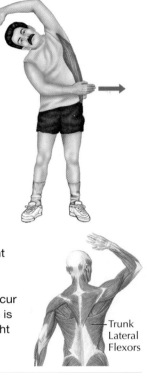

This exercise stretches the trunk lateral flexors. Stand with feet shoulder-width apart. Stretch left arm overhead to right. Bend to right at waist, reaching as far to right as possible with left arm; reach as far as possible to the left with right arm. Hold. Do not let trunk rotate or lower back arch. Repeat on opposite side. Note: this exercise is made more effective if a weight is held down at the side in the hand opposite the side being stretched. More stretch will occur if the hip on the stretched side is dropped and most of the weight is borne by the opposite foot.

Trunk Lateral Flexors

2. Trunk Lift

This exercise develops the muscles of the upper back and corrects round shoulders. Lie face down with hands clasped behind the neck. Pull the shoulder blades together, raising the elbows off the floor. Slowly raise the head and chest off the floor by arching the upper back. Return to the starting position. Repeat. For less resistance, hands may be placed under thighs. Caution: do not arch the lower back or neck. Lift only until the sternum (breastbone) clears the floor.

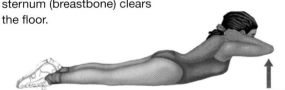

Variations: arms down at sides (easiest), hands by head, hands extended (hardest).

Trunk extensors

4. Supine Trunk Twist

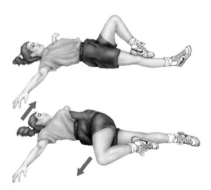

This exercise increases the flexibility of the spine and stretches the rotator muscles. Lie on your back with your arms extended at shoulder level. Place left foot on right knee cap. Twist the lower body by lowering left knee to touch floor on right. Turn head to left. Keep shoulders and arms on floor. Hold.

Trunk rotators

Table 9

Table 9 Exercises for the Trunk and Mobility

5. Lower Trunk Lift

This exercise develops low back and hip strength. Lie on your stomach on a bench or table with legs hanging over the edge. Have a partner stabilize the upper back or grasp the edges of the table with hands. Raise the legs parallel to the floor and lower them. Do not raise past the horizontal or arch the back. Suggested progression: (1) begin by alternating legs; (2) when you can do 25 reps, add ankle weights; (3) when you can do 25 reps, lift both legs simultaneously (no weights).

Erector spinae

Gluteus maximus

6. Press-Up (McKenzie Extension Exercise)

This exercise increases flexibility of the lumbar spine and restores normal lordotic curve, especially for people with a flat lumbar spine. Lie on your stomach with hands under the face. Slowly press up to a rest position on forearms. Keep pelvis on floor. Relax and hold 10 seconds. Repeat once. Do several times a day. Progress to gradually straightening the elbows while keeping the pubic bone on the floor. Caution: do not perform if you have lordosis or if you feel any pain or discomfort in the back or legs. Note: a prone press-up will feel good as a stretch after doing abdominal strength or endurance exercises. This relaxed lordotic position can be performed while standing. Place the hands in the small of the back and gently arch the back and hold. This should feel good after sitting for a long period with the back flat.

Stretching and Strengthening Exercises
for Round Shoulders

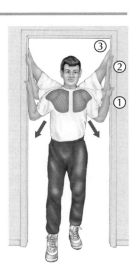 **Table 10**

These exercises are designed to stretch the muscles of the chest and strengthen the muscles that keep the shoulders pulled back in good alignment (scapular adduction).

1. Arm Lift

This exercise strengthens the scapular adductors. Lie on stomach with arms in reverse-T. Rest forehead on floor. Maintain the arm position and contract the muscles between the shoulder blades, lifting the arms as high as possible without raising head and trunk. Hold. Relax and repeat. Note: if the arms are first pressed against the floor before lifting, this becomes a PNF exercise and range of motion may be greater. Variation: this more advanced exercise is performed in the same way except the arms are extended overhead.

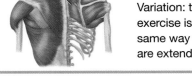

Rhomboids
Trapezius

2. Seated Rowing

This exercise strengthens the scapular adductors (rhomboid and trapezius). Sit facing pulley, feet braced and knees slightly bent. Grasp bar, palms down with hands shoulder-width apart. Pull bar to chest, keeping elbows high, and return.

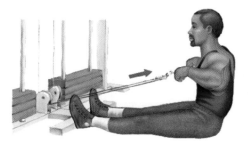

Rhomboids
Trapezius

3. Wand Exercise

This exercise stretches the muscles on the front of the shoulder joint. Sit with wand grasped at ends. Raise wand overhead. Be certain that the head does not slide forward into a "poke neck" position. Keep the chin tucked and neck straight. Bring wand down behind shoulder blades. Keep spine erect; hold. Hands may be moved closer together to increase stretch on chest muscles.

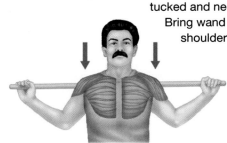

Pectoralis major

4. Pectoral Stretch

This exercise stretches the chest muscle (pectorals).

1. Stand erect in doorway with arms raised 45 degrees, elbows bent, and hands grasping door jambs, feet in front stride position. Press out on door frame, contracting the arms maximally for 3 seconds. Relax and shift weight forward on legs. Lean into doorway, so muscles on front of shoulder joint and chest are stretched. Hold.
2. Repeat with arms raised 90 degrees.
3. Repeat with arms raised 135 degrees.

(This exercise is not recommended for people with shoulder instability. Discontinue if it causes numbness in the arms or hands.)

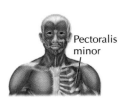

Pectoralis minor

Table 11

Table 11 Lumbar Stabilization Exercises with Stability Balls

These exercises are designed to help improve the ability of the back to stabilize and support the trunk. The physioballs provide a useful way to learn to balance the body in these positions.

1. Balancing

Contract abdominal muscles. Straighten one knee and raise opposite arm over head. Alternate sides. To increase difficulty, position ball farther from your body. Variation: slowly walk ball forward or backward with legs. Be careful not to arch back.

3. Wall Support

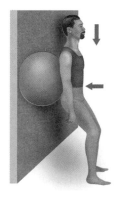

Stand against a wall with ball supporting low back. Contract abdominal muscles. Slowly bend knees 45 to 90 degrees and hold 5 seconds. Straighten knees and repeat. Raise both arms over head to increase difficulty.

2. Marching

Sit up straight with hips and knees bent 90 degrees. Contract abdominal muscles. Slowly raise one heel off the ground and opposite arm over head. Alternate sides. To increase difficulty, slowly raise one foot 2 inches from floor, alternating sides.

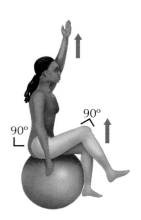

4. Stomach Roll

Lie prone over ball with abdominal region supported. Lower back and neck should be in neutral position with hands supported on floor directly under shoulders. Raise one leg off the floor while maintaining balance and a neutral spine. Alternate sides. To increase difficulty, raise one leg and opposite arm.

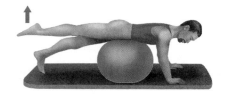

Lab Resource Materials: Healthy Back Tests

Chart 1 ▶ Healthy Back Tests

Physicians and therapists use these tests, among others, to make differential diagnoses of back problems. You and your partner can use them to determine if you have muscle tightness that may put you at risk for back problems. Discontinue any of these tests if they produce pain, numbness, or tingling sensations in the back, hips, or legs. Experiencing any of these sensations may be an indication that you have a low back problem that requires diagnosis by your physician. Partners should use *great caution* in applying force. Be gentle and listen to your partner's feedback.

Test 1—Back to Wall
Stand with your back against a wall with your head, heels, shoulders, and calves of legs touching the wall, as shown in the diagram. Flatten your neck and the hollow of your back by pressing your buttocks down against the wall. Your partner should just be able to place a hand in the space between the wall and the small of your back.

- If this space is greater than the thickness of his or her hand, you probably have lordosis with shortened lumbar and hip flexor muscles.

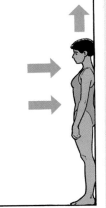

Test 2—Straight-Leg Lift
Lie on your back with hands behind your neck. The partner on your left should stabilize your right leg by placing his or her right hand on your knee. With the left hand, your partner should grasp your left ankle and raise your left leg as near to a right angle as possible. In this position (as shown in the diagram), your lower back should be in contact with the floor. Your right leg should remain straight and on the floor throughout the test.

- If your left leg bends at the knee, short hamstring muscles are indicated. If your back arches and/or your right leg does not remain flat on the floor, short lumbar muscles or hip flexor muscles (or both) are indicated. Repeat the test on the opposite side. (Both sides must pass in order to pass the test.)

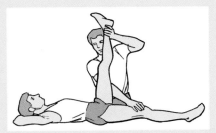

Test 3—Thomas Test
Lie on your back on a table or bench with your right leg extended beyond the edge of the table (approximately one-third of your thigh off the table). Bring your left knee to your chest and pull your thigh down tightly with your hands. Lower your right leg. Your lower back should remain flat against the table, as shown in the diagram. Your right thigh should be at table level or lower.

- If your right thigh lifts upward off the table while your left knee is hugged to your chest, a tight hip flexor (iliopsoas) on that side is indicated. Repeat on the opposite side. (Both sides must pass in order to pass the test.)

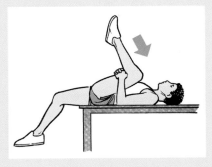

Test 4—Ely's Test*
Lie prone: flex your right knee. A partner should *gently* push your right heel toward your buttocks. Stop test when resistance or discomfort are felt.

- If your pelvis leaves the floor, your hip flexes, your knee fails to bend freely (135 degrees), or your heel fails to touch your buttocks, there is tightness in the quadriceps muscles. Repeat with your left leg. (Both sides must pass in order to pass the test.)

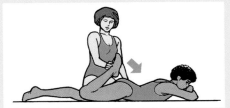

*Ely's test is suitable as a diagnostic test when performed one time. This test item is not a good exercise for regular use. It is important to follow directions carefully. If pain or discomfort occurs, stop the test.

Chart 1 ▶ Healthy Back Tests *(Continued)*

Test 5—Ober's Test

Lie on your left side with your left leg flexed 90 degrees at the hip and 90 degrees at the knee. A partner should place your right hip in neutral position (no flexion) and right knee in 90-degree flexion. Partner then allows the weight of the leg to lower it toward the floor.

- If there is no tightness in the iliotibial band (fascia and muscles on lateral side of leg), the knee touches the floor without pain and the test is passed. Repeat on the other side. (Both sides must pass in order to pass the test.)

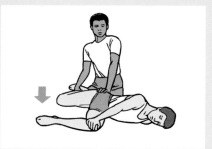

Test 6—Press-Up (Straight Arm)

Perform the press-up.

- If you can press to a straight-arm position, keeping your pubis in contact with the floor, and if your partner determines that the arch in your back is a continuous curve (not just a sharp angle at the lumbosacral joint), then there is adequate flexibility in spinal extension.

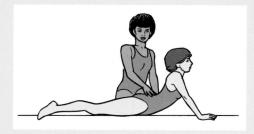

Test 7—Knee Roll

Lie supine with your knees and hips flexed 90 degrees, arms extended to the sides at shoulder level. Keep your knees and hips in that position and lower them to the floor on the right and then on the left.

- If you can accomplish this and still keep your shoulders in contact with the floor, then you have adequate rotation in the spine, especially at the lumbar and thoracic junction. (Both sides must pass in order to pass the test.)

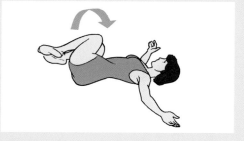

Test 8—Leg Drop Test*

Lie on your back on a table or on the floor with both legs extended overhead. Flatten your low back against the table or floor. Slowly lower your legs while keeping your back flat.

- If your back arches before you reach a 45-degree angle, your abdominal muscles are too weak. A partner should be ready to support your legs if needed to prevent your lower back from arching or strain to the back muscles.

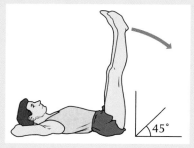

*The double leg drop is suitable as a diagnostic test when performed one time. It is not a good exercise to be performed regularly by most people. If it causes pain, stop the test.

Chart 2 ▶ Healthy Back Test Ratings

Classification	Number of Tests Passed
Excellent	7–8
Very good	6
Good	5
Fair	4
Poor	1–3

Lab 11A The Healthy Back Tests and Back/Neck Questionnaire

Name	Section	Date

Purpose: To self-assess your potential for back problems using the Healthy Back Tests and the back/neck questionnaire

Procedures

1. Answer the questions in the following back/neck questionnaire. Count your points for nonmodifiable factors, modifiable factors, and total score and record these scores in the Results section. Use Chart 1 to determine your rating for all three scores and record them in the Results section.
2. With a partner, administer the Healthy Back Tests to each other (see *Lab Resource Materials*). Determine your rating using Chart 2. Record your score and rating in the Results section. If you did not pass a test, list the muscles you should develop to improve on that test.
3. Complete the Conclusions and Implications section.

Risk Factor Questionnaire for Back and Neck Problems

Directions: Place an X in the appropriate circle after each question. Add the scores for each of the circles you checked to determine your modifiable risk, nonmodifiable risk, and total risk scores.

Nonmodifiable

1. Do you have a family history of osteoporosis, arthritis, rheumatism, or other joint disease? (0) No (1) Yes

2. What is your age? (0) <40 (1) 40–50 (2) 51–60 (3) 61+

3. Did you participate extensively in these sports when you were young: gymnastics, football, weight lifting, skiing, ballet, javelin, or shot put? (0) No (1) Some (3) Extensive

4. How many previous back or neck problems have you had? (0) None (1) 1 (2) 2 (5) 3+

Modifiable

5. Does your daily routine involve heavy lifting? (0) No (1) Some (3) A lot

6. Does your daily routine require you to stand for long periods? (0) No (1) Some (3) A lot

7. Do you have a high level of job-related stress? (0) No (1) Some (3) A lot

8. Do you sit for long periods of time (computer operator, typist, or similar job)? (0) No (1) Some (3) A lot

9. Does your daily routine require doing repetitive movements or holding objects (e.g., baby, briefcase, sales suitcase) for long periods of time? (0) No (1) Some (3) A lot

10. Does your daily routine require you to stand or sit with poor posture (e.g., sitting in a low car seat, reaching overhead with head tilted back)? (0) No (1) Some (3) A lot

11. What is your score on the Healthy Back Tests? (0) 6–7 (1) 5 (3) 4 (5) 0–3

12. What is your score on the posture test in Lab 11B? (0) 0–2 (1) 3–4 (3) 5–7 (5) 8+

Results

Tests	Pass	Fail	If you failed, what exercise should you do?
1. Back to wall	◯	◯	
2. Straight-leg lift	◯	◯	
3. Thomas test	◯	◯	
4. Ely's test	◯	◯	
5. Ober's test	◯	◯	
6. Press-up	◯	◯	
7. Knee roll	◯	◯	
8. Leg drop test	◯	◯	

Total [ ]

Chart 1 ▶ Back/Neck Questionnaire Ratings

Rating	Modifiable Score	Nonmodifiable Score	Total Score
Very high risk	7+	12+	19+
High risk	5–6	8–11	13–17
Average risk	3–4	4–7	7–11
Low risk	0–2	0–3	0–5

Chart 2 ▶ Healthy Back Tests Ratings

Classification	Number of Tests Passed
Excellent	7–8
Very good	6
Good	5
Fair	4
Poor	1–3

Back/Neck Questionnaire

Score [ ]   Rating [ ]

Back Tests

Score [ ]   Rating [ ]

Conclusions and Implications: In several sentences, discuss your need to do exercises for care of the back and neck. Include in your discussion whether you think your muscles are fit enough to prevent problems, the areas in which you are most likely to experience problems, and steps you might take to prevent future problems. Use your test results to answer.

Lab 11B Evaluating Posture

Name	**Section**	**Date**

Purpose: To learn to recognize postural deviations and thus become more posture conscious and to determine your postural limitations in order to institute a preventive or corrective program

Procedures

1. Wear as little clothing as possible (bathing suits are recommended) and remove shoes and socks.
2. Work in groups of two or three, with one person acting as the subject while partners serve as examiners; then alternate roles.
   a. Stand by a vertical plumb line.
   b. Using Chart 1 and Figure 1, check any deviations and indicate their severity (see points scale below).
   c. Total the score and determine your posture rating from the Posture Rating Scale (Chart 2).
3. If time permits, perform back and posture exercises (see Lab 11C).

Results

Record your posture score:

Record your posture rating from the Posture Rating Scale in Chart 2:

Chart 1 ▶ Posture Evaluation

Side View	Points	Back View	Points
Head forward	_____	Tilted head	_____
Sunken chest	_____	Protruding scapulae	_____
Round shoulders	_____	Symptoms of scoliosis	_____
		Shoulders uneven	_____
Kyphosis	_____	Hips uneven	_____
Lordosis	_____	Lateral curvature of spine (Adam's position)	_____
Abdominal ptosis	_____	One side of back high (Adam's position)	_____
Hyperextended knees	_____		
Body lean	_____		
		Total score	

Rate each using this point system:
- 0 = none
- 1 = slight
- 2 = moderate
- 3 = severe

Chart 2 ▶ Posture Rating Scale

Classification	Total Score
Excellent	0–2
Very good	3–4
Good	5–7
Fair	8–11
Poor	12 or more

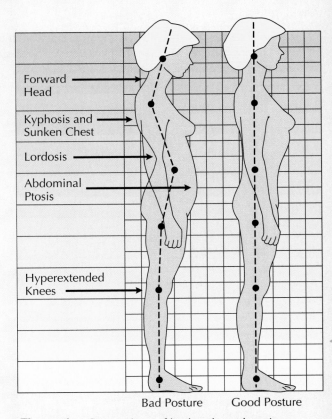

Forward Head

Kyphosis and Sunken Chest

Lordosis

Abdominal Ptosis

Hyperextended Knees

Bad Posture   Good Posture

Figure 1 ▶ Comparison of bad and good posture.

Conclusions and Implications

Were you aware of the deviations that were found?   Yes ◯   No ◯

1. List the deviations that were moderate or severe.

2. In several sentences, describe your current posture status. Include in this discussion your overall assessment of your current posture, whether you think you will need special exercises in the future, and the reasons your posture rating is good or not so good.

Lab 11C Planning and Logging Exercises: Care of the Back and Neck

Name	Section	Date

Purpose: To select several exercises for the back and neck that meet your personal needs and to self-monitor progress for one of these

Procedures

1. On Chart 1, check the tests from the Healthy Back Tests that you did *not* pass. Select at least one exercise from the group associated with those items. In addition, select several more exercises (a total of 8 to 10) that you think will best meet your personal needs. If you passed all of the items, select 8 to 10 exercises that you think will best prevent future back and neck problems. Check the exercises you plan to perform in Chart 1.
2. Perform each of the exercises you select 3 days in 1 week.
3. Keep a 1-week log of your actual participation using the last three columns in Chart 1. If possible, keep the log with you during the day. Place a check by each of the exercises you perform for each day, including ones that you didn't originally have planned. If you cannot keep the log with you, fill in the log at the end of the day. If you choose to keep a log for more than 1 week, make extra copies of the log before you begin.
4. Answer the question in the Results section.

Chart 1 ▶ Back and Neck Exercise Plan

Check the tests you failed.	✓	Place a check beside the exercises you plan to do. In the last three columns, check the exercises done and the days done.	✓	Day 1 Date:	Day 2 Date:	Day 3 Date:
1. Back to wall		Pelvic tilt				
		Bridging				
		Wall slide				
		Pelvic stabilizer				
2. Straight-leg lift		Back-saver hamstring stretch				
		Calf stretch				
3. Thomas test		Hip and thigh stretch				
4. Ely's test		Single knee-to-chest				
5. Ober's test		Lateral hip and thigh stretch				
6. Press-up		Upper trunk lift				
		Trunk lift				
7. Knee roll		Side bend				
		Supine trunk twist				
8. Leg drop test		Reverse curl				
		Crunch				
Choose other exercises for the neck and shoulders.		Chin tuck				
		Neck rotation				
		Arm lift				
		Pectoral stretch				

Results

Did you do 8 to 10 exercises at least 3 days in the week?　　Yes ◯　　No ◯

Conclusions and Interpretations

1. Do you feel that you will use back and neck exercises as part of your regular lifetime physical activity plan, either now or in the future? Use several sentences to explain your answer.

2. Discuss the exercises you did. What exercises would you continue to do and which ones would you change? Use several sentences to explain your answer.

Performance Benefits of Physical Activity

Health Goals for the year 2010

- Increase leisure-time physical activity.
- Increase adoption and maintenance of regular daily physical activity.
- Increase participation in vigorous forms of physical activity.
- Reduce steroid use, especially among young people.

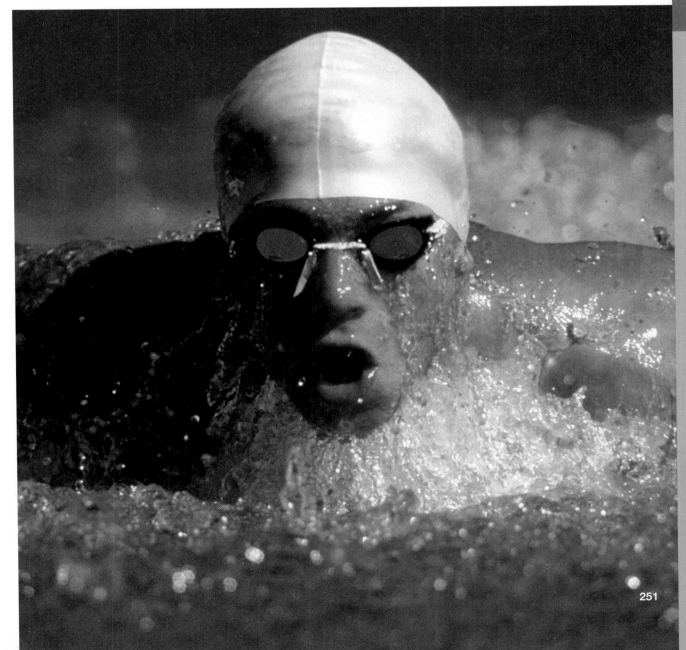

Specialized forms of training are needed to optimize adaptations to exercise and performance in sports.

Sports and competitive athletics provide opportunities for individuals to explore the limits of their ability and to challenge themselves in competition. Some individuals enjoy challenges associated with competitive aerobic activities, such as running, cycling, swimming, and triathlons. Others enjoy the challenges associated with competitive resistance training activities, such as powerlifting and bodybuilding. High-level performance is also a requirement for some types of work, such as fire safety, military service, and police work.

In this concept, specific attention is devoted to the methods used to train for high-level performance. Several types of training are discussed in detail, including endurance and speed training, specialized forms of resistance training, and other advanced training techniques, such as plyometrics, ballistic stretching, and functional balance training. Strategies for maximizing skill-related fitness and planning effective programs are also presented.

A full understanding of performance training requires a working knowledge of exercise physiology, an area of exercise science devoted to understanding how the body responds and adapts to exercise. The content provided in this concept provides a basic introduction to these principles and some practical guidelines for individuals interested in athletic performance.

High-Level Performance and Training Characteristics

Improving performance requires more specific training than the type needed to improve health. High levels of performance require good genetics, high levels of motivation, and a commitment to regular training. The amount of effort and training required to excel in sports, competitive athletics, or work requiring high-level performance is greater than the amount required for good health and wellness. Because adaptations to exercise are specific to the type of activity that is performed, training should be matched to the specific needs of a given activity.

High-level performance requires health-related, skill-related fitness and the specific motor skills necessary for the performance. To succeed in sports and certain jobs, high performance levels of health-related physical fitness are necessary, over and above what the normal person needs to enhance health. This is illustrated in Figure 1. **Training** (regular physical activity) builds health-related fitness to enhance health and high-level performance. This is why arrows in Figure 1 extend from health-related fitness to both health and high-level performance. High performance levels are not necessary for all people, only those who need exceptional performances. A distance runner needs exceptional cardiovascular fitness and muscular endurance, a lineman in football needs exceptional strength, and a gymnast needs exceptional flexibility.

Exceptional performance also requires high-level skill-related physical fitness and good physical and motor skills. It is important to understand that skill-related fitness and skills are not the same thing. Skill-related fitness components are abilities that help you learn skills faster and better, thus the arrow in Figure 1 from skill-related fitness to skills. Skills, on the other hand, are things such as throwing, kicking, catching, and hitting a ball. Practice enhances skills. Practicing the specific skills of a sport or a job is more productive to performance enhancement than more general drills associated with changing skill-related fitness.

Success in endurance sports requires a high aerobic capacity. For some performers, success depends on the ability to sustain activity for long periods of time without stopping. Distance run-

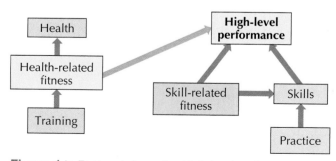

Figure 1 ▶ Factors influencing high-level performance.

ners, cyclists, and swimmers are good examples. These types of performers are in special need of high levels of cardiovascular fitness, or aerobic capacity. In aerobic exercise, adequate oxygen is available to allow the body to rebuild the high-energy fuel the muscles need to sustain performance. Aerobic exercise increases aerobic capacity (cardiovascular fitness) by enhancing the body's ability to supply oxygen to the muscles as well as their ability to use it. Slow-twitch muscle fibers are most suited for aerobic exercise, and these fibers adapt most to aerobic training. Any performance that involves sustained performance places special demands on the slow-twitch fibers and requires a high level of aerobic capacity (cardiovascular fitness). The best measure of cardiovascular fitness is $\dot{V}O_2$ max (see Concept 7).

Many types of high-level performance require anaerobic capacity. While all athletes benefit from a good level of aerobic fitness, success in many sports is determined more by speed, strength, and power. The sprinting, jumping, and powerful movements needed in most competitive sports are good examples. Strength competitions and sprint events in running, bicycling,

Web 02

and swimming also require short bursts of high-intensity activity. These activities require more energy than can be provided with aerobic metabolism. Anaerobic processes (i.e., processes that do not require oxygen) provide the additional energy needs, but a by-product of these processes (**lactic acid**) eventually causes the muscles to fatigue.

When you do anaerobic exercise the body cannot supply enough oxygen to sustain performance. So the body uses a high-energy fuel that the body has stored. When the high-energy fuel is used up, you cannot continue to perform. After the exercise you keep breathing fast and the heart continues to beat fast for a while, because the body needs to take in extra oxygen to rebuild the stores of the high-energy fuel used in anaerobic exercise. This is sometimes called **oxygen debt.** The body "borrows" oxygen that it cannot provide when it is using high-energy fuel during anaerobic exercise and then "pays back the debt" by supplying extra oxygen after the anaerobic exercise. Your body also breaks down lactic acid during the recovery period after anaerobic exercise. In some ways "borrowing" oxygen during anaerobic exercise, and paying back the oxygen debt later, is like using a credit card to borrow money that is paid back at a later time.

Athletes involved in anaerobic activities typically perform specialized forms of **anaerobic exercise** to help improve their bodies' ability to produce energy anaerobically and to tolerate higher levels of lactic acid. Using the credit card analogy, this is equivalent to the increases in available credit that are provided to customers that demonstrate that they can pay their credit card bills. Fast-twitch muscle fibers are used primarily during intense anaerobic activity and these fibers are more likely to adapt and respond to anaerobic exercise. Most sports require a combination of aerobic and anaerobic capacity, so it is important to conduct training that is most specific to the needs of a given activity.

Genetics can influence a person's potential for high-level performance. Each person inherits a unique genetic profile, which may predispose him or her to success in different sports and activities. A higher percentage of slow-twitch muscle fibers allow a person to adapt most effectively to aerobic exercise, while a higher percentage of fast-twitch muscle fibers will enhance adaptations from and performance in anaerobic exercise. Heredity

Training The type of physical activity performed by people interested in high-level performance—e.g., athletes, people in specialized jobs.

Lactic Acid Substance that results from the process of supplying energy during anaerobic exercise; a cause of muscle fatigue.

Oxygen Debt A term used to describe the body's ability to use high-energy fuel in anaerobic exercise without the presence of oxygen, and its ability to supply oxygen after the exercise to rebuild the supply of high-energy fuel.

Anaerobic Exercise *Anaerobic* means "in the absence of oxygen." Anaerobic exercise is performed at an intensity so great that the body's demand for oxygen exceeds its ability to supply it.

High-level performers need high-performance levels of fitness.

also influences the dimensions of skill-related fitness, such as balance, coordination, and reaction time, that enhance development of motor skills. The most successful performers are those who inherit good potential for health- and skill-related fitness, who train to improve their health-related fitness, and who do extensive practice to improve the skills associated with the specific activity in which they hope to excel.

Training for Endurance and Speed

Specific forms of training are needed to optimize endurance performance and speed. Speed and endurance are at opposite ends of the performance continuum. Speed events in running are as short as 100 meters, while endurance events, such as a marathon, last 26 miles. Middle-distance events, such as the mile run, fall between these extremes and present unique challenges, since it is important for athletes to have both speed and endurance. While these examples all involve running, the types of training needed for these events are very different.

One feature that is common in advanced training programs is the need to continually challenge the body. Involvement in regular physical activity will lead to increases in cardiovascular fitness in most people, but improvements are harder to achieve once a good level of fitness has been attained (the principle of diminishing returns). To maximize performance, it is necessary to perform more specific types of workouts that provide a greater challenge (overload) to the cardiovascular system. Serious athletes may exercise 6 or 7 days a week, but easier workouts are generally done after harder and more intense workouts. The hard workouts are generally very specific and are designed to challenge the body in different ways. Supplemental training to improve technique and efficiency are also used to enhance performance.

Long-slow distance training is important for endurance performance. Extended periods of aerobic exercise are needed to achieve high-level endurance performance. Athletes generally refer to this type of training as **long-slow distance (LSD) training.** Emphasis is placed on the overall duration or length of the exercise session rather than on speed. The reason for this is that specific adaptations take place within the muscles when used for long periods of time. These adaptations improve the muscles' ability to take up and use the oxygen in the bloodstream. Adaptations within the muscle cell also improve the body's ability to produce energy from fat stores. Long-slow distance training involves performances longer than the event for which you are performing but at a slower pace. For example, a mile runner will regularly perform 6- to 7-mile runs (at 50 to 60 percent of racing pace) to improve aerobic conditioning, even though the event is much shorter. A marathoner may perform runs of 20 miles or more to achieve even higher levels of endurance. Although this 20-mile distance is shorter than the marathon race distance, research suggests that ample adaptations occur from this volume of exercise. Excess mileage in this case may just wear the body down. Long-slow distance training should be performed once every 1 to 2 weeks, and a rest day is recommended on the subsequent day to allow the body to recover fully.

Improved anaerobic capacity can contribute to performance in activities considered to be aerobic. Many physical activities commonly considered to be aerobic—such as tennis, basketball, and racquetball—have an anaerobic component. These activities require periodic vigorous bursts of exercise. Regular anaerobic training will help you resist fatigue in these activities. Even participants in activities such as long-distance running can benefit from anaerobic training, especially if performance times or winning races is important. A fast start may be anaerobic, a sprint past an opponent may be anaerobic, and a kick at the end is certainly anaerobic. Anaerobic training can help prepare a person for these circumstances.

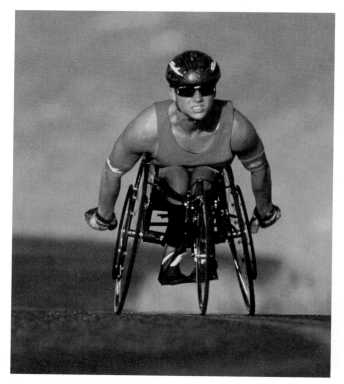

Interval training can be adapted for performers in a variety of activities.

🌐 **Interval training can be effective in building both aerobic and anaerobic capacity.** High-level performance requires high-level training. **Interval training** is commonly used by many competitive athletes. The premise behind interval training is that, by providing periodic rest, you can increase the overall intensity of the exercise session and provide a greater stimulus to the body. Interval training can be performed in different ways to achieve different training goals.

In aerobic interval training, the goal is to challenge the aerobic system to work near maximal levels for extended periods of time. Research suggests that a period of 4 to 6 minutes of activity is needed to cause the aerobic system to elicit maximal adaptations that will improve aerobic capacity (VO_2 max). The use of repeated mile runs at a faster than normal training pace would provide this type of challenge to the aerobic system. Alternately, shorter exercise bouts can be performed with brief rest periods to achieve the same goal. For example, a series of quarter-mile repeats with short rests is suitable as long as the total time at a high intensity is similar. In this case, the rest intervals must be short enough to only allow partial recovery between intervals.

Aerobic intervals are typically conducted at paces slower than the pace an individual would use in a race. An example of a schedule of aerobic interval training for a 10-km runner is illustrated in Table 1. To use the schedule, locate your typical 10-km time in the left-hand column. Perform 400-meter runs at the time specified in the "Pace" column. Repeat 20 times with intervals of 10 to 15 seconds between runs. Similar schedules can be developed with other activities, such as swimming and cycling.

In anaerobic interval training, the goal is to challenge the anaerobic energy systems. This is typically accomplished with repeated high-intensity bouts of activity. In response to this training, the body improves its ability to produce energy anaerobically and improves its ability to tolerate and remove lactic acid from the blood.

Anaerobic interval training can be performed with either short or long intervals. Short-interval workouts should use maximum speed with rest intervals lasting from 10 seconds to 2 minutes. These should be repeated 8 to 30 times. Long-interval training should use 90 to 100 percent speed, with rest intervals lasting from 3 to 15 minutes. These should be repeated 4 to 15 times. A sample short anaerobic interval program and a sample long interval running program are presented in Table 2. These plans can be modified for use with other types of activities.

Principles of interval training can be adapted for different activities. The principles of interval training can be integrated into workouts in less structured ways. Runners sometimes use *fartlek* training to break up their workouts. A fartlek training run incorporates bursts of higher-intensity running followed by recovery periods of lower intensity. The difference from interval training is that the intermittent bursts in fartlek training are dictated by the nature of the terrain or the feelings of the moment. The term is from a Swedish word meaning "speed play," because the unstructured nature is more relaxed than structured interval training.

Many competitive sports involve alternating bursts of high-intensity activity followed by periods of recovery. Basketball, for example, involves intermittent sprints and jumps interspersed with periods of short recovery. Similarly, tennis involves bursts of activity separated by

---

Table 1 ▶ Aerobic Interval Training Schedules for a 10-Kilometer Runner

Best 10-km Times (Min:Sec)	Reps	Distance (Meters)	Rest (Sec)	Pace (Min:Sec)
46:00	20	400	10–15	2:00
43:00	20	400	10–15	1:52
40:00	20	400	10–15	1:45
37:00	20	400	10–15	1:37
34:00	20	400	10–15	1:30

Source: Wilmore and Costill.

Table 2 ▶ Sample Anaerobic Interval Training Program (Moderate Intensity)

Short Intervals	Long Intervals
1. Do a flexibility and cardiovascular warm-up.	1. Do a flexibility and cardiovascular warm-up.
2. Run at 100% speed for 10 seconds (approximately 70–100 yards).	2. Run at 90% speed for 1 minute (approximately 300–500 yards).
3. Rest for 10 seconds by walking slowly.	3. Rest for 4 minutes by walking slowly.
4. Alternately repeat steps 2 and 3 until 20 runs have been completed.	4. Alternately repeat steps 2 and 3 until 5 runs have been completed.

Long-Slow Distance (LSD) Training Training technique that emphasizes long, slow distance. It is used by marathon runners and other endurance performers.

Interval Training A training technique often used for high-level aerobic and anaerobic training; uses repeated bouts of activity followed by rest to maximize the quality of the workout.

short recovery periods between points. To prepare for success in sports, it is important for athletes to incorporate intermittent interval-type training into their conditioning. Simulated games that require repeated sprints up and down the basketball court are a form of interval training specific to basketball players. Tennis players can incorporate a variety of forward and lateral movements into a high-intensity agility drill to improve conditioning for tennis.

Too much strength and flexibility training may impair endurance performance. The principle of specificity dictates that adaptations are specific to the type of training that is performed. While athletes should strive for a good balance of strength and flexibility, studies show that too much training in these areas can actually cause decreases in performance. Additional muscle mass from resistance training can reduce efficiency and impair performance. The use of weighted wristlets, ankles, or belts is also not recommended, as they may alter running mechanics and stride efficiency.

Flexibility has always been thought to be important for minimizing risks for injury, but recent studies have shown that running economy (the energy cost required to run a specific speed) is not as good in people with high flexibility as in those who have poorer flexibility. Because running economy is an advantage for distance running performance, this suggests that extra flexibility may actually reduce performance. The theory behind these findings is that stiffer muscle-tendon structures may help facilitate elastic energy return during running movements. This result shouldn't discourage you from stretching, but it does illustrate the complexities of high-level training. Regular stretching is still of value for most runners and endurance athletes.

Training for Strength and Muscular Endurance

Specific progressive resistance training programs are needed to achieve high-level muscular performance. A basic progressive resistance program for overall good health might involve performing a single exercise for each major muscle group two or three times a week. This level of training provides a regular stimulus to maintain healthy levels of muscular strength and endurance. However, many people enjoy challenging themselves to achieve higher levels of muscular performance. Olympic weight-lifting competitors use free weights and compete in two exercises: the snatch and the clean and jerk. Powerlifting competitors use free weights and compete in three lifts: the bench press, squat, and dead lift. Bodybuilding competitors use several forms of resistance training and are judged on muscular hypertrophy (large muscles) and **definition of muscle.** Performers in these activities and athletes in strength-related sports

need to use more advanced training methods to reach their full potential. The essential goal in high-level training is to provide the optimal stimulus, so that the muscles adapt in the desired way. Because the goals are clearly different for athletes interested in strength/power, muscular hypertrophy, or muscular endurance, it is important to follow appropriate programs. The essential aspects of these different training programs are described in the sections that follow. The basic concepts are summarized in Figure 2.

Performers training for high-level strength should use multiple sets with heavier weights. The best stimulus for strength gains is repeated lifts with very heavy loads. Guidelines for intermediate lifters call for multiple sets of 6 to 12 reps performed using 70 to 80 percent of 1RM values. The load and intensity guidelines are higher for advanced lifters (1 to 12 reps performed using 70 to 100 percent 1RM) because they may need to use a higher overload to get continued improvements. Rest intervals must be long (2 to 3 minutes) for high-intensity strength training to allow full recovery of the muscles between sets.

Strength/Power

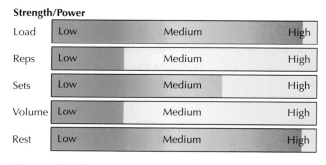

Hypertrophy/Size

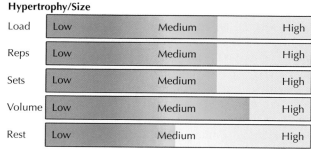

Muscular Endurance

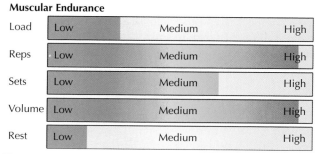

Figure 2 ▶ Differences in training stimulus for different resistance training programs.

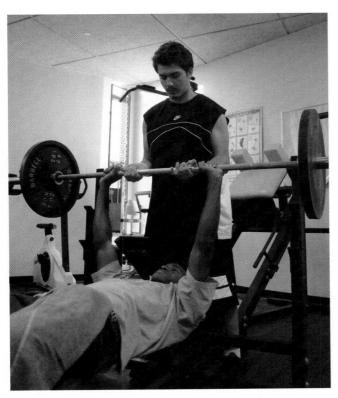

Strength training for high-level performance differs from strength training for health.

Multiple joint exercises, such as the bench press, have been found to be more effective in strength enhancement, since they allow a greater load to be lifted. The sequencing of exercises within a workout is also an important consideration for strength development. When training all major muscle groups in a workout, large muscle groups should be done before small muscle groups, and multiple-joint exercises should be done before single-joint ones.

Performers training for muscular endurance should emphasize many repetitions with lighter weights. Completing multiple sets of 10 to 25 repetitions is required to build endurance. Short rest periods of 1 to 2 minutes are recommended for high-repetition sets and periods of less than 1 minute should be used for lower-repetition sets. This challenges the muscles to perform repeatedly and with little or no rest. Variation in the order in which exercises are performed is also recommended to vary the stimulus. Intermediate lifters should aim for two to four times per week, but advanced lifters may perform up to six sessions per week if appropriate variation in muscle groups is used between workouts.

Web 04

Performers training for bulk and definition often use extra reps and/or sets. Bodybuilders are more interested in definition and hyper-

Web 05

trophy than in absolute strength. Gaining both size and definition requires a balance between strength and muscle endurance training. Most bodybuilders use 3 to 7 sets of 10 to 15 repetitions, rather than the 3 sets of 3 to 8 repetitions recommended for most weight lifters. Sometimes definition is difficult to obtain because it is obscured by fat. It should be noted that people with the largest-looking muscles are not always the strongest.

Training for cardiovascular fitness along with strength training can limit adaptations. The body adapts to the type of training that is performed. If too much endurance training is performed, the body tries to adapt to the needs of aerobic activity, and this makes it more difficult to gain muscle mass or achieve maximal increases in strength. The effect would only be an issue for competitive strength or power athletes and should not detract people from getting the important health benefits associated with moderate amounts of aerobic activity. Regular aerobic activity is considered essential for bodybuilders to help them reduce unwanted body fat.

Training for Power

Power is a combination of strength and speed, and it is both health-related and skill-related. Most experts classify power as a skill-related component of fitness because it is partially dependent on speed. On the other hand, power is also dependent on strength and can be classified as a health-related component to the extent that strength is involved. Thus, power falls somewhere between the two distinct groups of fitness attributes.

Some experts consider power to be the most functional mode in which all human motion occurs. Power is exceptionally important in sport activities such as hitting a baseball, blocking in football, putting the shot, and throwing the discus. Power is also essential for good vertical jumping—a movement critical for basketball and many other sports. A typical progressive resistance exercise program will build sufficient power for normal activities of daily living; however, people interested in high-level performance should consider using additional exercises that specifically develop power.

The stronger person is not necessarily the more powerful. Power is the amount of work per unit of time. To increase power, you must do more work in the same time or the same work in less time. If you extend your

Definition of Muscle The detailed external appearance of a muscle.

knee and move a 100-pound weight through a 90-degree arc in 1 second, you have twice as much power as a person who needs 2 seconds to complete the same movement. Power requires both strength and speed. Increasing one without the other limits power. Some power athletes (for example, football players) might benefit more by achieving less strength and more speed.

The principle of specificity applies to power development. If you need power for an activity in which you are required to move heavy weights, then you need to develop *strength-related power* by working against heavy resistance at slower speeds. If you need to move light objects at great speed, such as in throwing a ball, you need to develop *speed-related power* by training at high speeds with relatively low resistance. There must be trade-offs between speed and power because, the heavier the resistance, the slower the movement. Training adaptations are also specific to the type of training performed. Power exercises done at high speeds will help enhance muscular endurance, whereas power exercises that use heavy resistance at lower speeds will increase strength.

Performers who need explosive power to perform their events should use training that closely resembles those events. Jumpers, for example, should jump as a part of their training programs in order to learn correct timing and mechanics. If they use machines, it is better to use the leg press than a knee extension machine because the press more nearly resembles the leg action of the jump.

The performer's program should use similar speed, force, angle, and range of motion as the activity. However, if a performer is unable to do the specific skill because of weather or injury or is seeking variety, then plyometrics, isokinetics, and weight training (especially with free weights or pulleys if simulating a sport skill) are effective means of developing power.

Power training can be done with weight equipment, but care is needed to ensure safety and efficacy. Resistance training can be performed to optimize power development, but these movements are not recommended for beginning lifters. Studies have shown that heavy resistance training can actually decrease power unless training also includes some explosive movements. Current guidelines from the ACSM recommend heavy loading (85 to 100 percent of 1RM) to increase the force component of the power equation and light to moderate loading (30 to 60 percent of 1RM) performed at an explosive velocity to enhance the speed component of power. The guidelines recommend that a multiple set power program (three to six sets) be integrated within an overall strength training program. Exercises for power are most effectively done with free weights or pulleys to simulate sport-related movements more effectively. Isokinetic devices, such as isokinetic swim benches, may also be useful for enhancing sport-specific power.

Plyometrics may be useful in training for tasks or events requiring power. **Plyometrics** is an advanced training technique used by many athletes. It takes advantage of a quick prestretch prior to a movement to increase power. By repeatedly doing these movements in training, athletes can provide a greater stimulus to their muscles and improve their body's ability to perform power movements. Track and field athletes may do a hopping drill for 30 to 100 meters or alternate jumping from a box to the floor and back to the box (called depth jumping, drop jumping, or bounce loading). As the body lands, some of the major leg muscles lengthen in an eccentric contraction, then follow immediately with a strong concentric contraction as the legs push off for the next jump or stride. The prestretch of the muscle during landing adds an elastic recoil that provides extra force to the push-off (see Table 3).

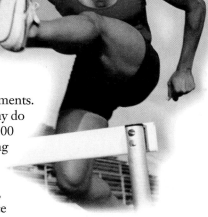

Plyometrics enhance power.

Plyometrics are used to apply the specificity principle to training for certain skills. Because eccentric exercise tends to result in more muscular soreness, it would be wise to proceed slowly with this type of training. It would also be important to have good flexibility before beginning a plyometrics program. Some safety guidelines for plyometrics are listed in Table 4.

Training for Balance and Flexibility

Functional balance training is used by some athletes to improve performance. Functional balance training involves the execution of skilled movements that promote balance and improve **proprioception**. The unique aspect of the movements is that they typically require movement and stabilization force production at the same time. In other words, one part of the body is in motion while another is stabilized. These actions essentially train the body's many somatic sensory organs to respond and adjust to different postures and positions—thereby improving balance. Functional balance training is frequently performed with exercise balls, balance boards, or Bosu® trainers (see

Table 3 ▶ Plyometric Exercise—a Technique for Developing Power

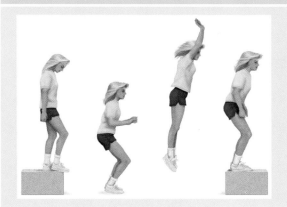

In this plyometric exercise, called the "depth jump," the athlete jumps off a box and then quickly bounds upward to land on another box. The first phase of the exercise involves an eccentric contraction (shortening of muscle fibers to slow the body during the landing phase). This is followed immediately by a concentric lengthening of muscle fibers to leap onto the next box. The recoiling of the fibers increases the force that can be applied to the muscles. Several repetitions of this type of exercise should be performed, followed by brief rests. Because of the eccentric contractions, plyometric exercises can promote greater amounts of muscle soreness, so it is important to work up to this gradually.

Table 4 ▶ Safety Guidelines for Plyometrics

- Plyometrics for growing teens should begin moderately and progress slowly, compared with plyometrics for adults.

- Progression should be gradual to avoid extreme muscle soreness.

- Adequate strength should be developed prior to plyometric training. (As a general rule, you should be able to do a half-squat with one-and-a-half times your body weight.)

- Get a physician's approval prior to doing plyometrics if you have a history of injuries or if you are recovering from injury to the body part being trained.

- The landing surface should be semiresilient, dry, and unobstructed.

- Shoes should have good lateral stability, be cushioned with an arch support, and have a nonslip sole.

- Obstacles used for jumping-over should be padded.

- The training should be preceded by a general and specific warm-up.

- The training sequence should
  - Precede all other workouts (while you are fresh)
  - Include at least one spotter
  - Be done no more than twice per week, with 48 hours' rest between bouts
  - Last no more than 30 minutes
  - (For beginners) include 3 or 4 drills, with 2 or 3 sets per drill, 10–15 reps per set and 1–2 minutes' rest between sets

Source: Adapted from Brittenham,

Concept 10). It is important to start slowly with easy movements and work up to more challenging positions and movements. This type of training is not recommended for people who have had recent orthopedic injuries, who have degenerative joint disease, or individuals with knee instability.

Stretching for performance may differ from stretching for good health. Static stretching is generally recommended for people interested in improving flexibility because it is both safe and effective. Ballistic stretching is appropriate for high-level performers because many of the motions of the activities in which they perform require ballistic movements. Nevertheless, it is recommended that ballistic stretching be performed after initiating the workout with static or PNF stretching.

The ballistic stretching phase should use stretches that closely approximate the performance activity. Examples of ballistic stretching exercises for specific performances are presented in Table 5 (page 260).

Training for High-Level Performance: Skill-Related Fitness and Skill

Good skill-related fitness is needed for success in many sports. As described in Concept 1, there are six primary components of skill-related fitness (agility, coordination, balance, reaction time, speed, and power).

Plyometrics A training technique used to develop explosive power. Referred to as "speed-strength training" in Eastern Europe and the former Soviet Union, where it originated, it consists of concentric-isotonic contractions performed after a prestretch or an eccentric contraction of a muscle.

Proprioception Awareness of body movements and orientation of the body in space; often used synonymously with *kinesthesis.*

Table 5 ▶ Examples of Ballistic Stretch to Enhance Performance

Ballistic Stretch for Throwing and Striking
This exercise can improve flexibility to aid one-handed throwing and striking skills (for example, racket sports forehand, backhand, and serve; baseball throw; or discus and shot put) and/or two-handed throwing or striking skills (for example, batting a softball or executing a golf drive or hammer throw). Assume a position at the end of the backswing for any skill listed above. A partner grasps hand(s) and resists movement while the performer turns the trunk away from the partner, making a series of gentle bouncing movements, attempting to rotate the trunk as if performing the skill. Alternate roles with the partner. Note: avoid overstretching by too vigorous bouncing. If no partner is available, use a door frame for resistance, or these sports actions can be practiced using elastic bands or inner tubes (attached to fixed objects) as resistance.

Ballistic Stretch for Golf Swing
This exercise is to improve flexibility for the golf swing. A similar exercise can be performed using one-handed throwing and striking skills (for example, racket sports forehand, backhand, and serve; baseball throw; or discus and shot put) and/or two-handed throwing or striking skills (for example, batting a softball or hammer throw). Stand and swing the club with or without a weight on the implement or on the wrist. Start by swinging backward and forward rhythmically and continuously. Gradually increase the speed and vigor of the swing to finally resemble the actual skill.

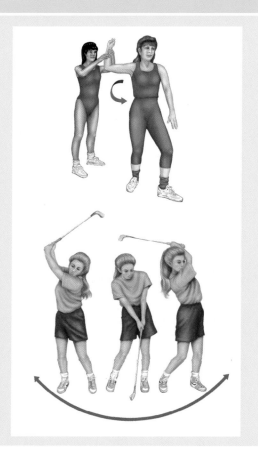

Possessing these attributes can make it easier to learn the skills that are important for many competitive sports. Balance and reaction time may be especially critical for hitting a baseball, considered by many to be the toughest skill in sports. Similarly, agility and coordination may help one master advanced dribbling skills for sports such as basketball or soccer. Because skill-related fitness can enhance performance in sports, it is often called **motor fitness** or **sports fitness.** Table 6 summarizes the general skill-related fitness requirements of 44 sport activities. In Lab 12A, you will evaluate your skill-related fitness and learn what activities you are most suited for.

An individual might possess ability in one area and not in another. For this reason, general motor ability probably does not really exist, and individuals do not have one general capacity for performing. Rather, the ability to play games or sports is determined by combined abilities in each of the separate skill-related components. However, some performers will probably be above average in many areas. The following are the key points about skill-related fitness.

- *Exceptional performers tend to be outstanding in more than one component of skill-related fitness.* Though people possess skill-related fitness in varying degrees, great athletes are likely to be above average in most, if not all, aspects. Indeed, exceptional athletes must be exceptional in many areas of skill-related fitness.

- *Excellence in one skill-related fitness component may compensate for a lack in another.* Each individual possesses a specific level of each skill-related fitness aspect. The performer should learn his or her other strengths and weaknesses in order to produce optimal performances. For example, a tennis player may use good coordination to compensate for lack of speed.

- *Excellence in skill-related fitness may compensate for a lack of health-related fitness when playing sports and games.* As you grow older, health-related fitness potential declines more rapidly than many components of skill-related fitness. You may use superior skill-related fitness to compensate. For example, a baseball pitcher who lacks the power to dominate hitters may rely on a pitch such as a knuckle ball, which is more dependent on coordination than on power.

Table 6 ▶ Skill-Related Requirements of Sports and Other Activities

Activity	Balance	Coordination	Reaction Time	Agility	Power	Speed
Archery	***	****	*	*	*	*
Backpacking	**	**	*	**	**	*
Badminton	**	****	***	***	**	***
Baseball/softball	***	****	****	***	****	***
Basketball	***	****	****	****	****	***
Bicycling	****	**	**	*	**	**
Bowling	***	****	*	**	**	**
Canoeing	***	***	**	*	***	*
Circuit training	**	**	*	**	***	**
Dance, aerobic	**	****	**	***	*	*
Dance, ballet	****	****	**	****	***	*
Dance, disco	**	***	**	****	*	**
Dance, modern	****	****	**	****	***	*
Dance, social	**	***	**	***	*	**
Fencing	***	****	****	***	***	****
Fitness calisthenics	**	**	*	***	**	*
Football	***	***	****	****	****	****
Golf (walking)	**	****	*	**	***	*
Gymnastics	****	****	***	****	****	**
Handball	**	****	***	****	***	***
Hiking	**	**	*	**	**	*
Horseback riding	***	***	**	***	*	*
Interval training	**	**	*	*	*	**
Jogging	**	**	*	*	*	*
Judo	***	****	****	****	****	****
Karate	***	****	****	****	****	****
Mountain climbing	****	****	**	***	***	*
Pool/billiards	**	***	*	**	**	*
Racquetball	**	****	***	****	**	***
Rope jumping	**	***	**	***	**	*
Rowing, crew	**	****	*	***	****	**
Sailing	***	***	***	***	**	*
Skating	****	****	**	***	**	***
Skiing, cross-country	**	****	*	***	****	**
Skiing, downhill	****	****	***	****	***	*
Soccer	**	****	***	****	***	***
Surfing	****	****	***	****	***	*
Swimming (laps)	**	***	*	***	**	*
Table tennis	**	***	***	**	**	**
Tennis	**	****	***	***	***	***
Volleyball	**	****	***	***	**	**
Walking	**	**	*	*	*	*
Waterskiing	***	****	*	***	**	*
Weight training	**	**	*	*	**	*

* = minimal needed; **** = a lot needed.

Guidelines for High-Performance Training

Overtraining is a common problem among athletes. Most Americans suffer from hypokinetic conditions resulting from too little activity. Athletes, on the other hand, often push themselves too hard in their pursuit of high-level performance and are susceptible to a variety of **hyperkinetic conditions.** Athletes who train too hard and do not allow adequate time for rest are susceptible to a hyperkinetic condition known as overload syndrome. This condition is characterized by fatigue, irritability, and sleep problems, as well as an increased risk for injuries. Performance is known to decline sharply in an overtrained status, and this can cause athletes to train even harder and become even more overtrained. Athletes should pay close attention to possible symptoms of overtraining and back off their training if they notice increased fatigue, lethargy, or unexpected decreases in their performance. Lab 12B will allow you to identify some of the symptoms of overtraining.

A useful physical indicator of overtraining is a slightly elevated morning heart rate (four or five beats more than normal values). Essentially, an elevated morning heart rate reveals that the body has had to work too hard to recover from the exercise and wasn't in its normal resting mode. To use this indicator, you should regularly monitor your resting heart rate prior to getting out of bed in the morning. Another indicator that is increasingly used by elite endurance athletes is compressed or reduced "heart rate variability." A lower beat to beat variability indicates fatigue or overtraining, since it reflects sympathetic dominance over the normally dominant parasympathetic system that exists during more rested states. Newer heart rate monitors provide an indicator of heart rate variability.

Rest and a history of regular exercise are important for reducing the risks for overuse injuries. Rest is a critical part of training programs for serious athletes. Adequate rest helps the body recover from the stress of vigorous training—it promotes the physiological adaptations that improve performance and reduces the likelihood of developing overuse injuries.

A history of regular exercise is also important for reducing risks for injury. Research conducted by the military has determined that recruits with a history of regular

Motor Fitness (Sports Fitness) Skill-related physical fitness.

Hyperkinetic Conditions Conditions caused by too much physical activity and/or insufficient rest.

exercise were less likely to get injured during basic training than recruits without this experience. This suggests that regular exercise can build up the strength and integrity of bones and joints and reduce the risk for injury. In other words, experienced athletes can perform higher levels of training without injury because they have built up a greater tolerance.

Periodization of training may help prevent overtraining. When a person trains for a single performance or perhaps several competitive events, such as games or matches during a sport season, he or she must plan carefully to reach peak performance at the right time and to avoid overtraining and injuries. Periodization is a modern concept of manipulating repetition, resistance, and exercise selection so there are periodic peaks and valleys during the training program. The peaks are needed to challenge the body, and the valleys are needed to allow the body to recover and adapt fully. Over the course of the season, there should be a gradual progression that allows the person to peak at just the right time. To accomplish this, training begins with an emphasis on base training, in which the volume of training is gradually increased (increasing reps or performing large numbers of sets). As the season progresses, the emphasis shifts to the intensity of training (going faster or lifting heavier weights). Because higher-intensity exercise requires more time for recovery, the volume of training should be reduced at these times. A key concept in periodization is to provide opportunities for the body to adapt and recover fully prior to competition. Thus, the phase immediately prior to competition (**tapering**) is characterized by a reduced volume and intensity of training. By applying periodization to their training, athletes are able to optimize performance and minimize the risks of overtraining (see Figure 3).

Athletes should be aware of various psychological disorders related to overtraining. Compulsive physical activity, often referred to as activity neurosis or exercise addiction, can be considered a hyperkinetic condition.

People with activity neurosis become irrationally concerned about their exercise regimen. They may exercise more than once a day, rarely take a day off, or feel the need to exercise even when ill or injured. One condition related to body neurosis is an obsessive concern for having an attractive body. Among females, it is usually associated with an extreme desire to be thin, whereas among males it is more often associated with an extreme desire to be muscular. The excessive desire to be fit or thin can negatively affect other aspects of life, threaten personal relationships, and contribute high amounts of stress. Anorexia nervosa, an eating disorder associated with an excessive drive to be thin, has frequently been associated with compulsive exercise.

Performance Trends and Ergogenic Aids

Athletes are driven to pursue the limits of human performance. Competition and the inherent challenges in sport have led athletes to strive continually to improve human performance. The Olympics, in fact, were founded on the principle of trying to go farther, higher, or faster and that same spirit drives modern Olympic athletes as well. Records drop as athletes learn better ways to train and better ways to perform. Table 7 compares Olympic records over the past 100+ years. An interesting observation from this comparison is that the improvements have been fairly consistent (17 to 42 percent) across types and distances of events. Advances in training, technology, and competition will continue to help athletes push for even faster records. The limits of human performance have al-

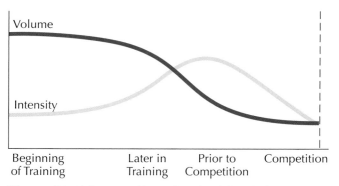

Figure 3 ▶ Volume and intensity of training during periodization.

Table 7 ▶ Trends in Olympic Records (1896–2004)				
Sport	**Event**	**1896**	**2004**	**% change**
Swimming	100 m (s)	82	48	41.5%
Track	100 m (s)	12	9.85	17.9%
	400 m (s)	54.2	44	18.8%
	800 m (m:s)	2:11	1:45	19.8%
	1,500 m (m:s)	4:33	3:34	21.6%
	Marathon (h:s)	2:59	2:10	26.8%
Field	High jump (m)	1.81	2.36	30.4%
	Long Jump (m)	6.35	8.59	35.3%

ways been intriguing. Will long jump records ever reach 10 m or will someone ever run a marathon in less than 2 hours? Only time will tell.

Many athletes look to ergogenic aids as an additional way to improve performance. Athletes are always looking for a competitive edge. In addition to pursuing rigorous training programs, many athletes look for alternative ways to improve their performance. Substances, strategies, and treatments designed to improve physical performance beyond the effects of normal training are collectively referred to as **ergogenic aids.** People interested in improving their appearance (including those with body neurosis) also abuse products they think will enhance their appearance. Ergogenic aids can be classified as mechanical, psychological, and physiological. Each category will be discussed in the subsequent sections.

Mechanical ergogenics may improve efficiency and performance. Mechanical ergogenic aids consist of equipment or devices that aid performance. Examples of mechanical ergogenic aids include oversized tennis racquets, more flexible poles for pole vaulting, spring-loaded ice skates (klap skates) for skating, lycra body suits for reducing drag in swimming and running, and carbon fiber bike frames to increase stiffness and force transmission. Consumers are presented with many options in the sport and fitness industry, and it is difficult to keep up with all the innovations.

While mechanical ergogenic aids may help maximize performance, the advantages provided by the latest high-tech innovations are probably only noticeable for highly elite athletes. For example, a recreational cyclist is not likely to appreciate (or need) an extremely light racing bicycle, but professional athletes in the Tour de France clearly benefit from having lighter and more efficient equipment. Similarly, a recreational athlete may not play any better with an expensive tennis racquet or new golf clubs, but expert players will notice and appreciate subtle differences in their equipment. Improving fitness and practicing skills will generally improve performance more than new equipment. Still, it is useful to stay abreast of changing technology in sport equipment and clothing that can make activity more enjoyable. An example is running and cycling clothing featuring microfiber or Cool Max technology that helps keep you cool and dry in hot conditions.

Psychological ergogenics improve concentration and focus during competitive activities. Many competitive activities require extreme levels of concentration and focus. Athletes who are able to maintain this mental edge during an event are at a clear advantage over athletes who cannot. Psychological ergogenics are strategies such as mental imagery and hypnosis, which have been shown to help athletes achieve peak performance.

Athletes are encouraged to use these psychological aids but to be wary of untested or unproven techniques, since quackery is prominent in this area.

Physiological ergogenics are designed to improve performance by enhancing biochemical and physiological processes in the body. Physiological ergogenics primarily are nutritional supplements that are thought to have a positive effect on various metabolic processes. Because the supplement industry is largely unregulated, many products are developed and marketed with little or no research to document their effects. These products prey on an athlete's lack of knowledge and concern over performance. Products with little or no evidence of benefits also have questionable safety, so consumers should be cautious.

Information about some of the more commonly used ergogenic aids follows. Additional information about ergogenic aids and links to performance are provided at Web09. Strategies for detecting quackery are presented in Concept 23.

- *Fluid replacement beverages and energy bars.* Fluid replacement beverages, such as Gatorade, Exceed, and Power Aide, contain carbohydrates needed for endurance exercise. People exercising for more than an hour can benefit from these supplements, and research shows that they can replace fluid lost in sweat at the same or a faster rate than water. Energy bars (e.g., Power Bars and Clif Bars), energy gels (e.g., GU), or energy chews (e.g., Clif Shot Blocks) also can provide valuable energy for extended endurance exercise. Consumers should be wary of other "energy" products that tout or promote energy without calories. These are simply stimulants or caffeine products.
- *Protein Supplements.* There is considerable interest among consumers about protein and amino acid supplements. Many strength athletes, in particular, believe strongly that extra protein in the diet can contribute to strength and muscle mass gains. As mentioned in Concept 10, the evidence does not support the contention that protein supplements are necessary for building strength and muscle mass among those who eat a healthy diet. However, deregulation of supplements and extensive advertising in magazines and on television have led many consumers to

Tapering A reduction in training volume and intensity prior to competition to elicit peak performance.

Ergogenic Aids Substances, strategies, and treatments that are intended to improve performance in sports or competitive athletics.

buy protein supplements resulting in great profits for sellers and a waste of money for buyers.

- *Creatine.* As described in Concept 10, creatine is a nutrient that is involved in the production of energy during intense exercise. The body produces it naturally from foods containing protein, but some athletes take creatine supplements (usually a powder that is dissolved into a liquid) to increase the amounts available in the muscle. The concept behind supplementation is that additional creatine intake enhances energy pro-

duction and therefore increases the body's ability to maintain force and delay fatigue. Some studies have shown improvements in performance and anaerobic capacity, but recent reviews indicate that the supplement may be effective only for athletes who are already well trained. Products containing creatine do not work by themselves; instead, they only help athletes maximize their training or performance during an event. Effects are not evident unless training is performed while taking the supplements.

Strategies for Action

Select activities that match your abilities. People differ in many factors, including skills and abilities that influence sports and athletic performance. You may be well suited to some sports but not to others. Behavioral scientists have also determined that perceptions of competence are important predictors of long-term exercise adherence. To give yourself the best chance of being successful in sports (and exercise involvement), it is important to choose activities that are well matched to your abilities. Lab 12A provides an assessment that will allow you to evaluate your levels of skill-related physical fitness. By referring to Table 6, you can determine the sports and activities that best match your individual abilities.

The assessments provided in Lab 12A are but a few of the many tests that can be done for each of the skill-related fitness parts. You may want to try other tests if you want more information about your abilities. If you have a personal desire to train for a specific sport or activity, but do not have a fitness profile that predicts success, you should not be deterred. Lab 12A will help you find an activity that you will enjoy and in which you have a good chance of success. People with good motivation, who persist in training, can often excel over others with greater ability.

Take time to plan and record your training sessions. Success in sports and competitive athletics requires careful planning and a lot of effort. To maximize your potential, it is important to take time to plan your training program. Coaches handle these tasks for many competitive athletes, but recreational athletes typically have to plan their own program. While you can contract with personal trainers to help with this task, adequate planning can be done by applying the principles described in this book. The key is to write a workout plan and keep careful records of your progress. This will allow you to monitor how your training program is progressing.

Get adequate rest and listen to your body. Because high-performance training can be quite intense, it is important to get adequate rest. Many athletes make the mistake of training too hard. An essential part of a good training program is rest. Without rest, the body does not have sufficient time to make the needed adaptations and overtraining syndrome can result. Lab 12B provides an assessment of overtraining to help you learn how to monitor for signs of overtraining.

Online Learning Center

www.mhhe.com/corbin7e
The Online Learning Center contains a variety of Web-based resources that will help you get the most out of this book and your course. In addition to the On the Web pages, there are video activities, interactive quizzes, application assignments, and a variety of other useful study aids. Log on to the URL above to access these resources.

Web Resources

Gatorade Sports Science Institute **www.gssiweb.com**
National Athletic Trainers Association **www.nata.org**
National Collegiate Athletic Association
        www.ncaa.org
National Strength and Conditioning Association
    www.nsca-cc.org
Special Olympics International **www.specialolympics.org**
United States Olympic Committee **www.usoc.org**
Women's Sports Foundation
    www.womenssportsfoundation.org

Technology Update
Applications of Nanotechnology and Chip Technology in Sports

Advances in material science have led to continued refinements in sporting goods technology. Materials in equipment have evolved from wood to metal or fiberglass and then to graphite and titanium. With each step, the materials have become lighter, stronger, and more durable. A new methodology known in industry as *nanotechnology* will further advance product development in sporting goods. The simplest way to explain nanotechnology is to view it as engineering on a scale of individual atoms. By working at this atomic level, it is possible to make materials that are both stronger *and* lighter. Carbon nanotubes, for example, are an engineered matrix of carbon molecules that creates a substance that is 100 times stronger than steel and one-sixth the weight. The use of this material will revolutionize much of the current sporting goods technology. Applications exist for improving a diverse array of equipment, including bikes, hockey sticks, softball bats, golf clubs, and ten-

nis rackets. Nanotechnology is even being used to develop golf balls that are more resistant to slices and hooks.

Refinements in computer chip technology also will likely have an impact on sports in the future. Most major running races and triathlons now use timing chips to keep track of split times and finishing times. The chips are attached to shoes and automatically communicate with sensors and computers to transmit the necessary information. A high-tech "smart ball," designed for accurate tracking of the ball's position, is undergoing testing for possible use in the World Cup and other major soccer events. When available, the chip in the ball will let the referee know if the ball is in bounds or out of bounds, or whether a goal has been scored or not. Eventually, this type of technology will be used in all ball sports that are dependent on accurate markings and placements. A logical application is in football to assist referees in determining the proper spot for the ball at the end of a play. Computer technology has revolutionized our lives in many ways and it will likely continue to influence the evolution of sports.

Suggested Readings

Additional reference materials for Concept 12 are available at Web11.

Web 11

Bahr, R., et al. 2003. Risk factors for sports injuries—A methodological approach. *British Journal of Sports Medicine* 37:384–392.

Barrett, S., et al. 2006. *Consumer Health: A Guide to Intelligent Decisions.* 8th ed. St. Louis: McGraw-Hill.

Bracko, M. R. 2002. Can stretching prior to exercise and sports improve performance and prevent injury? *ACSM's Health and Fitness Journal* 6(5):17–22.

Burke, E. 2003. *High-Tech Cycling.* 2nd ed. Champaign, IL: Human Kinetics.

Cobb, K. L. 2003. Disordered eating, menstrual irregularity and bone density in female runners. *Medicine and Science in Sports and Exercise* 35(5):711–719.

Dufek, J. S. 2002. Exercise variability: A prescription for overuse injury prevention. *ACSM's Health and Fitness Journal* 6(4):18–23.

Hootman, J. M., et al. 2001. Association among physical activity level, cardiorespiratory fitness, and risk of musculoskeletal injury. *American Journal of Epidemiology* 154(3):251–258.

Jones, A. M. 2002 Running economy is negatively related to sit and reach test performance in international-standard distance runners. *International Journal of Sports Medicine* 23(1):40–43.

Kraemer, W., et al. 2005. Progression and resistance training. *President's Council on Physical Fitness and Sports Research Digest* 6(3):1–8.

Kraemer, W. J., and N. A. Ratamess. 2004. Fundamentals of resistance training: Progression and exercise prescription. *Medicine and Science in Sports Exercise* 36(4):674–688.

Kraus, D. 2000. *Mastering Your Inner Game.* Champaign, IL: Human Kinetics.

Landry, G., and D. Bernhardt. 2003. *Essentials of Primary Care Sports Medicine.* Champaign, IL: Human Kinetics.

Manore, M., and J. Thompson. 2000. *Sport Nutrition for Health and Performance.* Champaign, IL: Human Kinetics.

Radcliffe, J., and R. Farebtinos. 2001. *High-Powered Plyometrics.* Champaign, IL: Human Kinetics.

Shiner, J., et al. 2005. Integrating low-intensity plyometrics into strength and conditioning programs. *Strength and Conditioning Journal* 27(6):10–20.

Uusitalo, A. L. 2001. Overtraining. *The Physician and Sportsmedicine* 29(5):35–50.

Volek, J. S. 2004. Influence of nutrition on responses to resistance training. *Medicine and Science in Sports and Exercise* 36(4):689–696.

Wescott, W. 2003. *Building Strength and Stamina.* 2nd ed. Champaign, IL: Human Kinetics.

Wilmore, J. H. 2003. Aerobic exercise and endurance. *The Physician and Sportsmedicine* 31(5):45–53.

Wilmore, J. H., and D. Costill. 2004. *Physiology of Sport and Exercise.* 3rd ed. Champaign, IL: Human Kinetics.

Yesalis, C. E., and M. S. Bahrke. 2005. Anabolic-androgenic steroids: Incidence of Use and Implications. *President's Council on Physical Fitness and Sports Research Digest* 5(5):1–8.

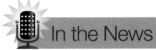

In the News

A Perspective on the Media Coverage of Sports

The Olympics provide the ultimate competitive environment for sports. Athletes train for years with dreams focused on qualifying and competing in the Olympics. The 2006 winter Olympic games in Turino, Italy, provided the usual share of excitement and thrills as athletes from across the world battled in an array of events. Much could be written about the prowess and skill of these incredible athletes, but an unwritten story is how athletes often have to handle defeat graciously. A troubling and unfortunate issue in sports is that newspaper and television reporters tend to place too much emphasis on winning. They focus on the medals that athletes *don't* win rather than on their effort and the inherent joy of competition. For example, snowboarder Lindsey Jacobellis was questioned over and over about her crash late in the Snowboard Cross event. She graciously handled the issue and acknowledged that she got "caught up in the moment." She should be congratulated both for her silver medal and for handling the questions in a positive manner.

Figure skater Sasha Cohen had an unfortunate fall early in her final skating performance but also recovered to win a silver medal. Instead of being congratulated for the way she finished her performance, Cohen was berated and questioned by the media about the fall. She commented how pleased she was with the way she responded (after the fall), but the interviewers then focused solely on whether she would come back in 4 years to redeem herself. She responded by saying that she simply loves skating and wants to continue competing to do her best. This is the real message of the Olympics.

Bode Miller received perhaps the most attention (and criticism) for his seemingly casual attitude and his comments about not needing to win to feel successful. He described his approach and attitude in frequent TV commercials but the media still seemed to label him as a failure for not winning any medals. Miller felt he gave his best in each event. He congratulated the other racers who had better races, and seemed at peace with his performance. In a final interview he commented, "The expectations were from other people. I'm comfortable with what I've accomplished, including at the Olympics. I came in here to race as hard as I could. That was my obligation to myself." His post-Olympics message was consistent with the philosophy he espoused well before the Olympics, but the media seemed to take his accepting attitude as an indication that he must not have given it his all. Instead of allowing Miller's message to communicate the true spirit of competition, the media reinforced the societal preoccupation with winning.

The point is that sports, including sports at the Olympics, are for the enjoyment of the participants. The authors encourage readers to focus on the intrinsic enjoyment of the sports and activities in which they choose to participate.

Lab Resource Materials: Skill-Related Physical Fitness

Important Note: Because skill-related physical fitness does not relate to good health, the rating charts used in this section differ from those used for health-related fitness. The rating charts that follow can be used to compare your scores with those of other people. You *do not* need exceptional scores on skill-related fitness to be able to enjoy sports and other types of physical activity; however, it is necessary for high-level performance. After the age of 30, you should adjust ratings by 1 percent per year.

Evaluating Skill-Related Physical Fitness

I. Evaluating Agility: The Illinois Agility Run

An agility course using four chairs 10 feet apart and a 30-foot running area will be set up as depicted in this illustration. The test is performed as follows:

1. Lie prone with your hands by your shoulders and your head at the starting line. On the signal to begin, get on your feet and run the course as fast as possible.
2. Your score is the time required to complete the course.

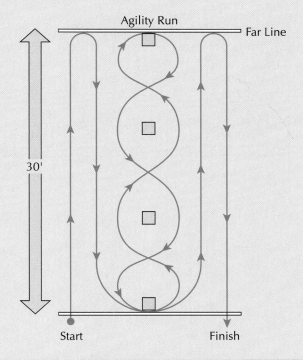

II. Evaluating Balance: The Bass Test of Dynamic Balance

Eleven circles (9 ½ inch) are drawn on the floor as shown in the illustration. The test is performed as follows:

1. Stand on the right foot in circle X. *Leap* forward to circle 1, then circle 2 through 10, alternating feet with each leap.
2. The feet must leave the floor on each leap and the heel may not touch. Only the ball of the foot and toes may land on the floor.
3. Remain in each circle for 5 seconds before leaping to the next circle. (A count of 5 will be made for you aloud.)
4. Practice trials are allowed.
5. The score is 50, plus the number of seconds taken to complete the test, minus the number of errors.
6. For every error, deduct 3 points each. Errors include touching the heel, moving the supporting foot, touching outside a circle, and touching any body part to the floor other than the supporting foot.

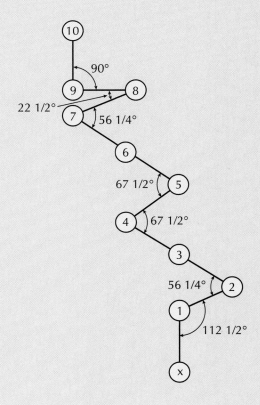

Chart 1 ▶ Agility Rating Scale

Classification	Men	Women
Excellent	15.8 or faster	17.4 or faster
Very good	16.7–15.9	18.6–17.5
Good	18.6–16.8	22.3–18.7
Fair	18.8–18.7	23.4–22.4
Poor	18.9 or slower	23.5 or slower

Source: Adams et al.

Chart 2 ▶ Balance Test Rating Scale

Rating	Score
Excellent	90–100
Very good	80–89
Good	60–79
Fair	30–59
Poor	0–29

Chart 3 ▶ Coordination Rating Scale

Classification	Men	Women
Excellent	14–15	13–15
Very good	11–13	10–12
Good	5–10	4–9
Fair	3–4	2–3
Poor	0–2	0–1

III. Evaluating Coordination: The Stick Test of Coordination

The stick test of coordination requires you to juggle three wooden sticks. The sticks are used to perform a one-half flip and a full flip, as shown in the illustrations.

1. *One-half flip.* Hold two 24-inch (½ inch in diameter) dowel rods, one in each hand. Support a third rod of the same size across the other two. Toss the supported rod in the air, so that it makes a half turn. Catch the thrown rod with the two held rods.
2. *Full flip.* Perform the preceding task, letting the supported rod turn a full flip.

The test is performed as follows:

1. Practice the half-flip and full flip several times before taking the test.
2. When you are ready, attempt a half-flip five times. Score 1 point for each successful attempt.
3. When you are ready, attempt the full flip five times. Score 2 points for each successful attempt.

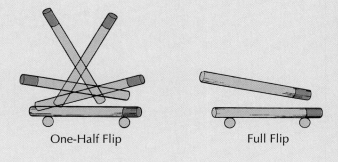

One-Half Flip   Full Flip

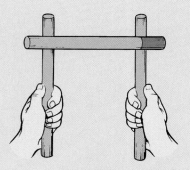

Hand Position

IV. Evaluating Power: The Vertical Jump Test

The test is performed as follows:

1. Hold a piece of chalk so its end is even with your fingertips.
2. Stand with both feet on the floor and your side to the wall and reach and mark as high as possible.
3. Jump upward with both feet as high as possible. Swing arms upward and make a chalk mark on a 5′ × 1′ wall chart marked off in half-inch horizontal lines placed 6 feet from the floor.
4. Measure the distance between the reaching height and the jumping height.
5. Your score is the best of three jumps.

Chart 4 ▶ Power Rating Scale

Classification	Men	Women
Excellent	25 ½″ or more	23 ½″ or more
Very good	21″–25″	19″–23″
Good	16 ½″–20 ½″	14 ½″–18 ½″
Fair	12 ½″–16″	10 ½″–14″
Poor	12″ or less	10″ or less

Metric conversions for this chart appear in Appendix A.

V. Evaluating Reaction Time: The Stick Drop Test

To perform the stick drop test of reaction time, you will need a yardstick, a table, a chair, and a partner to help with the test. To perform the test, follow this procedure:

1. Sit in the chair next to the table so that your elbow and lower arm rest on the table comfortably. The heel of your hand should rest on the table so that only your fingers and thumb extend beyond the edge of the table.
2. Your partner holds a yardstick at the top, allowing it to dangle between your thumb and fingers.
3. The yardstick should be held so that the 24-inch mark is even with your thumb and index finger. No part of your hand should touch the yardstick.
4. Without warning, your partner will drop the stick, and you will catch it with your thumb and index finger.
5. Your score is the number of inches read on the yardstick just above the thumb and index finger after you catch the yardstick.
6. Try the test three times. Your partner should be careful not to drop the stick at predictable time intervals, so that you cannot guess when it will be dropped. It is important that you react only to the dropping of the stick.
7. Use the middle of your three scores (for example: if your scores are 21, 18, and 19, your middle score is 19). The higher your score, the faster your reaction time.

Chart 5 ▶ Reaction Time Rating Scale

Classification	Score
Excellent	More than 21″
Very good	19″–21″
Good	16″–18 ¾″
Fair	13″–15 ¾″
Poor	Below 13″

Metric conversions for this chart appear in Appendix A.

VI. Evaluating Speed: 3-Second Run

To perform the running test of speed, it will be necessary to have a specially marked running course, a stopwatch, a whistle, and a partner to help you with the test. To perform the test, follow this procedure:

1. Mark a running course on a hard surface so that there is a starting line and a series of nine additional lines, each 2 yards apart, the first marked at a distance 10 yards from the starting line.

2. From a distance 1 or 2 yards behind the starting line, begin to run as fast as you can. As you cross the starting line, your partner starts a stopwatch.

3. Run as fast as you can until you hear the whistle, which your partner will blow exactly 3 seconds after the stopwatch is started. Your partner marks your location at the time when the whistle was blown.

4. Your score is the distance you were able to cover in 3 seconds. You may practice the test and take more than one trial if time allows. Use the better of your distances on the last two trials as your score.

Chart 6 ▶ Speed Rating Scale

Classification	Men	Women
Excellent	24–26 yards	22–26 yards
Very good	22–23 yards	20–21 yards
Good	18–21 yards	16–19 yards
Fair	16–17 yards	14–15 yards
Poor	Less than 16 yards	Less than 14 yards

Metric conversions for this chart appear in Appendix A.

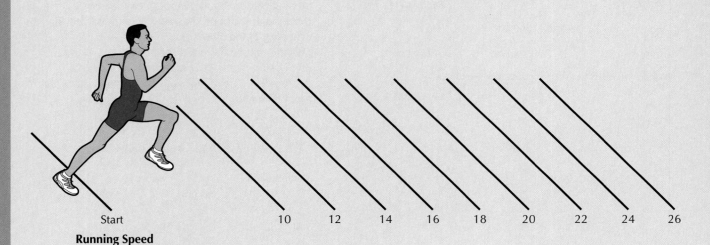

Start   10   12   14   16   18   20   22   24   26

Running Speed

Lab 12A Evaluating Skill-Related Physical Fitness

Name	**Section**	**Date**

Purpose: To help you evaluate your own skill-related fitness, including agility, balance, coordination, power, speed, and reaction time; this information may be of value in helping you decide which sports match your skill-related fitness abilities

Procedures

1. Read the direction for each of the skill-related fitness tests presented in *Lab Resource Materials.*
2. Take as many of the tests as possible, given the time and equipment available.
3. Be sure to warm up before and to cool down after the tests.
4. It is all right to practice the tests before trying them. However, you should decide ahead of time which trial you will use to test your skill-related fitness.
5. After completing the tests, write your scores in the appropriate places in the Results section.
6. Determine your rating for each of the tests from the rating charts in *Lab Resource Materials.*

Results

Place a check in the circle for each of the tests you completed.

Agility (Illinois run)　◯

Balance (Bass test)　◯

Coordination (stick test)　◯

Power (vertical jump)　◯

Reaction time (stick drop test)　◯

Speed (3-second run)　◯

Record your score and rating in the following spaces.

	Score	**Rating**	
Agility			(Chart 1)
Balance			(Chart 2)
Coordination			(Chart 3)
Power			(Chart 4)
Reaction time			(Chart 5)
Speed			(Chart 6)

Conclusions and Implications: In two or three paragraphs, discuss the results of your skill-related fitness tests. Comment on the areas in which you did well or did not do well, the meaning of these findings, and the implications of the results, with specific reference to the activities you will perform in the future.

Lab 12B Identifying Symptoms of Overtraining

Name	**Section**	**Date**

Purpose: To help you identify the symptoms of overtraining

Procedures

1. Answer the questions concerning overtraining syndrome in the Results section. If you are in training, rate yourself; if not, evaluate a person you know who is in training. As an alternative, you may evaluate a person you know who was formerly in training (and who experienced symptoms) or evaluate yourself when you were in training (if you trained for performance in the past).
2. Use Chart 1 (below) to rate the person (yourself or another person) who is (or was) in training.
3. Use Chart 2 (page 274) to identify some steps that you might take to treat or prevent overtraining syndrome.
4. Answer the questions in the Conclusions and Implications section.

Results

Answer "Yes" (place a check in the circle) to any of the questions relating to overtraining symptoms you (or the person you are evaluating) experienced.

○ 1. Has performance decreased dramatically in the last week or two?

○ 2. Is there evidence of depression?

○ 3. Is there evidence of atypical anger?

○ 4. Is there evidence of atypical anxiety?

○ 5. Is there evidence of general fatigue that is not typical?

○ 6. Is there general lack of vigor or loss of energy?

○ 7. Have sleeping patterns changed (inability to sleep well)?

○ 8. Is there evidence of heaviness of the arms and/or legs?

○ 9. Is there evidence of loss of appetite?

○ 10. Is there a lack of interest in training?

Chart 1 ▶ Ratings for Overtraining Syndrome

Number of "Yes" Answers	Rating
9–10	Overtraining syndrome is very likely present. Seek help.
6–8	Person is at risk for overtraining syndrome if it is not already present. Seek help to prevent additional symptoms.
3–5	Some signs of overtraining syndrome are present. Consider methods of preventing further symptoms.
0–2	Overtraining syndrome is not present, but attention should be paid to the few symptoms that do exist.

Conclusions and Implications

Chart 2 lists some of the steps that may be taken to help eliminate or prevent overtraining syndrome. Check the steps that you think would be (or would have been) most useful to the person you evaluated.

Chart 2 ▶ Steps for Treating or Preventing Overtraining Syndrome

○ 1. Consider a break from training.

○ 2. Taper the program to help reduce symptoms.

○ 3. Seek help to redesign the training program.

○ 4. Alter your diet.

○ 5. Evaluate other stressors that may be producing symptoms.

○ 6. Reset performance goals.

○ 7. Talk to someone about problems.

○ 8. Have a medical checkup to be sure there is no medical problem.

○ 9. If you have a coach, consider a talk with him or her.

○ 10. Add fluids to help prevent performance problems from dehydration.

Discuss overtraining syndrome in general. Elaborate on one or two of the steps in Chart 2 that you think would be (or would have been) most effective in treating or preventing overtraining syndrome for the person you evaluated.

Body Composition

Health Goals for the year 2010

- Increase proportion of adults who are at a healthy weight.
- Reduce proportion of adults who are obese.
- Reduce proportion of children and adolescents who are overweight or obese.

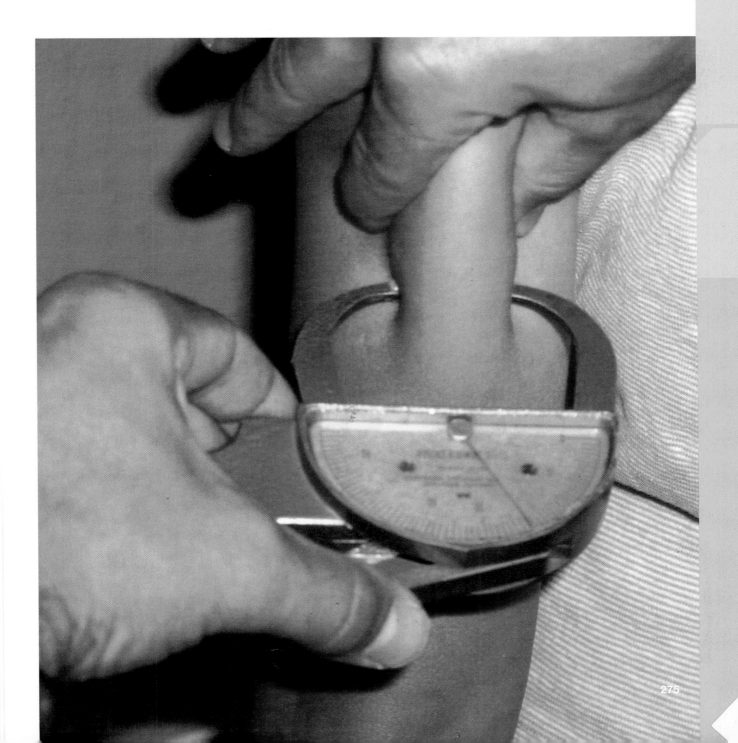

Possessing an optimal amount of body fat contributes to health and wellness.

The topic of overweight and obesity is in the news almost on a daily basis. Reports describe the health effects of obesity, the social and environmental factors that contribute to obesity, and the overall impact that it has on society. Despite considerable attention by the public health community and plenty of awareness by consumers, the prevalence of obesity has continued to increase. A recent study in *Journal of the American Medical Association* reported that nearly two–thirds (66 percent) of Americans are overweight and approximately one-third (32 percent) are considered to be obese (31 percent of men and 33 percent of women). The study also reported that approximately 17 percent of children and adolescents are overweight—rates that were found to be significantly greater than those reported just four years earlier.

The health implications of this obesity epidemic are hard to quantify and predict, but it is clear that obesity has become one of our greatest public health challenges. The problem is not unique to the United States, since similar trends are evident in almost all developed countries.

This concept describes issues associated with overweight and obesity as well as the health risks associated with being too lean. Developing a healthy body image and avoiding disordered patterns of eating are critical for optimal health and wellness. Bone health is another important parameter related to body composition. Strategies for building and maintaining healthy bones are also discussed in this concept.

Understanding and Interpreting Body Composition Measures

Body composition is considered a component of health-related fitness but can also be considered a component of metabolic fitness. Body composition is generally considered to be a health-related component of physical fitness. However, body composition is unlike the other parts of health-related physical fitness in that it is not a performance measure. Cardiovascular fitness, strength, muscular endurance, and flexibility can be assessed using movement or performance, such as running, lifting, or stretching. Body composition requires no movement or performance. This is one reason some experts prefer to consider body composition as a component of metabolic fitness. Whether you consider body composition to be a part of health-related or metabolic fitness, it is an important health-related factor.

Standards have been established for healthy levels of body fatness. Fat has important functions in the body and it is distributed naturally into different tissues and storage depots. The indicator of **percent body fat** is typically used to reflect the overall fat content of the body. This indicator takes into account differences in body size and allows recommendations to be made for healthy levels of body fatness.

A certain minimal amount of fat is needed to allow the body to function. This level of **essential fat** is necessary for temperature regulation, shock absorption, and the regulation of essential body nutrients, including vitamins A, D, E, and K. The exact amount of fat considered essential to normal body functioning has been debated, but most experts agree that males should possess no less than 5 percent and females no less than 10 percent. For females, an exceptionally low body fat percentage (**underfat**) is especially of concern. **Amenorrhea** may occur among women when fat levels fall too low. Low body fat levels, accompanied by amenorrhea, places a woman at risk for bone loss (osteoporosis). A body fat level below 10 percent is one of the criteria often used by clinicians for diagnosing eating disorders, such as anorexia nervosa.

Table 1 shows the health-related standards for body composition (percent body fat) for both males and females. Because individuals differ in their response to low fatness, a borderline range is provided above the essential fat (too low) zone. Values in this zone are not necessarily considered to be healthy but some individuals may seek to have lower body fat levels to enhance performance in certain sports. These levels can be acceptable for nonperformers if they can be maintained on a healthy diet and without overtraining. If symptoms such as amenorrhea, bone loss, and frequent injury occur, then levels of body fatness should be reconsidered, as should training techniques and eating patterns. For many people in training,

---

On the Web

www.mhhe.com/corbinweb

Web 01   Log on to this URL before reading this concept. See On the Web list of concepts. Click on the concept number you want to view. To access supplemental information, click on the number shown at each Web icon.

Table 1 ▶ Health-Related Standards for Body Fatness (Percent Body Fat) and Body Mass Index

	Too low	Borderline	Good fitness	Marginal	At risk	
Male	5 or less	6–9	10–20	21–25	26+	Body fatness (percent body fat)
Female	10 or less	11–16	17–28	29–35	36+	

	Too low	Borderline	Good fitness	Overweight*	Obesity*	
Male	12 or less	13–16	17–25	26–30	30+	Body mass Index (kg/m^2)
Female	12 or less	13–16	17–25	26–30	30+	

*Note: Based on international standards used for BMI classification

maintaining performance levels of body fatness is temporary; thus, the risk for long-term health problems is diminished.

Fat that is stored above essential fat levels is classified as **nonessential fat.** Just as percent body fat should not drop too low, it should not get too high. The healthy ranges for body fatness in males is between 10 and 20 percent while the healthy range for women is between 17 and 28 percent. These levels are associated with good metabolic fitness, good health, and wellness. The marginal zone includes levels that are above the healthy fitness zone but not quite into the range used to reflect **obesity.** The term *obesity* often carries negative connotations and stereotypes but it is important to understand that it is a clinical term that simply means excessively high body fat. Lab 13A will provide opportunities for you to assess your level of body fatness.

Health standards have been established for the Body Mass Index. The **Body Mass Index (BMI)** is a commonly used indicator of overweight and obesity in our society. It is easy to administer and can be used when studying large groups. Height and weight are used to calculate the BMI (see *Lab Resource Materials*). While the BMI is considered better than most height-weight tables as an indicator of overweight, it does have its limitations. Individuals who do regular physical activity and who possess considerable muscle mass may show up as overweight using the BMI. This is because muscle weighs more than fat, but height and weight measurements do not detect differences in muscle and fat in the body. The accepted international standard for defining overweight and obesity are the same for both men and women. BMI values over 25 are used to define **overweight** and values over 30 are used to define obesity. Table 1 provides additional information concerning BMI standards. In Lab 13B you will calculate your BMI and make comparisons to other body composition assessments.

Assessing body weight too frequently can result in making false assumptions about body composition changes. The most common way that people gauge their body composition is by periodic assessments of body weight. While occasional checks of weight (and BMI) can be helpful, frequent body weight measurements can provide incorrect information and lead to false assumptions.

Percent Body Fat The percentage of total body weight that is composed of fat.

Essential Fat The minimum amount of fat in the body necessary to maintain healthful living.

Underfat Too little of the body weight composed of fat (see Table 1).

Amenorrhea Absent or infrequent menstruation.

Nonessential Fat Extra fat or fat reserves stored in the body.

Obesity A clinical term for a condition that is characterized by an excessive amount of body fat (or extremely high BMI).

Body Mass Index (BMI) A measure of body composition using a height-weight formula. High BMI values have been related to increased disease risk.

Overweight A clinical term that implies higher than normal levels of body fat and potential risk for development of obesity.

For example, people vary in body weight from day to day and even hour to hour, based solely on their level of hydration. Short-term changes in weight are often due to water loss or gain, yet many people erroneously attribute the weight changes to their diet, a pill they have taken, or the exercise they recently performed. Monitoring your weight less frequently—once a week, for example—is more useful than taking daily or multiple daily measures because doing so is more likely to represent real changes in body composition. Weighing at the same time of day, preferably early in the morning, is best because it reduces the chances that your weight variation will be a result of body water changes. Of course, it is best to use body composition assessments in addition to those based on body weight if accurate evaluations are expected.

Methods Used to Assess Body Composition

Methods of body composition vary in accuracy and practicality. A number of techniques have been developed to assess body composition. Table 2 provides a summary of the effectiveness of these methods. The procedures vary in terms of practicality and accuracy, so it is important to understand the limitations of each method. It should be noted that even established techniques have potential for error.

Dual-energy absorptiometry (DXA) has emerged as the accepted "gold standard" measure of body composition. The DXA technique uses the attenuation of two energy sources in order to estimate the density of the body. A specific advantage of DXA is that it can provide whole body measurements of body fatness as well as amounts stored in different parts of the body. For the procedure, the person lies on a table and the machine scans up along the body. While some radiation

exposure is necessary with the procedure, it is quite minimal compared with X-ray and other diagnostic scans. Because the machine is quite expensive, this procedure is only found in medical centers and well-equipped research laboratories. The DXA (also called DEXA) procedure provides scientists with a highly accurate measure of body composition for research and a criterion measure that has been used to validate other, more practical measures of body composition.

Underwater weighing and Bod Pod are two highly accurate methods. Underwater weighing is another excellent method of assessing body fatness. Before the develpment of DXA it was considered to be the "gold standard" method of assessment. In this technique, a person is weighed in air and under water, and the difference in weight is used to assess the levels of body fatness. People with a lot of muscle, bone, and other lean tissue sink like a rock in water because muscle and other lean tissue are dense. Fat is less dense, so people with more fat tend to float in a water environment. People who weigh more underwater are more dense than those who weigh less in water. A limitation of this method is that participants must exhale all their air while submerged in order to obtain an accurate reading. Additional error from the estimations of residual lung volumes also tends to reduce the accuracy of this approach.

A relatively new device, called the Bod Pod, uses the same principles as underwater weighing, but relies on air displacement to assess body composition. Evidence suggests that it provides an acceptable alternative to underwater weighing and is particularly useful for special populations (obese older people and the physically challenged).

Skinfold measurements are the preferred, practical method of assessing body fatness. About one-half of the body's fat is located around the various body organs and in the muscles. The other half of the body's fat is located just under the skin, or in

Table 2 ▶ Ratings of the Validity and Objectivity of Body Composition Methods

Method	Precise	Objective	Accurate	Valid Equations	Overal Rating
Skinfold measurement	4.0	3.5	3.5	3.5	3.5
Bioelectric impedance	4.0	4.0	3.5	3.5	3.5
Circumferences	4.0	4.0	3.0	3.0	3.0
Body mass index (BMI)	5.0	5.0	1.5	1.5	2.0

Adapted from Lohman, Houtkooper, and Going.

Precise: can the same person get the same results time after time?

Accurate: do values compare favorably with underwater weighing?

5 = excellent; 4 = very good; 3 = good; 2 = fair; 1 = unacceptable.

Objective: can two people get the same results consistently?

Valid: is the formula accurate for predicting fat from measurements?

skinfolds (Figure 1). A skinfold is two thicknesses of skin and the amount of fat that lies just under the skin. By measuring skinfold thicknesses of various sites around the body, it is possible to estimate total body fatness (Figure 2). Skinfold measurements are often used because they are relatively easy to do. They are not nearly as costly as underwater weighing and other methods that require expensive equipment. Research-quality skinfold calipers cost more than $100 but consumer-models are available for less than $10 (see Web04 for more details).

In general, the more skinfolds measured, the more accurate the fatness estimate. However, measurements with two or three skinfolds have been shown to be reasonably accurate and can be done in a relatively short period. Two skinfold techniques are used in Lab 13A. You are encouraged to try both. With adequate training, most people can learn to use calipers to get a good estimate of fatness.

Bioelectric impedance analysis has become a practical alternative for body fatness assessment. Bioelectric impedance analysis ranks quite favorably for accuracy and has overall rankings similar to those of skinfold measurement techniques. The test can be performed quickly and is more effective for people high in body fatness (a limitation of skinfolds). The technique is based on measuring resistance to current flow. Electrodes are placed on the body and low doses of current are passed through the skin. Because muscle has greater water content than fat, it is a better conductor and has less resistance to current. The overall amount of resistance and body size are used to predict body fatness. Dehydration can bias the result and it is critical to not have measures taken within 3 to 4 hours after a meal. Accurate measures require the use of high-quality equip-

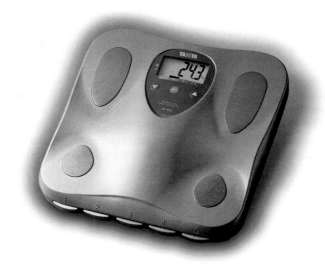

Bioelectric impedance scale

ment, but some commercially available "scales" provide estimates of body fatness that are based on the same principles. Instead of electrodes, you simply stand on metal plates that measure the current flow.

Infrared sensors are sometimes used to assess body fatness. Near-infrared interactance machines use the absorption of light to estimate body fatness. The technique was originally developed to measure the fat content of meats. Commercially available units for humans have not been shown to be effective for estimating body fat, and at least one company has faced sanctions from the government for selling an unapproved product. For this reason, this type of device is not included in Table 2.

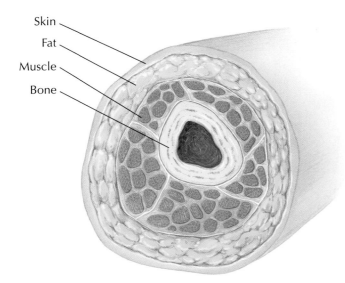

Figure 1 ▶ Location of body fat.

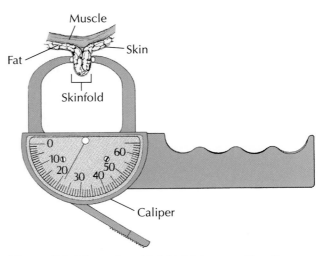

Figure 2 ▶ Measuring skinfold thickness with calipers.

BMI and other height-weight charts have limitations but are easy to use. BMI was previously described in an earlier section of this concept. As noted, it has its limitations. Height and weight charts can also be used to determine overweight, but like the BMI height-weight measures, are not particularly accurate in assessing body composition and body fatness. The BMI measure is more widely used and accepted because values correlate better with measures of body fatness. Mathematically, it is calculated with the following formula: BMI = [height (m) * height (m) / weight (kg)].

Because they are frequently used measures, it is important to know how to calculate and interpret your BMI and your "healthy weight range." Instructions and charts are provided in the *Lab Resource Materials*. Several BMI calculators and other online resources are available at Web06.

Health Risks Associated with Overfatness

Obesity contributes directly and indirectly to a number of major health problems. The diseases and medical complications associated with obesity are summarized in Figure 3. Collectively, the health-care dollars spent annually to treat medical complications associated with obesity have been estimated at over $100 billion. The biggest health burden is likely from the documented effect of obesity on risk for heart disease.

Prior to 1998, obesity was considered to be a secondary risk factor for heart disease. The reason for this was that the effects of obesity were thought to be mediated by other risk factors, such as high blood pressure and blood lipids. Because of the mounting evidence of the relation-

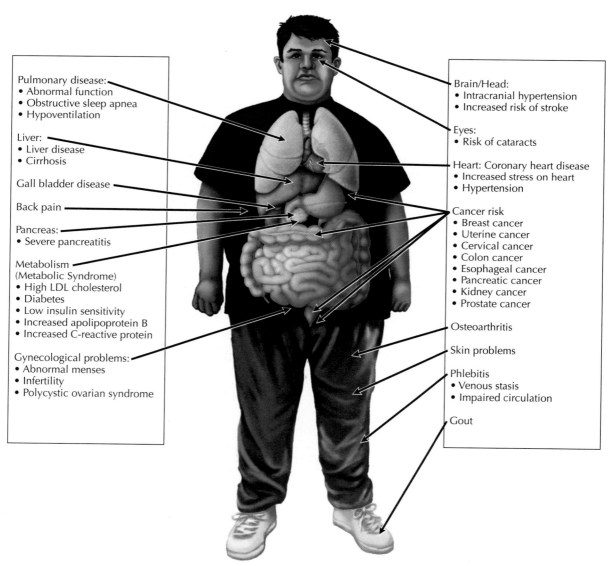

Figure 3 ▶ Diseases and medical complications associated with obesity.

ship of obesity to health risk, especially risk for heart disease, the American Heart Association classifies obesity as a primary risk factor, along with high blood lipids, high blood pressure, tobacco use, and sedentary living.

Heart disease is not the only disease associated with obesity. Diabetes is another leading killer that is associated with all components of metabolic fitness, including obesity. The incidence of diagnosis of this disease has increased sixfold in the past 40 years. Recent studies also indicate a significant increase in risk for various forms of cancer among the obese. High blood pressure, asthma, back pain, osteoarthritis, liver disease, pulmonary disease, pancreatitis, and gallbladder problems are associated with obesity (see Figure 3).

Obesity contributes to early death. In addition to the higher incidence of certain diseases and health problems, evidence shows that people who are moderately overfat have a 40 percent higher than normal risk of shortening their life span. More severe obesity results in a 70 percent higher than normal death rate.

Statistics indicate that underweight people also have a higher than normal risk for premature death. Though adequate evidence shows extreme leanness (e.g., anorexia nervosa) can be life threatening, underweight people may have lost weight because of a medical condition such as cancer. It appears that the medical problems are often the reason for low body weight rather than low body weight being the source of the medical problem. Most experts agree that people who are free from disease and who have lower than average amounts of body fat have a lower than average risk for premature death.

Physical fitness provides protection from the health risks of obesity. A general assumption in our society is that, if you are thin, you are probably fit and healthy and that, if you are overweight, you are unfit and unhealthy. A series of studies from the Aerobic Center Longitudinal Study (a large cohort study of patients from the Cooper Clinic in Dallas, Texas) have demonstrated that the health risks associated with overweight are greatly reduced by regular physical activity and reasonable levels of cardiovascular fitness (see Figure 4). In fact, the findings consistently show that active people who have a high BMI are at less risk than inactive people with normal BMI levels. Even high levels of body fatness may not be especially likely to increase disease risk if a person has good metabolic fitness as indicated by healthy blood fat levels, normal blood pressure, and normal blood sugar levels. It is when several of these factors are present at the same time that risk levels increase dramatically. For this reason, it is important to consider your cardiovascular and metabolic fitness levels before drawing conclusions about the effects of high body weight or high body fat levels on health and wellness. This information also points out the importance of periodically assessing your cardiovascular and metabolic fitness levels.

Excessive abdominal fat and excessive fatness of the upper body can increase the risk for various diseases. The location of body fat can influence the health risks associated with obesity. Fat in the upper part of the body is sometimes referred to as "Northern Hemisphere" fat, and a body type high in this type of fat is sometimes called the "apple" shape (see Figure 5). Upper body fat is also referred to as android fat because it is more characteristic of men than women. Postmenopausal women typically have a higher amount of upper body fat

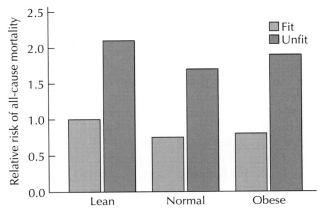

Figure 4 ▶ Risks of fatness vs. fitness.
Source: Lee, C. D., et al.

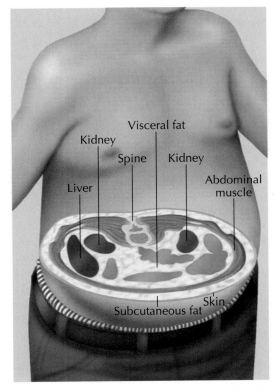

Figure 5 ▶ Visceral, or abdominal, fat is associated with increased disease risk.

than premenopausal women. Lower body fat, such as in the hips and upper legs, is sometimes referred to as "Southern Hemisphere" fat. This body type is sometimes called the "pear" shape. Lower body fat is also referred to as gynoid fat because it is more characteristic of women than men.

Body fat that is located in the core of the body is referred to as central fat or visceral fat. Visceral fat is located in the abdominal cavity (see Figure 5), as opposed to subcutaneous fat, which is located just under the skin. Though subcutaneous fat (skinfold measures) can be used to estimate body fatness, it is not a good indicator of central fatness. A useful indicator of fat distribution is the waist-to-hip circumference ratio (see *Lab Resource Materials*). A high waist circumference relative to hip circumference yields a high ratio indicative of high visceral fat. Visceral fat is associated with high blood fat levels as well as other metabolic problems. It is also associated with high incidence of heart attack, stroke, chest pain, breast cancer, and early death.

Part of the benefit of aerobic activity for health appears to be its ability to promote the preferential loss of abdominal body fat. Several recent studies have demonstrated that higher levels of activity and/or higher cardiorespiratory fitness are associated with lower levels of abdominal body fatness independent of body mass index. In other words, if one person who is fit and active has the same height and weight as a less active person, he or she will likely have a lower amount of abdominal fat. Abdominal body fat is considered to be more harmful than other forms. These studies provide a clear understanding of how fitness may protect against the health risks of obesity and improve overall health.

Health Risks Associated with Excessively Low Body Fatness

Web 08 **Excessive desire to be thin or low in body weight can result in health problems.** In western society, the near obsession with thinness has been, at least in part, responsible for eating disorders. Eating disorders, or altered eating habits, involve extreme restriction of food intake and/or regurgitation of food to avoid digestion. The most common disorders are anorexia nervosa, bulimia, and anorexia athletica. All of these disorders are most common among highly achievement-oriented girls and young women, although they affect virtually all segments of the population. Patterns of "disordered eating" are not the same as clinically diagnosed eating disorders. People who adopt disordered eating, however, tend to have a greater chance of developing an eating disorder.

Anorexia nervosa is the most severe eating disorder. If untreated, it is life threatening. Anorexics restrict food intake so severely that their bodies become emaciated. Among the many characteristics of anorexia nervosa are fear of maturity and inaccurate body image. The anorexic starves himself or herself and may exercise compulsively or use laxatives to prevent the digestion of food in an attempt to attain excessive leanness. The anorexic's self-image is one of being too fat, even when the person is too lean for good health. Assessing body fatness using procedures such as skinfolds and observation of the eating habits may help identify people with anorexia. Among anorexic girls and women, development of an adult figure is often feared. People with this disorder must obtain medical and psychological help immediately, as the consequences are severe. About 25 percent of those with anorexia do compulsive exercise in an attempt to stay lean. Anorexia is a very serious medical condition that deserves more discussion than can be provided in this book. For more information, visit Web08.

Bulimia is a common eating disorder characterized by bingeing and purging. Disordered eating patterns become habitual for many people with bulimia. They alternate between bingeing and purging. Bingeing means periodically eating large amounts of food at one time. A binge might occur after a relatively long period of dieting and often consists of junk foods containing empty calories. After a binge, the bulimic purges the body of the food by forced regurgitation or the use of laxatives. Another form of bulimia is bingeing on one day and starving on the next. The consequences of bulimia include serious mental, gastrointestinal, and dental problems. Bulimics may or may not be anorexic. It may not be possible to use measures of body fatness to identify bulimia, as the bulimic may be lean, normal, or excessively fat. For additional information, see Web08.

Anorexia athletica is a more recently identified eating disorder that appears to be related to participation in sports and activities that emphasize body leanness. Studies show that participants in sports such as gymnastics, wrestling, and bodybuilding and activities such as ballet and cheerleading are most likely to develop anorexia athletica. This disorder has many of the symptoms of anorexia nervosa, but not of the same severity. In some cases, anorexia athletica leads to anorexia nervosa.

Web 09 **Female athlete triad is an increasingly common condition among female athletes.** The female athlete triad is a collection of symptoms/conditions caused by poor eating habits and excessive training. The three health concerns (the triad) that characterize the condition are eating disorders, amenorrhea, and osteoporosis. The disordered eating patterns may be extreme, as in anorexia or bulimia, or less severe, as evidenced by poor eating habits. Because they are athletes, females with this condition are very active. Together, the poor eating habits and high levels of activity typically result in low body fat levels, altered menstrual cycles, and a corresponding reduction in the bone protective benefits of estrogen. Premature osteoporotic fractures can occur, and the lost opportunities to build higher bone density during youth increases the risk for problems later in life.

The female athlete triad is one of the more challenging conditions to treat because it often goes undetected. Once identified or diagnosed, it is hard to change because the three components of the triad are thought to be linked together pathophysiologically. The athlete is very serious about performance and has likely developed altered eating patterns to control body weight. Efforts to bring about change often result in resistance since the compulsion to be thin and perform well overrides other concerns such as eating well, moderating exercise, and having a normal menstrual cycle. Eating a well-balanced diet and moderating the frequency of exercise can help promote the natural return of menses. Hormone replacement therapy is also commonly prescribed to prevent the loss of bone density.

Many female athletes train extensively and have relatively low body fat levels but experience none of the symptoms of the triad. Eating well, training properly, using stress-management techniques, and monitoring health symptoms are the keys to their success.

Muscle dysmorphia is an emerging problem among male athletes. Muscle dysmorphia is characterized as a body dismorphic disorder in which a male becomes preoccupied with the idea that his body is not sufficiently lean and/or muscular. Athletes with this condition may be more inclined to use performance-enhancing drugs, to exercise while sick, to or have an eating disorder. Additional risks include depression and social isolation.

Fear of obesity is a less severe condition, but it can still have negative health consequences. Fear of obesity is most common among achievement-oriented teenagers who impose a self–restriction on caloric intake because they fear obesity. Consequences include stunting of growth, delayed puberty, delayed sexual development, and decreased physical attractiveness. It is important to avoid excessive eating and inactivity to prevent the problems associated with overfatness and obesity; however, an excessive concern for leanness can also result in serious health problems.

The Origin of Fatness

Obesity is a multifactorial disease that is influenced by both genetics and the environment. The evidence documenting a genetic component to human obesity is quite compelling. There is clear clustering of obesity within families, and studies have documented high concordance of body composition in monozygotic twins. Studies of adopted children have also demonstrated that there is an association between the BMI of adoptees and the biologic

parents but not between adoptees and adoptee parents. Despite the clear evidence, the role of genetic factors is still not well understood. Genetic mapping studies suggest that a number of genes may work in combination to influence susceptibility to obesity. These *susceptibility genes* may not lead directly to obesity but may predispose a person to overweight or obesity if exposed to certain environmental conditions. Key environmental factors that may trigger obesity genes are poor diet and lack of physical activity.

Thus, the prevailing model guiding obesity research is that complex genetic and environmental variables interact to increase potential risks for obesity. Genetic factors, by themselves, cannot account for the rapid changes in the prevalence of obesity because the gene pool does not change that rapidly. Future research will allow genetic and environmental data to be more fully integrated, so that the combined effects can be better understood.

Body weight is regulated and maintained through complex regulatory processes. Web 10 Some scholars have suggested that the human body type, or **somatotype,** is inherited. Clearly, some people have more difficulty than others controlling fatness, and this may be because of their somatotype and genetic predisposition. Regulatory processes appear to balance energy intake and energy expenditure so that body weight stays near a biologically determined **set-point.** The regulation is helpful for maintaining body weight but can be frustrating for people trying to lose weight. If a person slowly tries to cut calories, the body perceives an energy imbalance and initiates processes to protect the current body weight. The body can accommodate to a new, higher set-point if weight gain takes place over time, but there is greater resistance to adopting a lower set-point. Many people lose weight only to see the weight come back months later. One of the reasons that exercise is so critical for weight maintenance is that it may help in re-setting this set-point.

In recent years, the mechanisms involved in the regulation of the biological set-point have become better understood. The current view is that there are complex feedback loops among fatty tissues, the brain, and endocrine glands, such as the pancreas and the thyroid. A compound known as leptin plays a crucial role in altering appetite and in speeding up or slowing down the metabolism. Leptin levels rise during times of energy excess

Somatotype A term that refers to a person's individual body type. One researcher (Sheldon) suggested that there are three basic body types, ectomorph (linear), mesomorph (muscular), and endomorph (round).

Set-point A theoretical concept that describes the way the body protects current weight and resists change.

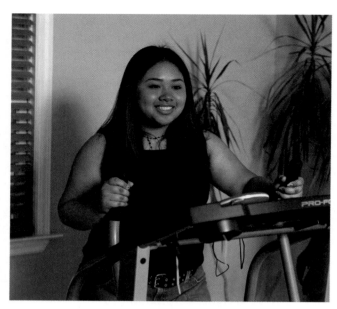

Physical activity can help in regulating body fatness.

in order to suppress appetite and levels fall when energy levels are low to stimulate appetite. Resistance to leptin has been hypothesized as a possible contributor to obesity. A number of other compounds also appear to be involved in the complex processes regulating energy balance. Problems with the thyroid gland can lead to impairments in metabolic regulation, but these do not contribute to overfatness in most people. Additional information on metabolic regulation of appetite and weight are available at Web10.

Fatness early in life leads to adult fatness. Research has documented that body composition levels tend to track through the life span. Although there are exceptions, individuals that are overweight or obese as children are more likely to be overweight or obese as adults. One explanation for this is that overfatness in children causes the body to produce more fat cells. Research has even suggested that the neonatal environment that the child is exposed to during development may also influence future risks for obesity. It appears that hormones and lipids circulating in the maternal blood can interact with genetic factors to establish metabolic conditions that contribute to overfatness. While these factors influence body composition, it is still possible to improve body composition by adopting healthy lifestyles.

Maintaining healthy levels of body fat is an important objective for children and adults. It was previously thought that only adult obesity was related to health problems, but it is now apparent that teens who are overfat are at a greater risk for heart problems and cancer than leaner peers. Obese children have been found to have symptoms of "adult-onset diabetes," indicating that the effects of obesity can impair health even for young people.

Changes in basal metabolic rate can be the cause of obesity. The amount of energy you expend each day must be balanced by your energy intake if you are to maintain your body fat and body weight over time. Your energy intake is determined solely by the **calories** you eat, while your energy expenditure is determined by a number of related factors. The **basal metabolic rate (BMR)** is the largest component of total daily energy expenditure. BMR is the amount of calories that are needed to maintain your body function under resting conditions. Other contributions to energy expenditure come from processing the food you eat and from the physical activity performed during the day.

BMR is highest during the growing years. The amount of food eaten increases to support this increased energy expenditure. When growing ceases, if eating does not decrease or activity level increase, fatness can result. Basal metabolism also decreases gradually as you grow older. One major reason for this is the loss of muscle mass associated with inactivity. Regular physical activity throughout life helps keep the muscle mass higher, resulting in a higher BMR. Evidence suggests that regular exercise can contribute in other ways to increased BMR. The higher BMR of active people helps them prevent overfatness, particularly in later life.

"Creeping obesity" is a problem as you grow older. People become less active and their BMR gradually decreases with age. Caloric intake does seem to decrease somewhat with age, but the decrease does not adequately compensate for the decreases in BMR and activity levels. For this reason, body fat increases gradually with age for the typical person (see Figure 6). This increase in fatness

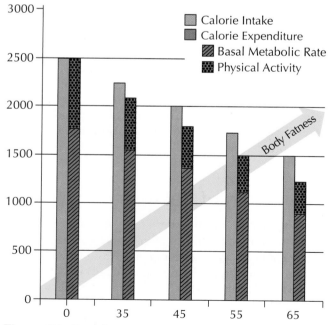

Figure 6 ▶ Creeping obesity.

over time is commonly referred to as "creeping obesity" because the increase in fatness is gradual. For a typical person, creeping obesity can result in a gain of 1/2 to 1 pound per year. People who stay active can keep muscle mass high and delay changes in BMR. For those who are not active, it is suggested that caloric intake decrease by 3 percent each decade after 25 so that by age 65 caloric intake is at least 10 percent less than it was at age 25. The decrease in caloric intake for active people need not be as great.

The Relationship between Physical Activity and Body Composition

A combination of regular physical activity and dietary restriction is the most effective means of losing body fat. Studies indicate that regular physical activity combined with dietary restriction is the most effective method of losing fat. **Diet** alone can contribute to weight loss, but much of this loss is actually lean tissue. When physical activity and diet are both used in a weight loss program, the same amount of weight may be lost but more of it is from fat. This is obviously beneficial for appearance and for participation in physical activity, but it can also help maintain resting metabolic rate at a higher level. This can contribute to further weight loss or facilitate weight maintenance. For optimal results, all weight loss programs should combine a lower caloric intake with a good physical exercise program. Thresholds of training and tar-

get zones for body fat reduction, including information for both physical activity and diet are presented in Table 3. A general guideline is to try to lose no more than 1–2 pounds a week. Because a pound of fat contains 3,500 calories, this requires a caloric deficit of approximately 500 calories per day. Individuals who are interested in maintaining body composition should aim for **caloric balance.** Individuals who want to increase lean body mass need to increase caloric intake while carefully increasing the intensity and duration of their physical activity (mainly muscular activity).

Physical activity that can be sustained for relatively long periods is considered the most effective for losing body fat. Physical activities from virtually any level of the physical activity pyramid can be effective

Calories Units of energy supplied by food; the quantity of heat necessary to raise the temperature of a kilogram of water 1°C (actually, a kilocalorie, but usually called a calorie for weight control purposes).

Basal Metabolic Rate (BMR) Energy expenditure in a basic, or rested, state.

Diet The usual food and drink for a person or an animal.

Caloric Balance Consuming calories in amounts equal to the number of calories expended.

Table 3 ▶ Threshold of Training and Target Zones for Body Fat Reduction

	Threshold of Training*		Target Zones*	
	Physical Activity	**Diet**	**Physical Activity**	**Diet**
Frequency	• To be effective, activity must be regular, preferably daily, though fat can be lost over the long term with almost any frequency that results in increased caloric expenditure.	• Reduce caloric intake consistently and daily. To restrict calories only on certain days is not best, though fat can be lost over a period of time by reducing caloric intake at any time.	• Daily moderate activity is recommended. For people who do regular vigorous activity, 3 to 6 days per week may be best.	• It is best to diet consistently and daily.
Intensity	• To lose 1 pound of fat, you must expend 3,500 calories more than you normally expend.	• To lose 1 pound of fat, you must eat 3,500 calories fewer than you normally eat.	• Slow, low-intensity aerobic exercise that results in no more than 1 to 2 pounds of fat loss per week is best.	• Modest caloric restriction resulting in no more than 1 to 2 pounds of fat loss per week is best.
Time	• To be effective, exercise must be sustained long enough to expend a considerable number of calories. At least 15 minutes per exercise bout are necessary to result in consistent fat loss.	• Eating moderate meals is best. Do not skip meals.	• Exercise durations similar to those for achieving aerobic cardiovascular fitness seem best. Exercise of 30 to 60 minutes in duration is recommended.	• Eating moderate meals is best. Skipping meals or fasting is not most effective.

*It is best to combine exercise and diet to achieve the 3,500-calorie imbalance necessary to lose a pound of fat. Using both exercise and diet in the target zone is most effective.

Table 4 ▶ Calories Expended per Hour in Various Physical Activities (Performed at a Recreational Level)*

Activity	Calories Used per Hour				
	100 lb. (46 kg)	120 lb. (55 kg)	150 lb. (68 kg)	180 lb. (82 kg)	200 lb. (91 kg)
Archery	180	204	240	276	300
Backpacking (40-lb. pack)	307	348	410	472	513
Badminton	255	289	340	391	425
Baseball	210	238	280	322	350
Basketball (half-court)	225	255	300	345	375
Bicycling (normal speed)	157	178	210	242	263
Bowling	155	176	208	240	261
Canoeing (4 mph)	276	344	414	504	558
Circuit training	247	280	330	380	413
Dance, aerobics	315	357	420	483	525
Dance, ballet (choreographed)	240	300	360	432	480
Dance, modern (choreographed)	240	300	360	432	480
Dance, social	174	222	264	318	348
Fencing	225	255	300	345	375
Fitness calisthenics	232	263	310	357	388
Football	225	255	300	345	375
Golf (walking)	187	212	250	288	313
Gymnastics	232	263	310	357	388
Handball	450	510	600	690	750
Hiking	225	255	300	345	375
Horseback riding	180	204	240	276	300
Interval training	487	552	650	748	833
Jogging (5 1/2 mph)	487	552	650	748	833
Judo/karate	232	263	310	357	388
Mountain climbing	450	510	600	690	750
Pool/billiards	97	110	130	150	163
Racquetball/paddleball	450	510	600	690	750
Rope jumping (continuous)	525	595	700	805	875
Rowing, crew	615	697	820	943	1025
Running (10 mph)	625	765	900	1035	1125
Sailing (pleasure)	135	153	180	207	225
Skating, ice	262	297	350	403	438
Skating, roller/inline	262	297	350	403	438
Skiing, cross-country	525	595	700	805	875
Skiing, downhill	450	510	600	690	750
Soccer	405	459	540	621	775
Softball (fast-pitch)	210	238	280	322	350
Softball (slow-pitch)	217	246	290	334	363
Surfing	416	467	550	633	684
Swimming (fast laps)	420	530	630	768	846
Swimming (slow laps)	240	272	320	368	400
Table tennis	180	204	240	276	300
Tennis	315	357	420	483	525
Volleyball	262	297	350	403	483
Walking	204	258	318	372	426
Waterskiing	306	390	468	564	636
Weight training	352	399	470	541	558

Source: Corbin and Lindsey.

*Locate your weight to determine the calories expended per hour in each of the activities shown in the table based on recreational involvement. More vigorous activity, as occurs in competitive athletics, may result in greater caloric expenditures.

in controlling body fatness because all physical activities expend calories. Among the most effective activities are those in the aerobic activity section of the pyramid because they can be done for relatively long periods of time. Lifestyle activities are also effective, if performed regularly for extended periods of time. Table 4 shows the caloric expenditures for 1 hour of involvement in various physical activities. Heavier people expend more calories than lighter people because more work is required to move larger bodies.

Popular books have claimed that vigorous activities are not effective in helping with body fat loss because they say vigorous activities burn less fat than less intense activities. Although this is true in theory, it has little practical meaning for most people. It is the total calories expended in your activity that counts. If you run for the same period of time that you walk, you will expend more calories in running.

Even though vigorous activity can be effective, it will not work if you do not do it regularly. For this reason, more vigorous activity may not be as effective as some less vigorous activities for certain people. For example, running at 10 miles per hour (a 6-minute mile) will cause a 150-pound person to expend 900 calories in 1 hour. Jogging about half as fast, or at 5 ½ miles per hour (approximately an 11-minute mile), will result in an expenditure of about 650 calories in the same amount of time. At first glance, the more vigorous exercise seems to be a better choice. But how many people can continue to run at a 10-mile-per-hour pace for a full hour? Each mile run at 10 miles per hour results in an expenditure of 90 calories,

whereas each mile run at 5 ½ miles per hour results in an expenditure of 118 calories. Per mile, you expend more calories in slow running. It takes longer to run a mile but, by the same token, you can also persist longer. The key is to expend as many calories as possible during each regular exercise period. Doing less vigorous activity for longer periods is better for fat control than doing very vigorous activities that can be done only for short periods. Nevertheless, several studies have shown that vigorous activity can be very effective for some people.

Strength training can be effective in maintaining a desirable body composition. Performing exercises from the strength and muscular endurance level of the physical activity pyramid can be effective in maintaining desirable body fat levels. People who do strength training increase their muscle mass (lean body mass). This extra muscle mass expends extra calories at rest, resulting in a higher metabolic rate. Also, people with more muscle mass expend more calories when doing physical activity.

Regular physical activity is critical for building and maintaining bone health. Weight-bearing forms of aerobic activity and muscular activity provide a positive stress on bones, which contributes to bone health. Peak bone mass occurs during the early adult years, so it is important for college students to remain active, so they can develop good bone density. Continued involvement in physical activity will delay the declines in bone density that typically occur with aging. This is particularly important for reducing the risks for osteoporosis later in life.

Strategies for Action

Doing a variety of self-assessments can help you make informed decisions about body composition. In Labs 13A and 13B, you will take various body composition self-assessments. It is important that you take all of the measurements and consider all of the information before making final decisions about your body composition. Each of the self-assessment techniques has its strengths and weaknesses, and you should be aware of these when making personal decisions. The importance you place on one particular measure may be different from the importance another person places on that measure because you are a unique individual and should use information that is more relevant for you personally.

Self-assessment information—especially body composition information—is personal and confidential. Body composition self-assessment information is personal and should be confidential. When performing the self-assessments, be aware of the following:

1. If doing a self-assessment around other people makes you self-conscious, do the measurement in private. If the measurement requires the assistance of another person, choose a person you trust and feel comfortable with.
2. Estimates of body composition from even the best techniques may be off by as much as 2 to 3 percent. The values should be interpreted only as estimates.
3. The formulas used to determine body fatness from skinfolds and other procedures are based on typical body types. Measurement will be larger for the very lean and people with higher than normal levels of fat.
4. Some measurements, such as the thigh skinfold, are hard to make on some people. This is one reason two different skinfold procedures are presented.
5. Self-assessments require skill. With practice, you can become skillful in making measurements. Your first few attempts will, no doubt, lack accuracy.

6. Use the same measuring device each time you measure (scale, calipers, measuring tape, etc.). This will assure that any measurement error is constant and will allow you to track your progress over time.

7. Once you have tried all of the self-assessments in Lab 13A, choose the ones you want to continue to do and use the same measurement techniques each time you do the measurements. Consider having your body composition assessed with some of the other techniques described in the concept.

Estimating your BMR can help you determine the number of calories you expend each day. In Lab 13C, you can estimate your BMR. This will give you an idea of how much energy you expend when you are resting. You can use this information together with the information about the energy you expend to help you balance the calories you consume with the calories you expend each day.

Logging your daily activities can help you determine the number of calories you expend each day. In Lab 13C, you will also log the activities you perform in a day. You can then determine your energy expenditure in these activities. You can combine this information with the information about your basal metabolism to determine your total daily energy expenditure.

Online Learning Center

www.mhhe.com/corbin7e
The Online Learning Center contains a variety of Web-based resources that will help you get the most out of this book and your course. In addition to the On the Web pages, there are video activities, interactive quizzes, application assignments, and a variety of other useful study aids. Log on to the URL above to access these resources.

Web Resources

American Anorexia/Bulimia Association
  www.aabainc.org
Web 12 ▮ Centers for Disease Control and Prevention BMI
   Information **http://www.cdc.gov/nccdphp/dnpa/bmi/adult_BMI/about_adult_BMI.htm**
Centers for Disease Control and Prevention Growth Chart
   Information **http://www.cdc.gov/growthcharts/**
Fat Control Inc., makers of calipers
   wellfarm@nfdc.net
FDA Consumer **www.fda.gov/fdac**
National Center for Health Statistics **www.cdc.gov/nchs**
National Heart Lung and Blood Institute (BMI Calculator)
  http://www.nhlbisupport.com/bmi/
North American Association for the Study of Obesity
   (NAASO) **www.naaso.org**
Partnership for Healthy Weight Management
  http://www.consumer.gov/weightloss/bmi.htm
Shape Up America **www.shapeup.org**
Surgeon General's Call to Reduce Overweight and Obesity
  http://www.surgeongeneral.gov/topics/obesity/

Technology Update
Obesity Gene Mapping

The problems associated with obesity have caused it to be one of the most active areas of health-related research. Governmental agencies and many health foundations have provided millions in funding to scientists who conduct work on obesity. One major area of funding is the isolation and mapping of the various genes and chromosomes that appear to play a role in obesity. This project has involved collaboration among researchers from many labs across the world. The project is far from complete but, to date, more than 430 genes, markers, and chromosomal regions have been linked with human obesity phenotypes. Technological advances in genetics research and Web-based communication have facilitated this type of collaboration. The electronic version of the genetic map with links to useful sites can be found at **http://obesitygene.pbrc.edu**.

Suggested Readings

Additional reference materials for Concept 13 are available at Web13.

Web 13 ▮

American College of Sports Medicine. 2001. Appropriate intervention strategies for weight loss and prevention of weight regain for adults. *Medicine and Science in Sports and Exercise* 33(12):2145–2156.

Bray, G. A. 2004. Obesity and the metabolic syndrome: Implications for dietetics practitioners. *Journal of the American Dietetics Association* 104(1).

Cancello, R., et al. 2004. Adiposity signals, genetic and body weight regulation in humans. *Diabetes and Metabolism* 30:215–227.

Christou, D. D., et al. 2005. Fatness is a better predictor of cardiovascular disease risk factor profile than aerobic fitness in healthy men. *Circulation* 111(15):1904–1914.

Cole, T. J., et al. 2000. Establishing a standard definition for child overweight and obesity worldwide: International survey. *British Medical Journal* 320:1240–1250.

Critser, G. 2003. *Fatland: How We Became the Fattest People in the World.* Boston: Houghton Mifflin.

Dong, L., et al. 2004. Activities contributing to total energy expenditure in the United States: Results from the NHAPS Study. *International Journal of Behavioral Nutrition and Physical Activity.* (www.ijbnpa.org/1/1/4)

Esco, M. R., M.S. Olson and H. N. Williford. 2005. Muscle dysmorphia: An emerging body image concern in men 27(6):76–79

Flegal, K. M., et al. 2006. Excess deaths associated with underweight, overweight, and obesity. *Journal of the American Medical Association* 293(15):1861–1867.

Finkelson, E. A., et al. 2004. State-level estimates of annual medical expenditures attributable to obesity. *Obesity Research* 12(1):18–24.

Franko, D. L., et al. 2005. Food, mood, and attitude: Reducing risk for eating disorders in college women. *Preventive Medicine* 24(6):

Hills, A. P., et al. 2006. Validation of the intensity of walking for pleasure in obese adults. *Preventive Medicine* 42(1):47–50.

Hellmich, N. 2006. Athlete's hunger to win fuels eating disorders. *USA Today* February 6:1A, 6A.

Institute of Medicine. 2004. *Preventing Childhood Obesity: Health in the Balance.* Washington, DC: Institute of Medicine.

Janssen, I., et al. 2004. Fitness alters the association of BMI and waist circumference with total and abdominal fat. *Obesity Research* 12(3):525–537.

Kuk, J. L., et al. 2006. Visceral fat is an independent predictor of all-cause mortality in men. *Obesity Research* 14:336–341

Levine, J. A., et al. Interindividual variation in posture allocation: Possible role in human obesity. *Science* 307:584–586.

Lohman, T. G. 2004. Seeing ourselves through the obesity epidemic. *President's Council on Physical Fitness and Sports Research Digest* 5(3):1–8.

Mayo, M. J. 2003. Exercise induced weight loss preferentially reduces abdominal fat. *Medicine and Science in Sports and Exercise* 35(2):207–213.

Mokdad, A. H., et al. 2004. Actual causes of death in the United States. *Journal of the American Medical Association* 29(10):1238–1246.

Nassis, et al. 2005. Aerobic exercise training improves insulin sensitivity without changes in body weight, body fat, adiponectin, and inflammatory markers in overweight and obese girls. *Metabolism* 54(11): 1472–1479.

Ogden, C. L., et al. 2004. Mean body weight, height, and BMI in the United States—1960–2002. *Advance Data from Vital Health Statistics* 347:1–20. (**www.cdc.gov/nchs**)

Ogden, C. L., et al. 2006 Prevalence of overweight and obesity in the United States, 1999–2004. *Journal of the American Medical Association* 293(13):1549–1555.

Pavkov, M. E., et al. 2006. Effect of youth-onset type 2 diabetes mellitus on incidence of end-stage renal disease and mortality in young and middle-aged Pima Indians. *Journal of the American Medical Association* 296(4):421–426.

Perusse, L., et al. The human obesity gene map: The 2004 update. *Obesity Research* 13(3):381–490.

Ribisl, P. M. 2004. Toxic "waist" dump: Our abdominal visceral fat. *ACSM's Health and Fitness Journal* 8(4):22–25.

van Dam, R. M., et al. 2006. The relationship between overweight in adolescence and premature death in women. *Annals of Internal Medicine* 145(2):91–97.

World Health Organization. 2004. *Global Strategy on Diet, Physical Act ivity and Health.* Geneva, Switzerland: WHO.

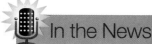

In the News

Mobile Workstations to Increase Energy Expenditure

The benefits of physical activity for weight control are well established, but many people still find it difficult to get the needed amount of activity for good health and weight maintenance. Researchers at the Mayo Clinic (led by Dr. Jim Levine) have been working on ways to reengineer activity into the typical activities of daily living. To test some of their ideas, Dr. Levine developed a mobile workstation that allows him to walk on a treadmill at very slow speeds (about ½ to 1 mph) while working on a computer and answering his phone. The adaptation allows him to expend far more calories per day than if he were sitting at his desk. The visibility from this project has helped increase awareness about the importance of small amounts of activity in the day. To expand the concept, his group established a partnership with local schools to test potential value of a similar active form of schooling for youth. Read more about Dr. Levine's research and learn more about his workstation at **http://cancercenter.mayo.edu/research/levine_lab/.**

Lab Resource Materials: Evaluating Body Fat

General Information about Skinfold Measurements

It is important to use a consistent procedure for "drawing up" or "pinching up" a skinfold and making the measurement with the calipers. The following procedures should be used for each skinfold site.

1. Lay the calipers down on a nearby table. Use the thumbs and index fingers of both hands to draw up a skinfold, or layer of skin and fat. The fingers and thumbs of the two hands should be about 1 inch apart, or 1/2 inch on each side of the location where the measurement is to be made.
2. The skinfolds are normally drawn up in a vertical line rather than a horizontal line. However, if the skin naturally aligns itself less than vertical, the measurement should be done on the natural line of the skinfold, rather than on the vertical.
3. Do not pinch the skinfold too hard. Draw it up so that your thumbs and fingers are not compressing the skinfold.
4. Once the skinfold is drawn up, let go with your right hand and pick up the calipers. Open the jaws of the calipers and place them over the location of the skinfold to be measured and 1/2 inch from your left index finger and thumb. Allow the tips, or jaw faces, of the calipers to close on the skinfold at a level about where the skin would be normally.
5. Let the reading on the calipers settle for 2 or 3 seconds; then note the thickness of the skinfold in millimeters.
6. Three measurements should be taken at each location. Use the middle of the three values to determine your measurement. For example, if you had values of 10, 11, and 9, your measurement for that location would be 10. If the three measures vary by more than 3 millimeters from the lowest to the highest, you may want to take additional measurements.

Skinfold Measurement Methods

You will be exposed to two methods of using skinfolds. The first method (FITNESSGRAM) uses the same sites for men and women. It was originally developed for use with school children but has since been modified for adults. The second method (Jackson-Pollock) is the most widely used method. It uses different sites for men and women and considers your age in estimating your body fat percentage. You are encouraged to try both methods.

Calculating Fatness from Skinfolds (FITNESSGRAM Method)

1. Sum the three skinfolds (triceps, abdominal, and calf) for men and women. Use horizontal abdominal measure.
2. Use the skinfold sum and your age to determine your percent fat using Chart 3. Locate your sum of skinfold in the left column at the top of the chart. Your estimated body fat percentage is located where the values intersect.
3. Use the Standards for Body Fatness (Chart 4) to determine your fatness rating.

FITNESSGRAM Locations (Men and Women)

Triceps

Make a mark on the back of the right arm, one-half the distance between the tip of the shoulder and the tip of the elbow. Make the measurement at this location.

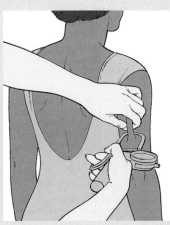

Abdominal

Make a mark on the skin approximately 1 inch to the right of the navel. Make a horizontal measurement.

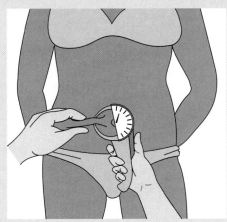

FITNESSGRAM Locations *(continued)*

Calf skinfold

Make a mark on the inside of the calf of the right leg at the level of the largest calf size (girth). Place the foot on a chair or other elevation so that the knee is kept at approximately 90 degrees. Make a vertical measurement at the mark.

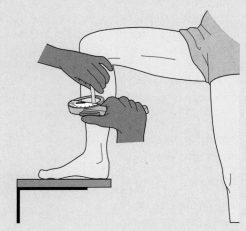

Self-Measured Triceps Skinfold

This measurement is made on the left arm so that the calipers can easily be read. Hold the arm straight at shoulder height. Make a fist with the thumb faced upward. Place the fist against a wall. With the right hand, place the calipers over the skinfold as it "hangs freely" on the back of the tricep (halfway from the tip of the shoulder to the elbow).

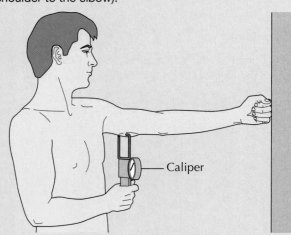

Caliper

Chart 1 ▶ Percent Fat Estimates for Sum of Triceps, Abdominal, and Calf Skinfolds

Men		Women	
Sum of Skinfolds	Percent Fat	Sum of Skinfolds	Percent Fat
8–10	3.2	23–25	16.8
11–13	4.1	26–28	17.7
14–46	5.0	29–31	18.5
17–19	6.0	32–34	19.4
20–22	6.0	35–37	20.2
23–25	7.8	38–40	21.0
26–28	8.7	41–43	21.9
29–31	9.7	44–46	22.7
32–34	10.6	47–49	23.5
35–37	11.5	50–52	24.4
38–40	12.5	53–55	25.2
41–43	13.4	56–58	26.1
44–46	14.3	59–61	26.9
47–49	15.2	62–64	27.7
50–52	16.2	65–67	28.6
53–55	17.1	68–70	29.4
56–58	18.0	71–73	30.2
59–61	18.9	74–76	31.1
62–64	19.9	77–79	31.9
65–67	20.8	80–82	32.7
68–70	21.7	83–85	33.6
71–73	22.6	86–88	34.4
74–76	23.6	89–91	35.5
77–79	24.5	92–94	36.1
80–82	25.4	95–97	36.9
83–85	26.4	98–100	37.8
86–88	27.3	101–103	38.6
89–91	28.2	104–106	39.4
92–94	29.1	107–109	40.3
95–97	30.1	110–112	41.1
98–100	31.0	113–115	42.0
101–103	31.9	116–118	42.8
104–106	32.8	119–121	43.6
107–109	33.8	122–124	44.5
110–112	34.7	125–127	45.3
113–115	35.6	128–130	46.1
116–118	36.6	131–133	47.0
119–121	37.5	134–136	47.8
122–124	38.4	137–139	48.7
125–127	39.3	140–142	49.5

Chart 2 ▶ Standards for Body Fatness (Percent Body Fat)

	Too Low	Borderline	Good Fitness (Healthy)	Marginal	Overfat
	Below Essential Fat Levels	Unhealthy for Many People	Optimal for Good Health	Associated with Some Health Problems	Unhealthy
Males	No less than 5%	6–9%	10–20%	21–25%	>25%
Females	No less than 10%	11–16%	17–28%	29–35%	>35%

Calculating Fatness from Skinfolds (Jackson-Pollock Method)

1. Sum three skinfolds (tricep, iliac crest, and thigh for women; chest, abdominal [vertical], and thigh for men).
2. Use the skinfold sum and your age to determine your percent fat using Chart 1 for men and Chart 2 for women. Locate your sum of skinfold in the left column and your age at the top of the chart. Your estimated body fat percentage is located where the values intersect.
3. Use the Standards for Body Fatness (Chart 2) to determine your fatness rating.

Jackson-Pollock Locations (Women)

Triceps

Same as FITNESSGRAM (see page 292).

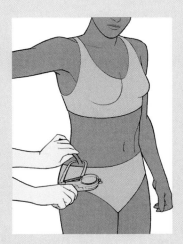

Iliac crest

Make a mark at the top front of the iliac crest. This skinfold is taken diagonally because of the natural line of the skin.

Thigh

Make a mark on the front of the thigh midway between the hip and the knee. Make the measurement vertically at this location.

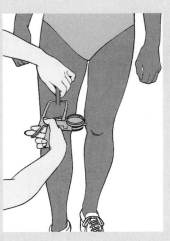

Jackson-Pollock Locations (Men)

Chest

Make a mark above and to the right of the right nipple (one-half the distance from the midline of the side and the nipple). The measurement at this location is often done on the diagonal because of the natural line of the skin.

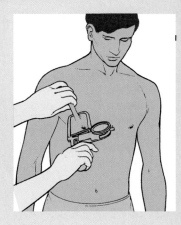

Abdominal

Make a mark on the skin approximately 1 inch to the right of the navel. Make a vertical measure for the Jackson-Pollock Method and horizontally for the Fitnessgram method.

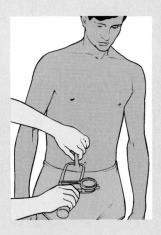

Thigh

Same as for women.

Chart 3 ▶ Percent Fat Estimates for Women (Sum of Triceps, Iliac Crest, and Thigh Skinfolds)

Sum of Skinfolds (mm)	Age to the Last Year								
	22 and Under	23 to 27	28 to 32	33 to 37	38 to 42	43 to 47	48 to 52	53 to 57	Over 57
23–25	9.7	9.9	10.2	10.4	10.7	10.9	11.2	11.4	11.7
26–28	11.0	11.2	11.5	11.7	12.0	12.3	12.5	12.7	13.0
29–31	12.3	12.5	12.8	13.0	13.3	13.5	13.8	14.0	14.3
32–34	13.6	13.8	14.0	14.3	14.5	14.8	15.0	15.3	15.5
35–37	14.8	15.0	15.3	15.5	15.8	16.0	16.3	16.5	16.8
38–40	16.0	16.3	16.5	16.7	17.0	17.2	17.5	17.7	18.0
41–43	17.2	17.4	17.7	17.9	18.2	18.4	18.7	18.9	19.2
44–46	18.3	18.6	18.8	19.1	19.3	19.6	19.8	20.1	20.3
47–49	19.5	19.7	20.0	20.2	20.5	20.7	21.0	21.2	21.5
50–52	20.6	20.8	21.1	21.3	21.6	21.8	22.1	22.3	22.6
53–55	21.7	21.9	22.1	22.4	22.6	22.9	23.1	23.4	23.6
56–58	22.7	23.0	23.2	23.4	23.7	23.9	24.2	24.4	24.7
59–61	23.7	24.0	24.2	24.5	24.7	25.0	25.2	25.5	25.7
62–64	24.7	25.0	25.2	25.5	25.7	26.0	26.2	26.4	26.7
65–67	25.7	25.9	26.2	26.4	26.7	26.9	27.2	27.4	27.7
68–70	26.6	26.9	27.1	27.4	27.6	27.9	28.1	28.4	28.6
71–73	27.5	27.8	28.0	28.3	28.5	28.8	28.0	29.3	29.5
74–76	28.4	28.7	28.9	29.2	29.4	29.7	29.9	30.2	30.4
77–79	29.3	29.5	29.8	30.0	30.3	30.5	30.8	31.0	31.3
80–82	30.1	30.4	30.6	30.9	31.1	31.4	31.6	31.9	32.1
83–85	30.9	31.2	31.4	31.7	31.9	32.2	32.4	32.7	32.9
86–88	31.7	32.0	32.2	32.5	32.7	32.9	33.2	33.4	33.7
89–91	32.5	32.7	33.0	33.2	33.5	33.7	33.9	34.2	34.4
92–94	33.2	33.4	33.7	33.9	34.2	34.4	34.7	34.9	35.2
95–97	33.9	34.1	34.4	34.6	34.9	35.1	35.4	35.6	35.9
98–100	34.6	34.8	35.21	35.3	35.5	35.8	36.0	36.3	36.5
101–103	35.3	35.4	35.7	35.9	36.2	36.4	36.7	36.9	37.2
104–106	35.8	36.1	36.3	36.6	36.8	37.1	37.3	37.5	37.8
107–109	36.4	36.7	36.9	37.1	37.4	37.6	37.9	38.1	38.4
110–112	37.0	37.2	37.5	37.7	38.0	38.2	38.5	38.7	38.9
113–115	37.5	37.8	38.0	38.2	38.5	38.7	39.0	39.2	39.5
116–118	38.0	38.3	38.5	38.8	39.0	39.3	39.5	39.7	40.0
119–121	38.5	38.7	39.0	39.2	39.5	39.7	40.0	40.2	40.5
122–124	39.0	39.2	39.4	39.7	39.9	40.2	40.4	40.7	40.9
125–127	39.4	39.6	39.9	40.1	40.4	40.6	40.9	41.1	41.4
128–130	39.8	40.0	40.3	40.5	40.8	41.0	41.3	41.5	41.8

Source: Baumgartner and Jackson.

Note: Percent fat calculated by the formula by Siri. Percent fat = $[(4.95/BD) - 4.5] \times 100$, where BD = body density.

Chart 4 ▶ Percent Fat Estimates for Men (Sum of Thigh, Chest, and Abdominal Skinfolds)

Sum of Skinfolds (mm)	Age to the Last Year								
	22 and Under	23 to 27	28 to 32	33 to 37	38 to 42	43 to 47	48 to 52	53 to 57	Over 57
8–10	1.3	1.8	2.3	2.9	3.4	3.9	4.5	5.0	5.5
11–13	2.2	2.8	3.3	3.9	4.4	4.9	5.5	6.0	6.5
14–16	3.2	3.8	4.3	4.8	5.4	5.9	6.4	7.0	7.5
17–19	4.2	4.7	5.3	5.8	6.3	6.9	7.4	8.0	8.5
20–22	5.1	5.7	6.2	6.8	7.3	7.9	8.4	8.9	9.5
23–25	6.1	6.6	7.2	7.7	8.3	8.8	9.4	9.9	10.5
26–28	7.0	7.6	8.1	8.7	9.2	9.8	10.3	10.9	11.4
29–31	8.0	8.5	9.1	9.6	10.2	10.7	11.3	11.8	12.4
32–34	8.9	9.4	10.0	10.5	11.1	11.6	12.2	12.8	13.3
35–37	9.8	10.4	10.9	11.5	12.0	12.6	13.1	13.7	14.3
38–40	10.7	11.3	11.8	12.4	12.9	13.5	14.1	14.6	15.2
41–43	11.6	12.2	12.7	13.3	13.8	14.4	15.0	15.5	16.1
44–46	12.5	13.1	13.6	14.2	14.7	15.3	15.9	16.4	17.0
47–49	13.4	13.9	14.5	15.1	15.6	16.2	16.8	17.3	17.9
50–52	14.3	14.8	15.4	15.9	16.5	17.1	17.6	18.1	18.8
53–55	15.1	15.7	16.2	16.8	17.4	17.9	18.5	18.2	19.7
56–58	16.0	16.5	17.1	17.7	18.2	18.8	19.4	20.0	20.5
59–61	16.9	17.4	17.9	18.5	19.1	19.7	20.2	20.8	21.4
62–64	17.6	18.2	18.8	19.4	19.9	20.5	21.1	21.7	22.2
65–67	18.5	19.0	19.6	20.2	20.8	21.3	21.9	22.5	23.1
68–70	19.3	19.9	20.4	21.0	21.6	22.2	22.7	23.3	23.9
71–73	20.1	20.7	21.2	21.8	22.4	23.0	23.6	24.1	24.7
74–76	20.9	21.5	22.0	22.6	23.2	23.8	24.4	25.0	25.5
77–79	21.7	22.2	22.8	23.4	24.0	24.6	25.2	25.8	26.3
80–82	22.4	23.0	23.6	24.2	24.8	25.4	25.9	26.5	27.1
83–85	23.2	23.8	24.4	25.0	25.5	26.1	26.7	27.3	27.9
86–88	24.0	24.5	25.1	25.5	26.3	26.9	27.5	28.1	28.7
89–91	24.7	25.3	25.9	25.7	27.1	27.6	28.2	28.8	29.4
92–94	25.4	26.0	26.6	27.2	27.8	28.4	29.0	29.6	30.2
95–97	26.1	26.7	27.3	27.9	28.5	29.1	29.7	30.3	30.9
98–100	26.9	27.4	28.0	28.6	29.2	29.8	30.4	31.0	31.6
101–103	27.5	28.1	28.7	29.3	29.9	30.5	31.1	31.7	32.3
104–106	28.2	28.8	29.4	30.0	30.6	31.2	31.8	32.4	33.0
107–109	28.9	29.5	30.1	30.7	31.3	31.9	32.5	33.1	33.7
110–112	29.6	30.2	30.8	31.4	32.0	32.6	33.2	33.8	34.4
113–115	30.2	30.8	31.4	32.0	32.6	33.2	33.8	34.5	35.1
116–118	30.9	31.5	32.1	32.7	33.3	33.9	34.5	35.1	35.7
119–121	31.5	32.1	32.7	33.3	33.9	34.5	35.1	35.7	36.4
122–124	32.1	32.7	33.3	33.9	34.5	35.1	35.8	36.4	37.0
125–127	32.7	33.3	33.9	34.5	35.1	35.8	36.4	37.0	37.6

Source: Baumgartner and Jackson.

Note: Percent fat calculated by the formula by Siri. Percent fat = [(4.95/BD) − 4.5] × 100, where BD = body density.

Calculating Fatness from Self-Measured Skinfolds

1. Use either the Jackson-Pollock or Fitnessgram method but make the measures on yourself rather than have a partner do the measures. When doing the triceps measure, use the self-measurement technique for men and women. (See page 292)
2. Calculate fatness using the methods described previously.

Height-Weight Measurements

1. *Height*—Measure your height in inches or centimeters. Take the measurement without shoes, but add 2.5 centimeters or 1 inch to measurements, as the charts include heel height.
2. *Weight*—Measure your weight in pounds or kilograms without clothes. Add 3 pounds or 1.4 kilograms because the charts include the weight of clothes. If weight must be taken with clothes on, wear indoor clothing that weighs 3 pounds, or 1.4 kilograms.
3. Determine your frame size using the elbow breadth. The measurement is most accurate when done with a broad-based sliding caliper. However, it can be done using skinfold calipers or can be estimated with a metric ruler. The right arm is measured when it is elevated with the elbow bent at 90 degrees and the upper arm horizontal. The back of the hand should face the person making the measurement. Using the calipers, measure the distance between the epicondyles of the humerus (inside and outside bony points of the elbow). Measure to the nearest millimeter (1/10 centimeter). If a caliper is not available, place the thumb and the index finger of the left hand on the epicondyles of the humerus and measure the distance between the fingers with a metric ruler. Use your height and elbow breadth in centimeters to determine your frame size (Chart 5); you need not repeat this procedure each time you use a height and weight chart.

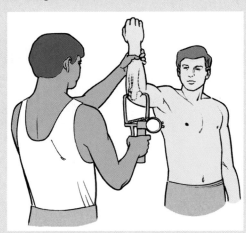

4. Use Chart 6 to determine your healthy weight range. The new healthy weight range charts do not account for frame size. However, you may want to consider frame size when determining a personal weight within the healthy weight range. People with a larger frame size typically can carry more weight within the range than can those with a smaller frame size.

Chart 5 ► Frame Size Determined from Elbow Breadth (mm)

Height	Elbow Breadth (mm)		
	Small Frame	Medium Frame	Large Frame
Males			
5′2″ or less	<64	64–72	>72
5′3″–5′6 ½″	<67	67–74	>74
5′7″–5′10 ½″	<69	69–76	>76
5′11″–6′2 ½″	<71	71–78	>78
6′3″ or less	<74	74–81	>81
Females			
4′10 ½″ or less	<56	56–64	>64
4′11″–5′2 ½″	<58	58–65	>65
5′3″–5′6 ½″	<59	59–66	>66
5′7″–5′10 ½″	<61	61–68	>69
5′11″ or less	<62	62–69	>69

Source: Metropolitan Life Insurance Company.

Height is given including 1-inch heels.

Chart 6 ► Healthy Weight Ranges for Adult Women and Men

Women			Men		
Height			Height		
Feet	Inches	Pounds	Feet	Inches	Pounds
4	10	91–119	5	9	129–169
4	11	94–124	5	10	132–174
5	0	97–128	5	11	136–179
5	1	101–132	6	0	140–184
5	2	104–137	6	1	144–189
5	3	107–141	6	2	148–195
5	4	111–146	6	3	152–200
5	5	114–150	6	4	156–205
5	6	118–155	6	5	160–211
5	7	121–160	6	6	164–216
5	8	125–164			

Source: U.S. Department of Agriculture and Department of Health and Human Services.

Chart 7 ▶ Body Mass Index (BMI)

Height	100	105	110	115	120	125	130	135	140	145	150	155	160	165	170	175	180	185	190	195	200	205	210	215	220	225	230	235	240	245	250
5'0"	20	21	21	22	23	24	25	26	27	28	29	30	31	32	33	34	35	36	37	38	39	40	41	42	43	44	45	46	47	48	49
5'1"	19	20	21	22	23	24	25	26	26	27	28	29	30	31	32	33	34	35	36	37	38	39	40	41	42	43	43	44	45	46	47
5'2"	18	19	20	21	22	23	24	25	26	27	27	28	29	30	31	32	33	34	35	36	37	37	38	39	40	41	42	43	44	45	46
5'3"	18	19	19	20	21	22	23	24	25	26	27	27	28	29	30	31	32	33	34	35	35	36	37	38	39	40	41	42	43	43	44
5'4"	17	18	19	20	21	21	22	23	24	25	26	27	27	28	29	30	31	32	33	33	34	35	36	37	38	39	39	40	41	42	43
5'5"	17	17	18	19	20	21	22	22	23	24	25	26	27	27	28	29	30	31	32	32	33	34	35	36	37	37	38	39	40	41	42
5'6"	16	17	18	19	19	20	21	22	23	23	24	25	26	27	27	28	29	30	31	31	32	33	34	35	36	36	37	38	39	40	40
5'7"	16	16	17	18	19	20	20	21	22	23	23	24	25	26	27	27	28	29	30	31	31	32	33	34	34	35	36	37	38	38	39
5'8"	15	16	17	17	18	19	20	21	21	22	23	24	24	25	26	27	27	28	29	30	30	31	32	33	33	34	35	36	36	37	38
5'9"	15	16	16	17	18	18	19	20	21	21	22	23	24	24	25	26	27	27	28	29	30	30	31	32	32	33	34	35	35	36	37
5'10"	14	15	16	17	17	18	19	19	20	21	22	22	23	24	24	25	26	27	27	28	29	29	30	31	32	32	33	34	34	35	36
5'11"	14	15	15	16	17	17	18	19	20	20	21	22	22	23	24	24	25	26	26	27	28	29	29	30	31	31	32	33	33	34	35
6'0"	14	14	15	16	16	17	18	18	19	20	20	21	22	22	23	24	24	25	26	26	27	28	28	29	30	31	31	32	33	33	34
6'1"	13	14	15	15	16	16	17	18	18	19	20	20	21	22	22	23	24	24	25	26	26	27	28	28	29	30	30	31	32	32	33
6'2"	13	13	14	15	15	16	17	17	18	19	19	20	21	21	22	22	23	24	24	25	26	26	27	28	28	29	30	30	31	31	32
6'3"	12	13	14	14	15	16	16	17	17	18	19	19	20	21	21	22	22	23	24	24	25	26	26	27	27	28	29	29	30	31	31
6'4"	12	13	13	14	15	15	16	16	17	18	18	19	19	20	21	21	22	23	23	24	24	25	26	26	27	27	28	29	29	30	30

Weight

- ■ Low
- ■ Normal (good fitness zone)
- □ Overweight
- □ Obese

Body Mass Index (BMI)

Use the steps listed below or use Chart 7 to calculate your BMI.

1. Divide your weight in pounds by 2.2 to determine your weight in kilograms.
2. Multiply your height in inches by 0.0254 to determine your height in meters.
3. Square your height in meters (multiply your height in meters by your height in meters).
4. Divide your weight in kilograms from step 1 by your height in meters squared from step 3.
5. If you use these steps to determine your BMI, use the Rating Scale for Body Mass Index (Chart 8) to obtain a rating for your BMI.

Chart 8 ▶ Rating Scale for Body Mass Index (BMI)

Classification	BMI
Obese (high risk)	Over 30
Overweight	25–30
Normal (good fitness zone)	17–24.9
Low	Less than 17

Note: An excessively low BMI is not desirable. Low BMI values can be indicative of eating disorders and other health problems. The government rating for marginal is overweight.

Formula

$$BMI = \frac{\text{weight in kilograms}}{(\text{height in meters})^2}$$

Determining the Waist-to-Hip Circumference Ratio

The waist-to-hip circumference ratio is recommended as the best available index for determining risk for disease associated with fat and weight distribution. Disease and death risk are associated with abdominal and upper body fatness. When a person has high fatness and a high waist-to-hip ratio, additional risks exist. The following steps should be taken in making measurements and calculating the waist-to-hip ratio.

1. Both measurements should be done with a nonelastic tape. Make the measurements while standing with the feet together and the arms at the sides, elevated only high enough to allow the measurements. Be sure the tape is horizontal and around the entire circumference. Record scores to the nearest millimeter or 1/16th of an inch. Use the same units of measure for both circumferences (millimeters or 1/16th of an inch). The tape should be pulled snugly but not to the point of causing an indentation in the skin.

2. *Waist measurement*—Measure at the natural waist (smallest waist circumference). If no natural waist exists, the measurement should be made at the level of the umbilicus. Measure at the end of a normal inspiration.

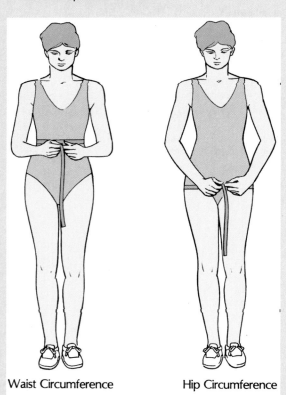

Waist Circumference   Hip Circumference

Note: Using a partner or mirror will aid you in keeping the tape horizontal.

3. *Hip measurement*—Measure at the maximum circumference of the buttocks. It is recommended that you wear thin-layered clothing (such as a swimming suit or underwear) that will not add significantly to the measurement.

4. Divide the hip measurement into the waist measurement or use the waist-to-hip nomogram (Chart 9) to determine your waist-to-hip ratio.

5. Use the Waist-to-Hip Ratio Rating Scale (Chart 10) to determine your rating for the waist-to-hip ratio.

Chart 9 ▶ Waist-to-Hip Ratio Nomogram

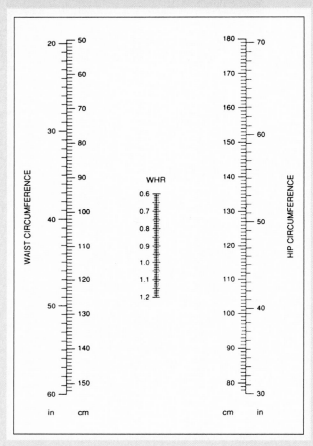

Chart 10 ▶ Waist-to-Hip Ratio Rating Scale

Classification	Men	Women
High risk	>1.0	>0.85
Moderately high risk	0.90–1.0	0.80–0.85
Lower risk	<0.90	<0.80

Lab 13A Evaluating Body Composition: Skinfold Measures

Name	**Section** **Date**

Purpose: To estimate body fatness using two skinfold procedures; to compare measures made by an expert, by a partner, and by self-measurements; to learn the strengths and weaknesses of each technique; and to use the results to establish personal standards for evaluating body composition

General Procedures: Follow the specific procedures for the two self-assessment techniques. If possible, have one set of measurements made by an expert (instructor) for each of the two techniques. Next, work with a partner you trust. Have the partner make measurements at each site for both techniques. Finally, make self-measurements for each of the sites. If you are just learning a measurement technique, it is important to practice the skills of making the measurement. If you do measurements over time, use the same instrument (if possible) each time you measure. If your measurements vary widely, take more than one set until you get more consistent results.

If you have had an underwater weighing, a bioelectric impedance measurement, a near-infrared interactance measure, or some other body fatness measurement done recently, record your results below.

Measurement Technique	% Body Fat	Rating
1.		
2.		

Skinfold Measurements (Jackson-Pollock Method)

Procedures for Jackson-Pollock Method

1. Read the directions for the Jackson-Pollock Method measurements in *Lab Resource Materials.*
2. If possible, observe a demonstration of the proper procedures for measuring skinfolds at each of the different locations before doing partner or self-measurements.
3. Make expert, partner, and self-measurements (see *Lab Resource Materials*). When doing the self-measure of the triceps, use the self-measurement technique described in *Lab Resource Materials* (women only).
4. Record each of the measurements in the Results section.
5. Calculate your body fatness from skinfolds by summing the appropriate skinfold values (chest, thigh, and abdominal for men; triceps, iliac crest, and thigh for women). Using your age and the sum of the appropriate skinfolds, determine your body fatness using Charts 1 and 2 in *Lab Resource Materials*.
6. Rate your fatness using Chart 4 in *Lab Resource Materials*.

Results for Jackson-Pollock Method

Skinfolds by an Expert (If Possible)

Male

Chest

Thigh

Abdominal

Sum

% body fat

Rating

Female

Triceps

Iliac crest

Thigh

Sum

% body fat

Rating

Skinfolds by Partner

Male

Chest

Thigh

Abdominal

Sum

% body fat

Rating

Female

Triceps

Iliac crest

Thigh

Sum

% body fat

Rating

Self-Measurements

Male

Chest

Thigh

Abdominal

Sum

% body fat

Rating

Female

Triceps

Iliac crest

Thigh

Sum

% body fat

Rating

Make a check by the statements that are true about your measurements.

- [ ] The person doing measurements has experience with these three skinfold measurements.

- [ ] Self-measurements were practiced until measurements became consistent.

- [ ] Results of several trials for each measure are consistent (do not vary more than 2–3 mm).

- [ ] You are not exceptionally low or exceptionally high in body fat.

The more checks you have, the more likely your measurements are accurate.

Skinfold Measurements (Fitnessgram Method)

Procedures for Fitnessgram Method

1. Read the directions for the Fitnessgram measurements in *Lab Resource Materials.*
2. Use the procedures as for the Fitnessgram Method using the triceps, abdominal, and calf sites described in *Lab Resource Materials.* When doing the self-measure of the triceps, use the self-measurement technique shown earlier.
3. Calculate your body fatness from skinfolds by summing the appropriate skinfold values (same for both men and women). Using the sum of the appropriate skinfolds, determine your body fatness using Chart 3 in *Lab Resource Materials.*
4. Rate your fatness using Chart 4 in *Lab Resource Materials.*

Results for Fitnessgram Method

Skinfolds by an Expert (If Possible)

Triceps

Abdominal

Calf

Sum

% body fat

Rating

Skinfolds by Partner

Triceps

Abdominal

Calf

Sum

% body fat

Rating

Self-Measurements

Triceps

Abdominal

Calf

Sum

% body fat

Rating

Make a check by the statements that are true about your measurements.

☐ The person doing measurements has experience with these three skinfold measurements.

☐ Self-measurements were practiced until measurements became consistent.

☐ Results of several trials for each measure are consistent (do not vary more than 2–3 mm).

☐ You are not exceptionally low or exceptionally high in body fat.

The more checks you have, the more likely your measurements are accurate.

Conclusions and Implications

In the space provided below, discuss your current body composition based on the two skinfold procedures and any other measures of body fatness you did. Note any discrepancies in the measurements and discuss which of the measurements you think provide the most useful information. To what extent do you think you need to alter your level of body fatness?

Lab 13B Evaluating Body Composition: Height, Weight, and Circumference Measures

Name	**Section**	**Date**

Purpose: To assess body composition using a variety of procedures, to learn the strengths and weaknesses of each technique, and to use the results to establish personal standards for evaluating body composition

General Procedures: Follow the specific procedures for the three self-assessment techniques. If possible, work with a partner you trust to help with measurements that you have difficulty making on yourself. If you are just learning a measurement technique, it is important to practice the skills of making the measurement. If you do measurements over time, use the same instrument (if possible) each time you measure. If your measurements vary widely, take more than one set until you get more consistent results. If possible, have an expert make measurements on you using these procedures.

Height and Weight Measurements

Procedures

1. Read the directions for height and weight measurements in *Lab Resource Materials.*
2. Determine your healthy weight range using Chart 6 in *Lab Resource Materials.* You may want to use your elbow breadth (Chart 5). People with a smaller frame size should typically weigh less than those with a larger frame size within the healthy weight range. You may need the assistance of a partner to make the elbow breadth measurement.
3. Record your scores in the Results section.

Results

Weight ☐   Healthy weight range ☐

Height ☐

Make a check by the statements that are true about your measurements.

☐   You are confident in the accuracy of the scale you used.

☐   You are confident that the height technique is accurate.

The more checks you have, the more likely your measurements are accurate.
If you are a very active person with a high amount of muscle, use this method with caution.

Body Mass Index

Procedures

1. Use the height and weight measures from above.
2. Determine your BMI score by using Chart 7 or the directions in *Lab Resource Materials.* Determine your rating using Chart 8.
3. Record your score and rating in the Results section.

Results

Body mass index ☐   Rating ☐

If you are a very active person with a high amount of muscle, use this method with caution.

Waist-to-Hip Ratio

Procedures

1. Measure your waist and hip circumferences using the procedures in *Lab Resource Materials*.
2. Divide your hip circumference into your waist circumference or use Chart 9 in *Lab Resource Materials* to calculate your waist-to-hip ratio.
3. Determine your rating using Chart 10 in *Lab Resource Materials*.
4. Record your scores in the Results section.

Results

Waist circumference [ ]

Hip circumference [ ]

Waist-to-hip ratio [ ]   Rating [ ]

Make a check by the statements that are true about you.

[ ] I am a male 5′9″ or less and have a waist girth of 34 inches or more.

[ ] I am a male 5′10″ to 6′4″ and have a waist girth of 36 inches or more.

[ ] I am a male 6′5″ or more and have a waist girth of 38 inches or more.

[ ] I am a female 5′2″ or less and have a waist girth of 29 inches or more.

[ ] I am a female 5′3″ to 5′10″ and have a waist girth of 31 inches or more.

[ ] I am a female 5′11″ or more and have a waist girth of 33 inches or more.

If you checked one of the boxes above, the waist-to-hip ratio is especially relevant for you.

Conclusions and Implications

In the space below, discuss your results for the height, weight, and circumference procedures. Note any discrepancies in the measurements. Indicate the strengths and weaknesses of the various methods. Which of the measures do you think provided you with the most useful information? If you also did the skinfold measures (Lab 13A), discuss your body composition based on all the information you have collected (skinfolds and height, weight, and circumference measures).

Lab 13C Determining Your Daily Energy Expenditure

Name	Section	Date

Purpose: To learn how many calories you expend in a day

Procedures

1. Estimate your basal metabolism using step 1 in the Results section. First determine the number of minutes you sleep.
2. Monitor your activity expenditure for 1 day using Chart 1 (page 307). Record the number of 5-, 15-, and 30-minute blocks of time you perform each of the different types of physical activities (e.g., if an activity lasted 20 minutes, you would use one 15-minute block and one 5-minute block). Be sure to distinguish between moderate (Mod) and vigorous (Vig) intensity in your logging. If you perform an activity that is not listed, specify the activity on the line labeled "Other" and estimate if it is moderate or vigorous. You may want to keep copies of Chart 1 for future use. One extra copy is provided.
3. Sum the total number of minutes of moderate and vigorous activity. Determine your calories expended during moderate and vigorous activity using steps 2 and 3.
4. Determine your nonactive minutes using step 4. This is all time that is not spent sleeping or being active.
5. Determine your calories expended in nonactive minutes using step 5.
6. Determine your calories expended in a day using step 6.

Results

Daily Caloric Expenditure Estimates

Step 1:

Basal calories = .0076 × [Body wt. (lbs.)] × [Minutes of sleep] = [Basal calories] (A)

Step 2:

Calories (moderate activity) = .036 × [Body wt. (lbs.)] × [Minutes of moderate activity] = [Calories in moderate activity] (B)

Step 3:

Calories (vigorous activity) = .053 × [Body wt. (lbs.)] × [Minutes of vigorous activity] = [Calories in vigorous activity] (C)

Step 4:

Minutes (nonactive) = 1,440 min − [Minutes of sleep] − [Minutes of moderate activity] − [Minutes of vigorous activity] = [Nonactive minutes]

Step 5:

Calories (rest and light activity) = .011 × [Body wt. (lbs.)] × [Nonactive minutes] = [Calories in other activities] (D)

Step 6:

Calories expended (per day) = [ ] (A) + [ ] (B) + [ ] (C) + [ ] (D) = [**Daily calories**]

Answer the following questions about your daily caloric expenditure estimate.

Yes	No	
☐	☐	Were the activities you performed similar to what you normally perform each day?
☐	☐	Do you think your daily estimated caloric expenditure is an accurate estimate?
☐	☐	Do you think you expend the correct number of calories in a typical day to maintain the body composition (body fat level) that is desirable for you?

Conclusions and Interpretations: In several paragraphs, discuss your daily caloric expenditure. Comment on your answers to the preceding questions. In addition, comment on whether you think you should modify your daily caloric expenditure for any reason.

Chart 1 ▶ Daily Activity Log

Day of Monitoring:				
Physical Activity Category	**5 Minutes**	**15 Minutes**	**30 Minutes**	**Minutes**
Lifestyle Activity	1 2 3 4 5 6	1 2 3 4 5 6	1 2 3	
Dancing (general) — Mod				
Gardening — Mod				
Home repair/maintenance — Mod				
Occupation — Mod				
Walking/hiking — Mod				
Other: — Mod				
Aerobic Activity	1 2 3 4 5 6	1 2 3 4 5 6	1 2 3	
Aerobic dance (low-impact) — Mod / Vig				
Aerobic machines (rowing, stair, ski) — Mod / Vig				
Bicycling — Mod / Vig				
Running — Mod / Vig				
Skating (roller/ice) — Mod / Vig				
Swimming (laps) — Mod / Vig				
Other: — Mod / Vig				
Sport/Recreation Activity	1 2 3 4 5 6	1 2 3 4 5 6	1 2 3	
Basketball — Mod / Vig				
Bowling/billiards — Mod				
Golf — Mod				
Martial arts (judo, karate) — Mod / Vig				
Racquetball/tennis — Mod / Vig				
Soccer/hockey — Mod / Vig				
Softball/baseball — Mod				
Volleyball — Mod / Vig				
Other: — Mod				
Flexibility Activity	1 2 3 4 5 6	1 2 3 4 5 6	1 2 3	
Stretching — Mod				
Other: — Mod				
Strengthening Activity	1 2 3 4 5 6	1 2 3 4 5 6	1 2 3	
Calisthenics (push-ups/sit-ups) — Mod				
Resistance exercise — Mod				
Other: — Mod				

Minutes of moderate activity ☐

Minutes of vigorous activity ☐

Total minutes of activity ☐

Chart 2 ▶ Daily Activity Log

Lab 13C

Determining Your Daily Energy Expenditure

Day of Monitoring:					
Physical Activity Category		**5 Minutes**	**15 Minutes**	**30 Minutes**	**Minutes**
Lifestyle Activity		1 2 3 4 5 6	1 2 3 4 5 6	1 2 3	
Dancing (general)	Mod				
Gardening	Mod				
Home repair/maintenance	Mod				
Occupation	Mod				
Walking/hiking	Mod				
Other:	Mod				
Aerobic Activity		1 2 3 4 5 6	1 2 3 4 5 6	1 2 3	
Aerobic dance (low-impact)	Mod				
	Vig				
Aerobic machines (rowing, stair, ski)	Mod				
	Vig				
Bicycling	Mod				
	Vig				
Running	Mod				
	Vig				
Skating (roller/ice)	Mod				
	Vig				
Swimming (laps)	Mod				
	Vig				
Other:	Mod				
	Vig				
Sport/Recreation Activity		1 2 3 4 5 6	1 2 3 4 5 6	1 2 3	
Basketball	Mod				
	Vig				
Bowling/billiards	Mod				
Golf	Mod				
Martial arts (judo, karate)	Mod				
	Vig				
Racquetball/tennis	Mod				
	Vig				
Soccer/hockey	Mod				
	Vig				
Softball/baseball	Mod				
Volleyball	Mod				
	Vig				
Other:	Mod				
Flexibility Activity		1 2 3 4 5 6	1 2 3 4 5 6	1 2 3	
Stretching	Mod				
Other:	Mod				
Strengthening Activity		1 2 3 4 5 6	1 2 3 4 5 6	1 2 3	
Calisthenics (push-ups/sit-ups)	Mod				
Resistance exercise	Mod				
Other:	Mod				

Minutes of moderate activity ☐

Minutes of vigorous activity ☐

Total minutes of activity ☐

Nutrition

Health Goals for the year 2010

- Promote health and reduce chronic disease associated with dietary factors and weight.

- Increase proportion of people who eat healthy snacks.

- Increase proportion of people who eat no more than 30 percent of calories as fat.

- Increase proportion of people who eat no more than 10 percent of calories as saturated fat.

- Increase proportion of people who eat at least five servings of vegetables and fruits daily.

- Increase proportion of people who eat at least six servings of grain products daily.

- Increase proportion of people who meet the dietary recommendation for calcium.

- Reduce proportion of people who consume excess sodium.

- Reduce incidence of iron deficiency and anemia (especially children and women).

- Increase proportion of worksites that offer nutrition and/or weight-management classes.

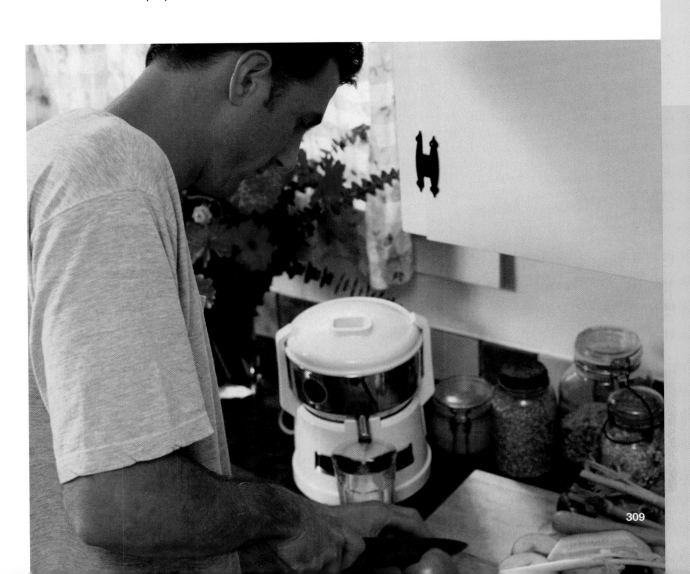

The amount and kinds of food you eat affect your health and wellness.

The importance of good nutrition for optimal health is well established. Eating patterns have been related to four of the seven leading causes of death, and poor nutrition increases the risks for numerous diseases, including heart disease, obesity, stroke, diabetes, hypertension, osteoporosis, and many cancers (e.g., colon, prostate, mouth, throat, lung, and stomach). The links to cancer are probably not fully appreciated in today's society, but the American Cancer Society estimates that 35 percent of cancer risks are related to nutritional factors. In addition to these health risks, proper nutrition can enhance the quality of life by improving appearance and enhancing the ability to carry out work and leisure-time activity without fatigue.

Most people believe that nutrition is important but still find it difficult to maintain a healthy diet. One reason is that foods are usually developed, marketed, and advertised for convenience and taste rather than for health or nutritional quality. Another reason is that many individuals have misconceptions about what constitutes a healthy diet. Some of these misconceptions are propagated by so-called experts with less than impressive credentials and those with commercial interests. Others are created by the confusing, and often contradictory, news reports about new nutrition research. In spite of the fact that nutrition is an advanced science, many questions remain unanswered. This concept reviews important national guidelines and recommendations for healthy eating. The significance of essential dietary nutrients are also described along with strategies for adopting and maintaining a healthy diet.

Guidelines for Healthy Eating

National dietary guidelines provide a sound plan for good nutrition. The U.S. Department of Agriculture (USDA) and the Department of Health and Human Services (DHHS) recently published new dietary guidelines intended to help consumers make healthier food choices. Federal law requires that these guidelines be updated every 5 years to incorporate new research findings. The latest guidelines (2005) include many of the same recommendations as past guidelines but emphasize a more personalized, behavioral approach to nutrition. A new food pyramid (*MyPyramid*) was released with the Guidelines to help consumers remember and apply the key points in the guidelines (see Figure 1). A web-based assessment tool called *MyPyramid Tracker* was also released to help consumers monitor their diet and activity behaviors (see Web01 and Technology Update section).

The revised MyPyramid model was designed to convey the key nutrition principles described in the guidelines. The colored bars on the model represent the different food groups (grains, vegetables, fruits, oils, milk, and meat/beans) and the importance of eating a variety of foods. The width of the bars in this figure is proportional to the amount of each food group that should be consumed. This principle of proportionality is conceptually similar to the presentation in the old food guide pyramid, which depicted grains on the bottom level, fruits and vegetables on the second layer, protein sources on the third layer, and fats on the top layer. The tapering of the bars from bottom to top is intended to illustrate the principle of moderation in food choices. The wider base at the bottom stands for the healthier options which should be the base of the diet, while the narrower area at the top stands for the foods (those with more added fat and sugar) that should be consumed less often. This helps people learn to balance sweet treats with other healthier food choices.

The new USDA nutrition guidelines also emphasize the importance of daily physical activity (60 minutes a day). The steps and the person climbing them on the left of MyPyramid serve as a specific reminder of the importance of physical activity in energy balance. People who are more active (higher up on the stairway) can typically get away with eating more of the high-calorie foods near the top of the pyramid because they can burn off the excess calories. As described in previous concepts, each of the components in the physical activity pyramid provides important health benefits. To illustrate this, the labels from the activity pyramid are superimposed on the steps of the MyPyramid image in Figure 1.

The revised dietary guidelines provide specific suggestions for eating healthier. A criticism of the previous food guide pyramid is that distinctions were not

On the Web

www.mhhe.com/corbinweb

Web 01 ▾ Log on to this URL before reading this concept. See On the Web list of concepts. Click on the concept number you want to view. To access supplemental information, click on the number shown at each Web icon.

KEY PRINCIPLES		MAIN MESSAGES

KEY PRINCIPLES

- **Physical Activity**
  represented by steps
- **Moderation**
  represented by narrowing
  of each food group from
  bottom to top
- **Personalization**
  represented by person
- **Proportionality**
  represented by different
  widths—the widths suggest
  how much a person should
  choose from each group
- **Variety**
  symbolized by the different
  colors, which represent the
  five food groups

MyPyramid
STEPS TO A HEALTHIER YOU

FLEXIBILITY EXERCISES
MUSCLE FITNESS EXERCISES
SPORTS & RECREATION
ACTIVE AEROBICS
LIFESTYLE

MAIN MESSAGES

- Make 1/2 your grains "whole"
- Vary your veggies
- Focus on fruits
- Know your fats
- Eat calcium rich foods
- Go lean on protein

GRAINS   VEGETABLES   FRUITS   MILK   MEAT & BEANS

Figure 1 ▶ MyPyramid presents a combination of nutrition guidelines and emphasis on daily physical activity.

Source: Adapted from the USDA 2005 MyPyramid (www.mypyramid.com) by Corbin, Welk, and LeMasurier.

made to denote differences in the quality of foods in each segment of the pyramid. There are clear differences in the quality of various foods containing carbohydrates, fats, and proteins, and it is important to make healthier selections when possible. The revised dietary guidelines describe a healthy diet as one that meets the following criteria: *1.* Emphasizes fruits, vegetables, whole grains, and fat-free or low-fat milk and milk products; *2.* Includes lean meats, poultry, fish, beans, eggs, and nuts; and *3.* Is low in saturated fats, trans fats, cholesterol, salt (sodium), and added sugars. A few specific guidelines are provided to help consumers make better choices within each food category:

- *Make half your grains whole.* Whole grains provide more nutrients and more fiber than processed grains.
- *Vary your veggies.* Variety is recommended to ensure adequate amounts of different nutrients.
- *Focus on fruits.* Fruits are valuable sources of vitamins, minerals, and phytochemicals that contribute to good health.
- *Know your fats.* The consumption of trans fat and saturated fat are discouraged, but other forms of fat are considered beneficial in moderation.
- *Get your calcium-rich foods.* The importance of calcium from dairy products is highlighted to promote bone health.
- *Go lean with protein.* Lean meats and poultry are recommended, as are alternative sources of protein (e.g., beans, nuts).

National dietary recommendations provide a target zone for healthy eating. About 45 to 50 nutrients in food are believed to be essential for the body's growth, maintenance, and repair. These are

Web 02

classified into six categories: carbohydrates (and fiber), fats, proteins, vitamins, minerals, and water. The first three provide energy, which is measured in calories. Specific dietary recommendations for each of the six nutrients are presented later in this concept.

National guidelines, specifying the nutrient requirements for good health, are developed by the Food and Nutrition Board of the National Academy of Science's Institute of Medicine. **Recommended Dietary Allowance (RDA)** historically was used to set recommendations for nutrients, but the complexity of dietary interactions prompted the board to develop a more comprehensive and functional set of dietary intake recommendations. These broader guidelines, referred to as **Dietary Reference Intake (DRI),** include RDA values when adequate scientific information is available and estimated **Adequate Intake (AI)** values when sufficient data aren't available to establish a firm RDA. The

Recommended Dietary Allowance (RDA) Dietary guideline that specifies the amount of a nutrient needed for almost all of the healthy individuals in a specific age and gender group.

Dietary Reference Intake (DRI) Appropriate amounts of nutrients in the diet (AI, RDA, and UL).

Adequate Intake (AI) Dietary guideline established experimentally to estimate nutrient needs when sufficient data are not available to establish an RDA value.

Table 1 ► Dietary Reference Intake (DRI), Recommended Dietary Allowance (RDA), and Tolerable Upper Intake Level (UL) for Major Nutrients

B-Complex Vitamins	DRI/RDA		UL	Function
	Males	Females		
Thiamin (mg/day)	1.2	1.1	ND	Co-enzyme for carbohydrates and amino acid metabolism
Riboflavin (mg/day)	1.3	1.1	ND	Co-enzyme for metabolic reactions
Niacin (mg/day)	16	14	35	Co-enzyme for metabolic reactions
Vitamin B-6 (mg/day)	1.3	1.3	100	Co-enzyme for amino acid and glycogen reactions
Folate (µg/day)	400	400	1,000	Metabolism of amino acids
Vitamin B-12 (µg/day)	2.4	2.4	ND	Co-enzyme for nucleic acid metabolism
Pantothenic acid (mg/day)	5*	5*	ND	Co-enzyme for fat metabolism
Biotin (µg/day)	30*	30*	ND	Synthesis of fat, glycogen, and amino acids
Choline (mg/day)	550*	425*	3,500	Precursor to acetylcholine
Antioxidants and Related Nutrients				
Vitamin C (mg/day)	90	75	2,000	Co-factor for reactions, antioxidant
Vitamin E (mg/day)	15	15	1,000	Undetermined, mainly antioxidant
Selenium (µg/day)	55	55	400	Defense against oxidative stress
Bone-Building Nutrients				
Calcium (mg/day)	1,000*	1,000*	2,500	Muscle contraction, nerve transmission
Phosphorus (mg/day)	700	700	3,000	Maintenance of pH, storage of energy
Magnesium (mg/day)	400–420	310–320	350	Co-factor for enzyme reactions
Vitamin D (µg/day)	5*	5*	50	Maintenance of calcium and phosphorus levels
Fluoride (mg/day)	4*	3*	10	Stimulation of new bone formation
Micronutrients and Other Trace Elements				
Vitamin K (µg/day)	120*	90*	ND	Blood clotting and bone metabolism
Vitamin A (µg/day)	900	700	3,000	Vision, immune function
Iron (mg/day)	8	18	45	Component of hemoglobin
Zinc (mg/day)	11	8	40	Component of enzymes and proteins
Energy and Macronutrients				
Carbohydrates (45–65%)	130 g	130 g	ND	Energy (only source of energy for the brain)
Fat (20–35%)	ND	ND	ND	Energy, vitamin carrier
Protein (10–35%)	.8 g/kg	.8 g/kg	ND	Growth and maturation, tissue formation
Fiber (g/day)	38 g/day*	25 g/day*	ND	Digestion, blood profiles

Note: These values reflect the dietary needs generally for adults aged 19–50 years. Specific guidelines for other age groups are available from the Food and Nutrition Board of the National Academy of Sciences (www.iom.edu). Values labeled with an asterisk (*) are based on Adequate Intake (AI) values rather than the RDA values; ND = not determined.

DRI values also include **Tolerable Upper Intake Level (UL),** which reflects the maximum, or highest, level of daily intake a person can consume without adverse effects on health (see Table 1). The guidelines make it clear that, although too little of a nutrient can be harmful to health, so can too much. In many ways, the RDAs can be considered threshold values similar to the threshold of training values for physical activity. The target zone for healthy eating would range from the RDA/AI values to the UL values (see Figure 2).

A unique aspect of the DRI values is that they are categorized by function and classification in order to facilitate awareness of the different roles that nutrients play in the diet. Specific guidelines have been developed for B-complex vitamins; vitamins C and E; bone-building nutrients, such as calcium and vitamin D; micronutrients, such as iron and zinc; and the class of macronutrients that includes carbohydrates, fats, proteins, and fiber. Table 1 includes the DRI values (including the UL values) for most of these nutrients.

Another unique aspect of the DRI values is that they were designed to accommodate individualized eating patterns. The recommended DRI values for protein ranges from 10 to 35 percent, while the DRI values for fat ranges from 20 to 35 percent. These ranges are much broader than previous recommendations from the USDA in previous versions of the dietary guidelines. According to the Institute of Medicine (IOM), this broader range was established to "help people make healthy and more realistic choices based on their own food preferences." The recommended DRI distributions for carbohydrates, fats, and proteins are shown in Figure 3.

The quantity of nutrients recommended varies with age and other considerations; for example, young children need more calcium than adults and pregnant women and postmenopausal women need more calcium than other women. Accordingly, Dietary Reference Intakes, including RDAs, have been established for several age/gender groups. In this book, the values used are appropriate for most adult men and women.

Food labels provide consumers with detailed information to help them make good food choices. Food labels describe the overall nutrient content of foods. They list the calorie content per serving and specify the amount of carbohydrates, fats, and protein in the food. The label also provides separate listings of saturated fat, cholesterol, sodium, sugar, and fiber content. For each listing, a % Daily Value calculation is provided to help consumers see how the food contributes to overall daily requirements (assuming a 2,000-calories-per-day diet).

A change in labeling laws in 2006 led to some additions to labels. Food manufacturers are now required to list trans fat content on the Nutrition Facts portion of food labels (see Figure 4, page 314). This action was prompted by the clear scientific evidence that trans fats are more likely to cause atherosclerosis and heart disease than are other types of fat. The requirement has forced companies to reconfigure their labels but, more important, the action has prompted companies to look for ways to remove excess trans fats from products. Companies realize that the label will shift consumer choices toward foods with lower trans fat content, so food manufacturers have worked to remove trans fat from their products or decrease it. The FDA estimates that, through greater awareness and changes in food products, the labeling regulations will

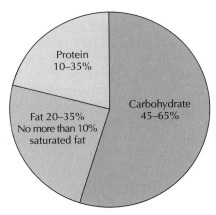

Figure 3 ▶ Dietary Reference Intake values.

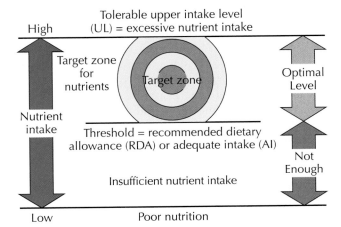

Figure 2 ▶ Dietary Reference Intake: a target zone for healthy eating.

Tolerable Upper Intake Level (UL) Maximum level of a daily nutrient that will not pose a risk of adverse health effects for most people.

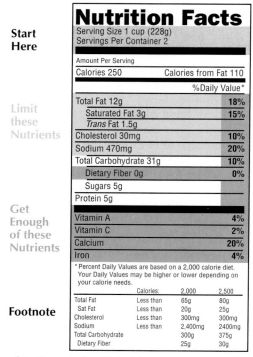

Start Here

Limit these Nutrients

Get Enough of these Nutrients

Footnote

Figure 4 ▶ Sample food label for macaroni and cheese.
Source: U.S. Food and Drug Administration.

help prevent 600 to 1,200 cases of coronary heart disease and 250 to 500 deaths each year.

Reading food labels can help you be more aware of what you are eating and can help you make healthier choices in your daily eating. In particular, paying attention to the amounts of saturated fat, trans fat, and cholesterol posted on food labels will help you make heart-healthy food choices. When comparing similar food products, combine the grams (g) of saturated fat and trans fat and look for the lowest combined amount. The listing of % Daily Value (% DV) can also provide useful information. Foods low in saturated fat and cholesterol generally have % DV values less than 5 percent while foods high in saturated fat and cholesterol have values greater than 20 percent (% DV values are not yet available for trans fat).

Dietary Recommendations for Carbohydrates

Complex carbohydrates should be the principal source of calories in the diet.
Web 04 Carbohydrates have gotten a bad rap in recent years due to the hype associated with low-carbohydrate diets. Carbohydrates have been unfairly implicated as a cause of obesity. The suggestion that they cause insulin to be released and that insulin, in turn, causes the body to

take up and store excess energy as fat is overly simplistic and doesn't take into account differences in types of carbohydrates. Simple sugars (such as sucrose, glucose, and fructose) found in candy and soda lead to quick increases in blood sugar and tend to promote fat deposition. Complex carbohydrates (e.g., bread, pasta, rice), on the other hand, are broken down more slowly and do not cause the same effect on blood sugar. They contribute valuable nutrients and fiber in the diet and should constitute the bulk of a person's diet. Lumping simple and complex carbohydrates together is not appropriate, since they are processed differently and have different nutrient values.

A number of low-carb diet books have used an index known as the glycemic index (GI) as the basis for determining if foods are appropriate in the diet. Foods with a high GI value produce rapid increases in blood sugar, while foods with a low GI value produce slower increases. While this seems to be a logical way to categorize carbohydrates, it is misleading, since it doesn't take into account the amount of carbohydrates in different servings of a food. A more appropriate indicator of the effect of foods on blood sugar levels is called the glycemic load. Carrots, for example, are known to have a very high GI value but the overall glycemic load is quite low. The carbohydrates from most fruits and vegetables exhibit similar properties.

While there is merit in trying to reduce excessive consumption of simple sugars, excess calories are only problematic if caloric intake is larger than caloric expenditure. Carbohydrates are the body's preferred form of energy for physical activity, and the body is well equipped for processing extra carbohydrates. Athletes and other active individuals typically have no difficulty burning off extra energy from carbohydrates. Sugar consumption, among people with an adequate diet, is also not associated with major chronic diseases. Increasing carbohydrates in the diet is more desirable than supplementing protein or consuming higher amounts of fat.

Dietary fiber is not considered a separate dietary nutrient, but it is considered to be
Web 05 **important for overall good nutrition and health.** Studies clearly demonstrate that diets high in complex carbohydrates and **fiber** are associated with a low incidence of coronary heart disease, stroke, and some forms of cancer. Long-term studies indicate that high-fiber diets may also be associated with a lower risk for diabetes mellitus, diverticulosis, hypertension, and gallstone formation. It is not known whether these health benefits are directly attributable to high dietary fiber or other effects associated with the ingestion of vegetables, fruits, and cereals.

The American Dietetics Association has released a position statement on dietary fiber that summarizes the health benefits and importance of fiber in a healthy diet.

It points out that a fiber-rich diet is lower in energy density, often has a lower fat content, is larger in volume, and is richer in micronutrients, all of which have beneficial health effects. Evidence for health benefits has become strong enough that the FDA has stated that specific beneficial health claims can be made for specific dietary fibers. The National Cholesterol Education Program has also recommended dietary fiber as part of overall strategies for treating high cholesterol in adults.

In the past, clear distinctions were made between soluble fiber and insoluble fiber because they appeared to provide separate effects. Soluble fiber (typically found in fruits and oat bran) was more frequently associated with improving blood lipid profiles, while insoluble fiber (typically found in grains) was mainly thought to help speed up digestion and reduce risks for colon and rectal cancer. Difficulties in measuring these compounds in typical mixed diets has led a National Academy of Sciences Panel to recommend eliminating distinctions between soluble and insoluble fibers and instead to use a broader definition of fiber.

Currently, few Americans consume the recommended amounts of dietary fiber. The average intake of dietary fiber is about 15 g/day, which is much lower than the recommended 25–35 g/day. Foods in the typical American diet contain little, if any, dietary fiber, and servings of commonly consumed grains, fruits, and vegetables contain only 1–3 g of dietary fiber. Therefore, individuals have to look for ways to ensure that they get sufficient fiber in their diet. A number of supplements are available to help consumers increase the fiber content of their diet.

Fruits and vegetables are essential for good health. Fruits and vegetables are a valuable source of dietary fiber, are packed with vitamins and minerals, and contain many additional phytochemicals, which may have beneficial effects on health. The International Agency of Research on Cancer (IARC), an affiliate of the World Health Organization, did a comprehensive review on the links between dietary intake of fruits and vegetables and cancer. It concluded that both human studies and animal experimental studies "indicate that a higher intake of fruits and vegetables is associated with a lower risk of various types of cancer." The clearest evidence of a cancer-protective effect from eating more fruits is for stomach, lung, and esophageal cancers. A higher intake of vegetables is associated with reduced risks for cancers of the esophagus and colon-rectum. Overall, 1 in 10 cancers are estimated to be due to insufficient intake of fruits and vegetables. This evidence—plus the evidence of the beneficial effects of fruits and vegetables on other major diseases, such as heart disease—indicates that individuals should strive to increase their intake of these foods. The "5 a day" nutrition program sponsored by the National Cancer Institute aims to increase awareness of the importance of eating at least five fruits and vegetables a day. The guidelines in the food guide pyramid recommend up to nine servings for optimal health.

Some recommendations can be followed to assure healthy amounts of carbohydrates in the diet. The following list summarizes the key recommendations in the 2005 dietary guidelines for carbohydrate content in the diet:

- Choose fiber-rich fruits, vegetables, and whole grains often.
- Choose and prepare foods and beverages with little added sugars or caloric sweeteners.
- Reduce the incidence of dental caries by practicing good oral hygiene and consuming sugar- and starch-containing foods and beverages less frequently.

The following guidelines will help you implement these recommendations:

- Eat at least 3 ounces of whole-grain cereals, breads, crackers, rice, or pasta every day. One ounce is about 1 slice of bread, 1 cup of breakfast cereal, or ½ cup of cooked rice or pasta. Look to see that grains such as wheat, rice, oats, and corn are referred to as "whole" in the list of ingredients.
- Eat more dark green vegetables, such as broccoli, kale, and other dark, leafy greens; orange veggies, such as carrots, sweet potatoes, pumpkin, and winter squash; and beans and peas, such as pinto beans, kidney beans, black beans, garbanzo beans, split peas, and lentils.
- Eat a variety of fruits—whether fresh, frozen, canned, or dried—rather than fruit juice for most of your fruit choices. For a 2,000-calorie diet, you will need 2 cups of fruit each day (for example, one small banana, one large orange, and ¼ cup of dried apricots or peaches).

Dietary Recommendations for Fat

Fat is an essential nutrient and is an important energy source. Humans need some fat in their diet because fats are carriers of vitamins A, D, E, and K. They are a source of essential linoleic acid, they make food taste better, and they provide a concentrated form of calories, which serve as an important source of energy during moderate to vigorous exercise. Fats have more than twice the calories per gram as carbohydrates.

Fiber Indigestible bulk in foods that can be either soluble or insoluble in body fluids.

There are several types of dietary fat. **Saturated fats** come primarily from animal sources, such as red meat, dairy products, and eggs, but they are also found in some vegetable sources, such as coconut and palm oils. **Unsaturated fats** are of two basic types: polyunsaturated and monounsaturated. Polyunsaturated fats are derived principally from vegetable sources, such as safflower, cottonseed, soybean, sunflower, and corn oils (omega-6 fats), and cold-water fish sources, such as salmon and mackerel (omega-3 fats). Monounsaturated fats are derived primarily from vegetable sources, including olive, peanut, and canola oil.

Saturated fat is associated with an increased risk for disease. Excessive total fat in the diet (particularly saturated fat) is associated with atherosclerotic cardiovascular diseases and breast, prostate, and colon cancer, as well as obesity. Excess saturated fat in the diet contributes to increased cholesterol and increased low-density lipoprotein (LDL) cholesterol in the blood. For this reason, no more than 10 percent of your total calories should come from saturated fats.

Unsaturated fats are generally considered to be less likely to contribute to cardiovascular disease, cancer, and obesity than saturated fats. Polyunsaturated fats can reduce total cholesterol and LDL cholesterol, but they also decrease levels of high-density lipoprotein (HDL) cholesterol. Monounsaturated fats, on the other hand, have been shown to decrease total cholesterol and LDL cholesterol without an accompanying decrease in the desirable HDL. Omega-3 fatty acids found in cold-water fish have been shown to reduce triglycerides, but it isn't clear if this alters cholesterol levels.

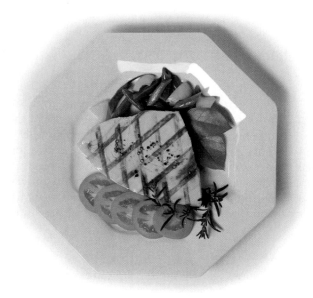

Broiled foods have less fat than fried foods.

Humans produce their own cholesterol, even when dietary cholesterol is limited. Still, high dietary cholesterol can increase the risk for atherosclerosis and coronary heart disease. Principal sources of dietary cholesterol are organ meats, some shellfish, and egg yolks.

The past dietary guidelines recommended a diet low in saturated fat and cholesterol but moderate in total fat. This distinction makes it clear that excess saturated fat is the main concern and acknowledges that some fat is necessary in the diet. The revised guidelines do not explicitly use this terminology but it remains a sound way to view dietary recommendations for these types of fat.

Trans fats and hydrogenated vegetable oils should be minimized in the diet. For decades, Web 08 the public has been cautioned to avoid saturated fats and foods with excessive cholesterol. Many people switched from using butter to margarine because it is made from vegetable oils that are unsaturated and contain no cholesterol. The hydrogenation process used to convert oils into solids, however, is known to produce trans fat, which is just as harmful as saturated fats, if not more so. Trans fats are known to cause increases in LDL cholesterol and have been shown to contribute to the buildup of atherosclerotic plaque. Because of these effects, it is important to try to minimize consumption of trans fats in your diet.

A number of margarines have been developed that have little or no **trans fatty acids** (e.g., Smart Balance). Because food labels now include trans fat content, manufacturers are experimenting with ways of cutting the amount of trans fats in other food products that include hydrogenated vegetable oil. New types of oils are showing promise because they require little or no hydrogenation. Lays recently switched from cottonseed oil to sunflower oil to help eliminate trans fats from Fritos, Tostitos, and Cheetos.

Consumers appear to be responding to messages about the need to reduce the fat content of their diet. A large national survey conducted by the International Food Information Council (IFIC) indicated that 50 percent of adults are trying to cut down on saturated fat and 44 percent are trying to consume less fat. As more and more consumers shift their eating patterns, other food companies will follow with healthier options.

Fat substitutes and neutraceuticals in food products may reduce fat consumption and Web 09 **lower cholesterol.** Olestra is a synthetic fat substitute in foods that passes through the gastrointestinal system without being digested. Thus, foods cooked with Olestra have fewer calories. For example, a chocolate chip cookie baked in a normal way would have 138 calories, but an Olestra cookie would have 63. To date, studies examining the effects of Olestra use have not noted any harmful effects. Still, some consumer groups warn that the promotion of Olestra-containing products may make individuals more likely to snack on less energy-dense snack foods. They also express concern that Olestra inhibits absorption of many naturally occurring antioxidants that have been shown to have many beneficial effects on health.

Several other new products offer potential to modify the amount and effect of dietary fat in our diets. The first is a naturally occurring compound included in several margarines (Benecol and Take Control). The active ingredient in this compound (sitostanol ester) comes from pine trees and has been shown to reduce total and LDL cholesterol in the blood. Several clinical trials have confirmed that these margarines are both safe and effective in lowering cholesterol levels. The products must be used regularly to be effective and may be useful only in individuals with high levels of cholesterol. Food products that contain these medically beneficial compounds are often referred to as neutraceuticals or functional foods because they are a combination of pharmaceuticals and food. Debate continues as to whether this type of product will be regulated by the FDA as a drug or will be classified as a food supplement and not be regulated by FDA. Decisions on these products will, no doubt, influence the way similar neutraceuticals will be regulated in the future.

Some recommendations can be followed to assure healthy amounts of fat in the diet. The following list summarizes the key recommendations in the 2005 dietary guidelines for fat content of the diet:

- Consume less than 10 percent of calories from saturated fatty acids and less than 300 mg/day of cholesterol, and keep trans fatty acid consumption as low as possible.
- Keep total fat intake between 20 to 35 percent of calories, with most fats coming from sources of polyunsaturated and monounsaturated fatty acids, such as fish, nuts, and vegetable oils.
- When selecting and preparing meat, poultry, dry beans, and milk or milk products, make choices that are lean, low-fat, or fat-free.
- Limit intake of fats and oils high in saturated and/or trans fatty acids, and choose products low in such fats and oils.

The following guidelines will help you implement these recommendations:

- Substitute lean meat, fish, poultry, nonfat milk, and other low-fat dairy products for high-fat foods.
- Reduce intake of fried foods, especially those cooked in saturated fats (often true of fast-food restaurants), desserts with high levels of fat (many cookies and cakes), and dressings with high-fat ingredients.
- Limit dietary intake of foods high in cholesterol, such as egg yolks, organ meats, and shellfish.

- Use monounsaturated or polyunsaturated fats for cooking.
- Limit the amount of trans fatty acids in the diet and in cooking.
- Though two or three servings of fish per week may be prudent because of its content of omega-3 polyunsaturated oils, there is not sufficient evidence to endorse a fish oil dietary supplement.
- Be careful of the total elimination of a single food source from the diet. For example, the elimination of meat and dairy products could result in iron or calcium deficiency, especially among women and children.

Dietary Recommendations for Proteins

Web 10 **Protein is the basic building block for the body, but dietary protein constitutes a relatively small amount of daily caloric intake.** Proteins are often referred to as the building blocks of the body because all body cells are made of protein. Proteins are formed from 20 different **amino acids.** More than 100 proteins are made of amino acids. Eleven of these amino acids can be synthesized from other nutrients, but 9 **essential amino acids** must be obtained directly from the diet. Certain foods, called complete proteins, contain all of the essential amino acids, along with most of the others. Examples of complete proteins are meat, dairy products, and fish. Incomplete proteins contain some, but not all, of the essential amino acids. Examples of incomplete proteins are beans, nuts, and rice.

Saturated Fats Dietary fats that are usually solid at room temperature and come primarily from animal sources.

Unsaturated Fats Monounsaturated or polyunsaturated fats that are usually liquid at room temperature and come primarily from vegetable sources.

Trans Fatty Acids Fats that result when liquid oil has hydrogen added to it to make it more solid. Hydrogenation transforms unsaturated fats so that they take on the characteristics of saturated fats, as is the case for margarine and shortening.

Amino Acids The 20 basic building blocks of the body that make up proteins.

Essential Amino Acids The nine basic amino acids that the human body cannot produce and that must be obtained from food sources.

One way to identify amino acids is the *-ine* at the end of their name. For example, arginine and lysine are two of the amino acids. Only 3 of the 20 amino acids do not have the *-ine* suffix. They are aspartic acid, glutamic acid, and tryptophan.

All of the amino acids can be obtained from food and are essential to good health (see Figure 5). Most experts agree that there are no known benefits and some possible risks to consuming diets exceptionally high in animal protein. Certain cancers and coronary heart disease risk have been associated with high dietary intake of animal protein. Researchers are not certain whether the increased risk of contracting these diseases is because of the protein itself or because diets high in animal protein are also high in fat. High-protein diets are also damaging on the kidneys, as the body must process a lot of extra nitrogen. Excessive protein intake can lead to urinary calcium loss, which can weaken bones and lead to osteoporosis.

Because of problems associated with excessive protein intake and health problems encountered by people who have used protein supplements, supplements are not recommended. In fact, many of the more serious health problems resulting from the consumption of dietary supplements are associated with excessive protein intake. More information concerning high-protein diets and protein supplements is included later in this concept and in Concept 15.

Vegetarian diets may provide sufficient protein but care must be used. Vegetarian diets provide ample sources of protein as long as a variety of protein-rich food sources are included in the diet. According to the American Dietetics Association, well-planned vegetarian diets "are appropriate for all stages of the life cycle, including during pregnancy, and lactation," and can "satisfy the nutrient needs of infants, children, and adolescents." You can get enough protein as long as the variety and amounts of foods consumed are adequate. **Vegans** must supplement the diet with vitamin B-12 because this vitamin's only source is animal foods. **Lacto-ovo vegetarians** do not have the same concerns. The guidelines also emphasize the need for vegans to take care that, especially for children, adequate vitamin D and calcium are contained in the diet because most people get these nutrients from milk products.

People who eat a variety of foods, including meat, dairy products, eggs, and plants rich in protein, virtually always eat more protein than the body needs. Eating various foods assures that all essential amino acids are consumed.

Some recommendations can be followed to assure healthy amounts of protein in the diet. The following list summarizes the key recommendations in the 2005 dietary guidelines for protein content in the diet:

- Of the three major nutrients that provide energy, protein should account for the smallest percentage of total calories consumed (see Figure 3).
- Protein in the diet should meet the RDA of 0.8 gram per kilogram (2.2 pounds) of a person's desirable weight. This is about 36 grams for a 100-pound person.
- Generally, protein in the diet should not exceed twice the RDA (1.6 grams per kilogram of a person's desirable weight).
- Vegetarians must be especially careful to eat combinations of foods that assure an adequate intake of essential amino acids, and vegans should supplement their diets with vitamin B-12.

The following guidelines will help you implement these recommendations:

- Consume at least two servings a day of lean meat, fish, poultry, and dairy products (especially those low in fat content) or adequate combinations of foods, such as beans, nuts, grains, and rice.
- Dietary supplements of protein, such as tablets and powders, are not recommended.

Dietary Recommendations for Vitamins

Adequate vitamin intake is necessary for good health and wellness, but excessive vitamin intake is not necessary and can be harmful. Consuming foods containing the minimum RDA of each of the vitamins is essential to the prevention of disease and maintenance

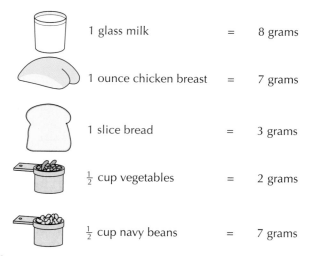

1 glass milk	=	8 grams
1 ounce chicken breast	=	7 grams
1 slice bread	=	3 grams
½ cup vegetables	=	2 grams
½ cup navy beans	=	7 grams

Figure 5 ▶ Protein content of various foods.
Source: Williams, M.

Table 2 ▶ Top 10 Antioxidant All-Stars

	C (mg)	Beta-Carotine (mg)	E (mg)	Folacin (mg)
Broccoli (½ cup cooked)	49	0.7	0.9	53
Cantaloupe (1 cup cubed)	68	3.1	0.3	17
Carrot (1 medium)	7	12.2	0.3	10
Kale (½ cup cooked)	27	2.9	3.7	9
Mango (1 medium)	57	4.8	2.3	31
Pumpkin (½ cup canned)	5	10.5	1.1	15
Red bell pepper (½ cup raw)	95	1.7	0.3	8
Spinach (½ cup cooked)	9	4.4	2.0	131
Strawberries (1 cup)	86	— — —	0.3	26
Sweet potato (1 medium, cooked)	28	14.9	5.5	26
Adult RDA or suggested intake	60	5–6	8–10	180–200

Runners-up: brussels sprouts, all citrus fruits, tomatoes, potatoes, other berries, other leafy greens (dandelion, turnip, and mustard greens; swiss chard; arugula), cauliflower, green pepper, asparagus, peas, beets, and winter squash

Source: University of California at Berkeley Wellness Letter.

of good health (see Table 1). Consuming foods high in carotinoid and retinoid is recommended because these foods are associated with the reduced risk for some forms of cancer. Carotinoid- and retinoid-rich foods, such as green and yellow vegetables (e.g., carrots and sweet potatoes), contain high amounts of vitamin A. Diets high in vitamin C (e.g., citrus fruits and vegetables) and vitamin E (e.g., green, leafy vegetables) are also associated with reduced risk for cancer, and one study indicated that diets high in vitamin E are associated with reduced risk for heart disease. It has been hypothesized that vitamins C and E and carotinoid-rich foods act as **antioxidants,** which help prevent cancer and other forms of disease.

Surprisingly, several large-scale studies have shown either no benefit from beta-carotene supplements or possible negative effects. Another study of over 20,000 people failed to find health benefits associated with taking a daily mixture of antioxidants, including vitamin E (600 IU), vitamin C (250 mg), and beta-carotene (20 mg). The individuals in the study had no lower risk for heart disease than participants taking a placebo. Additional studies are needed to confirm these findings in other populations, so some experts still recommend vitamin E supplements.

Although supplements have not proven to be highly effective, the benefits of antioxidants for good health are clear. It is now accepted that there may be other ben-

eficial substances in foods that have not been isolated or that must be consumed naturally. The initial studies suggesting the possible benefits of antioxidants were based on studies that compared the amounts of fruits and vegetables consumed, so the best bet is to include more fruits and vegetables in your diet. This is the recommendation in the Dietary Guidelines for Americans. Some foods that are especially rich in vitamins and minerals are considered nutritional "all-stars" and make good dietary choices (see Table 2).

Vegans Strict vegetarians, who not only exclude all forms of meat from the diet but, also exclude dairy products and eggs.

Lacto-Ovo Vegetarians Vegetarians who include dairy and eggs in the diet.

Antioxidants Vitamins that are thought to inactivate "activated oxygen molecules," sometimes called free radicals. Free radicals are naturally created by human cells but are also caused by environmental factors, such as smoke and radiation. Free radicals may cause cell damage that leads to diseases of various kinds. Antioxidants may inactivate the free radicals before they do their damage.

Fortification of foods has been used to ensure adequate vitamin intake in the population. National policy requires many foods to be fortified—milk is fortified with vitamin D, low-fat milk with vitamins A and D, and margarine with vitamin A. These foods were selected because they are common food sources for growing children. Many common grain products are fortified with folic acid because low folic acid levels increase the risk for birth defects in babies. Fortification is considered essential, since more than half of all women do not consume adequate amounts of folic acid in the diet during the first months of gestation (before most women even realize they are pregnant). Research has clearly demonstrated the value of fortification. One study showed that neural tube defects are 19 percent less likely today than in 1996 (prior to fortification). Though factors other than fortification may have contributed to this decline, the study supports the benefits of fortification for improving nutritional intakes.

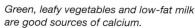 **Taking a daily multiple vitamin supplement may be a good idea.** Sometimes supplements are needed to meet specific nutrient requirements for specific groups. For example, older people may need a vitamin D supplement if they get little exposure to sunlight, and iron supplements are often recommended for pregnant women. Vitamin supplements at or below the RDA are considered safe; however, excess doses of vitamins can cause health problems. For example, excessively high amounts of vitamin C are dangerous for the 10 percent of the population who inherit a gene related to health problems. Excessively high amounts of vitamin D are toxic, and mothers who take too much vitamin A risk birth defects in unborn children.

Eating a variety of foods should ensure an adequate amount of vitamins in the diet, but most people have an inadequate diet. Vitamin intake is especially poor in individuals who avoid certain foods (e.g., limit fats or carbohydrates) or who make poor food choices (e.g., eat a lot of processed foods or few fruits and vegetables). Therefore, a daily multivitamin may be a good way to ensure adequate

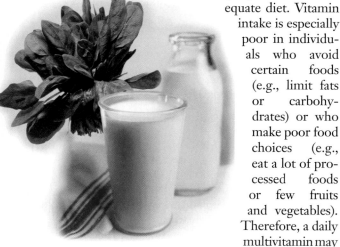
Green, leafy vegetables and low-fat milk are good sources of calcium.

Table 3 ▶ Issues to Consider Regarding the Use of Vitamin and Mineral Supplements

- Limit the use of supplements unless warranted because of a health problem or a specific lack of nutrients in the diet.

- If you decide that supplementation is necessary, select a multivitamin/mineral supplement that contains micronutrients in amounts close to the recommended levels (e.g., "one-a-day"-type supplements).

- If your diet is deficient in a particular mineral (e.g., calcium or iron), it may be necessary to also incorporate dietary sources or an additional mineral supplement, since most multivitamins do not contain the recommended daily amount of minerals.

- Choose supplements that provide between 50 and 100 percent of the AI or RDA and avoid those that provide many times the recommended amount. The use of supplements that hype "megadoses" or vitamins and minerals can increase the risk for some unwanted nutrient interactions and possible toxic effects.

- Buy supplements from a reputable company and look for supplements that carry the U.S. Pharmocopoeia (USP) notation (www.usp.org).

Source: Manore.

vitamin intake. A highly publicized article in the *Journal of the American Medical Association* encouraged physicians to recommend daily multivitamin supplements as a normal part of their patient counseling. Some guidelines for selecting supplements are presented in Table 3.

Some recommendations can be followed to assure healthy amounts of vitamins in the diet. Vitamins in the amounts equal to the RDAs should be included in the diet each day. The following guidelines will help you implement this recommendation:

- A diet containing the food servings recommended for carbohydrates, proteins, and fats will more than meet the RDA standards.
- Extra servings of green and yellow vegetables, citrus and other fruits, and other nonanimal food sources high in fiber, vitamins, and minerals are wise (especially foods from the nutrition all-stars).
- People who eat a sound diet as described in this concept do not need a vitamin supplement, but taking a daily multivitamin is a sound dietary practice. The guidelines suggested in Table 3 should be considered before taking any supplement.
- People with special needs should seek medical advice before selecting supplements and should inform medical personnel as to the amounts and content of all supplements (vitamin and other).

Dietary Recommendations for Minerals

Adequate mineral intake is necessary for good health and wellness, but excessive mineral intake is not necessary and can be harmful. Like vitamins, minerals have no calories and provide no energy for the body. They are important in regulating various bodily functions. Two particularly important minerals are calcium and iron. Calcium is important to bone, muscle, nerve, blood development and function and has been associated with reduced risk for heart disease. Iron is necessary for the blood to carry adequate oxygen. Other important minerals are phosphorus, which builds teeth and bones; sodium, which regulates water in the body; zinc, which aids in the healing process; and potassium, which is necessary for proper muscle function.

RDAs for minerals are established to determine the amounts of each necessary for healthy daily functioning. A sound diet provides all of the RDA for minerals. Evidence indicating that some segments of the population may be mineral-deficient have led to the establishment of health goals identifying a need to increase mineral intake for some segments of the population.

A National Institutes of Health (NIH) consensus statement indicates that a large percentage of Americans fail to get enough calcium in their diet and emphasizes the need for increased calcium—particularly for pregnant women, postmenopausal women, and people over 65, who need 1,500 mg/day, which is higher than previous RDA amounts. The NIH has indicated that a total intake of 2,000 mg/day of calcium is safe and that adequate vitamin D in the diet is necessary for optimal calcium absorption to take place. Though getting these amounts in a calcium-rich diet is best, calcium supplementation for those not eating properly seems wise. Many multivitamins do not contain enough calcium for some classes of people, so some may want to consider additional calcium. Check with your physician or a dietitian before you consider a supplement because individual needs vary.

Another concern is iron deficiency among very young children and women of childbearing age. Low iron levels may be a special problem for women taking birth control pills because the combination of low iron levels and birth control pills has been associated with depression and generalized fatigue. Eating the appropriate number of servings from the food guide pyramid provides all the minerals necessary for meeting the RDA for minerals. Nutrition goals for the nation emphasize the importance of adequate servings of foods rich in calcium, such as green, leafy vegetables and milk products; adequate servings of foods rich in iron, such as beans, peas, spinach, and meat; and reduced salt in the diet.

Some recommendations can be followed to assure healthy amounts of minerals in the diet. The following list includes basic recommendations for mineral content in the diet:

- Minerals in amounts equal to the RDAs should be consumed in the diet each day.
- In general, a calcium dietary supplement is not recommended for the general population; however, supplements (up to 1,000 mg/day) may be appropriate for adults who do not eat well. For postmenopausal women, a calcium supplement is recommended (up to 1,500 mg/day for those who do not eat well). A supplement may also be appropriate for people who restrict calories, but RDA values should not be exceeded unless the person consults with a registered dietitian or a physician.
- Salt should be limited in the diet to no more than 4 to 6 grams per day, and even less is desirable (3 grams). Three grams equals 1 teaspoon of table salt.

The following guidelines will help you implement these recommendations:

- A diet containing the food servings recommended for carbohydrates, proteins, and fats will more than meet the RDA standards.
- Extra servings of green and yellow vegetables, citrus and other fruits, and other nonanimal sources of foods high in fiber, vitamins, and minerals are recommended as a substitute for high-fat foods.

Dietary Recommendations for Water and Other Fluids

Water is a critical component of a healthy diet. Though water is not in the food guide pyramid because it contains no calories, provides no energy, and provides no key nutrients, it is crucial to health and survival. Water is a major component of most of the foods you eat, and more than half of all body tissues are composed of it. Regular water intake maintains water balance and is critical to many important bodily functions. Though a variety of fluid-replacement beverages are available for use during and following exercise, replacing water is the primary need.

Beverages other than water are a part of many diets, but some beverages can have an adverse effect on good health. Coffee, tea, soft drinks, and alcoholic beverages are often substituted for water in the diet. Too much caffeine consumption has been shown to cause symptoms such as irregular heartbeat in some people. Tea has not been shown to have similar effects, though this may be because tea drinkers typically consume less volume than coffee drinkers, and tea has less caffeine per cup than coffee. Many soft drinks also have caffeine, though drip coffee typically contains two to three times the caffeine of a typical cola drink.

Excessive consumption of alcoholic beverages can have negative health implications because the alcohol often replaces nutrients. Excessive alcohol consumption is associated with increased risk for heart disease, high blood pressure, stroke, and osteoporosis. Long-term excessive alcoholic beverage consumption leads to cirrhosis of the liver and to increased risk for hepatitis and cancer. Alcohol consumption during pregnancy can result in low birth weight, fetal alcoholism, and other damage to the fetus. The National Dietary Guidelines indicate that alcohol used in moderation can "enhance the enjoyment of meals" and is associated with a lower risk for coronary heart disease for some individuals.

Some recommendations can be followed to assure healthy amounts of water and other fluids in the diet. The following list includes basic recommendations for water and other fluids in the diet:

- In addition to foods containing water, the average adult needs about eight glasses (8 ounces each) of water every day. Active people and those who exercise in hot environments require additional water.
- Coffee, tea, and soft drinks should not be substituted for sources of key nutrients, such as low-fat milk, fruit juices, or foods rich in calcium.
- Limit daily servings of beverages containing caffeine to no more than three.
- Limit sugared soft drinks; they contain empty calories.
- If you are an adult and you choose to drink alcohol, do so in moderation. The dietary guidelines for Americans indicate that moderation means no more than one drink per day for women and no more than two drinks per day for men (one drink equals 12 ounces of regular beer, 5 ounces of wine [small glass], or one average-size cocktail [1.5 ounces of 80-proof alcohol]).

Sound Eating Practices

Consistency (with variety) is a good general rule of nutrition. Eating regular meals every day, including a good breakfast, is wise. Many studies have shown breakfast to be an important meal, in which one-fourth of the day's calories should be consumed. Skipping breakfast impairs performance because blood sugar levels drop in the long period between dinner the night before and lunch the following day. Eating every 4 to 6 hours is wise.

Moderation is a good general rule of nutrition. Just as too little food can cause problems, so can excessive intake of various nutrients. More is not always better. Moderation in food choices is advised.

You do not have to permanently eliminate foods that you really enjoy, but some of your favorite foods may not be among the best of choices. Enjoying special foods on occasion is part of moderation. The key is to limit food choices high in empty calories.

Considerable evidence indicates that portion sizes have increased in recent years. Large portions are featured in advertising campaigns to lure customers. Cafeteria-style restaurants (and others) sometimes offer all you can eat for a specific price, encouraging large portions. Reducing portion size is very important when eating out and at home (see Concept 15 for more information).

Minimizing your reliance on fast foods is a sound eating practice. Many Americans rely on fast foods as part of their normal diet. Unfortunately, many fast foods are poor nutritional choices. Many hamburgers are high in fat. French fries are high in fat because they are usually cooked in saturated fat. Even choices deemed to be more nutritious, such as chicken or fish sandwiches, are often high in fat and calories because they are cooked in fat and covered with high-fat/high-calorie sauces. Minimizing consumption of fast food can help you avoid excess calories and fat. Nutritional analyses for various fast foods are presented in Appendix D. Fast foods are also discussed in more detail in Concept 15.

See Table 4 for a list of fat content in restaurant meals. Each of the meals in the table contains over 1,000 calories (about 50 percent of daily needs) and more than 1.5 days' worth of saturated fat intake. Minimizing consumption of fast foods can greatly improve overall nutrition patterns.

Minimize your consumption of overly processed foods and foods high in saturated fat or hydrogenated fats. Many foods available in grocery stores have been highly processed to enhance shelf life and convenience. In many cases, the processing of foods removes valuable food nutrients and includes other additives that may compromise overall nutrition. Processing of grains, for example, typically removes the bran and germ layers, which contain fiber and valuable minerals. In regard to additives, there has been considerable attention on the possible negative effects of high fructose corn syrup, as well as the pervasive use of hydrogenated vegetable oils containing trans fatty acids. One way to enhance overall nutrition is to minimize your reliance on processed foods. Table 5 compares food quality in each of the main food categories. To the extent possible, you should aim to choose foods in the "more desirable" category instead of those in the "less desirable" category.

Healthy snacks can be an important part of good nutrition. Snacking is not necessarily bad. For people interested in losing weight or maintaining their current weight, small snacks of appropriate foods can help fool the appetite. For people interested in gaining weight, snacks

Table 4 ▶ Fat and Cholesterol Content of Some Typical Restaurant Meals

Food Option	Calories	Total Fat (g)	Saturated Fat (g)
Prime rib, caesar salad, loaded baked potato	2,210	151	78
Fettuccini alfredo, salad with dressing, garlic bread	2,210	146	57
Burger King Double Whopper with cheese, king fries, king soft drink	2,050	95	43
Fried seafood combo with fries, coleslaw, two biscuits	2,170	130	39
BBQ baby back ribs, French fries, coleslaw	1,530	99	36
Starbucks white chocolate mocha (20 oz.), cinnamon scone	1,130	51	31
Lasagna, salad with dressing, garlic bread	1,670	102	30
Denny's meat lovers skillet, two slices of toast with margarine	1,420	105	28
KFC Extra Crisp Chicken, potato wedges, biscuit	1,420	89	28
Beef burrito, refried beans, sour cream, guacamole	1,640	79	28

Source: Adapted from Jacobson and Hurley.

provide additional calories. For people trying to maintain or lose weight, the calories consumed in snacks will probably necessitate limiting the calories consumed at meals. The key is proper selection of the foods for snacking.

As with your total diet, the best snacks are nutritionally dense. Too many snacks are high in calories, fats, simple sugar, and salt. Check the content of snacks. Even foods sold as "healthy snacks," such as granola bars, are often high in fat and simple sugar. Some common snacks, such as chips, pretzels, and even popcorn, may be high in salt and may be cooked in fat.

Some suggestions for healthy snacks include ice milk (instead of ice cream), fresh fruits, vegetable sticks, popcorn not cooked in fat and with little or no salt, crackers, and nuts with little or no salt.

Nutrition and Physical Performance

Some basic dietary guidelines exist for active people. In general, the nutrition rules described in this concept apply to all people, whether active or sedentary, but some additional nutrition facts are important for exercisers and athletes. Because active people often expend calories in amounts considerably above normal, they need extra calories in their diet. To avoid excess fat and protein, complex carbohydrates should constitute as much as 70 percent of total caloric intake. A higher amount of protein is generally recommended for active individuals (1.2 grams per kg of body weight) because some protein is used as an energy source during exercise. Extra protein is obtained in the additional calories consumed. While the IOM range of 10–35 percent allows a

Table 5 ▶ Comparing the Quality of Similar Food Products

Food Product	Less Desirable Option	More Desirable Option	Benefit of More Desirable Option in Nutrition Quality
Bread	White bread	Wheat bread	More fiber
Rice	White rice	Brown rice	More fiber
Juice	Sweetened juice	100% juice	More fiber and less fructose corn syrup
Fruit	Canned	Fresh	More vitamins, more fiber, less sugar
Vegetables	Canned	Fresh	More vitamins, less salt
Potatoes	French fries	Baked potato	Less saturated fat
Milk	2% milk	Skim milk	Less saturated fat
Meat	Hamburger	Lean beef	Less saturated fat
Oils	Vegetable oil	Canola oil	More monounsaturated fat
Snack food	Fried chips	Baked chips	Less fat/calorie content, less trans fat

"broader range" of choice, intake above 15 percent is not typically necessary.

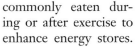 **Carbohydrate loading and carbohydrate replacement during exercise can enhance sustained aerobic performances.** Athletes and vigorously active people must maintain a high level of readily available fuel, especially in the muscles. Adequate complex carbohydrate consumption is the best way to assure this.

Prior to an activity that will require extended duration of physical performance (more than 1 hour in length, such as a marathon), **carbohydrate loading** can be useful. Carbohydrate loading is accomplished by resting 1 or 2 days before the event and eating a higher than normal amount of complex carbohydrates. This helps build up maximum levels of stored carbohydrate (**glycogen**) in the muscles and liver so it can be used during exercise. The key in carbohydrate loading is not necessarily to overeat but, rather, to eat a higher percentage of carbohydrates than normal.

Ingesting carbohydrate beverages during sustained exercise can also aid performance by preventing or forestalling muscle glycogen depletion. Drinking fluids that have no more than 6 to 8 percent sugar helps prevent dehydration and replenishes energy stores. Fluid-replacement drinks containing 6 to 8 percent carbohydrates are very helpful in preventing dehydration and replacing energy stores. A number of companies also make concentrated carbohydrate gels that deliver carbohydrates (generally 80 percent complex, 20 percent simple) in a format the body can absorb quickly for energy. Examples are PowerGel and Gu. Energy bars, such as Powerbars and Clif bars, are also commonly eaten during or after exercise to enhance energy stores.

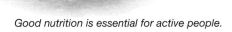

Good nutrition is essential for active people.

The Powerbar version provides about 100 calories of carbohydrates derived from maltodextrin, brown rice, and oat bran to provide a slow release of energy during exercise. The various carbohydrate supplements have been shown to be effective for exercise sessions lasting over an hour and are good for replacing glycogen stores after exercise. Studies show that consuming carbohydrates 15 to 30 minutes following exercise can aid in rapid replenishment of muscle glycogen, which may enhance future performance or training sessions.

These supplements have little benefit for shorter bouts of exercise. Because they contain considerable calories, they are not recommended for individuals primarily interested in weight control.

The timing may be more important than the makeup of a pre-event meal. If you are racing or doing high-level exercise early in the morning, eat a small meal prior to starting. Eat about 3 hours before competition or heavy exercise to allow time for digestion. Generally, athletes can select foods on the basis of experience, but easily digested carbohydrates are best. Generally, fat intake should be minimal because fat digests more slowly; proteins and high-cellulose foods should be kept to a moderate amount prior to prolonged events to avoid urinary and bowel excretion. Drinking 2 or 3 cups of liquid will ensure adequate hydration.

Consuming simple carbohydrates (sugar, candy) within an hour or two of an event is not recommended because it may cause an insulin response, resulting in weakness and fatigue, or it may cause stomach distress, cramps, or nausea.

People who are interested in enhancing physical performance are especially subject to nutrition quackery. A food or nutrition product thought to enhance performance is considered to be an **ergogenic aid.** Many so-called ergogenic aids can be classified as quack products because they do not enhance performance as promised and are exceptionally expensive. In some cases, so-called performance-enhancing supplements are dangerous to health and wellness (see Concept 6 for more information on ergogenic aids).

Legislation designed to regulate food supplements has not been effective in protecting the consumer. The Dietary Supplements Health and Education Act was passed in 1994. Many experts considered it to be a compromise between health food manufacturers who wanted no regulation of dietary supplements (such as vitamins, minerals, proteins, and herbs) and those who wanted strict control of these substances. Many nutrition experts now feel that the act is responsible for an explosion in the sales of products that have not been proven to be effective (see Concept 24).

Strategies for Action

An analysis of your current diet is a good first step in making future decisions about what you eat. Many experts recommend keeping a log of what you eat over an extended period of time so you can determine the overall quality of your diet. In Lab 14A, you will have an opportunity to analyze your diet over several days. In addition to computing the amount of carbohydrates, fats, and proteins, you will also be able to monitor your consumption of fruits and vegetables. A number of online tools and personal software programs can make dietary calculations for you and provide a more comprehensive report of nutrient intake. Whether you use a web-based tool or a paper and pencil log doesn't really matter—the key is to learn how to monitor and evaluate the quality of your diet.

Making small changes in diet patterns can have a big impact. Experts in nutrition emphasize the importance of making small changes in your diet over time rather than trying to make comprehensive changes at one time. Try cutting back on sweets or soda. Simply adding a bit more fruit and vegetables to your diet can lead to major changes in overall diet quality. In Lab 14B, you will be given the opportunity to compare a "nutritious diet" to a "favorite diet." Analyzing two daily meal plans will help you get a more accurate picture as to whether foods you think are nutritious actually meet current healthy lifestyle goals.

Online Learning Center

www.mhhe.com/corbin7e
The Online Learning Center contains a variety of Web-based resources that will help you get the most out of this book and your course. In addition to the On the Web pages, there are video activities, interactive quizzes, application assignments, and a variety of other useful study aids. Log on to the URL above to access these resources.

Web Resources

Web 14
American College of Sports Medicine **www.acsm.org**
American Dietetic Association **www.eatright.org**
Berkeley Nutrition Services **www.nutritionquest.com**
Center for Nutrition Policy and Promotion
   www.usda.gov/cnpp
Center for Science in the Public Interest **www.cspinet.org**
Food and Drug Administration (FDA) **www.fda.gov**
Food Safety Database **www.foodsafety.gov**
Institute of Medicine **www.iom.edu**
International Food Information Council **www.ific.org**
MyPyramid Website **www.mypyramid.gov**
National Academy of Sciences **www.nas.edu**
National Nutrition Summit Database
   www.nlm.nih.gov/pubs/cbm/nutritionsummit.html
Nutrition.gov **www.nutrition.gov**
Office of Dietary Supplements **http://ods.od.nih.gov**
USDA Food and Nutrition Information Center
   www.nal.usda.gov/fnic
U.S. Department of Agriculture (USDA) **www.usda.gov**

Technology Update
MyPyramid Tracker

The MyPyramid model was developed to help promote healthy eating. To aid people in using MyPyramid, the Center for Nutrition Policy and Promotion (CNPP) within the U.S. Department of Agriculture (USDA) has developed a new and powerful web-based assessment and tracking tool. This tool, known as MyPyramid Tracker, has a number of interactive features that are worth trying out. A detailed computerized diet assessment allows you to determine the nutrient quality and calorie content of your diet. A physical activity assessment allows you to determine total daily energy expenditure. Together, these assessments allow you to determine if your diet and activity patterns are in balance (i.e., whether calories in = calories out). You can also establish a personal profile that allows you to track eating and activity patterns over time. To get started, go to the following website: **http://www.mypyramidtracker.gov/** and register to receive a free UserID and password.

Carbohydrate Loading The extra consumption of complex carbohydrates in the days prior to sustained performance.

Glycogen A source of energy stored in the muscles and liver necessary for sustained physical activity.

Ergogenic Aid In this concept, a nutritional supplement claimed by its promoters to improve performance.

Suggested Readings

Additional reference materials for Concept 14 are available at Web15.

Web 15

Fletcher, R. H., and K. M. Fairfield. 2002. Vitamins for chronic disease prevention in adults: Clinical applications. *Journal of the American Medical Association* 287(23):3127–3130.

Food and Nutrition Board, Institute of Medicine. 2002. *Dietary Reference Intakes for Energy, Carbohydrates, Fiber, Fat, Protein, and Amino Acids (Macronutrients).* Washington, DC: National Academy Press.

Franko, D. L., et al. 2005. Food, mood, and attitude: Reducing risk for eating disorders in college women. *Health Psychology* 24(6):586–593.

Gaesser, G. A. 2002. *Big Fat Lies: The Truth about Your Weight and Your Health.* Carlsbad, CA: Gurze Books.

Giddings, S. S., et al. 2005. American Heart Association; American Academy of Pediatrics. Dietary recommendations for children and adolescents: A guide for practitioners: Consensus statement of the American Heart Association. *Circulation* 112:2061–2075.

Goldberg, J. P., et al. 2004. The obesity crisis: Don't blame it on the pyramid. *Journal of the American Dietetic Association* 104(7):1141–1147.

Jacobson, M. F., and J. Hurley. 2002. *Restaurant Confidential.* New York: Workman.

Lichtenstein, A. H., et al. 2006. Diet and lifestyle recommendations revision 2006: A scientific statement from the American Heart Association Nutrition Committee. *Circulation* 114:82–96. Available online at http://circ.ahajournals.org/cgi/content/full/114/1/82.

Manore, M. M. 2003. Cultivating good nutrition habits: How can we maintain a healthy body weight throughout life? *ACSM's Health and Fitness Journal* 7(3):24–25.

Manore, M. M. 2003. New Dietary Reference Intakes set for energy, carbohydrates, fiber, fat, fatty acids, cholesterol, proteins, and amino acids. *ACSM's Health and Fitness Journal* 7(1):25–27.

Manore, M. M. 2004. Nutrition and physical activity: Fueling the active individual. *President's Council on Physical Fitness and Sports Research Digest* 5(1):1–8.

Manore, M. M., S. I. Barr, and G. E. Butterfield. 2001. Position of the American Dietetic Association: Nutrition and athletic performance. *Journal of the American Dietetic Association* 5(1):1543–1556.

Millen, A. E., et al. 2004. Use of vitamin, mineral, nonvitamin, and nonmineral supplements in the United States: The 1987, 1992, and 2000 National Health Interview Survey results. *Journal of the American Dietetic Association* 104(8):942–950.

Schlosser, E. 2001. *Fast Food Nation: The Dark Side of the All-American Meal.* New York: Houghton Mifflin.

Spence, K. and K. Beals. Eating for the health of it: Dietary interventions for reducing disease risk. *ACSM's Fit Society Page.* Summer, 2006, 1–9. Available at ACSM website.

Weinstein, S. J., et al. 2004. Healthy eating index scores are associated with blood nutrient concentrations in the third national health and nutrition examination survey. *Journal of the American Dietetic Association* 104(4):576–584.

In the News

American Heart Association Recommendations

Just as the USDA updates its dietary guidelines periodically, so does the American Heart Association (AHA). Its new 2006 recommendations for diet and lifestyles have been updated from the previous statement released in 2000. The recommendations emphasize the importance of healthy eating and regular physical activity (energy balance) in maintaining a healthy body weight, and in maintaining healthy blood sugar and blood fat levels as well as a healthy blood pressure. Similar to the new USDA recommendations discussed earlier in this concept, the AHA recommendations include eating a diet rich in vegetables, fruits, whole grains, high-fiber foods, and fish (especially oil fish). It is recommended that saturated fat be limited to 7 percent or less of total diet, trans fats to 1 percent or less, and cholesterol to less than 300 mg/day. Non-fat (skim) or low-fat (1%) dairy products are recommended to help meet fat intake goals. Other foods to be limited in the diet include added sugars, packaged foods high in salt (sodium), and alcohol. Special attention should be paid to knowing the content of foods, especially those prepared outside the home and in which you have little input into the contents. http://circ.ahajournals.org/cgi/content/full/114/1/82

Lab 14A Nutrition Analysis

Name	Section	Date

Purpose: To learn to keep a dietary log, to determine the nutritional quality of your diet, to determine your average daily caloric intake, and to determine necessary changes in eating habits

Procedures

1. Record your dietary intake for 2 days using the Daily Diet Record sheets (see pages 329–330). Record intake for 1 weekday and 1 weekend day. You may wish to make copies of the record sheet for future use.
2. Include the actual foods eaten and the amount (size of portion in teaspoons, tablespoons, cups, ounces, or other standard units of measurement). Be sure to include all drinks (coffee, tea, soft drinks, etc.). Include *all* foods eaten, including sauces, gravies, dressings, toppings, spreads, and so on. Determine your caloric consumption for each of the 2 days. Use the Calorie Guide to Common Foods in Appendix C or visit the Healthy Eating Index at **www.cnpp.usda.gov/mypyramidtracker.htm.**
3. List the number of servings from each food group by each food choice.
4. Estimate the proportion of complex carbohydrate, simple carbohydrate, protein, and fat in each meal and in snacks, as well as for the total day.
5. Answer the questions in Chart 1 (page 328), using information for a typical day based on the Daily Diet Record sheets. Score 1 point for each "yes" answer on Chart 1. Use Chart 2 (page 328) to rate your dietary habits. Circle the appropriate rating.

Results

Record the number of calories consumed for each of the 2 days.

Weekday [   ] calories   Weekend [   ] calories

Conclusions and Implications: In several sentences, discuss your diet as recorded in this lab. Explain any changes in your eating habits that may be necessary. Comment on whether the days you surveyed are typical of your normal diet.

Chart 1 ► Dietary Habits Questionnaire

Yes No   Answer questions based on a typical day (use your Daily Diet Records to help).

1. Do you eat three normal-sized meals?
2. Do you eat a healthy breakfast?
3. Do you eat lunch regularly?
4. Does your diet contain 45 to 65 percent carbohydrates with a high concentration of fiber?*
5. Are less than one-fourth of the carbohydrates you eat simple carbohydrates?
6. Does your diet contain 10 to 35 percent protein?*
7. Does your diet contain 20 to 35 percent fat?*
8. Do you limit the amount of saturated fat in your diet (no more than 10 percent)?
9. Do you limit salt intake to acceptable amounts?
10. Do you get adequate amounts of vitamins in your diet without a supplement?
11. Do you typically eat 6 to 11 servings from the bread, cereal, rice, and pasta group of foods?
12. Do you typically eat 3 to 5 servings of vegetables?
13. Do you typically eat 2 to 4 servings of fruits?
14. Do you typically eat 2 to 3 servings from the milk, yogurt, and cheese group of foods?
15. Do you typically eat 2 to 3 servings from the meat, poultry, fish, beans, eggs, and nuts group of foods?
16. Do you drink adequate amounts of water?
17. Do you get adequate minerals in your diet without a supplement?
18. Do you limit your caffeine and alcohol consumption to acceptable levels?
19. Is your average caloric consumption reasonable for your body size and for the amount of calories you normally expend?

Total number of "yes" answers

*Based on USDA standards.

Chart 2 ► Dietary Habits Rating Scale

Score	Rating
18–19	Very good
15–17	Good
13–14	Marginal
12 or less	Poor

Daily Diet Record

Day 1

Breakfast Food	Amount (cups, tsp., etc.)	Calories	Food Servings				Estimated Meal Calorie %
			Bread/Cereal	Fruit/Veg.	Milk/Meat	Fat/Sweet	
							☐ % Protein
							☐ % Fat
							☐ % Complex carbohydrate
							☐ % Simple carbohydrate
							100% Total
Meal Total	✕						

Lunch Food	Amount (cups, tsp., etc.)	Calories	Food Servings				Estimated Meal Calorie %
			Bread/Cereal	Fruit/Veg.	Milk/Meat	Fat/Sweet	
							☐ % Protein
							☐ % Fat
							☐ % Complex carbohydrate
							☐ % Simple carbohydrate
							100% Total
Meal Total	✕						

Dinner Food	Amount (cups, tsp., etc.)	Calories	Food Servings				Estimated Meal Calorie %
			Bread/Cereal	Fruit/Veg.	Milk/Meat	Fat/Sweet	
							☐ % Protein
							☐ % Fat
							☐ % Complex carbohydrate
							☐ % Simple carbohydrate
							100% Total
Meal Total	✕						

Snack Food	Amount (cups, tsp., etc.)	Calories	Food Servings				Estimated Snack Calorie %
			Bread/Cereal	Fruit/Veg.	Milk/Meat	Fat/Sweet	
							☐ % Protein
							☐ % Fat
							☐ % Complex carbohydrate
							☐ % Simple carbohydrate
							100% Total
							Estimated Daily Total Calorie %
Meal Total							☐ % Protein
Daily Totals	✕						☐ % Fat
		Calories	Servings	Servings	Servings	Servings	☐ % Complex carbohydrate
							☐ % Simple carbohydrate
							100% Total

Daily Diet Record

Day 2

Breakfast Food	Amount (cups, tsp., etc.)	Calories	Food Servings				Estimated Meal Calorie %
			Bread/Cereal	Fruit/Veg.	Milk/Meat	Fat/Sweet	
							☐ % Protein
							☐ % Fat
							☐ % Complex carbohydrate
							☐ % Simple carbohydrate
							100% Total
Meal Total							

Lunch Food	Amount (cups, tsp., etc.)	Calories	Food Servings				Estimated Meal Calorie %
			Bread/Cereal	Fruit/Veg.	Milk/Meat	Fat/Sweet	
							☐ % Protein
							☐ % Fat
							☐ % Complex carbohydrate
							☐ % Simple carbohydrate
							100% Total
Meal Total							

Dinner Food	Amount (cups, tsp., etc.)	Calories	Food Servings				Estimated Meal Calorie %
			Bread/Cereal	Fruit/Veg.	Milk/Meat	Fat/Sweet	
							☐ % Protein
							☐ % Fat
							☐ % Complex carbohydrate
							☐ % Simple carbohydrate
							100% Total
Meal Total							

Snack Food	Amount (cups, tsp., etc.)	Calories	Food Servings				Estimated Snack Calorie %
			Bread/Cereal	Fruit/Veg.	Milk/Meat	Fat/Sweet	
							☐ % Protein
							☐ % Fat
							☐ % Complex carbohydrate
							☐ % Simple carbohydrate
							100% Total
Meal Total							
Daily Totals		Calories	Servings	Servings	Servings	Servings	

Estimated Daily Total Calorie %

☐ % Protein
☐ % Fat
☐ % Complex carbohydrate
☐ % Simple carbohydrate
100% Total

Lab 14B Selecting Nutritious Foods

Name	**Section**	**Date**

Purpose: To learn to select a nutritious diet, to determine the nutritive value of favorite foods, and to compare nutritious and favorite foods in terms of nutrient content

Procedures

1. Select a favorite breakfast, lunch, and dinner from the foods list in Appendix D. Include between-meal snacks with the nearest meal. If you cannot find foods you would normally choose, select those most similar to choices you might make.
2. Select a breakfast, lunch, and dinner from foods you feel would make the most nutritious meals. Include between-meal snacks with the nearest meal.
3. Record your "favorite foods" and "nutritious foods" on page 332. Record the calories for proteins, carbohydrates, and fats for each of the foods you choose.
4. Total each column for the "favorite" and the "nutritious" meals.
5. Determine the percentages of your total calories that are protein, carbohydrate, and fat by dividing each column total by the total number of calories consumed.
6. Comment on what you learned in the Conclusions and Implications section.

Results: Record your results below. Calculate percent of calories from each source by dividing total calories into calories from each food source (protein, carbohydrates, or fat).

Food Selection Results

	Favorite Foods		Nutritious Foods	
Source	**Calories**	**% of Total Calories**	**Calories**	**% of Total Calories**
Protein				
Carbohydrates				
Fat				
Total 100%		100%		100%

Conclusions and Implications: In several sentences, discuss the differences you found between your nutritious diet and your favorite diet. Discuss the quality of your nutritious diet as well as other things you learned from doing this lab.

"Favorite" versus "Nutritious" Food Choices for Three Daily Meals

Breakfast Favorite	Food Choices				Breakfast Nutritious	Food Choices			
Food No.	Cal.	Pro. Cal.	Car. Cal.	Fat Cal.	Food No.	Cal.	Pro. Cal.	Car. Cal.	Fat Cal.
Totals					Totals				

Lunch Favorite	Food Choices				Lunch Nutritious	Food Choices			
Food No.	Cal.	Pro. Cal.	Car. Cal.	Fat Cal.	Food No.	Cal.	Pro. Cal.	Car. Cal.	Fat Cal.
Totals					Totals				

Dinner Favorite	Food Choices				Dinner Nutritious	Food Choices			
Food No.	Cal.	Pro. Cal.	Car. Cal.	Fat Cal.	Food No.	Cal.	Pro. Cal.	Car. Cal.	Fat Cal.
Totals					Totals				
Daily Totals (Calories)					Daily Totals (Calories)				
Daily % of Total Calories					Daily % of Total Calories				

Managing Diet and Activity for Healthy Body Fatness

Health Goals for the year 2010

- Increase prevalence of a healthy weight.
- Reduce prevalence of overweight.
- Increase proportion of people who meet national dietary guidelines.
- Increase adoption and maintenance of daily physical activity.
- Increase teaching about nutrition and physical activity.

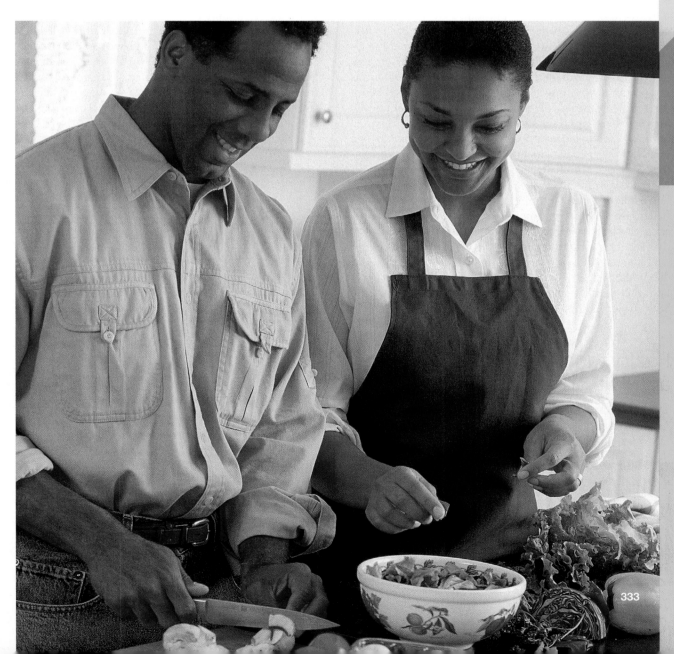

Various management strategies for eating and performing physical activity are useful in achieving and maintaining optimal body composition.

The fact that more than 67 percent of the American adult population is classified as overweight is clear evidence that weight control is a vexing problem for the majority of the population. Most Americans recognize the importance of the problem and want to correct it. In fact, a recent national survey by the International Food Information Council (IFIC) reported that nearly two-thirds of Americans were either very concerned or somewhat concerned about their weight.

Too often, the focus is on appearance rather than health and on weight loss rather than fat loss. In attempts to lose weight, the dietary (energy intake) side of the energy balance equation is typically emphasized. Evidence suggests that the energy expenditure side of the equation is just as important, if not more so. Despite the documented benefits, few people trying to lose weight report being physically active. A state-based survey determined that approximately one-half of individuals trying to lose weight do not engage in any physical activity and only 15 percent report exercising regularly. The challenges many people experience with weight control may be an indirect reflection of the challenges people face in trying to be more active. Although being physically active cannot ensure that you will become as thin as you desire, it may allow you to attain a body size that is appropriate for your genetics and body type.

The focus in this concept is on lifestyle patterns (both diet and physical activity) that will assist with losing body fat rather than weight. Guidelines for maintaining healthy body fat levels over time are also presented.

Factors Influencing Weight and Fat Control

Subtle changes in diet and activity patterns can have major effects on body weight and body fatness. Experts have concluded that the recent trends in obesity are due in large part to environmental influences that make it difficult to manage body fat levels. The term *obesigenic* has been used to describe the elements of our environment that collectively promote eating and inactivity. The model in Figure 1 shows the various aspects of the obesigenic environment and how they influence the energy balance equation.

The essence of the model is that we are continually confronted with environments that make it easy to consume large quantities of energy-dense food. We also live in an environment in which most physical tasks are no longer necessary and people have less apparent time available for active recreation. Small increases in energy intake combined with small decreases in energy expenditure lead to the storage of fat. Awareness of these environmental influences is important if we desire to maintain a healthy body fat level and weight.

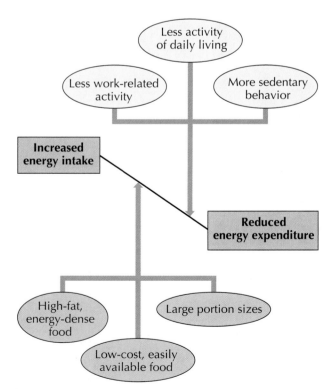

Figure 1 ▶ Factors contributing to increased energy intake and reduced energy expenditure.

Source: Model adapted from Hill et al.

On the Web

www.mhhe.com/corbinweb

Web 01 Log on to this URL before reading this concept. See On the Web list of concepts. Click on the concept number you want to view. To access supplemental information, click on the number shown at each Web icon.

Physical activity contributes to energy balance in a number of ways. By maintaining an active lifestyle, you can burn off extra calories, keep your body's metabolism high, and prevent the decline in basal metabolic rate that typically occurs with aging (due to reduced muscle mass). All types of physical activity can be beneficial for weight control. Since aerobic exercise can be maintained for a long period, it allows you to expend large numbers of calories and therefore is the best type of physical activity for fat loss and maintenance. Strength training can contribute to weight control by increasing muscle mass and helping increase metabolic rate.

New evidence suggests that minimizing inactivity may be just as important as getting sufficient amounts of activity. Scientists at the Mayo clinic have coined the term *non-exercise activity thermogenesis (NEAT)* to refer to the energy expenditure that results from unintentional or very low-intensity movements throughout the day. They contend that lower levels of NEAT may contribute to lower overall levels of energy expenditure and increases in overweight and obesity. NEAT may account for about 15 percent of total daily energy expenditure in very sedentary individuals and up to 50 percent in highly active persons or those with active jobs. Numerous labor-saving devices, such as escalators, moving sidewalks, motorized lawn mowers, and golf carts contribute in small but important ways to a less active lifestyle.

Inactivity, lower amounts of work-related activity, and less activity of daily living can all contribute to reduced energy expenditure and weight (fat) gain (see Figure 1). For effective weight management, it is important to look for ways to add activity back into your lifestyle (see Concept 6 for suggestions).

Awareness and dietary restraint are needed to avoid excess caloric intake. Consumers are able to buy food almost anywhere. For example, convenience stores and food courts in malls allow people to snack more readily during the day. To provide more apparent value to consumers, restaurants and convenience stores have continued to provide larger portion sizes. Terms such as *super sizing* and *Value Meals* are commonly used to entice customers to buy larger servings than they really need. Typical value sized orders of French fries contain over 600 calories. Similarly, consumers can purchase soft drinks in volumes up to 64 ounces rather than a standard 12- to 16-ounce drink. Choosing normal-sized meals and drinks is one way to avoid excess calories in your diet (see Figure 2).

In response to increasing pressure from consumer groups and public health advocates, many restaurants have started to provide healthier alternatives on menus. McDonald's recently announced a major nutrition labeling effort as part of its Balanced, Active Lifestyle campaign. Improved labeling and healthier options, such as fruit, salads, and water, will help consumers make health-

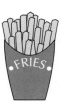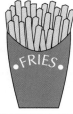

Size	Small	Large	Super Size
Calories (kcal)	450	540	610

Figure 2 ▶ Comparison of added calories in different sizes of French fries.

ier choices. While progress is evident on some fronts, similar movements pull consumers toward gluttony and excess. Hardee's advertisements proudly tout the merits of the Thickburger, which contains two, 1/3-pound patties and over 1,400 calories. Dietary restraint is clearly needed to avoid the excess energy intake that can occur from easy access to high-calorie foods (see Figure 1).

Guidelines for Losing Body Fat

Following appropriate weight loss guidelines is important for the best long-term results. There is considerable misinformation about diet and weight loss strategies. The information leads many people to use unsafe or ineffective weight loss supplements or to follow inappropriate exercise programs. Fat, weight, and body proportions are all factors that can be changed, but people often set goals that are impossible to achieve. Starting with small goals and aiming for reasonable rates of weight loss (1–2 pounds a week) are recommended. Setting unrealistic goals may result in eating disorders, failure to meet goals, or failure to maintain weight loss over time. Table 1 provides a summary of weight loss guidelines from the American College of Sports Medicine (ACSM).

Behavioral goals are more effective than outcome goals. Researchers have shown that setting **outcome goals,** or goals that set a specific amount of weight or fat loss (or gain), can be discouraging. If a **behavioral goal**

Outcome Goals Statements of intent to achieve a specific test score or a specific standard associated with good health or wellness—for example, "I will lower my body fat level by 3 percent."

Behavioral Goal A statement of intent to perform a specific behavior (changing a lifestyle) for a specific period of time—for example, "I will reduce the calories in my diet by 200 a day for the next four weeks."

Table 1 ▶ Guidelines for Weight Loss Treatment

Questions about Weight Loss	Recommendations
Who should consider weight loss?	Individuals with a BMI of >25 or in the marginal or overfat zone *should consider* reducing their body weight—especially if it is accompanied by abdominal obesity. Individuals with a BMI of >30 *are encouraged to seek* weight loss treatment.
What types of goals should be established?	Overweight and obese individuals should target reducing their body weight by a minimum of 5–10% and should aim to maintain this long-term weight loss.
What about maintenance?	Individuals should strive for long-term weight maintenance and the prevention of weight regain over the long term, especially when weight loss is not desired or when attainment of ideal body weight is not achievable.
What should be targeted in a weight loss program?	Weight loss programs should target both eating and exercise behaviors, as sustained changes in both behaviors has been associated with significant long-term weight loss.
How should diet be changed?	Overweight and obese individuals should reduce their current intake by 500–1,000 kcal/day to achieve weight loss (<30% of calories from fat). Individualized level of caloric intake should be established to prevent weight regain after initial loss.
How should activity be changed?	Overweight and obese individuals should progressively increase to a minimum of 150 minutes of moderate-intensity physical activity per week for health benefits. However, for long-term weight loss, the program should progress to higher amounts of activity (e.g., 200–300 minutes per week or >2,000 kcal/week).
What about resistance exercise?	Resistance exercise should supplement the endurance exercise program for individuals who are undertaking modest reductins in energy intake to lose weight.
What about using drugs for weight loss?	Pharmacotherapy (medicine/drugs) for weight loss should be used only by individuals with a BMI >30 or those with excessive body fatness. Weight loss medications should be used only in combination with a strong behavioral intervention that focuses on modifying eating and exercise behaviors.

Source: American College of Sports Medicine.

of eating a reasonable number of calories per day and expending a reasonable number of calories in exercise is met, outcome goals will be achieved. Most experts believe that behavioral goals work better than weight or fat loss goals, especially in the short term.

Changes in eating patterns can be effective in fat loss. For successful weight loss or maintenance of healthy weight, it is important to adopt healthy behaviors that can be maintained over time. The following list highlights a few suggested dietary habits that may be helpful.

Web 03

- Restrict calories in moderate amounts per day rather than make large reductions in daily caloric intake.
- Eat less fat. Research shows that reduction of the fat in the diet results not only in fewer calories consumed (fats have more than twice the calories per gram as carbohydrates or proteins) but in greater body fat loss as well.
- Severely restrict **empty calories,** which provide little nutrition and can account for an excessive amount of your daily caloric intake. Examples of these foods are candy (often high in simple sugar) and potato chips (often fried in saturated fat).

- Increase complex carbohydrates. Foods high in fiber, such as fresh fruits and vegetables, contain few calories for their volume. They are nutritious and filling, and they are especially good foods for a fat loss program.
- Learn the difference between craving and hunger. Hunger is a physiological phenomenon that is a result of the body's need to supply energy to sustain life. A craving is simply a desire to eat something, sometimes a food you do not particularly like. When you feel the urge to eat, you may want to ask yourself, Is this real hunger or a craving? Hunger is accompanied by growling of the stomach and is most likely to occur after long periods without food. If you have the urge to eat soon after a meal, it is probably from craving, not hunger.
- Develop personal habits that can help you make better dietary choices when eating at restaurants, work, and special occasions. Making good selections when purchasing and preparing food is also important. See Table 2 for suggestions.

Extreme diets are not likely to be effective. Diets that require severe caloric restriction and exercise programs that require exceptionally large caloric expenditure can

Table 2 ▶ Guidelines for Healthy Shopping and Eating in a Variety of Settings

Guidelines for Shopping	• Shop from a list to avoid the purchase of foods that contain empty calories and other foods that will tempt you to overeat. • Shop with a friend to avoid buying unneeded foods. For this technique to work, the other person must be sensitive to your goals. In some cases, a friend can have a bad, rather than a good, influence. • Shop on a full stomach to avoid the temptations of snacking on and buying junk food. • Check the labels for contents of foods to avoid foods that are excessively high in fat or saturated fat.
Guidelines for How You Eat	• When you eat, do nothing else but eat. If you watch television, read, or do some other activity while you eat, you may be unaware of what you have eaten. • Eat slowly. Taste your food. Pause between bites. Chew slowly. Do not take the next bite until you have swallowed what you have in your mouth. Periodically take a longer pause. Be the last one finished eating. • Do not eat food you do not want. Some people do not want to waste food, so they clean their plate even when they feel full. • Follow an eating schedule. Eating at regular meal times can help you avoid snacking. Spacing meals equally throughout the day can help reduce appetite. • Leave the table after eating to avoid taking extra, unwanted bites and servings. • Eat meals of equal size. Some people try to restrict calories at one or two meals to save up for a big meal. • Eating several *small* meals helps you avoid hunger (fools the appetite) and this may help prevent over-eating. • Avoid second servings. Limit your intake to one moderate serving. If second servings are taken, make them one-half the size of first servings. • Limit servings of salad dressings and condiments (e.g., catsup). These are often high in fat and calories and can amount to greater caloric consumption than is expected.
Guidelines for Controlling the Home Environment	• Store food out of sight. Avoid containers that allow you to see food. It is especially important to limit the accessibility of foods that tempt you and foods with empty calories. Foods that are out of sight are out of mouth. • Do your eating in designated areas only. Designate areas such as the kitchen and dining room as eating areas, so you do not snack elsewhere. It is especially easy to eat too much while watching television. • If you snack, eat foods high in complex carbohydrates and low in fats, such as fresh fruits and carrot sticks. • Freeze leftovers. Leftover foods are often tempting to eat. Freezing them so that it takes preparation to eat them will help you avoid temptation.
Guidelines for Controlling the Work Environment	• Take food from home rather than eating from vending machines or catering trucks. • Do not eat while working but take your lunch as a break. Do something active during other breaks. For example, take a walk. • Avoid sources of food provided by co-workers—for example, food in work rooms, such as birthday cakes, or candy in jars. • Have drinking water or low-calorie drinks available to substitute for snacks.
Guidelines for Eating on Special Occasions	• Practice ways to refuse food. Knowing exactly what to say will help you not get talked into eating something you do not want. • Eat before you go out, so you are not as hungry at parties and events. • Do not stand near food sources and distract yourself if tempted to eat when you are not really hungry. • Limit servings of nonbasic parts of the meal. It is easy to consume large numbers of calories on alcohol, soft drinks, appetizers, and desserts. Limit these items.
Guidelines for Eating Out at Restaurants	• Try to make healthy selections from the menu. Choose chicken without skin, fish, or lean cuts of meat. Grilled or broiled options are better than fried. Choose healthier options for dessert, as many decadent desserts can have more calories than the whole dinner. • Limit the use of sauces and condiments, such as butter, margarine, catsup, mayonnaise, and salad dressings. Asking for the condiments on the side allows you to determine how much to put on. • Do not feel compelled to eat everything on your plate. Many restaurants serve exceptionally large portions to try to please the customers. • Order à la carte rather than full meals to avoid multiple courses and servings. • Avoid super sizing your meals if eating at fast-food restaurants, as this can add unwanted calories.

be effective in fat loss over a short period but are seldom maintained for a lifetime. Studies show that extreme programs for weight control, designed to "take it off fast," result in long-term success rates of less than 5 percent. Research shows one reason extremely low-calorie diets

Empty Calories Calories in foods considered to have little or no nutritional value.

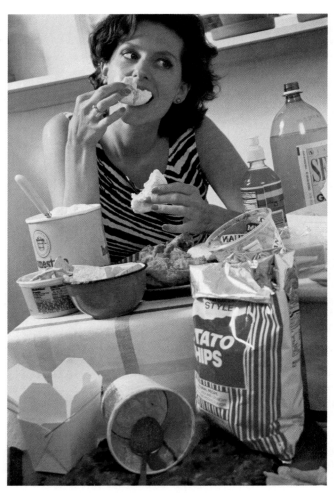

Foods with empty calories have few nutrients and often are relatively high in colorie content.

are ineffective is that they may promote "calorie sparing." When caloric intake is 800 to 1,000 or less, the body protects itself by reducing basal and resting metabolism levels (sparing calories). This results in less fat loss, even though the caloric intake is very low.

A common strategy in fad diets is to warn dieters not to eat carbohydrates. Because water is required to store carbohydrates, reductions in carbohydrate intake leads to reductions in water storage—and weight. The person who restricts carbohydrates may see a reduction in "weight" (not fat!) and assume that the diet worked when it didn't.

A combination of physical activity and a healthy diet is the best approach for long-term weight control. One major advantage of emphasizing both physical activity and dietary changes is that physical activity can help maintain the metabolic rate and prevent the decline that occurs with calorie sparing. Studies have

shown that programs that include both diet and physical activity promote greater loss of body fat than programs based solely on dietary changes. The total weight loss from the programs may be about the same, but a larger fraction of the weight comes from fat when physical activity is included. In contrast, programs based solely on diet result in greater loss of lean muscle tissue.

A healthy diet and regular physical activity are the keys for long-term weight control. Small changes, such as eating a few hundred calories less per day or walking for 30 minutes every day, can make a big difference over time. The important point is to strive for permanent changes that can be maintained in a normal daily lifestyle. Fad diets cannot be maintained for long periods; therefore, the individual usually regains any weight lost. Constant losing and gaining, known as "yo-yo" dieting, is counterproductive and may lead to negative changes in the person's metabolism and unwanted shifts in sites of fat deposition. When in doubt, avoid programs that promise fast and easy solutions, extreme diets that favor specific foods or eating patterns, and any product that makes unreasonable claims about easy ways to stimulate your metabolism or "melt away fat."

Low-carbohydrate diets are not a good choice for long-term weight control. Low carbohydrate diets were in vogue just a few years ago but their popularity has dropped off. The surge in popularity was fueled by some studies that showed that they were effective in reducing weight and lipid levels of extremely obese people. Experts were surprised by the findings but still did not support or endorse the use of low-carb diets for weight loss by the general population. The media generally portrayed results from the low-carb diets in a very positive light and swayed many consumers, but critical analyses have shown that these types of diets offer no advantage over more balanced eating plans that emphasize healthy food choices and moderation. In a 7-year study of diet and weight change published in the *Journal of the American Medical Association*, a low-carb diet plan was found to be ineffective for long-term weight loss and a low-fat/high-carb diet was not found to contribute to weight gain. A key finding of the study was that women who ate the least amount of fat lost the most weight. Vegetable intake was also positively correlated with weight loss. These reports confirm that reducing fat content is still one of the keys to weight loss and weight maintenance.

While the hype about low-carbohydrate diets was clearly not warranted, recent studies have shown that the higher protein content in some of these diet plans may have acted to inhibit appetite. This could explain why studies reported inconsistent findings. The emphasis on animal protein in the Atkins diet is problematic because of the high saturated fat and cholesterol content, but increased consumption of other sources of protein may prove beneficial for some people. The current dietary guidelines support a broader range of intakes for protein (10 to 35 percent of total calories) than previous guidelines (approximately 15 percent).

Low "glycemic load" diets may be a more sensible alternative to low-carbohydrate diets. A positive outcome of the low-carb craze is that it sensitized Americans to the problems of consuming too much sugar. During the low-fat craze of the early 1990s, people assumed that they could eat anything they wanted as long as it didn't have fat in it. The popularity of "fat-free" cookies and desserts skyrocketed as consumers sought ways to consume snack foods without feeling guilty. Then the pendulum swung the other way and consumers appeared to be avoiding carbohydrates with the same vigor. Both low-fat and low-carb diets are probably too restrictive when followed to extremes.

Many experts have begun to recommend less restrictive diets that manage excessive carbohydrate intake without compromising important benefits from other foods.

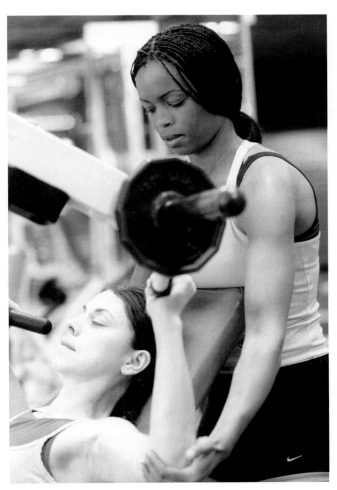

Resistance training helps you gain lean body mass (muscle).

For example, there is overwhelming research documenting important health benefits associated with consuming fruits, vegetables, legumes, and sufficient amounts of fiber. Because these foods have a low glycemic load, they are not prone to the same problems as simple carbohydrates. There is also clear evidence of harm associated with the excessive consumption of saturated fat advocated by some diet plans and potential benefits associated with the consumption of monounsaturated fats. A more sensible diet plan minimizes saturated fats while including heart healthy oils. This type of diet provides the vitamins, minerals, and fiber that are typically lacking in most low-carb diets. The emphasis on healthy forms of polyunsaturated and monounsaturated fats also makes this type of diet easier to adhere to than traditional low-fat diet plans. By emphasizing the quality of carbohydrates, fats, and proteins, consumers should be able to make dietary choices that contribute to weight control and good health. This type of diet plan is emphasized in the revised MyPyramid model and the new dietary guidelines. See Concept 14 for more information.

Developing a regular eating plan is important for weight maintenance. A number of studies have suggested that individual eating patterns may be associated with obesity. One study found that breakfast skipping, meals eaten away from home, and frequent episodes of eating during the day are associated with obesity—even after controlling for total caloric intake. These results highlight the importance of establishing regular patterns of eating.

Some prescription medicines may help some obese individuals curb their appetite.
Web 05 Only two prescription drugs (Sibutramine and Orlistat) have been approved by the FDA to help patients curb appetite and lose weight. Sibutramine (used in the product Meridia) acts by inhibiting the reuptake of the neurotransmitters serotonin and noradrenaline, which regulate hunger. By keeping the levels high, the body doesn't have as high a hunger response. Orlistat (used in Xenical) enhances weight loss by inhibiting the body's absorption of fat. Studies have confirmed that it can help patients lose more weight, but a limitation is that is also blocks the absorption of important fat-soluble vitamins (A, D, E and K, as well as beta-carotene). Both of these pharmacotherapy treatments are considered to be adjuncts to lifestyle modification and are used only with obese patients (BMI > 30) or overweight adults with other comorbidities (e.g., diabetes or hypertension). A lower-dose over-the-counter version of Xenical is currently being considered by the FDA.

Artificial sweeteners and fat substitutes may help but cannot be considered a "sure
Web 06 **cure" for body fat problems.** Artificial sweet-

eners are frequently used in soft drinks and food to reduce the calorie content. Because they have few or no calories, these supplements were originally expected to help people with weight control. However, since they were introduced, the general public has not eaten fewer calories and more people are now overweight than before they were introduced. Studies suggest that people consuming these products end up consuming just as many calories per day as people consuming products with real sugar or sweeteners.

As described in Concept 14, a variety of artificial fat substitutes (e.g. orlistat) are now used to reduce fat content in foods. Potato chips and other fried foods cooked in these products as well as baked goods using these products have less fat and fewer calories. If you eat no more food than usual and substitute foods made with these products, you will consume fewer calories and less fat. Experts worry that consumers will not eat the same amount of foods with these fake fats but will feel they can eat more because the fake fats contain fewer calories and less fat.

Dietary supplements and products containing stimulants should be avoided. Because long-term weight control is difficult, many individuals seek simple solutions from various nonprescription weight loss products. The most common additive in dietary supplements has been the stimulant ephedra (or the herbal equivalent, Ma Huang). Many negative reactions and multiple deaths have been attributed to the use of ephedra, and this has led the FDA to ban the sale and use of any products containing this compound. A concern among public health officials is that many products do not accurately label the contents of their supplements. A report in the *Journal of the American Medical Association* indicated that over 50 percent of the ephedra supplements tested by the FDA failed to list the ephedra content or had amounts 20 percent or higher than listed on the label. Manufacturers of supplements have recently started selling "ephedra-free" supplements that use other stimulants. A commonly used alternative compound is known as "bitter orange," and this supplement has also been shown to present similar health risks. Consumers should be wary of dietary supplements, due to the unregulated nature of the industry. See Concept 23 to learn how to interpret the diverse array of health information in the print and web media.

Guidelines for Gaining Muscle Mass

Young people often have difficulty in gaining weight or muscle mass. Typically, those most likely to have difficulty gaining weight are age 10 to 20. The reason for this is that more calories are required to maintain weight during the growing years than in adulthood. They have probably been told more than once that they will not have trouble gaining weight when they grow older. This is true for most people, but it is of little consolation to those who want to gain weight now. During adolescence, most people begin to gain weight, including muscle mass that can be enhanced with regular exercise. Excessive eating to gain weight (especially during adolescence) is not without its problems. The body requires more caloric intake during the teen years because the body is growing. A person who develops a habit of high caloric intake during this time may have a difficult time controlling fatness when the demands on the body are less. Most people who want to gain weight want to gain lean body tissue. Only those who have body fat percentages less than what is considered to be essential for good health need to gain body fat.

Changes in the frequency and composition of meals are important to gain muscle mass. To increase muscle mass, the body requires a greater caloric intake. The challenge is to provide enough extra calories for the muscle without excess amounts going to fat. An increase of 500 to 1,000 calories a day will help most people gain muscle mass over time. Smaller, more frequent meals are best for weight gain, since they tend to keep the metabolic rate high. The majority of extra calories should come from complex carbohydrates. Breads, pasta, rice, and fruits such as bananas are good sources. Granola, nuts, juices (grape and cranberry), and milk also make good high-calorie, healthy snacks. High-protein diets and diet supplements are not particularly effective if you maintain a normal diet. High-fat diets can result in weight gain but may not be best for good health, especially if they are high in saturated fat. If weight gain does not occur over a period of weeks and months with extra calorie consumption, medical assistance may be necessary.

Physical activity is important in gaining muscle mass. Regular strength training can aid in weight gain. The stimulus from this form of exercise causes the body to increase protein synthesis, which allows the body to gain muscle mass. Of course, the body requires higher caloric intake to form this new muscle tissue.

Excessive aerobic exercise may actually make it difficult to gain weight. Although some regular aerobic exercise is necessary for health and cardiovascular fitness, it may be necessary to limit aerobic exercise if weight gain is the goal. Studies have shown that extensive aerobic training can even cause a reduction in muscle mass. When one is training to gain weight, aerobic exercise expending no more than 3,500 calories per week is probably best.

Knowing about guidelines for controlling body fat is not as important as following them. The guidelines in this concept work only if you use them. In Lab 15A, you will identify guidelines that may help you in the future.

Recordkeeping is important in meeting fat control goals and making moderation a part of your normal lifestyle. Studies have shown that it is easy to fool yourself when determining the amount of food you have eaten or the amount of exercise you have done. Once fat control goals have been set, whether for weight loss, maintenance, or gain, it is important to keep records of your behavior. Keeping a diet log and an exercise log can help you monitor your behavior and maintain the lifestyle necessary to meet your goals. A log can also help you monitor changes in weight and body fat levels. But remember, care should be taken to avoid too much emphasis on short-term weight changes. Lab 15B will help you learn about the actual content of fast foods, so you can learn to make better choices when eating out.

The support of family and friends can be of great importance in balancing caloric intake and caloric expenditure. They can also help in adopting and maintaining healthy eating practices and assist in following the guidelines presented in this concept. They can help you change and adhere to healthy eating practices, provide support, and help the person adhere to guidelines presented in this concept. Unfortunately friends and family can sometimes "try too hard" to help. This can have the opposite effect of that intended if it is perceived as an attempt to control the person's behavior. Encouragement and support rather than control of behavior is the key.

Group support can be one of the best reinforcers of proper eating and exercise behavior. Group support is beneficial to many individuals who are attempting to change their behavior. Groups such as Overeaters Anonymous and Weight Watchers help those who need the support of peers in attaining and maintaining desirable fat levels for a lifetime.

Psychological strategies can be of assistance in eating and exercising to attain and maintain a desirable level of body fat. Adopting healthy lifestyle habits often requires the use of behavioral skills and some degree of discipline. The following list provides tips on maintaining weight control efforts.

- Avoid food fantasies. Sometimes the thought of food is what causes overeating. Practice restructuring your thought process to something other than food fantasies. Use mental imagery to create a mind's-eye view of something you enjoy other than food. When food fantasies occur, you may want to exercise or engage in an activity that refocuses your attention.
- Avoid weight fantasies. Sometimes the thought of being excessively thin or muscular occurs. By itself, this may not be bad. If, however, it causes you to become discouraged and makes your goals seem unattainable, it is bad. When weight fantasies occur, do an activity to redirect your focus of attention or imagine something other than the weight fantasy.
- Avoid **negative self-talk.** One type of negative self-talk occurs when a person starts self-criticism for not meeting a goal. For example, if a person is determined not to eat more than one serving of food at a party but fails to meet this goal, he or she might say, "It's no use stopping now; I've already blown it." It is not too late. Anyone can fail to meet goals. Negative self-talk makes it easy to fail in the future. A more appropriate response is **positive self-talk,** such as "I'm not going to eat anything else tonight; I can do it."

Web Resources

Web 08

American Dietetic Association **www.eatright.org**
Berkeley Nutrition Sciences **www.nutritionquest.com**
Center for Science in the Public Interest
   www.cspinet.org
Fast Food Facts: Interactive Food Finder **www.olen.com/food**
Meals Online **www.my-meals.com**
Office of Dietary Supplements **http://ods.od.nih.gov**
USDA Food and Nutrition Information Center
   www.nal.usda.gov/fnic

Online Learning Center

www.mhhe.com/corbin7e
The Online Learning Center contains a variety of Web-based resources that will help you get the most out of this book and your course. In addition to the On the Web pages, there are video activities, interactive quizzes, application assignments, and a variety of other useful study aids. Log on to the URL above to access these resources.

Negative Self-Talk Self-defeating discussions with yourself focusing on your failures rather than your successes.

Positive Self-Talk Telling yourself positive, encouraging things that help you succeed in accomplishing your goals.

Suggested Readings

Web 09

Additional reference materials for Concept 15 are available at Web09.

American College of Sports Medicine. 2001. Appropriate intervention strategies for weight loss and prevention of weight regain for adults. *Medicine and Science in Sports and Exercise* 33(12):2145–2156.

Foster, G. D., et al. 2003. A randomized trial of a low-carbohydrate diet for obesity. *New England Journal of Medicine* 348(21):2082–2090.

Frank, L. D. 2004. Obesity relationships with community design, physical activity, and time spent in cars. *American Journal of Preventive Medicine* 27(2):87–96.

Howard, B. V., et al. 2006. Low fat dietary pattern and weight change over 7 years. *Journal of the American Medical Association* 295(1):39–49.

Jakicic, J. M. and A. D. Otto. 2005. Motivating change: Modifying eating and exercise behaviors for weight management. *ACSM's Health and Fitness Journal* 9(1):6–12.

Kruskall, L. J. 2006. Portion distortion. Sizing up food servings. *ACSM's Health and Fitness Journal* 10(3):8–14.

Miller, G. D. 2005. Your clients are what they eat: Balancing weight with diet 2005. *ACSM's Health and Fitness Journal* 9(1):13–18.

Riebe, R., et al. 2005. Long-term maintenance of exercise and healthy eating behaviors in overweight adults. *Preventive Medicine* 40(6):769–778.

Samaha, F. F., et al. 2003. A low-carbohydrate as compared with a low-fat diet in severe obesity. *New England Journal of Medicine* 348(21):2074–2081.

Schlosser, E. 2001. *Fast Food Nation: The Dark Side of the All-American Meal.* New York: Houghton Mifflin.

Winett, R. A., et al. 2005. Long-term weight gain prevention: A theoretically based Internet approach. *Preventive Medicine* 41(2):629–641.

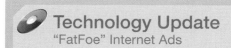

Technology Update
"FatFoe" Internet Ads

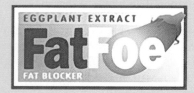

The Federal Trade Commission (FTC) has decided to fight fire with fire. It has started to post ads for a new weight loss product called FatFoe on the Internet. It makes the *same promises* as other products ("wouldn't it be nice to have the trim, shapely figure you've always wanted without having to diet or exercise? NOW—FINALLY—YOU CAN!"). It also makes some of the *same guarantees* ("FatFoe™ is GUARANTEED to work for everyone—regardless of how much you eat, regardless of how much you'd like to lose.").

One feature makes this ad different. When consumers try to click on the Web site to order or learn more, they are informed that the ad is completely bogus. The FTC is using this ad to promote awareness about how to spot fraudulent weight loss products. Go to the FatFoe Web site to learn how to spot fraudulent weight loss products (**http://wemarket4u.net/fatfoe/**).

In the News

Nutrition Policies Aimed at Promoting Healthier Diets

The epidemic of obesity has led to many public health efforts to promote healthy lifestyle behaviors.

A law passed as part of the federal school lunch assistance program has required schools to adopt formal wellness policies that specify what foods can be provided in lunches and in vending machines. The policies also stipulate the type, amount, and extent of physical activity programming in schools (e.g., physical education, recess, and after-school programs). A unique and beneficial aspect of the policy is that it stipulates that each district establish a local wellness council to help support physical activity and nutrition programming and policies.

Another new policy initiative is an agreement by soft drink manufacturers to stop providing full-calorie soft drinks in public schools by the year 2010. This agreement was negotiated and coordinated by the Clinton Foundation to help reduce the access to soft drinks (and marketing) during school. The agreement was likely facilitated by concerns that it may prove difficult and costly to comply with the new vending requirements in each school. These are just a few of the examples of new policies related to nutrition and health.

Lab 15A Selecting Strategies for Managing Eating

Name   Section   Date

Purpose: To learn to select strategies for managing eating to control body fatness

Procedures

1. Read the strategies listed in Chart 1.
2. Make a check in the box beside 5 to 10 of the strategies that you think will be most useful to you.
3. Answer the questions in the Conclusions and Implications section.

Chart 1 ▶ Strategies for Managing Eating to Control Body Fatness

✔	**Check 5 to 10 strategies that you might use in the future.**
	Shopping Strategies
	Shop from a list.
	Shop with a friend.
	Shop on a full stomach.
	Check food labels.
	Consider foods that take some time to prepare.
	Methods of Eating
	When you eat, do nothing but eat. Don't watch television or read.
	Eat slowly.
	Do not eat food you do not want.
	Follow an eating schedule.
	Do your eating in designated areas, such as kitchen or dining room only.
	Leave the table after eating.
	Avoid second servings.
	Limit servings of condiments.
	Limit servings of nonbasics, such as dessert, breads, and soft drinks.
	Eat several meals of equal size rather than one big meal and two small ones.
	Eating in the Work Environment
	Take your own food to work.
	Avoid snack machines.
	If you eat out, plan your meal ahead of time.
	Do not eat while working.
	Avoid sharing foods from co-workers, such as birthday cakes.
	Have activity breaks during the day.
	Have water available to substitute for soft drinks.
	Have low-calorie snacks to substitute for office snacks.

✔	**Check 5 to 10 strategies that you might use in the future.**
	Eating on Special Occasions
	Practice ways to refuse food.
	Avoid tempting situations.
	Eat before you go out.
	Don't stand near food sources.
	If you feel the urge to eat, find someone to talk to.
	Strategies for Eating Out
	Limit deep-fat fried foods.
	Ask for information about food content.
	Limit use of condiments.
	Choose low-fat foods (e.g., skim milk, low-fat yogurt).
	Choose chicken, fish, or lean meat.
	Order á la carte.
	If you eat desserts, avoid those with sauces or toppings.
	Eating at Home
	Keep busy at times when you are at risk of overeating.
	Store food out of sight.
	Avoid serving food to others between meals.
	If you snack, choose snacks with complex carbohydrates, such as carrot sticks or apple slices.
	Freeze leftovers to avoid the temptation of eating them between meals.

Conclusions and Implications

1. In several sentences, discuss your need to use strategies for effective eating. Do you need to use them? Why or why not?

2. In several sentences, discuss the effectiveness of the strategies contained in Chart 1. Do you think they can be effective for people who have a problem controlling their body fatness?

3. In several sentences, discuss the value of using behavioral goals versus outcome goals when planning for fat loss.

Lab 15B Evaluating Fast-Food Options

Name		**Section**	**Date**

Purpose: To learn about the energy and fat content of fast food and how to make better choices when eating at fast-food restaurants

Procedures

1. Using Appendix B, select a fast-food restaurant and a typical meal you might order there.
2. Record the total calories, fat calories, saturated fat intake, and cholesterol for each food item.
3. Sum up the totals for the meal in Chart 2.
4. Record recommended daily values by selecting an amount from Chart 1. Estimate should be based on your estimated needs for the day.
5. Compute the percentage of the daily recommended amounts that you consume in the meal by dividing recommended amounts (step 4) into meal totals (step 3). Record percent of recommended daily amounts in Chart 2.
6. Answer the questions in the Conclusions and Implications section.

Chart 1 ▶ Recommended Daily Amounts of Fat, Saturated Fat, Cholesterol, and Sodium

	2,000 kcal	3,000 kcal
Total fat	65 g	97.5 g
Saturated fat	20 g	30 g
Cholesterol	300 mg	450 mg
Sodium	2,400 mg	3,600 g

Results

Chart 2 ▶ Listing of Foods Selected for the Meal

Food Item	Total Calories	Total Fat (g)	Saturated Fat (g)	Cholesterol (mg)
1.				
2.				
3.				
4.				
5.				
6.				
Total for meal (sum up each column)				
Recommended daily amount (record your values from Chart 1)				
% of recommended daily amount (record your % of recommended)				

Conclusions and Implications:

1. Describe how often you eat at fast-food restaurants and indicate whether you would like to reduce how much fast food you consume.

2. Were you surprised at the amount of fat, saturated fat, and cholesterol in the meal you selected?

3. What could you do differently at fast-food restaurants to reduce your intake of fat, saturated fat, and cholesterol?

Stress and Health

Health Goals for the year 2010

- Improve mental health and ensure access to appropriate, quality mental health services.

- Increase mental health treatment, including treatment for depression and anxiety disorders.

- Increase mental health screening and assessment.

- Reduce suicide and suicide attempts, especially among young people.

- Increase availability of worksite stress-reduction programs.

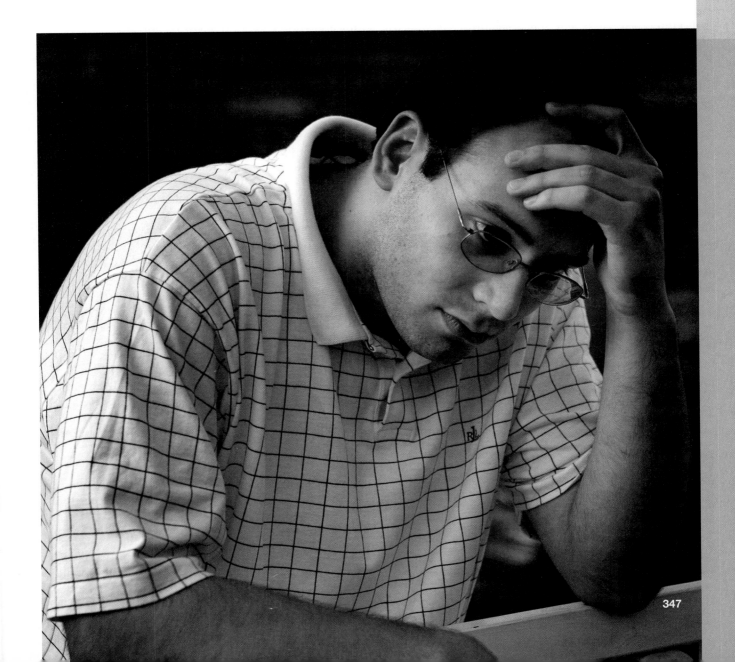

347

Mental and physical health are affected by an individual's ability to adapt to stress.

Stress affects everyone to some degree. In fact, approximately 67 percent of adults indicate that they experience "great stress" at least 1 day a week. **Stressors** come in many forms, and even positive life events can increase our stress levels.

At moderate levels, stress can motivate us to reach our goals and keep life interesting. However, when stressors are severe or chronic, our bodies may not be able to adapt successfully. Stress can compromise immune functioning, leading to a host of diseases of **adaptation.** In fact, stress has been linked to between 50 and 70 percent of all illnesses. Further, stress is associated with negative health behaviors, such as alcohol and other drug use, and to psychological problems, such as depression and anxiety. Although all humans have the same physiological system for responding to stress, stress reactivity varies across individuals. In addition, the way we think about or perceive stressful situations has a significant impact on how our bodies respond. Thus, there are large individual differences in responses to stress.

This concept will review the causes and consequences of stress. Figure 1 illustrates the many factors involved in individual reactions to stress. First, the sources of stress, (stressors) such as daily hassles and major life events, will be described. Then the physiological responses to stress and the impact of these effects on physical and mental health will be reviewed. Finally, individual differences in physiological and cognitive responses to stress and the implications of these individual differences for health and wellness will be discussed.

Sources of Stress

The first step in managing stress is to recognize the causes and to be aware of the symptoms. You need to recognize the factors in your life that cause stess. Identify the things that make you feel "stressed-

out." Everything from minor irritations, such as traffic jams, to major life changes, such as births, deaths, or job loss, can be a stressor. A stress overload of too many demands on your time can make you feel that you are no longer in control. You may feel so overwhelmed that you become depressed. Recognizing the causes and effects of stress is important for learning how to manage it.

Stress has a variety of sources. There are many kinds of stressors. Environmental stressors include heat, noise, overcrowding, climate, and terrain. Physiological stressors are such things as drugs, caffeine, tobacco, injury, infection or disease, and physical effort.

Emotional stressors are the most frequent and important stressors. Some people refer to these as psychosocial stressors. These include life-changing events, such as a change in work hours or line of work, family illnesses, deaths of relatives or friends, and increased responsibilities. In school, pressures such as grades, term papers, and oral presentations induce stress. A national study of daily experiences indicated that more than 60 percent of all stressful experiences fall into a few areas (see Table 1).

Stressors vary in severity. Because stressors vary in magnitude and duration, many experts categorize them by severity. Major stressors create major emotional turmoil or require tremendous amounts of adjustment. This category includes personal crises (e.g., major health problems or death in the family, divorce/separation, financial problems, legal problems) and job/school-related pressures or major age-related transitions (e.g., college, marriage, career, retirement). Minor stressors are generally viewed as shorter-term or less severe. This category includes events or problems such as traffic hassles, peer/work relations, time pressures, and family squabbles. Major stressors can alter daily patterns of stress and impair our ability to handle the minor stressors of life, while minor stressors can accumulate and create more significant problems. It is important to be aware of both types of stressors.

Negative, ambiguous, and uncontrollable events are usually the most stressful. Although stress can come from both positive and negative events, negative ones generally cause more distress because negative stressors usually have harsher consequences and little benefit. Positive stressors, on the other hand, usually have enough benefit to make them worthwhile. For example,

On the Web

www.mhhe.com/corbinweb

Web 01   Log on to this URL before reading this concept. See On the Web list of concepts. Click on the concept number you want to view. To access supplemental information, click on the number shown at each Web icon.

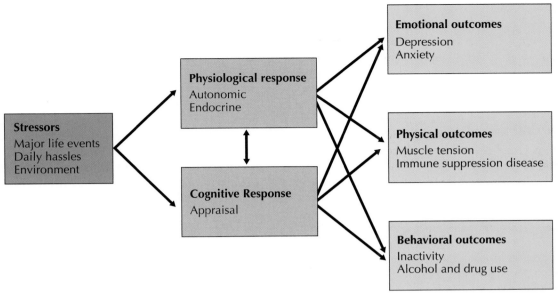

Figure 1 ▶ Reactions to stress.

although the stress of getting ready for a wedding may be tremendous, it is not as bad as the negative stress associated with losing a job.

Table 1 ▶ Ten Common Stressors in the Lives of College Students and Middle-Aged Adults

College Students	Middle-Aged Adults
1. Troubling thoughts about the future	1. Concerns about weight
2. Not getting enough sleep	2. Health of a family member
3. Wasting time	3. Rising prices of common goods
4. Inconsiderate smokers	4. Home maintenance (interior)
5. Physical appearance	5. Too many things to do
6. Too many things to do	6. Misplacing or losing things
7. Misplacing or losing things	7. Yard work or outside home maintenance
8. Not enough time to do the things you need to do	8. Property, investments, or taxes
9. Concerns about meeting high standards	9. Crime
10. Being lonely	10. Physical appearance

Source: Kanner, et al.

Ambiguous stressors are harder to accept than are more clearly defined problems. In most cases, if the cause of a stressor or problem can be identified, active measures can be taken to improve the situation. For example, if you are stressed about a project at work or school, you can use specific strategies to help you complete the task on time. Stress brought on by a relationship with friends or co-workers, on the other hand, may be harder to understand. In some cases, it is not possible to determine the primary source or cause of the problem. These situations are more problematic because fewer clear-cut solutions exist.

Another factor that makes events stressful is a lack of control. Stress brought on by illness, accidents, or natural disasters fit into this category. Because little can be done to change the situation, these events leave us feeling powerless. If the stressor is something that can be dealt with more directly, efforts at minimizing the stress are likely to be effective.

Stress The nonspecific response (generalized adaptation) of the body to any demand made on it in order to maintain physiological equilibrium. This positive or negative response results from emotions that are accompanied by biochemical and physiological changes directed at adaptation.

Stressors Things that place a greater than routine demand on the body or evoke a stress reaction.

Adaptation The body's efforts to restore normalcy.

The nature and magnitude of stressors change during the life span. Depending on your perspective, some periods in life are more stressful than others, but each phase has its own challenges and experiences. Some argue that adolescence represents the most stressful time of life. Drastic changes in a person's body and numerous psychosocial challenges must be overcome. College provides additional mental challenges as well as financial pressures and the pressures of living independently. During the early adult years, tremendous pressures and responsibilities force you to juggle career and family obligations. Late adulthood presents still other new challenges, such as coping with declining functioning or illness. Although the nature of the stressor changes, the presence of stress remains consistent.

College presents unique challenges and stressors. For college students, schoolwork can be a full-time job, and those who have to work outside of school must handle the stresses of both jobs. Although the college years are often thought of as a break from the stresses of the real world, college life has its own stressors. Obvious sources of stress include taking exams, speaking in public, and becoming comfortable with talking to professors. Students are often living independently of family for the first time while negotiating new relationships—with roommates, dating partners, and so on. Young people entering college are also faced with a less structured environment and with the need to control their own schedules. Though this environment has a number of advantages, students are faced with a greater need to manage their stress effectively.

In addition to the traditional challenges of college, the new generation of students faces stressors that were not typical for college students in the past. According to the American Council on Education, only 40 percent of today's college students enroll full-time immediately after high school. Once in college, more students now work to support their studies, and many go back to school after spending time in the working world. These students are likely to have additional pressures not characteristic of the typical college student. Further, more of today's students are the first in their families to go to college. This may place additional pressure on these students to succeed. Perhaps as a result of some of these factors, rates of mental health problems among college students have increased dramatically (see Figure 2). A study from the American College Health Association indicated that 10 percent of college students are diagnosed with depression. In another study, 53 percent of students reported feeling depressed at some point during their college careers and 9 percent reported considering suicide. Although more people are receiving care for mental health problems than in the past, the vast majority are still not receiving adequate care. University counseling centers are typically understaffed and unable to handle the increasing number of college students seeking mental health services.

Reactions to Stress

All people have a general reaction to stress. In the early 1900s, Walter Cannon identified the fight-or-flight response to threat. According to his model, the body reacts to a threat by preparing to either fight or flee the situation. The body prepares for either option through the activation of the **sympathetic nervous system (SNS).** When the SNS is activated, epinephrine (adrenaline) and norepinephrine are released to focus attention on the task at hand. Heart rate and blood pressure increase to deliver oxygen to the muscles and essential organs, the eyes take in more light to increase visual acuity, and more sugar is released into the bloodstream to increase energy level. At the same time, nonessential functions like digestion and urine production are slowed. Figure 3 depicts some of the many physiological changes that occur during this process. Once the immediate threat has passed, the **parasympathetic nervous system (PNS)** takes over in an attempt to restore the body to homeostasis and conserve resources. The PNS largely reverses the changes initiated by the SNS (e.g., slows heart rate and returns blood from the muscles and essential organs to the periphery).

Sometimes the fight-or-flight or SNS response is essential to survival but, when invoked inappropriately or excessively, it may be more harmful than the effects of the original stressor. Hans Selye, another prominent scientist, was the first to recognize the potential negative consequences of this response. Selye suggested that this system could be invoked by mental as well as physical threats and that the short-term benefits might lead to long-term negative consequences. Based on these ideas, Selye described the general adaptation syndrome, which

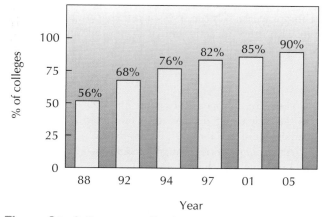

Figure 2 ▶ Colleges reporting increased psychological problems.

Source: R. Gallagher.

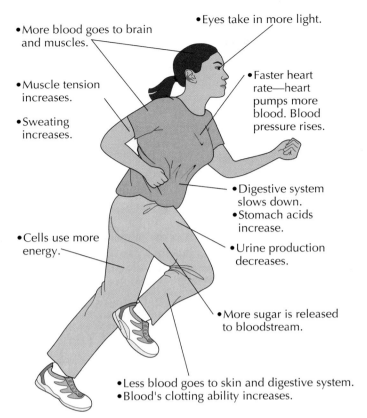

- More blood goes to brain and muscles.
- Eyes take in more light.
- Muscle tension increases.
- Faster heart rate—heart pumps more blood. Blood pressure rises.
- Sweating increases.
- Digestive system slows down.
- Stomach acids increase.
- Cells use more energy.
- Urine production decreases.
- More sugar is released to bloodstream.
- Less blood goes to skin and digestive system.
- Blood's clotting ability increases.

Figure 3 ▶ Physical symptoms of stress.

Table 2 ▶ The Three Stages in the General Adaptation Syndrome

Stage 1: Alarm Reaction
Any physical or mental trauma triggers an immediate set of reactions that combat the stress. Because the immune system is initially depressed, normal levels of resistance are lowered, making us more susceptible to infection and disease. If the stress is not severe or long-lasting, we bounce back and recover rapidly.

Stage 2: Resistance
Eventually, sometimes rather quickly, we adapt to stress, and we tend to become more resistant to illness and disease. The immune system works overtime during this period, keeping up with the demands placed on it.

Stage 3: Exhaustion
Because the body is not able to maintain homeostasis and the long-term resistance needed to combat stress, we invariably experience a drop in resistance level. No one experiences the same resistance and tolerance to stress, but everyone's immunity at some point collapses following prolonged stress reactions.

Source: Health News Network.

explains how the autonomic nervous system reacts to stressful situations and the conditions under which the system may break down (Table 2). The term *general* highlights the similarities in response to stressful situations across individuals. Seyle's work led him to be referred to as the "father of stress."

Although chronic activation of the SNS is still believed to be important in the development of physical disease, other important systems in the body are also involved. For example, the hypothalamic-pituitary-adrenal (HPA) axis is activated during stress, leading to the release of corticotropin-releasing hormone (CRH) and secondary activation of the pituitary gland. The pituitary releases a chemical called adrenocorticotropic hormone (ACTH) which ultimately causes the release of an active stress hormone called cortisol. With chronic exposure to stress, the HPA system can become dysregulated. Both over- and under-activation of the HPA-axis is associated with risk for negative health outcomes.

Individuals respond differently to stress. Individuals exposed to high levels of stress are most at risk for negative health consequences. At the same time, not everyone exposed to severe or chronic stress will experience negative outcomes. Those with positive health outcomes despite high levels of stress are said to be "resilient" and have been the subject of study. There is obviously more to the stress-illness relationship than the total number or severity of stressors. What makes an individual more or less susceptible to negative stress-related outcomes?

Two important areas in which individuals differ are stress reactivity and stress appraisals. Stress reactivity is the extent to which the sympathetic nervous system, or fight-or-flight system, is activated by a stressor, whereas stress appraisals are an individual's perceptions of a stressor and the person's resources for managing stressful situations. These individual differences are partly due to inherited predispositions and partly due to our unique histories of experiencing and attempting to cope with stress. Recognizing these individual differences has important implications for our well-being because knowledge of our own response to stressful situations can increase our awareness of the impact of stress and can provide information that may lead to more effective stress management.

Sympathetic Nervous System (SNS) The component of the autonomic nervous system that responds to stressful situations by initiating the fight-or-flight response.

Parasympathetic Nervous System (PNS) The component of the autonomic nervous system that helps bring the body to a resting state following stressful experiences.

Everyone has an optimal level of arousal. We all need sufficient stress to motivate us to engage in activities that make our lives meaningful. Otherwise, we would be in a state of **hypostress,** which leads to apathy, boredom, and less than optimal health and wellness. An example of hypostress is a person working on an assembly line. Because the same task is repeated without variation, the level of stimulation is quite low and might lead to a state of boredom and job dissatisfaction. It has also been suggested that increased rates of property crime in the summer months might be due to hypostress because adolescents are out of school and have insufficient stress or stimulation due to the lack of school-related activities. In fact, a certain level of stress, called **eustress,** is experienced positively. In contrast, **distress** is a level of stress that compromises performance and well-being. Each of us possesses a system that allows us to mobilize resources when necessary and that seeks to find a homeostatic level of arousal (see Figure 4). Although we all have an optimal level of arousal, the optimal level varies considerably. What one person finds stressful another may find exhilarating. Stress mobilizes some to greater efficiency, while it confuses others. For example, riding a roller coaster is thrilling for some people, but for others it is a stressful and unpleasant experience.

Level of arousal exists on a continuum with all possible gradations, but the extreme ends of the spectrum illustrate the marked differences across individuals. At one end of the continuum are those who find even moderate levels of arousal stressful or anxiety-provoking. Behavior-

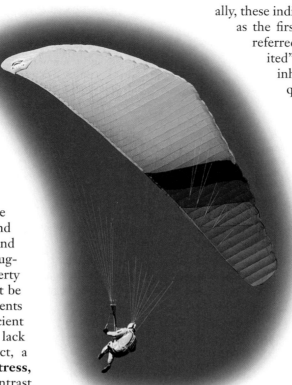

One person's stress is another's pleasure.

ally, these individuals can be identified as early as the first year of life and are generally referred to as temperamentally "inhibited" or "withdrawn." Although an inhibited individual may function quite well in the right environment, such a person is susceptible to a number of emotional disorders, including anxiety and depression.

At the other end of the continuum are those who prefer a very high level of arousal. The characteristics associated with an increased enjoyment of highly stimulating situations include sensation seeking, novelty seeking, and impulsivity. Although individuals with high levels of these characteristics may be able to withstand higher levels of stress, they are also at increased risk for unhealthy lifestyles (e.g., alcohol, nicotine, and other drug use; unprotected sexual behavior; aggressiveness) and the associated health consequences.

Stress Responses and Health

Chronic or repetitive acute stress can lead to fatigue and can cause or exacerbate a variety of health problems. Some stress persists only as long as the stressor is present. For example, job-related stress caused by a challenging project generally subsides once that project is complete. In contrast, exposure to chronic stress or repeated exposure to acute stress may lead to a state of fatigue. Fatigue may result from lack of sleep, emotional strain, pain, disease, or a combination of these factors. Both **physiological fatigue** and **psychological fatigue** can result in a state of exhaustion, with resultant physical and mental health consequences. Chronic stress has been linked to health maladies that plague individuals on a daily basis, such as headaches, indigestion, insomnia, and the common cold. In fact, one study concluded that out-of-control stress is the leading preventable source of increased health-care cost in the workforce, roughly equivalent to the costs of the health problems related to smoking.

Even illnesses with a substantial genetic component, such as cardiovascular disease and depression, have been linked to stress. One model (the diathesis-stress

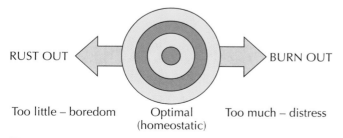

RUST OUT ⟵   ⟶ BURN OUT

Too little – boredom   Optimal   Too much – distress
(homeostatic)

Figure 4 ▶ Stress target zone.

model) suggests that individuals with a genetic, or biological, predisposition for a particular illness will express that illness only when environmental stresses are sufficient. Hypertension is a good example. Although there is a strong genetic component to hypertension, not all individuals with a genetic risk will experience the condition.

Excessive stress reduces the effectiveness of the immune system. In addition to preparing the body for fight or flight, the stress-related activation of the SNS and the HPA axis slow down the functioning of the immune response. In the face of an immediate threat, mobilizing resources that will help in the moment is more important to the body than preventing or fighting infection. As a result, if the stress response is chronically activated, high levels of adrenaline and cortisol continue to tell the body to mobilize resources at the expense of immune functioning. The suppression of immune function by the stress response can lead to a host of both short-term and long-term health consequences. In the short term, stress can lead to increased risk for the common cold and make existing conditions, such as allergies or asthma worse. In the long term, persistently elevated levels of stress increase risk for gastrointestinal problems and heart disease. Elevated blood pressure and cholesterol levels associated with chronic stress may account for the increased risk for heart disease.

Stress can have mental and emotional effects. The challenges caused by psychosocial stress may lead to a variety of mental and emotional effects. In the short term, stress can impair concentration and attention span. Anxiety is an emotional response to stress characterized by apprehension. Because the response usually involves expending a lot of nervous energy, anxiety can lead to fatigue and muscular tension.

Anxiety may persist long after a stressful experience. For example, many who were living in New Orleans when Hurricane Katrina struck in 2005 may continue to experience distress related to this event years later. In some cases, traumatic experiences lead to posttraumatic stress disorder (PTSD). Symptoms of PTSD include flashbacks of the traumatic event, avoidance of situations that remind the person of the event, emotional numbing, and increased level of arousal.

People who are excessively stressed are also more likely to be depressed than people who have optimal amounts of stress in their lives. Health-care costs for depressed people are 70 percent higher than for those who are not. Research has shown that drugs commonly prescribed to reduce depression can be effective in many cases. However, drugs do not get to the source of the life stressors that cause depression, and many have negative side effects.

Stress can alter both positive and negative lifestyles. Stress can cause people to adopt nervous habits, such as biting their nails. It can also cause normally calm people to become irritable and short-tempered. Other behavioral responses to stress include altered eating and sleeping patterns, smoking, and the use of alcohol and other drugs. In addition to increased tendencies for negative behavior, stress can result in engaging in fewer positive behaviors, such as regular physical activity and sufficient sleep.

Reactions to stress depend on one's appraisal of both the event and the subsequent physiological response. Stressors by themselves generally do not cause problems unless they are perceived as stressful. Appraisal usually involves consideration of the consequences of the situation (primary appraisal) and an evaluation of the resources available to cope with the situation (secondary appraisal). If one sees a stressor as a challenge that can be tackled, one is likely to respond in a more positive manner than if the stressor is viewed as an obstacle that cannot be overcome.

The events that occurred on September 11, 2001, provide a vivid example of the very different reactions that people have to the same or similar stressors. Everyone who witnessed these events, in person or on television, was profoundly impacted. At the same time, individual reactions varied dramatically. Most felt overwhelming sadness, many felt extreme anger, others felt hopeless or desperate, and yet others felt lost or confused. Undoubtedly, there were some that were simply too shocked to process their emotional experience at all. With time, most Americans began to experience a wave of additional emotions, such as hope, patriotism, courage, and determination. Others were less quick to experience these positive emotions and many developed anxiety, depression, or posttraumatic stress disorder. All of these emotions were

---

Hypostress Insufficient levels of stress leading to boredom or apathy.

Eustress Positive stress, or stress that is mentally or physically stimulating.

Distress Negative stress, or stress that contributes to health problems.

Physiological Fatigue A deterioration in the capacity of the neuromuscular system as a result of physical overwork and strain; also referred to as true fatigue.

Psychological Fatigue A feeling of fatigue, usually caused by such things as lack of exercise, boredom, or mental stress, that results in a lack of energy and depression; also referred to as subjective or false fatigue.

reactions to the same stressful events. Although a number of factors contributed to these individual differences (e.g., proximity to New York City or personal relationships with individuals who lost their lives), differences in appraisals of the events were probably responsible for much of the variability.

In addition to the appraisal of the event, one's appraisal of the body's response to an event is important. The way in which bodily sensations are interpreted has a significant impact on how one will react emotionally and behaviorally. For example, public speaking is a situation that leads to significant autonomic arousal for most people. Those who handle these situations well probably recognize that these sensations are normal and may even interpret them as excitement about the situations. In contrast, those who experience severe and sometimes debilitating anxiety are probably interpreting the same sensations as indicators of fear, panic, and loss of control. The combination of individual differences in stress reactivity and appraisals may lead to characteristic ways of responding to stress that either confer risk or protect against risk for physical and mental health problems. In fact, several different patterns of behavior (or personality styles) have been clearly identified. These patterns have been shown to influence stress responses and associated health outcomes.

Type A and Type D Personality may increase risk for negative health outcomes. The best known "personality" style associated with risk for negative health outcomes is the **Type A** behavior pattern. Several decades ago psychologists Friedman and Rosenman identified a subgroup of goal-oriented or "driven" patients who they believed were at increased risk based on their pattern of behavior. These individuals demonstrated a sense of time urgency, were highly competitive, and had a tendency to experience and express anger and hostility under conditions of stress. In contrast, individuals with the Type B behavior pattern were relatively easy going, and less reactive to stress. Although early research on Type A behavior demonstrated increased risk for heart disease, it now appears that certain aspects of the Type A behavior pattern pose greater risk than others. In particular, hostility and anger appear to be consistently associated with risk for cardiovascular disease. Although most studies have not found time urgency or competitiveness predictive of risk for cardiovascular disease, a recent study found that people who scored highly on a measure of impatience were nearly twice as likely to have high blood pressure relative to individuals lower on this trait. At the same time, there is evidence that certain aspects of the Type A behavior pattern (other than hostility) lead to higher levels of achievement and an increased sense of personal accomplishment. Although the type A behavior pattern has often been referred to as Type A personality, it was

not the intention of those who developed the concept to identify a "personality type." In contrast, the more recently identified **Type D,** or "distressed," personality is associated with two well-defined personality characteristics based on personality theory. Individuals with Type D personality are characterized by high levels of "negative affectivity" or negative emotion, and "social inhibition," or the tendency not to express negative emotions in social interactions. The combination of these characteristics appears to comprise risk for cardiovascular disease and other negative health outcomes. Converging evidence from recent research on both Type A and Type D has led some to conclude that negative affectivity, in general, is a more important risk for negative health outcomes than any emotion in particular. In other words, anger and hostility (Type A), as well as anxiety and depressed mood (Type D), pose a health risk.

Some characteristics may improve responses to stress and promote positive health outcomes. Several general styles of reacting to stress have been shown to be associated with more favorable health profiles and health outcomes. Examples include hardiness, optimism, and an internal locus of control.

Hardiness

Hardiness is a collection of characteristics that have been associated with more favorable reactions to stressful situations. Individuals possessing hardiness have been found to appraise and respond to stress in more favorable ways than people without it. Research in a college population indicates that individuals who have high levels of hardiness are at reduced risk for illness, due to the way they perceive stress and the coping mechanisms they use in response to stressful situations. The dimensions of hardiness are

Commitment: Although stress cannot be avoided, a sense of commitment to your life and your aspirations can make stress more tolerable. Hardy individuals possess a strong sense of commitment and are willing to put up with adversity to keep pushing toward their desired goals.

Challenge: Hardy individuals see new responsibilities and situations as challenges rather than stressors. With this perspective, new situations become opportunities for growth rather than chances for failure.

Control: Rather than easily giving up when situations seem out of control, hardy individuals find ways to assume control over their problems. Being proactive rather than reactive is an effective strategy for combating stress. It is important to acknowledge that many stressors may be out of your control. In these cases it may be necessary to use other coping strategies.

Optimism

Research supports the idea that **optimism** relates to psychological well-being. Positive emotion may also be an effective coping mechanism for managing acute stress. Positive moods seem to help undo the effects of negative emotion. For example, positive moods have been shown to undo some of the cardiovascular effects associated with negative emotions. Positive moods may also help individuals effectively use additional coping strategies to manage stress.

Locus of Control

People with an internal **locus of control** generally believe that they have the capacity to impact the outcomes of stressful events. In contrast, individuals with an external locus of control generally believe that outcomes are determined by factors other than personal control (e.g., luck, fate, powerful others). You can evaluate your own locus of control in Lab 16C.

An individual's locus of control can have a significant impact on how he or she responds to a stressful situation Research has consistently found that having an internal locus of control is associated with better health outcomes. People with an internal locus of control are more likely to take steps to address the problems that created the stress, rather than avoiding the problem. Those with an external locus of control are more likely to use passive methods for managing stress. In addition, an external locus of control is related to higher perceived levels of stress, lower job satisfaction, and poorer school achievements.

Interestingly, locus of control in the United States has become increasingly external over the past 40 years. A recent study found that the average college student had a more external locus of control than 80 percent of college students in the early 1960s. The authors concluded that these changes were due to increased levels of alienation from society accompanied by increases in cynicism and individualism. They further suggested that increases in external locus of control may have contributed to increases in levels of depression, anxiety, and other negative outcomes.

Although an internal locus of control generally promotes health, this is not always the case. This truth is apparent in depressed individuals with a pessimistic explanatory style. They believe that their failures are due to internal factors, squarely placing the control of these events within themselves. Even though they believe stressors are under their control, they don't believe in their ability to initiate change. Thus, for an internal locus of control to be beneficial to well-being, it must be combined with the belief that one is capable of making changes to prevent future problems. The belief in one's ability to reach a desired goal is often referred to as **self-efficacy.**

Type A Personality The personality type characterized by impatience, ambition, and aggression; Type A personalities may be more susceptible to the effects of stress but may also be more able to cope with stress.

Type D Personality The personality type characterized by high levels of negative emotion and the tendency to withhold expression of these emotions.

Hardiness A collection of personality traits thought to make a person more resistant to stress.

Optimism The tendency to have a positive outlook on life or a belief that things will work out favorably.

Locus of Control The extent to which we believe the outcomes of events are under our control (internal locus) or outside our personal control (external locus).

Self-Efficacy The belief in one's ability to take action that will lead to the attainment of a goal.

Strategies for Action

Learning stress management skills can help you respond more effectively to stress. Personality characteristics have been associated with both positive and negative health outcomes. The following are some obvious questions based on this information: "Can a person change his or her personality?" "Can a pessimist become an optimist?" "Can someone develop an internal locus of control or become a more hardy individual?" Although overall personality structure has proven somewhat resistant to change, it is certainly possible to change both the physiological and the cognitive responses and the resulting emotional, physi-

cal, and behavioral outcomes depicted in Figure 1 at the beginning of this concept. Learning and practicing effective stress-management techniques will help you handle stress better and will contribute to improved health and wellness.

Self-assessments of stressors in your life can be useful in managing stress. You will have the opportunity to evaluate your stress levels using the Life Experience Survey; to assess your hardiness, a characteristic associated with effectively coping with stress; and to evaluate your locus of control in the labs that follow.

Online Learning Center

Web Resources

Web 04

American Institute of Stress **www.stress.org**
International Stress Management Association **www.isma.org**
Medicinenet.com **www.emedicinenet.com/stress/article.htm**
Medline Plus Health Information from the National Library of Medicine **www.medlineplus.gov/stress.html**
National Center for Post Traumatic Stress Disorder **www.ncptsd.org**
National Institute for Occupational Safety and Health **www.cdc.gov/niosh/stresswk.html**
National Mental Health Information Center **www.mentalhealth.samhsa.gov**
Stress and Health **www.stress-and-health.com**
Ulifeline: The online behavioral support system for young adults **www.ulifeline.org**

Suggested Readings

Additional reference materials for Concept 16 are available at Web05.

Web 05

Benson, H. 2006. Mind-Body Pioneer. *Psychology Today*. Available on the Web at www.psychologytoday.com, click stress.

Blonna, R. 2007. *Coping with Stress in a Changing World*. 4th ed. New York: McGraw-Hill.

Fusilier, M., and M. R. Manning. 2005. Psychosocial predictors of health status revisited. *Journal of Behavioral Medicine* 28:347–358.

Greenberg, J. S. 2006. *Comprehensive Stress Management*. 9th ed. New York: McGraw-Hill.

Technology Update
New Technology for Monitoring Stress Hormones

The stress hormone cortisol has been shown to have a significant impact on physical health. Although there is currently no fast, easy way to monitor cortisol levels in humans, this may change in the near future. Researchers have developed a method for quickly testing salivary cortisol levels using a procedure much like that used in pregnancy tests. A plastic device contains a window that produces colored lines when saliva is applied. The first line is a test line, and the second line indicates low cortisol levels. Researchers are currently working on ways to estimate actual cortisol levels using this technology. This development would make it possible to easily monitor one of the most important stress-related hormones.

Maddux, J. E. 2002. Self-efficacy: The power of believing you can. In C. R. Snyder and S. J. Lopez (eds.). *Handbook of Positive Psychology*. New York: Oxford University Press.

Matthews, K. A. 2005. Psychological perspectives on the development of coronary heart disease. *American Psychologist* 60:783–796.

Pederson, S. S. and J. Denollet. 2003. Type D personality, cardiac events, and impaired quality of life: A review. *European Journal of Cardiovascular Prevention and Rehabilitation* 10:241–248.

Seligman, M. E. 1998. *Learned Optimism: How to Change Your Mind and Your Life*. New York: Pocket Books.

Selye, H. 1978. *The Stress of Life*. 2nd ed. New York: McGraw-Hill.

Tsigos, C., and G.P. Chrousos. 2002. Hypothalamic-pituitary-adrenal axis, neuroendocrine factors and stress. *Journal of Psychosomatic Research* 53(4):865–871.

Twinge, J. M., L. Zhang, and C. Im. 2004. It's beyond my control: A cross temporal meta-analysis of increasing externality of locus of control. 1960–2002. *Personality and Social Psychology Review* 8:308–319.

Williams, R. and V. Williams. 1999. *Anger Kills: 17 Strategies for Controlling Hostility That Can Harm You* New York: HarperCollins.

 In the News

Stress and the Aging Process

A new study provides scientific evidence to support a link between stress and accelerated aging. Researchers found that stress leads to more rapid deterioration of the chromosomes that normally decrease in number during the aging process. Telomeres are DNA-protein complexes located at the end of chromosomes; they promote stability. Telomerase is an enzyme that protects the chromosome by preserving telomere length. The researchers found that, the longer women had been caring for a sick child (a cause of chronic stress), the shorter their telomeres and the lower their levels of telomerase. As a result, at the cellular level, these women were prematurely aging. In addition to being important theoretically, this research has implications for early identification of the negative consequences of stress. Telomere length and telomerase levels may serve as markers for future health risk, allowing early identification and intervention with individuals experiencing chronic stress.

Lab 16A Evaluating Your Stress Level

Name	Section	Date

Purpose: To evaluate your stress during the past year and determine its implications

Procedures

1. Complete the Life Experience Survey based on your experiences during the past year. This survey lists a number of life events that may be distressful or eustressful. Read all of the items. If you did not experience an event, leave the box blank. In the box after each event that you did experience, write a number ranging from –3 to +3 using the scale described in the directions. Extra blanks are provided to write in positive or negative events not listed. Some items apply only to males or females. Items 48 to 56 are only for current college students.
2. Add all of the negative numbers and record your score (distress) in the Results section. Add the positive numbers and record your score (eustress) in the Results section. Use all of the events in the past year.
3. Find your scores on Chart 1 and record your ratings in the Results section.
4. Interpret the results by discussing the conclusions and implications in the space provided.

Results

Sum of negative scores [ ] (distress)   Rating on negative scores [ ]

Sum of positive scores [ ] (eustress)   Rating on positive scores [ ]

Chart 1 ▶ Scale for Life Experiences and Stress

	Sum of Negative Scores (Distress)	Sum of Positive Scores (Eustress)
May need counseling	14+	
Above average	9–13	11+
Average	6–8	9–10
Below average	<6	<9

Scoring the Life Experience Survey

1. Add all of the negative scores to arrive at your own distress score (negative stress).
2. Add all of the positive scores to arrive at a eustress score (positive stress).

Conclusions and Implications: In several sentences, discuss your current stress rating and its implications.

Life Experience Survey

Directions: If you did not experience an event, leave the box next to the event empty. If you experienced an event, enter a number in the box based on how the event impacted your life. Use the following scale:

Extremely negative impact	= −3
Moderately negative impact	= −2
Somewhat negative impact	= −1
Neither positive nor negative impact	= 0
Somewhat positive impact	= +1
Moderately positive impact	= +2
Extremely positive impact	= +3

1. Marriage

2. Detention in jail or comparable institution

3. Death of spouse

4. Major change in sleeping habits (much more or less sleep)

5. Death of close family member:

   a. Mother

   b. Father

   c. Brother

   d. Sister

   e. Child

   f. Grandmother

   g. Grandfather

   h. Other (specify) _____

6. Major change in eating habits (much more or much less food intake)

7. Foreclosure on mortgage or loan

8. Death of a close friend

9. Outstanding personal achievement

10. Minor law violation (traffic ticket, disturbing the peace, etc.)

11. *Male:* Wife's/girlfriend's pregnancy

    Female: Pregnancy

12. Changed work situation (different working conditions, working hours, etc.)

13. New job

14. Serious illness or injury of close family member:

    a. Father

    b. Mother

    c. Sister

    d. Brother

    e. Grandfather

    f. Grandmother

    g. Spouse

    h. Child

    i. Other (specify) _____

15. Sexual difficulties

16. Trouble with employer (in danger of losing job, being suspended, demoted, etc.)

17. Trouble with in-laws

18. Major change in financial status (a lot better off or a lot worse off)

19. Major change in closeness of family members (decreased or increased closeness)

20. Gaining a new family member (through birth, adoption, family member moving in, etc.)

21. Change of residence

22. Marital separation from mate (due to conflict)

23. Major change in church activities (increased or decreased attendance)

24. Marital reconciliation with mate

25. Major change in number of arguments with spouse (a lot more or a lot fewer arguments)

26. *Married male:* Change in wife's work outside the home (beginning work, ceasing work, changing to a new job)

    Married female: Change in husband's work (loss of job, beginning new job, retirement, etc.)

27. Major change in usual type and/or amount of recreation

28. Borrowing more than $10,000 (buying a home, business, etc.)

29. Borrowing less than $10,000 (buying car or TV, getting school loan, etc.)

30. Being fired from job

31. *Male:* Wife/girlfriend having abortion

    Female: Having abortion

32. Major personal illness or injury

33. Major change in social activities, such as parties, movies, visiting (increased or decreased participation)

34. Major change in living conditions of family (building new home, remodeling, deterioration of home or neighborhood, etc.)

35. Divorce

36. Serious injury or illness of close friend

37. Retirement from work

38. Son or daughter leaving home (due to marriage, college, etc.)

39. Ending of formal schooling

40. Separation from spouse (due to work, travel, etc.)

41. Engagement

42. Breaking up with boyfriend/girlfriend

43. Leaving home for the first time

44. Reconciliation with boyfriend/girlfriend

Other recent experiences that have had an impact on your life: list and rate.

45. _____

46. _____

47. _____

For Students Only

48. Beginning new school experience at a higher academic level (college, graduate school, professional school, etc.)

49. Changing to a new school at same academic level (undergraduate, graduate, etc.)

50. Academic probation

51. Being dismissed from dormitory or other residence

52. Failing an important exam

53. Changing a major

54. Failing a course

55. Dropping a course

56. Joining a fraternity/sorority

Source: Sarason, Johnson, and Siegel.

Lab 16B Evaluating Your Hardiness and Locus of Control

Name	Section	Date

Purpose: To evaluate your level of hardiness and locus of control and to help you identify the ways in which you appraise and respond to stressful situations

Procedures

1. Complete the Hardiness Questionnaire and the Locus of Control Questionnaire. Make an X over the circle that best describes what is true for you personally.
2. Compute the scale scores and record the values in the Results section.
3. Evaluate your scores using the Rating chart (Chart 1) and record your ratings in the Results section.
4. Interpret the results by answering the questions in the Conclusions and Implications section.

Hardiness Questionnaire

	Not True	Rarely True	Sometimes True	Often True	Score
1. I look forward to school and work on most days.	1	2	3	4	
2. Having too many choices in life makes me nervous.	4	3	2	1	
3. I know where my life is going and look forward to the future.	1	2	3	4	
4. I prefer to not get too involved in relationships.	4	3	2	1	
Commitment Score, Sum 1–4					
5. My efforts at school and work will pay off in the long run.	1	2	3	4	
6. I just have to trust my life to fate to be successful.	4	3	2	1	
7. I believe that I can make a difference in the world.	1	2	3	4	
8. Being successful in life takes more luck and good breaks than effort.	4	3	2	1	
Control Score, Sum 5–8					
9. I would be willing to work for less money if I could do something really challenging and interesting.	1	2	3	4	
10. I often get frustrated when my daily plans and schedule get altered.	4	3	2	1	
11. Experiencing new situations in life is important to me.	1	2	3	4	
12. I don't mind being bored.	4	3	2	1	
Challenge Score, Sum 9–12					

Locus of Control Questionnaire

					Score
13. Hard work usually pays off.	1	2	3	4	
14. Buying a lottery ticket is not worth the money.	1	2	3	4	
15. Even when I fail I keep trying.	1	2	3	4	
16. I am usually successful in what I do.	1	2	3	4	
17. I am in control of my own life.	1	2	3	4	
18. I make plans to be sure I am successful.	1	2	3	4	
19. I know where I stand with my friends.	1	2	3	4	
Locus of Control, Sum 13–19					

359

Results

Hardiness

Commitment score [ ]   Commitment rating [ ]

Control score [ ]   Control rating [ ]

Challenge score [ ]   Challenge rating [ ]

Hardiness score [ ]   Hardiness rating [ ]

Locus of Control

Locus of Control score [ ]   Locus of Control rating [ ]

Chart 1 ▶ Rating Chart

Rating	Individual Hardiness Scale Scores	Total Hardiness Score	Locus of Control Score
High	14–16	40–48	24–28
Moderate	10–13	30–39	12–23
Low	<10	<30	<12

Conclusions and Implications

1. In several sentences, discuss your commitment, control and challenge ratings, as well as your overall hardiness rating. Are they what you expected? Do you think they are true indications of you hardiness? Explain.

2. In several sentences, discuss your locus of control rating. Is it what you expected (a high rating indicates an internal locus of control)? Do you think your rating is a realistic indicator of your locus of control? Explain.

Stress Management, Relaxation, and Time Management

Health Goals for the year 2010

- Improve mental health and ensure access to appropriate, quality mental health services.

- Increase mental health treatment, including treatment for depression and anxiety disorders.

- Increase mental health screening and assessment.

- Reduce suicide and suicide attempts, especially among young people.

- Increase availability of worksite stress-reduction programs.

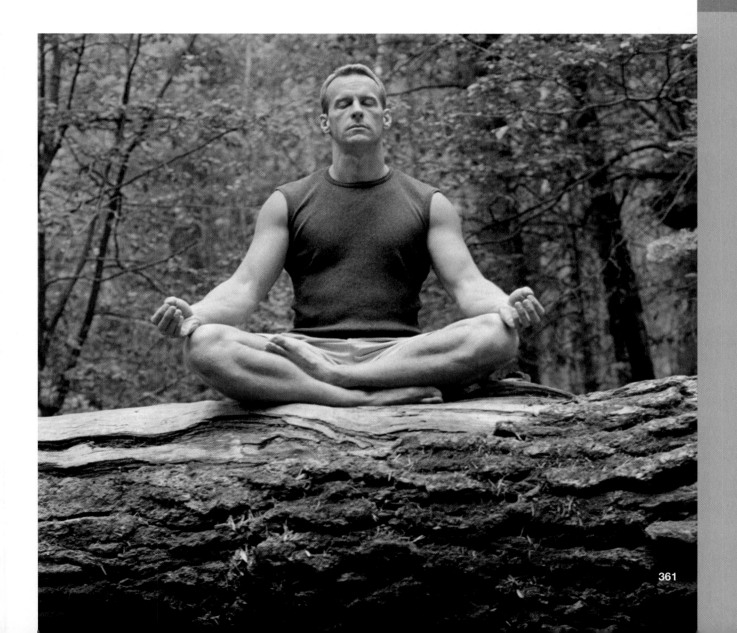

Although stress cannot be avoided, proper stress-management techniques can help reduce the impact of stress in your life.

As outlined in Concept 16, we all experience stress on a daily basis and must find ways to manage stress effectively. We can do many things to prevent excessive levels of stress, including exercising regularly, getting sufficient sleep, and allowing time for recreation. Effective time management is essential for balancing work and other activities. Despite our best efforts, stressful situations will occur and we must find a way to deal with them. Later in this concept, three effective methods for managing stress will be described.

Physical Activity and Stress Management

Regular activity and a healthy diet can help you adapt to stressful situations. An individual's capacity to adapt is not a static function but fluctuates as situations change. The better your overall health, the better you can withstand the rigors of tension without becoming susceptible to illness or other disorders. Physical activity is especially important because it conditions your body to function effectively under challenging physiological conditions.

Physical activity can provide relief from stress and aid muscle tension release. Physical activity has been found to be effective at relieving stress, particularly white-collar job stress. Studies show that regular exercise decreases the likelihood of developing stress disorders and reduces the intensity of the stress response. It also shortens the time of recovery from an emotional trauma. Its effect tends to be short-term, so one must continue to exercise regularly for it to have a continuing effect. Aerobic exercise is believed to be especially effective in

reducing anxiety and relieving stress (though other activities are also good). Whatever your choice of exercise, it is likely to be more effective as an antidote to stress if it is something you find enjoyable.

The relation between physical activity and the stress response remains unclear. Physical activity is associated with a physiological response that is similar, in many ways, to the body's response to psychosocial stressors. Further, individuals who are physically fit have a reduced physiological response to exercise. Presumably, someone who is physically fit would also have a reduced response to psychosocial stressors. Research supports this hypothesis indicating that regular exercise reduces physiological reactivity to nonexercise stressors.

Recent studies have attempted to clarify the role of exercise in stress reactivity by more clearly specifying the physiological systems activated by exercise-related stress and nonexercise-related stress. The body's physiological response consists of both a sympathetic nervous system response and an endocrine response. According to one study, the sympathetic nervous system response to exercise is immediate, while the endocrine response to exercise is delayed. In contrast, the endocrine response to psychosocial stressors is usually immediate. Such differences in responses suggest that more complex models may be necessary to understand the role of exercise in protecting against psychosocial stress.

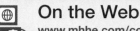 **Physical activity can improve mental health.** The physical health benefits of exercise have been well established for some time. Research suggests that the benefits of exercise extend beyond the physical and into the realm of mental health. Exercise can reduce anxiety, aid in recovery from depression, and assist in efforts to eliminate negative health behaviors, such as smoking.

- *Physical activity can reduce anxiety.* Evidence shows that physical activity leads to reductions in anxiety in nonclinical samples. One study found that exercise may also be effective in reducing anxiety among individuals with panic disorder. An aerobic exercise program led to reductions in panic symptoms relative to a control group. Although exercise was not as effective as medication, it may be a useful addition to other treatment methods for anxiety disorders.

On the Web
www.mhhe.com/corbinweb
Web 01 Log on to this URL before reading this concept. See On the Web list of concepts. Click on the concept number you want to view. To access supplemental information, click on the number shown at each Web icon.

- *Physical activity can reduce depression.* A randomized clinical trial compared antidepressant medication and aerobic exercise with a combined antidepressant and exercise condition in the treatment of major depressive disorder. The aerobic exercise group fared as well as the other two at the end of treatment. In addition, the patients who only exercised were less likely to have a remission to depression at a 6-month follow-up. The individuals in the exercise condition possibly felt more responsible for the improvements in their condition, and this increase in self-efficacy led to better long-term outcomes. The results of this clinical trial are consistent with evidence reported in a review of 30 studies on exercise and depression, which found that those who exercise are less depressed than those who do not exercise.
- *Physical activity can aid in changing behaviors related to health.* One study tested vigorous physical activity as an adjunct to a cognitive-behavioral smoking cessation program for women. The results indicated that women who received the exercise intervention were able to sustain continuous abstinence from smoking for a longer period of time relative to those who did not receive the exercise intervention. Women in the exercise condition also gained less weight during smoking cessation. It is not yet clear how exercise facilitates smoking cessation and reductions in other health risk behaviors, such as alcohol use. Exercise-related decreases in stress and increases in positive mood may be responsible. In addition, one study found that acute bouts of exercise reduced the severity of withdrawal symptoms and decreased craving for a cigarette in smokers.

These points are merely a brief listing of the data now supporting the mental health benefits of exercise. A review of the literature on exercise and psychiatric disorders suggests that exercise may also be effective in reducing problem behaviors among those with developmental disabilities and may serve as an adjunct in treatments for schizophrenia, conversion disorder, and alcohol dependence. In addition, it is important to note that exercise may lead to better overall psychological functioning in the general population.

Stress, Sleep, and Recreation

Stress can be both a cause and a consequence of impaired sleep. In order to function effectively and adapt effectively to stressful situations, one must get adequate sleep. Although the number of hours needed varies from person to person, the average adult needs between 7 and 8 hours of sleep per night. Research suggests that teenagers and young adults (i.e., those in their early twenties) may need slightly more sleep. Unfortunately, many

in these age groups do not obtain this extra amount of sleep. With insufficient sleep, many people resort to caffeine to stay awake, leading to an endless cycle of deficient sleep and caffeine usage. This disturbed sleep pattern can compromise health and wellness.

Sleep and stress may interact to increase risk for other conditions. Evidence suggests that people who do not get enough sleep are at risk for obesity. One study reported that those who get less than 5 hours of sleep a night have a 50 percent greater risk of obesity than those who get 7 to 9 hours of sleep. Getting enough sleep can help keep weight under control, help reduce stress levels, and increase productivity. Some guidelines for good sleep are presented in Table 1.

All work and no play can lead to poor mental and physical health. Between 1860 and 1990, the number of hours typically spent working in industrialized countries decreased relatively dramatically. While that trend has continued in most countries, work hours in the United States have increased during the past two decades (see

---

Table 1 ▶ Guidelines for Good Sleep

- Be aware of the effects of medications. Some medicines, such as weight loss pills and decongestants, contain caffeine, or other ingredients that interfere with sleep.
- Avoid tobacco use. Nicotine is a stimulant and can interfere with sleep.
- Avoid excess alcohol use. Alcohol may make it easier to get to sleep but may be a reason you wake up at night and are unable to get back to sleep.
- You may exercise late in the day, but do not do vigorous activity right before bedtime.
- Sleep in a room that is cooler than normal.
- Avoid hard-to-digest foods late in the day, as well as fatty and spicy foods.
- Avoid large meals late in the day or right before bedtime. A light snack before bedtime should not be a problem for most people.
- Avoid too much liquid before bedtime.
- Avoid naps during the day.
- Go to bed and get up at the same time each day.
- Do not study, read, or engage in other activities in your bed. You want your brain to associate your bed with sleep, not with activity.
- If you are having difficulty falling asleep, do not stay in bed. Get up and find something to do until you begin to feel tired and then go back to bed.

Figure 1). A major reason for this increase is that more people now hold second jobs than in the past. Also, some jobs of modern society have increasing rather than decreasing time demands. For example, many medical doctors and other professionals work more hours than the 35 to 44 hours that most people work. Nearly three times as many married women with children work full-time now, as compared with 1960.

Experts have referred to young adults as the "overworked Americans" because they work several jobs and maintain dual roles (full-time employment coupled with normal family chores), or they work extended hours in demanding professional jobs. A Gallup poll showed that the great majority of adults have "enough time" for work, chores, and sleep but not enough time for friends, self, spouse, and children. When time is at a premium, the factors most likely to be negatively affected are personal health, relationships with children, and marriage or romantic relationships.

Work pressures can be stressful. This suggests a need to manage time effectively and to find activities that are enjoyable during free time.

Free time is important to the average person. Most people say that free time is important, but surveys indicate that more than half of all adults feel that they get too little of it. Many adults report that they get too little time for **recreation** or to simply relax and "do nothing."

Recreation and leisure are important contributors to wellness (quality of life). **Leisure** is time spent "doing things we just want to do" or "doing nothing." Recreation, on the other hand, is often purposeful. Leisure and recreation can contribute to stress reduction and wellness, though leisure activities are not done specifically to achieve these benefits.

The value of recreation and leisure in the busy lives of people in Western culture is evidenced by the emphasis public health officials place on the availability and accessibility of recreational facilities in the future.

To achieve wellness and stress-reduction benefits, recreation should provide a sense of play. **Play** is done of one's own free will and most often for fun or intrinsic rather than extrinsic reasons. Activities performed for material things, such as trophies and medals, can be considered recreational as long as the principal reason for doing the activity is a sense of fun and playfulness. If the activity is done primarily for extrinsic reasons, it may not provide wellness benefits and is probably not true recreation. For example, playing golf to impress the boss is an extrinsic reason that may increase life stress rather than decrease it.

There are many meaningful types of recreation. If fitness is the goal, recreational activities involving moderate to vigorous physical activity should be chosen. Involvement in nonphysical activities also constitutes recreation. For example, reading is an activity that can contribute significantly to other wellness dimensions, such as emotional/mental and spiritual. Passive involvement (spectating) is a third type of participation.

Passive participation has been criticized by some people who feel that active participation is an important ingredient of meaningful recreation. Experts point out that spectating can be refreshing and meaningful. For example, watching a good play qualifies as meaningful recreation and can be true leisure. Likewise, active participation in community theater can be meaningful recreation. To achieve the wellness benefits of recreation, liberal participation and meaningful passive involvement (spectating) are encouraged.

Time Management

Effective time management helps you adapt to the stresses of modern living. Lack of time is cited by both the general public and experts as a source of stress and a reason for failing to implement healthy lifestyle changes. For college students, managing time is critical to academic success as well as overall well-being. In one study of college students, higher levels of perceived control over time were associated with lower levels of stress and higher levels of academic performance, problem-solving ability, and health. In another study, better time management was more protective against academic stress than was satisfaction with leisure activities. Thus, gaining a sense of control over your time may have important academic and health benefits. The following strategies may help you learn to manage your time more effectively.

- *Know how you spend your time.* Where does your time go? The answer to this question is the first step toward better time management. Most of us are not fully aware of how we spend our time. If you carry a note-

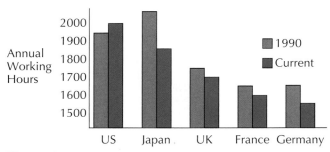

Figure 1 ▶ Average annual working hours of five nations.
Source: Organization for Economic Cooperation and Development.

book and write down what you are doing and how long it takes, you can find out exactly where the time goes. You probably need to do this for at least a week. After you complete this exercise, you will know where you need to spend more time. Just as important, monitoring your time will help you identify where you could spend less time. Some common areas where people spend too much time are socializing (in person, by phone, or via e-mail), watching television, playing video games, surfing the Internet, and doing busywork. Lab 17A will give you a chance to evaluate your current use of time.

- *Set goals and deadlines.* In addition to knowing how you spend your time, it is important to know what things need to get done. This includes everything from small tasks that need to get done today to important long-term goals. When setting goals, make sure they are attainable and that the time frame for completing them is reasonable. Some tasks may be more easily accomplished if they are broken down into a series of smaller tasks, each with its own deadline. Setting deadlines for the completion of goals will increase the likelihood that you will follow through.

- *Prioritize.* Many people feel that there are not enough hours in the day to do everything that needs to be done. The truth is that they are probably right. If you think about all of the things that have to get done, it can seem unmanageable. That is why it is important to prioritize. Certain things need to get done now, others might be able to wait until next week, and still others might wait longer without significant problems. People often busy themselves with things that do not need to get done immediately while putting off the things that do. The ABC approach is one advocated by many time-management experts as a way to prioritize tasks effectively. Create three lists of things you need to do, with list A including the most urgent tasks and list C containing the least urgent. See Table 2 for a brief description of the ABC approach.

- *Write it down.* When things are not too busy, it may be possible to remember what you need to do and when you need to do it without writing it down. During busy times, though, trying to remember everything can lead to big problems. One of the most important steps in effective time management is to write things down. This includes keeping a daily planner to remember your schedule, calendars (weekly and/or monthly) to remember important events and deadlines, and a to-do list (or several using the ABC approach) to help you remember your goals and priorities. Computers and other digital organizers allow you to keep all of this information in one place.

- *Include recreational activities in your schedule in addition to your responsibilities.* Although it may seem that scheduling fun takes away from the enjoyment, you may not find this to be the case. By scheduling your free time,

you can fully enjoy it rather than worrying about other things you "should" be doing.

- *Make the most of the time you have.* To get the most out of your time, it is important to know when you do your best work and under what conditions. If you are sharpest in the morning, schedule the most important work to be done during this time. If you study most effectively when you are alone in a quiet place, schedule your studying at a time when you can create that environment. It is also important not to let time that could be productive go to waste. Keep materials with you that will allow you to take advantage of small periods of time (e.g., between classes).

Table 2 ▶ The ABC System for Time Management	
Level of Importance	Description
A	*A tasks* are those that *must* be done, and soon. When accomplished, A tasks may yield extraordinary results. Left undone, they may generate serious, unpleasant, or disastrous consequences. Immediacy is what an A priority task is all about.
B	*B tasks* are those that *should* be done soon. While not as pressing as A tasks, they're still important. They can be postponed, but not for too long. Within a brief time, though, they can easily rise to A status.
C	*C tasks* are those that *could* be done These tasks could be put off without creating dire consequences. Some can linger in this category almost indefinitely. Others—especially those tied to distant completion dates—will eventually rise to A or B levels as the deadline approaches.

Source: Mancini, M.

Recreation *Recreation* means creating something anew. In this book, it refers to something that you do for amusement or for fun to help you divert your attention and to refresh yourself (re-create yourself).

Leisure Time that is free from the demands of work. Leisure is more than free time; it is also an attitude. Leisure activities need not be means to ends (purposeful) but are ends in themselves.

Play Activity done of one's own free will. The play experience is fun and intrinsically rewarding, and it is a self-absorbing means of self-expression. It is characterized by a sense of freedom or escape from life's normal rules.

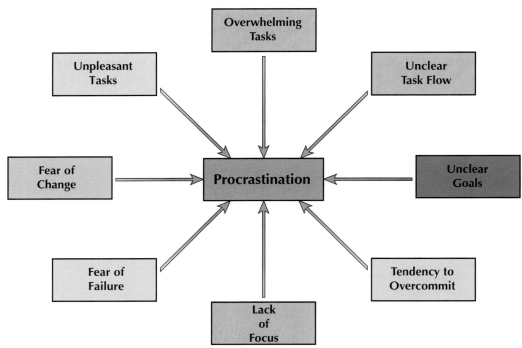

Figure 2 ▶ Causes of procrastination.

Source: Mancini, M.

- *Avoid procrastination.* Virtually all of us procrastinate at one time or another but, for many, procrastination can significantly decrease performance and increase stress. A number of causes of procrastination have been identified, including both internal and external influence (see Figure 2). Understanding the causes of procrastination can help you find ways to prevent it in the future. Strategies such as the ABC approach should also help you limit procrastination by getting you to work on the things that are most important first. One of the simplest solutions to procrastination is simply to "get started." The first step toward completing a project is often the most difficult. Once people take the first step, they often find that the task becomes easier, so get started on projects as soon as possible, even if you spend only a short time working.

- *Self-assessment of time management can help you improve your ability to manage your time effectively.* Monitoring your progress in time management is helpful in two important ways. First, it allows you to see the progress you have made. Success is rewarding in and of itself, but you might also consider rewarding yourself with something tangible when you first start out. For example, you might treat yourself to a nice dinner if you finish an important project on time. Monitoring also helps you identify areas in need of further improvement, so that you can adapt your plan to improve your chances of success.

Coping with Stress

Unresolved stress poses the greatest physical and emotional danger. Although some stressors are short-lived, many stressors persist over a long period of time. The ability to adapt, or cope with these stressors, largely determines their ultimate effect. If effective **coping** strategies are used, the effects of a stressful situation can be more tolerable. In many cases, reasonable solutions or compromises can be found. On the other hand, if ineffective coping strategies are used, problems may become even worse. This can lead to more stress and more severe outcomes. Although stress cannot be avoided, it can be managed. Effective stress management is a skill that contributes to both health and quality of life.

Stress management training has been shown to improve both physical and mental health outcomes in a variety of populations. For example, a recent study found that stress management training for patients with ischemic heart disease resulted in improved cardiovascular function, decreased depression, and lower levels of general distress. These improvements were comparable to those obtained by regular exercise. In addition, stress management might actually improve academic performance. A recent study of secondary students between the ages of 15 and 16 found that stress management training led to performance on a standardized test equivalent to an improvement of one letter grade. Although stress management approaches vary in their focus, they typically address multiple domains of the stress response including emotional, behavioral, cognitive, and physiological. The coping strategies defined in the section that follows will address each of these components of stress and provide concrete ways in which you can manage these aspects of stress in your own life. Many of the approaches described are standard components of stress management training programs.

Stress management training focuses on teaching active coping strategies. Active coping strategies are those that attempt to directly affect the source of the stress or to effectively manage the individuals' reactions

to stress. In contrast, passive coping strategies attempt to direct attention away from the stressor. Active coping strategies can be classified into three basic categories including **emotion-focused coping,** a**ppraisal-focused coping,** and **problem-focused coping.** These coping strategies target the emotional and physiological, behavioral, and cognitive aspects of stress, respectively (see Table 3). Emotion-focused coping strategies attempt to regulate the emotions resulting from stressful events. In contrast, problem-focused strategies are aimed at changing the source of the stress. Appraisal-focused coping strategies are based on changing the way one perceives the stressor or changing one's perceptions of resources for effectively managing stress. While each of these strategies is effective in various circumstances, **avoidant coping** strategies, such as ignoring or escaping the problem, are likely to be ineffective for almost everyone.

Concept 16 described the characteristics associated with positive health outcomes, including hardiness, optimism, and internal locus of control. Not surprisingly, individuals with these characteristics tend to engage more effectively in problem-focused, emotion-focused, and appraisal-focused coping and they are less likely to engage in avoidant coping. Thus, if you want to reap the health benefits of individuals with these characteristics, learning to use problem-, emotion-, and appraisal-focused coping strategies is a good place to start.

Coping with most stress requires a variety of thoughts and actions. Stress forces the body to work under less than optimal conditions, yet this is the time when we need to function at our best. Effective coping may require some efforts to regulate the emotional aspects of the stress and other efforts to solve the problem. For example, if you are experiencing stress over grades in school, you have to accept your current grades and take active steps to improve them. Your appraisal of your

Table 3 ▶ Strategies for Stress Management	
Category	**Description**
Emotion-Focused Strategies	**Strategies That Minimize the Emotional and Physical Effects of the Situation**
• Relaxing	• Using relaxation techniques to reduce the symptoms of stress
• Exercising	• Using physical activity to reduce the symptoms of stress
• Seeking passive social support	• Talking with someone about what you are experiencing or accepting sympathy and understanding
• Praying	• Looking for spiritual guidance to provide comfort
Appraisal-Focused Strategies	**Strategies That Alter Perceptions of the Problem or Your Ability to Cope Effectively with the Problem**
• Cognitive restructuring	• Changing negative or automatic thoughts leading to unnecessary distress
• Seeking knowledge or practicing skills	• Finding ways to increase your confidence in your ability to cope
Problem-Focused Strategies	**Strategies That Directly Seek to Solve or Minimize the Stressful Situation**
• Systematic problem solving	• Making a plan of action to solve the problem and following through to make the situation better
• Being assertive	• Standing up for your own rights and values while respecting the opinions of others
• Seeking active social support	• Getting help or advice from others who can provide specific assistance for your situation
Avoidant Coping Strategies	**Strategies That Attempt to Distract the Individual from the Problem**
• Ignoring	• Refusing to think about the situation or pretending no problem exists
• Escaping	• Looking for ways to feel better or to stop thinking about the problem, including eating or using nicotine, alcohol, or other drugs

Coping A person's constantly changing cognitive and psychological efforts to manage stressful situations.

Emotion-Focused Coping The method of adapting to stress that is based on regulating the emotions that cause or result from stress.

Appraisal-Focused Coping The method of adapting to stress that is based on changing your perceptions of stress and your resources for coping.

Problem-Focused Coping The method of adapting to stress that is based on changing the source or cause of stress.

Avoidant Coping Seeking immediate, temporary relief from stress through distraction or self-indulgence (i.e., the use of alcohol, tobacco, or other drugs.)

past performance and the likelihood of improving your performance in the future will significantly impact how you respond to the situation. It does no good to worry about past events. Instead, it is important to look ahead for ways to solve the problems at hand. Coping with this situation may, therefore, require the use of all three effective coping strategies.

Emotion-Focused Coping Strategies

Relaxation technique and/or coping strategies can help in relieving stress. When you are aware of what stress does to your body, you can do something to relieve those symptoms immediately, as well as on a regular and more long-term basis. Although there is no magical cure for stress or tension, various therapeutic approaches may be effective in helping you handle stress. These approaches can slow your heart and respiration rate, relax tense muscles, clear your mind, and help you relax mentally and emotionally. Perhaps most important, these techniques can improve your outlook and help you cope better with the stressful situation. In Lab 17C, you will perform a progressive relaxation program. Performing Lab 17C only once will not prepare you to use relaxation techniques effectively. Remember, you must practice learning to relax.

Some treatments are less desirable than others because they act only as "crutches" or "fire extinguishers" and do not get at the root of the problem. Hypnosis may lead to fantasy and dependency. Alcoholic beverages, tranquilizers, and painkillers may give temporary relief and may be prescribed by a physician as part of treatment, but they do not resolve the problem and may even mask symptoms or cause further problems, such as addiction. Drugs do not provide a long-term solution to chronic stress or tension, and, contrary to vitamin and mineral advertisements, supplementing the diet with vitamin C or so-called stress vitamin formulations has no proven benefits.

Various conscious relaxation techniques exist. Conscious relaxation techniques reduce stress and tension by directly altering the symptoms. When you are stressed, heart rate, blood pressure, and muscle tension all increase to help your body deal with the challenge. Conscious relaxation techniques reduce these normal effects and bring the body back to a more relaxed state. Most techniques use the "three *R*s" of relaxation to help the body relax: (1) reduce mental activity, (2) recognize tension, and (3) reduce respiration. Detailed descriptions and examples are available at Web03. Brief descriptions follow.

Web 03

- *Deep Breathing.* One of the quickest ways to experience relaxation is through deep breathing. There are many versions of deep breathing exercises. For example, first inhale deeply through your nose for about 4 seconds, making sure that your abdomen rises when you are inhaling. Next let the air out slowly through your mouth (for about 8 seconds, or twice as long as the inhalation). Repeating these steps for several minutes can help control the body's reaction to stress. See Table 4 for detailed instructions on diaphragmatic breathing.

- *Mental Imagery.* Although it is not always possible to leave a stressful situation and go somewhere peaceful and relaxing, you can accomplish the same goal by using mental imagery. This approach involves imagining a pleasant image or scene that you associate with relaxation, such as a peaceful lake or stream. The goal is to imagine the scene as completely as possible using all of your senses. For example, you might imagine seeing and hearing the stream and smelling the flowers growing along the banks of the stream. Many relaxation approaches combine deep breathing with mental imagery to maximize the relaxation response. The main advantage of these approaches is that they can be used in any setting, and they take very little time to induce a relaxation response. For example, you might combine deep breathing and mental imagery while at school or work and reduce your stress level in as little as 5 minutes.

- *Jacobson's progressive relaxation method.* You must be able to recognize how a tense muscle feels before you can voluntarily release the tension. In this technique, contract the muscles strongly and then relax. Relax each of the large muscles first and later the small ones. Gradually reduce the contractions in intensity until no movement is visible. The emphasis is always placed on detecting the feeling of tension as the first step in "letting go," or "going negative." Jacobson, a pioneer in

Table 4 ▶ Diaphragmatic Breathing

This exercise will help improve your awareness of using deep abdominal breathing over shallower, chest-type breathing. To begin, lie on your back with your knees bent and feet on the floor. Place your right hand over your abdomen and your left hand over your chest. Your hands will be used to monitor breathing technique. Slowly inhale through your nose by allowing the abdomen to rise under your right hand. Concentrate on expanding your abdomen for 4 seconds. Continue inhaling another 2 seconds, allowing your chest to rise under your left hand. Exhale through your mouth in reverse order (for about 8 seconds, or twice as long as inhalation). Relax your chest first feeling it sink beneath your left hand and then your abdomen allowing it to sink beneath your right hand. Repeat four or five times. Discontinue if you become light-headed.

muscle relaxation research, emphasized the importance of relaxing eye and speech muscles, because he believed these muscles trigger the reactions of the total organism more than other muscles. A sample contract-relax exercise routine for relaxation is presented in Lab 17C.

- *Autogenic (autosuggestive) relaxation training.* Although any self-induced relaxation technique can be properly called autogenic, this term is typically associated with a specific type of relaxation training that involves the repetition of preselected words or phrases, such as "My hand feels heavy." This approach has been used to focus on the heaviness of limbs, the warmth of limbs, heart rate regulation, respiratory rate and depth regulation, and coolness in the forehead. Although this approach takes considerable practice, those who are skilled in this technique have demonstrated the ability to alter bodily states leading to relaxation.

- *Biofeedback.* Biofeedback training uses machines that monitor certain physiological processes of the body and that provide visual or auditory evidence of what is happening to normally unconscious bodily functions. The evidence, or feedback, is then used to help you decrease these functions. When combined with autogenic training, subjects have learned to relax and reduce the electrical activity in their muscles, lower blood pressure, decrease heart rate, change their brainwaves, and decrease headaches, asthma attacks, and stomach acid secretion.

- *Stretching and rhythmical exercises.* People who work long hours at a desk can release tension by getting up frequently and stretching, by taking a brisk walk, or by performing "office exercises." Exercising to music or to a rhythmic beat has been found to be relaxing and even hypnotic. One popular activity that uses stretching and rhythmic exercise (as well as breathing techniques) is Yoga. Many find Yoga beneficial in reducing stress, and research has found both physical and mental health benefits associated with Yoga.

Prayer and mindful meditation can help you cope with stress and daily problems. In addition to managing the body's physical response to stress, one must deal with the impact of stress on thoughts and emotions. Although relaxation strategies may also impact these dimensions, additional approaches may be necessary to adequately manage these aspects of the stress response.

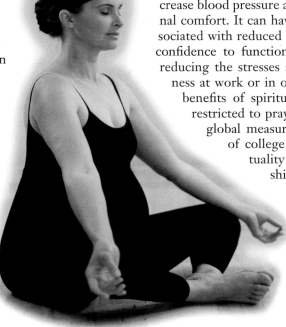

Prayer and mediation can reduce physical symptoms of stress and can help you cope.

Examples include prayer and mindful meditation.

- *Prayer.* Studies have shown that prayer can decrease blood pressure and can be a source of internal comfort. It can have other calming effects associated with reduced distress. It can also provide confidence to function more effectively, thereby reducing the stresses associated with ineffectiveness at work or in other situations. The health benefits of spirituality do not appear to be restricted to prayer, however. Using a more global measure of spirituality, one study of college students found that spirituality moderated the relationship between stress and health outcomes. For those low in spirituality, stress was associated with higher levels of negative emotion and physical symptoms of illness. Among those higher in spirituality, the link between stress and health outcomes was much weaker.

- *Mindfulness meditation.* While most relaxation techniques seek to distract attention away from distressing emotions, mindfulness meditation encourages the individual to experience fully his or her emotions in a nonjudgmental way. The individual is encouraged to bring full attention to the internal and external experiences that are occurring "in the moment." John Kabat-Zinn, founder of the Stress Reduction Clinic at the University of Massachusetts, has generated considerable enthusiasm for this technique, which is based on ancient Buddhist philosophy. Mindfulness training has been incorporated into empirically validated psychotherapies, and a number of self-help books provide additional information about the technique (see *Suggested Readings*).

Appraisal-Focused Coping Strategies (Cognitive Restructuring)

Changing your way of thinking can help you cope. Research suggests that you can reduce stress by changing the way you think. Although appraisal-focused coping has received considerably less attention than emotion- and problem-focused coping as an adaptive way to manage stress, there is evidence to suggest that this approach can be equally effective. In a study of workplace stress and health, a cognitive-behavioral intervention that targeted appraisal of stress was slightly more effective than a behavioral coping skills intervention that combined emotion- and problem-focused coping strategies. Thus, the way you think about stressful situations can be as important as how you respond to them. At one time or another, virtually all people have distorted thinking, which can create unnecessary stress. Distorted thinking is also referred to as negative or automatic thinking. To alleviate stress, it can be useful to recognize some of the common types of distorted thinking. If you can learn to recognize distorted thinking, you can change the way you think and often reduce your stress levels. Some common types of distorted thinking are listed in Table 5.

If you have ever used any of the 10 types of distorted thinking described in Table 5, you may find it useful to consider different methods of "untwisting" your thinking. Using the strategies for untwisting your thinking can be useful in changing negative thinking to positive thinking (see Table 6, page 371).

If you really want to change your way of thinking to avoid stress, you may have to practice the guidelines outlined in Table 6. To do this, you can think of a recent situation that caused stress. Describe the situation on paper, and see if you used distorted thinking in the situation (see Table 5). If so, write down which types of distorted thinking you used. Finally, determine if any of the guidelines in Table 6 would have been useful. If so, write down the strategy you could have used. When a similar situation arises, you will be prepared to deal with the stressful situation. Repeat this technique, using several situations that have recently caused stress.

Problem-Focused Coping Strategies

Problem-focused coping is most effective in dealing with controllable stressors. While emotion- and appraisal-focused coping may be the most effective means for coping with situations beyond one's control, a problem under personal control may be best addressed by taking action to solve the problem.

Problem solving and assertiveness can help you cope. Each stressful situation has unique circumstances and meaning to the individual. For this reason it is impossible to offer specific information about the best stress management strategy without knowing the source of the stress and how it is affecting a specific person. However, it is possible to offer a framework for consistently responding to difficult situations. A technique called systematic problem solving provides an excellent framework. This approach has been shown to improve the likelihood of problem resolution.

The first step is brainstorming, generating every possible solution to the problem. During this stage, you

Table 5 ▶ Types of Distorted Thinking

Type	Description
1. All-or-none thinking	You look at things in absolute, black-and-white categories.
2. Overgeneralization	You view a negative event as a never-ending pattern of defeat.
3. Mental filter	You dwell on the negatives and ignore the positives.
4. Discounting the positives	You insist that your accomplishments and positive qualities don't count.
5. Jumping to conclusions	(a) Mind reading—you assume that others are reacting negatively to you when there is no definite evidence of this. (b) Fortune telling—you arbitrarily predict that things will turn out badly.
6. Magnification or minimization	You blow things out of proportion or shrink their importance inappropriately.
7. Emotional reasoning	You reason from how you feel: "I feel like an idiot, so I must be one." "I don't feel like doing this, so I'll put it off."
8. Should statements	You criticize yourself or other people with "shoulds" or "shouldn'ts." "Musts," "oughts," and "have tos" are similar offenders.
9. Labeling	You identify with your shortcomings. Instead of saying, "I made a mistake," you tell yourself, "I am a jerk," "a fool," or "a loser."
10. Personalization and blame	You blame yourself for something that you weren't entirely responsible for, or you blame other people and overlook ways that your own attitudes and behaviors might have contributed to the problem.

Source: Burns, D. D.

Table 6 ▶ Ten Ways to Untwist Your Thinking

Way	Description
1. Identify the distortion.	Write down your negative thoughts, so you can see which of the 10 types of distorted thinking you are involved in. This will make it easier to think about the problem in a more positive and realistic way.
2. Examine the evidence.	Instead of assuming that your negative thought is true, if you feel you never do anything right, you can list several things that you have done successfully.
3. Use the double standard method.	Instead of putting yourself down in a harsh, condemning way, talk to yourself in the same compassionate way you would talk to a friend with a similar problem.
4. Use the experimental technique.	Do an experiment to test the validity of your negative thought. For example, if, during an episode of panic you become terrified that you are about to die of a heart attack, you can jog or run up and down several flights of stairs. This will prove that your heart is healthy and strong.
5. Think in shades of gray.	Although this method might sound drab, the effects can be illuminating. Instead of thinking about your problems in all-or-none extremes, evaluate things on a range from 0 to 100. When things do not work out as well as you had hoped, think about the experience as a partial success, rather than a complete failure. See what you can learn from the situation.
6. Use the survey method.	Ask people questions to find out if your thoughts and attitudes are realistic. For example, if you believe that public speaking anxiety is abnormal and shameful, ask several friends if they have ever felt nervous before giving a talk.
7. Define terms.	When you label yourself "inferior," "a fool," or "a loser," ask, "What is the definition of 'a fool'?" You will feel better when you see that there is no such thing as a fool or a loser.
8. Use the semantic method.	Simply substitute language that is less colorful or emotionally loaded. This method is helpful for "should" statements. Instead of telling yourself "I *shouldn't* have made that mistake," you can say, "It would be better if I hadn't made that mistake."
9. Use re-attribution.	Instead of automatically assuming you are "bad" and blaming yourself entirely for a problem, think about the many factors that may have contributed to it. Focus on solving the problem instead of using up all your energy blaming yourself and feeling guilty.
10. Do a cost-benefit analysis.	List the advantages and disadvantages of a feeling (such as getting angry when your plane is late), a negative thought (such as "No matter how hard I try, I always screw up"), or a behavior pattern (such as overeating and lying around in bed when you are depressed). You can also use the cost-benefit analysis to modify a self-defeating belief, such as "I must always be perfect."

Source: Burns, D. D.

should not limit the solutions you generate in any way. Even silly and impractical solutions should be included. After you have generated a comprehensive list, you can narrow your focus by eliminating any solutions that do not seem reasonable. When you have reduced the number of solutions to a reasonable number (four or five), carefully evaluate each option. You should consider the potential costs and benefits of each approach to aid in making a decision. Once you decide on an approach, carefully plan the implementation of the strategy. This includes anticipating anything that might go wrong and being prepared to alter your plan as necessary.

In some cases, directly addressing the source of stress involves responding assertively. For example, if the source of stress is an employer placing unreasonable demands on your time, the best solution to the problem may involve talking to your boss about the situation. This type of confrontation is difficult for many people concerned about being overly aggressive. However, you can stand up for yourself without infringing on the rights of others.

Many people confuse assertiveness with aggression, leading to passive responses in difficult situations. An aggressive response intimidates others and fulfills one's own needs at the expense of others. In contrast, an assertive response protects your own rights and values while respecting the opinions of others.

Once you are comfortable with the idea of responding assertively, you may want to practice or role-play assertive responses before trying them in the real world. With a friend you trust, practice responding assertively. Your friend may provide valuable feedback about your approach, and the practice may increase your self-efficacy for responding and your expectancies for a positive outcome.

Social Support and Stress Management

Social support is important for effective stress management. **Social support** has been found to play an important role in coping with stress, and it has been linked to faster recovery from various medical procedures. In one study of athletic injuries, people who were the most stressed were injured more often, and those who had the poorest support system were the most likely to be injured. Although the mechanism for these effects is not understood, it is clear that social support plays a major role in stress management. Social support can assist in emotion-focused and problem-focused forms of coping. Friends and family can provide concrete advice that helps to solve a problem, and they can provide moral support and encouragement.

Social support may be particularly important for women. Women may be particularly likely to seek and provide social support when stressed. A paradigm called the "tend or befriend" model suggests that women have a unique stress response. Women respond to stress by tending to others (nurturing) and affiliating with a social group (befriending). This response is helpful in protecting offspring and reducing the risk for the negative health consequences of stress.

Social support has various sources. Everyone needs someone to turn to for support when feeling overwhelmed. Support can come from friends, family members, clergy, a teacher, a coach, or a professional counselor. Different sources provide different forms of support. Even pets have been shown to be a good source of social support, with consequent health and quality of life benefits. The goal is to identify and nurture relationships that can provide this type of support. In turn, it is important to look for ways to support and assist others.

There are many types of social support. Social support has three main components: informational, material, and emotional. Informational (technical) support includes tips, strategies, and advice that can help a person get through a specific stressful situation. For example, a parent, friend, or co-worker may offer insight into how he or she once resolved similar problems. Material support is direct assistance to get a person through a stressful situation—for example, providing a loan to help pay off a short-term debt. Emotional support is encouragement or sympathy that a person provides to help another cope with a particular challenge.

Regardless of the type of support, it is important that it fosters autonomy. Social support that helps you to become more self-reliant because of increased feelings of competence is best for developing autonomy. Social support that is controlling or leads to dependence on another person does not lead to autonomy and may increase rather than decrease stress over time.

Obtaining good social support requires close relationships. Although we live in a social environment, it is often difficult to ask people for help. Sometimes the nature and severity of our problems may not be apparent to others. Other times, friends may not want to offer suggestions or insight because they do not want to appear too pushy. To obtain good support, it is important to develop quality personal relationships with several individuals. Research on the effects of social support indicates that the quality, not the quantity, of social support leads to better health outcomes. A high-quality social support system is particularly important during times of high stress.

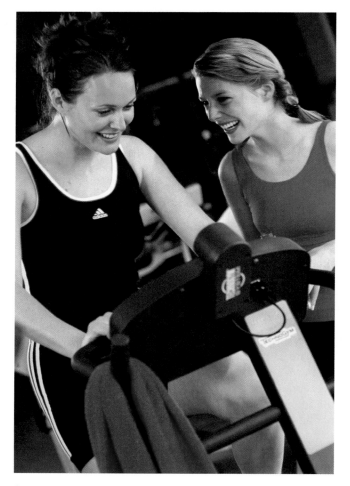

Social support is important for stress management and for maintaining an exercise program.

Strategies for Action

Several practical steps can help you identify and manage your stress. This concept is dedicated to strategies and skills for preventing, managing, and coping with stress. It is important to understand that, for strategies to be effective, they must be used regularly. Several practical steps that you can take are described in the following list.

- *Self-assess your stress levels.* Making self-assessments such as those in Labs 16A, 16B, and 16C can help you identify the sources and the magnitude of stress in your life.
- *Adopt coping strategies.* Consistent with the information presented in this concept, learning about and using a variety of emotion-focused, appraisal-focused, and problem-focused strategies will help you manage stress in your daily life.
- *Manage time effectively.* Lab 17A can help you understand your current time use patterns and help you develop a schedule that will allow you to focus on your priorities.
- *Evaluate strategy effectiveness.* Lab 17B is designed to help you assess the effectiveness of the various coping strategies you adopt. It will also provide a basis for altering strategies to manage your stress levels more effectively. Lab 17C will help you to relax tense muscles, an emotion-focused coping strategy. Lab 17D will help you evaluate your current social support system.

Online Learning Center

www.mhhe.com/corbin7e
The Online Learning Center contains a variety of Web-based resources that will help you get the most out of this book and your course. In addition to the On the Web pages, there are video activities, interactive quizzes, application assignments, and a variety of other useful study aids. Log on to the URL above to access these resources.

Web Resources

Web 04

American Institute of Stress **www.stress.org**
American Psychological Association **www.apa.org**
International Stress Management Association
   www.stress-management-isma.org
Mental Health Resources **www.mentalhealth.about.com**
National Institute of Mental Health **www.nimh.nih.gov**
National Mental Health Information Center
   www.mentalhealth.samhsa.gov
Time Management for College Students
   www.time-management-for-students.com

Suggested Readings

Web 05

Additional reference materials for Concept 17 are available at www.mhhe.com/fit_well/web19 Click 05.

Bernardi, L., et al. 2001. Effect of rosary prayer and Yoga mantras on autonomic cardiovascular rhythms: Comparative study. *British Medical Journal* 323:1446–1449.

Blonna, R. 2007. *Coping with Stress in a Changing World.* 4th ed. New York: McGraw-Hill.

Technology Update
Online Therapy

You have probably heard of online college courses, but are you familiar with online therapy? Interventions for treating panic disorder, post-traumatic stress disorder, and eating disorders are increasingly being delivered via the Internet. This wave of Internet-based interventions has also targeted those without psychological disorders. For example, one study evaluated the effectiveness of an Internet-based stress-management program that included training in relaxation techniques, problem-solving skills, time management, and cognitive restructuring. Relative to a control group, reductions in perceived stress, anxiety, and depression were observed in the group who participated in the Internet-based program.

Blumenthal, J. A., et al. 2006. Effects of exercise and stress management training on markers of cardiovascular risk in patients with ischemic heart disease: A randomized controlled trial. *Journal of the American Medical Association* 293:1626–1634.

Caspi, A., et al. 2003. Influence of life stress on depression. *Science* 301(5631):386–389.

Craft, L. L. 2003. Potential mechanisms for the antidepressant effects of exercise. *Medicine and Science in Sports and Exercise* 35(5):S216.

Social Support The behavior of others that assists a person in addressing a specific need.

Diener, E., et al. 2002. Subjective well-being: The science of happiness and life satisfaction. In C. R. Snyder and S. J. Lopez (eds.). *Handbook of Positive Psychology.* New York: Oxford University Press.

Girdano, D., D. Dosek, and G. Everly. 2005. *Controlling Stress and Tension.* 7th ed. Needham Heights, MA: Benjamin Cummings.

Greenberg, J. S. 2006. *Comprehensive Stress Management.* 9th ed. New York: McGraw-Hill.

Grossman, P., et al. 2004. Mindfulness-based stress reduction and health benefits: A meta-analysis. *Journal of Psychosomatic Medicine* 57:35–43.

Jacobson, E. 1978. *You Must Relax.* New York: McGraw-Hill.

Jason, L. A., and G. S. Glenwick. 2002. *Innovative Strategies for Promoting Health and Mental Health Across the Life Span.* New York: Springer.

Keogh, E., F. W. Bond, and P. E. Flaxman. 2006. Improving academic performance and mental health through a stress management intervention: Outcomes and mediators of change. *Behaviour Research and Therapy* 44:339–357.

Mancini, M. 2003. *Time Management.* New York: McGraw-Hill.

Nolen-Hoeksema, S. 2003. *Women Who Think Too Much.* New York: Henry Holt.

O'Keefe, E. J., and D. S. Berger. 2007. *Self-management for college students: The ABC approach.* 3rd ed. Hyde Park, NY: Partridge Hill.

Paterson, R. J. 2000. *The Assertiveness Workbook: How to Express Your Ideas and Stand Up for Yourself at Work.* Oakland, CA: New Harbinger.

Penedo, F. J., and J. R. Dahn. 2005. Exercise and well-being: A review of mental and physical health benefits associated with physical activity. *Current Opinion in Psychiatry* 18:189–193.

Romas, J. A., and M. Sharma. 2004. *Practical Stress Management.* 3rd ed. Needham Heights, MA: Benjamin Cummings.

Romas, J. A., and M. Sharma. 2007. *Practical Stress Management: A Comprehensive Workbook for Managing Change and Promoting Health.* 4th ed. San Francisco: Benjamin Cummings.

Seligman, M. E. 1998. *Learned Optimism: How to Change Your Mind and Your Life.* New York: Pocket Books.

Shapiro, S. L., et al. 2002. Meditation and positive psychology. In C. R. Snyder and S. J. Lopez (eds.). *Handbook of Positive Psychology.* New York: Oxford University Press.

Smith, J. C. 2002. *Stress Management: A Comprehensive Handbook of Techniques and Strategies.* New York: Springer.

Snyder, C. R. (ed.). 2001. *Coping with Stress: Effective People and Processes.* New York: Oxford University Press.

Snyder, C. R., and S. J. Lopez (eds.). 2002. *Handbook of Positive Psychology.* New York: Oxford University Press.

U.S. Department of Health and Human Services. November 2000. *Healthy People 2010.* 2nd ed. With *Understanding and Improving Health and Objectives for Improving Health.* 2 vols. Washington, DC: U.S. Government Printing Office.

Williams, R., and V. Williams. 1999. *Anger Kills: 17 Strategies for Controlling Hostility That Can Harm You.* New York: HarperCollins.

 In the News

Exercise and Mindfulness

Exercise and mindfulness have been shown to improve the functioning of individuals with various forms of psychiatric disorders. Recent studies suggest that these approaches might also improve psychological functioning in adolescents and adults who do not have psychological disorders. For example, a recent study of adolescents without diagnosable levels of depressive symptoms found that exercise levels were inversely related with depressive symptoms. A study in adults with ischemic heart disease showed that individuals assigned to an aerobic exercise condition had decreased symptoms of depression and lower levels of distress. The consensus from this research is that exercise is associated with enhanced mood, decreased stress responsivity, and higher self-esteem. Mindfulness, defined as a state of self-awareness where an individual seeks to experience fully his or her emotions in a non-judgemental way, has also demonstrated significant benefits. A mindfulness-based stress-reduction program led to significant decreases in mood disturbance in medical students. In another study, mindfulness meditation led to a 26 percent decrease in the effects of daily stressors, a 44 percent decrease in psychological distress, and a 46 percent decrease in medical symptoms. Mindfulness-based interventions have been shown to produce mental health benefits for a variety of medical populations, including patients with fibromyalgia, cancer, and coronary artery disease. Exercise and mindfulness have been known to provide important mental benefits, but these studies demonstrate that benefits are possible even for those without clinical levels of anxiety and depression.

Lab 17A Time Management

Name	Section	Date

Purpose: To learn to manage time to meet personal priorities

Procedures

1. Follow the four steps outlined below.
2. Complete the Conclusions and Implications section.

Results

Step 1: Establishing Priorities

1. Check the circles that reflect your priorities in the list below. Add priorities as necessary.
2. Rate each of the priorities you checked. Use a 1 for highest priority, 2 for moderate priority, and 3 for low priority.

Check Priorities	Rating	Check Priorities	Rating	Check Priorities	Rating
◯ More time with family		◯ More time with boy/girlfriend		◯ More time with spouse	
◯ More time for leisure		◯ More time to relax		◯ More time to study	
◯ More time for work success		◯ More time for physical activity		◯ More time to improve myself	
◯ More time for other recreation		◯ Other _____		◯ Other _____	

Step 2: Monitor Current Time Use

1. On the following daily calendar, keep track of daily time expenditure.
2. Write in exactly what you did for each time block.

7–9 A.M.	9–11 A.M.	11 A.M.–1 P.M.	1–3 P.M.
3–5 P.M.	**5–7 P.M.**	**7–9 P.M.**	**9–11 P.M.**

Step 3: Analyze Your Current Time Use

Where can I spend less time? (Write below.)

Where do I need to spend more time? (Write below.)

Step 4: Make a Schedule: Write in Your Planned Activities for the Day

7–9 A.M.	9–11 A.M.	11 A.M.–1 P.M.	1–3 P.M.
3–5 P.M.	5–7 P.M.	7–9 P.M.	9–11 P.M.

Conclusions and Implications: In several sentences, discuss how you might modify your schedule to find more time for important priorities.

Lab 17B Evaluating Coping Strategies

Name	Section	Date

Purpose: To learn how to use appropriate coping strategies that work best for you

Procedures

1. Think of five recent stressful experiences that caused you some concern, anxiety, or distress. Describe these situations in Chart 1. Then use Chart 2 to make a rating for changeability, severity, and duration. Assign one number for each category for each situation.
2. In Chart 3, place a check for each coping strategy that you used in coping with each of the five situations you described.
3. Answer the questions in the Conclusions and Implications section.

Results

Chart 1 ▶ Stressful Situations

Think of five different stressful situations. Appraise each situation and assign a score (changeability, severity, duration) using the scale in Chart 2.

Briefly describe the situation.	Changeability	Severity	Duration
1.			
2.			
3.			
4.			
5.			

Chart 2 ▶ Appraisal of the Stressful Situations

Use this chart to rate the five situations you described in Chart 1. Assign a number for changeability, severity, and duration for each situation in Chart 1.

	1	2	3	4	5
Was the situation changeable?	Completely within my control	Mostly within my control	Both in and out of my control	Mostly out of my control	Completely outside of my control
What was the severity of the stress?	Very minor	Fairly minor	Moderate	Fairly major	Very major
What was the duration of the stress?	Short-term (weeks)	Moderately short	Moderate (months)	Moderately long	Long (months to year)

Chart 3 ▶ Coping Strategies

Directions: Think about your response to the five stressful situations you recently experienced and check the strategies that you used in each situation.

Coping Strategy	Situation 1	Situation 2	Situation 3	Situation 4	Situation 5
1. I apologized or corrected the problem as best I could.					
2. I ignored the problem and hoped that it would go away.					
3. I told myself to forget about it and grew as a person from the experience.					
4. I tried to make myself feel better by eating, drinking, or smoking.					
5. I prayed or sought spiritual meaning from the situation.					
6. I expressed anger to try to change the situation.					
7. I took active steps to make things work out better.					
8. I used music, images, or deep breathing to help me relax.					
9. I tried to keep my feelings to myself and kept moving forward.					
10. I pursued leisure or recreational activity to help me feel better.					
11. I talked to someone who could provide advice or help me with the problem.					
12. I talked to someone about what I was feeling or experiencing.					

Conclusions and Implications: In several sentences, discuss the coping strategies you used. What were the ones you used the most? Are these the ones you typically use? Were they effective? Would you consider other strategies in the future?

Lab 17C Relaxation Exercises

Name	**Section**	**Date**

Purpose: To gain experience with specific relaxation exercises and to evaluate their effectiveness.

Procedures

1. Choose two of the relaxation exercises included in Chart 1 of this lab (see page 380) and read through the written instructions until you have a basic understanding of the exercises. Think through the specific aspects of the exercise until you have the process figured out.
2. Find a quiet place to try one of the exercises and follow the procedures as best you can. It is not possible to provide detailed instructions but the information should be sufficient to give you a basic understanding of the exercises.
3. One another day try a different exercise.
4. Answer the questions in the Results section. Then complete the Conclusions and Implications section.

Results

1. Which of the two exercises did you try (list them below).

2. Have you done either of the exercises before? ◯ Yes ◯ No

3. Was one relaxation exercise more effective better suited to you than the others? Which one?

Conclusions and Implications

In several sentences, discuss whether or not you feel that relaxation exercises will be a part of your wellness program. In what ways might you benefit from relaxation training? If you do not think you have a problem with relaxation, explain why.

Chart 1 ▶ Descriptions of Relaxation Exercises

A. Progressive Relaxation

Progressive relaxation uses active (conscious) mechanisms to achieve a state of relaxation. The technique involves alternating phases of muscle contraction (tension) and muscle relaxation (tension release). Muscle groups are activated one body segment at a time, incorporating all regions of the body by the end of the routine. Begin by lying on your back in a quiet place with eyes closed. Alternately contract and relax each of the muscles below—following the procedures described below. Begin with the dominant side of the body first; repeat on the nondominant side.

1. Hand and forearm—Make a fist.
2. Biceps—Flex elbows.
3. Triceps—Straighten arm.
4. Forehead—Raise your eyebrows and wrinkle forehead.
5. Cheeks and nose—Wrinkle nose and squint.
6. Jaws—Clench teeth.
7. Lips and tongue—Press lips together and tongue to roof of mouth, teeth apart.
8. Neck and throat—Tuck chin and push head backward against floor (if lying) or chair (if sitting).
9. Shoulder and upper back—Hunch shoulders to ears.
10. Abdomen—Suck abdomen inward.
11. Lower back—Arch back.
12. Thighs and buttocks—Squeeze buttocks together, push heels into floor (if lying) or chair rung (if sitting).
13. Calves—Pull instep and toes toward shins.
14. Toes—curl toes.

Muscle contraction phase: Inhale as you contract the designated muscle for 3-5 seconds. Use only a moderate level of tension.

Muscle relaxation phase: Exhale, relaxing the muscle and releasing tension for 6-10 seconds. Think of relaxation words such as warm, calm, peaceful, and serene.

Relax every muscle in your body at end of the exercise.

B. Autogenic Relaxation

This type of relaxation utilizes passive (subconscious) mechanisms to achieve relaxation. Lie down on your back with the body fully supported. Proceed through the following six stages by focusing on the sensation indicated. Repeat each phrase three times (per body area) before proceeding to the next stage.

1. "My right arm is heavy." (Repeat for each arm/leg)
2. "My right arm is warm." (Repeat for each arm/leg)
3. "My heart rate is regular and calm."
4. "My breathing is calm and relaxed."
5. "My solar plexus (abdomen) is warm.
6. "My forehead is cool."

Continue focusing on the phrases and images of these stages for 20 minutes.

C. Diapraghmatic Breathing

This exercise will help improve awareness of using deep abdominal breathing over shallower chest-type breathing. To begin, lie on your back with knees bent and feet on the floor. Place your right hand over your abdomen and left hand over your chest. Your hands will be used to monitor breathing technique. Slowly inhale through the nose by allowing the abdomen to rise under your right hand. Concentrate on expanding the abdomen for 4 seconds. Continue inhaling another 2 seconds allowing the chest to rise under your left hand. Exhale through your mouth in reverse order (for about 8 seconds or twice as long as inhalation). Relax the chest first feeling it sink beneath the left hand and then the abdomen allowing it to sink beneath the right hand. Repeat 4-5 times. Discontinue of you become light-headed. See Page 368 for additional details.

D. Show Gun

This is a form of Chi Gun, a Chinese meditation technique. The basic principles of Tai Chi are to maintain balance, use the entire body to achieve movement, unite movement with awareness (mind) and breathing (chi), and to keep the body upright Tai Chi involves holding the body in specific positions or "forms". To execute the basic form, stand straight, feet shoulder width apart and parallel with one another. You knees should be bent and turned outward slightly with knees over the foot. Your hands on belly button with palms facing body (men place hands right on left and women left on right), fingers are straight, spread slightly and relaxed.

1. Bring arms in front of body at a 30 degree angle to the plane of the back, palms face downward. Reach up to shoulder height with arms moving up and to the sides. (Breathe in allowing belly to move out as you raise arms upward).
2. When hands reach shoulder height, turn palms up and move hands to head allowing wrists to drop down. Imagine energy (chi) to flow from palms to top of head. (Continue breathing in).
3. Imagine energy flowing down through a central line of the body. Follow the energy with hands, point fingers toward one another, palms down, move arms downward in front of the midline of face and chest. (Breathe out as arms lower.)
4. Two inches bellow belly button stop, cross palms and move hands together.
5. Lower hands toward sides. (Complete breathing out.)
6. Repeat.

Lab 17D Evaluating Levels of Social Support

Name		Section	Date

Purpose: To evaluate your level of social support and to identify ways that you can find additional support.

Procedures

1. Answer each question in Chart 1 by placing a check in the box below Not True, Somewhat True, or Very True. Place the number value of each answer in the score box to the right.
2. Sum the scores (in the smaller boxes) for each question to get subscale scores for the three social support areas.
3. Record your three subscores in the results section on the next page. Total your subscores to get a total social support score.
4. Determine your ratings for each of the three social support subscores and for your total social support score using Chart 2 on the next page.
5. Answer the questions in the Conclusions and Implications section.

Chart 1 ▶ Social Support and Locus of Control Questionnaire

The first nine questions assess various aspects of social support. Base your answer on your actual degree of support, not on the type of support that you would like to have. Place a check in the space that best represents what is true for you.

Social Support Questions	Not True 1	Somewhat True 2	Very True 3	Score
1. I have close personal ties with my relatives.				
2. I have close relationships with a number of friends.				
3. I have a deep and meaningful relationship with a spouse or close friend.				
Access to social support score:				
4. I have parents and relatives who take the time to listen and understand me.				
5. I have friends or co-workers whom I can confide in and trust when problems come up.				
6. I have a nonjudgmental spouse or close friend who supports me when I need help.				
Degree of social support score:				
7. I feel comfortable asking others for advice or assistance.				
8. I have confidence in my social skills and enjoy opportunities for new social contacts.				
9. I am willing to open up and discuss my personal life with others.				
Getting social support score:				

Results

Scores and Ratings

(Use Chart 2 to obtain ratings.)

Access to social support score [   ]   Rating [   ]

Degree of social support score [   ]   Rating [   ]

Getting social support score [   ]   Rating [   ]

Total social support score [   ]   Rating [   ]
(sum of three scores)

Chart 2 ▶ Rating Scale for Social Support

Rating	Item Scores	Total Score
High	8–9	24–27
Moderate	6–7	18–23
Low	Below 6	Below 18

Conclusions and Implications

1. In several sentences, discuss your overall social support. Do you think your scores and ratings are a true representation of your social support?

[ ]

2. In several sentences, describe any changes you think you should make to improve your social support system. If you do not think change is necessary, explain why.

[ ]

The Use and Abuse of Tobacco

Health Goals for the year 2010

- Reduce disease, disability, and death related to tobacco use and exposure to secondhand smoke.

- Reduce initiation of tobacco use among youth.

- Reduce tobacco use.

- Reduce exposure to secondhand smoke.

- Increase tobacco-free environments.

- Increase tobacco-use cessation attempts.

- Eliminate tobacco ads that influence youth and young adults.

- Increase average age of first tobacco use by adolescents and young adults.

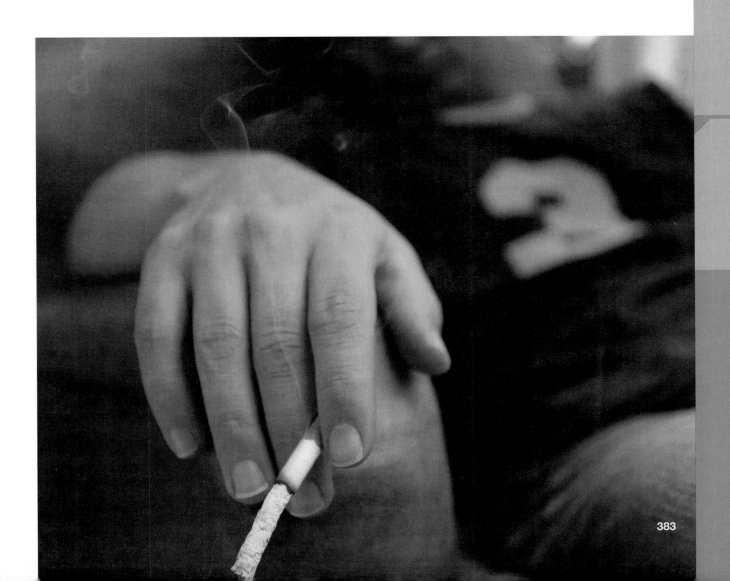

Concept 18

Tobacco use is the number one cause of preventable disease and is associated with the leading causes of death in our culture.

Tobacco is the number one cause of preventable mortality in the United States. It is linked to most of the leading causes of death and it leads to various other chronic conditions. Rates of smoking in the United States have decreased in recent decades due to better awareness and a changed social norm concerning smoking and tobacco use. Despite the progress, smoking is still a major public health problem. Today, 44.5 million adults in the United States smoke (23.4 percent of men and 18.5 percent of women). The majority of smokers (70 percent) would prefer to quit but find freeing themselves from the grip of nicotine addiction too difficult. This concept will review the health risks of tobacco use and provide practical guidelines for quitting.

Tobacco and Nicotine

Tobacco and its smoke contain over 400 noxious chemicals, including 200 known poisons and 50 carcinogens. Tobacco smoke contains both gases and particulates. During one phase of burning tobacco (the gaseous phase), a variety of gases dangerous to humans are released. The most dangerous is carbon monoxide. This gas binds onto hemoglobin in the bloodstream and thereby limits how much oxygen can be carried in the bloodstream. As a result, less oxygen is supplied to the vital organs of the body. While not likely from smoking, overexposure to carbon monoxide can be fatal.

The other phase of burning tobacco is the particulate phase. This phase releases a variety of particulates that contain a variety of carbon-based compounds referred to as tar. Many of these compounds are known to be **carcinogens.** Cigarettes have nearly 2,000 times more benzene

On the Web
www.mhhe.com/corbinweb

Web 01 Log on to this URL before reading this concept. See On the Web list of concepts. Click on the concept number you want to view. To access supplemental information, click on the number shown at each Web icon.

contamination than the Perrier water that was recalled years ago because it had benzene levels that were above health standards. Nicotine is also inhaled during the particulate phase of smoking. Nicotine is a highly addictive and poisonous chemical (often used in insecticides). It has a particularly broad range of influence and is a potent psychoactive **drug** that affects the brain and alters mood and behavior.

Nicotine is the addictive component of tobacco. When smoke is inhaled, the nicotine reaches the brain in 7 seconds, where it acts on highly sensitive receptors and provides a sensation that brings about a wide variety of responses throughout the body. At first, heart and breathing rates increase. Blood vessels constrict, peripheral circulation (especially to the hands and feet) slows down, and blood pressure increases. New users may experience dizziness, nausea, and headache. Then feelings of tension and tiredness are relieved.

After a few minutes, the feeling wears off and a rebound, or **withdrawal,** effect occurs. The smoker may feel depressed and irritable and have the urge to smoke again. **Physical dependence** occurs with continued use. Nicotine is one of the most addictive drugs known, even more addictive than heroin or alcohol.

Smokeless chewing tobacco is as addictive (and maybe more so) as smoking and produces the same kind of withdrawal symptoms on quitting. Chewing tobacco comes in a variety of forms, including loose leaf, twist, and plug forms. Rather than being smoked, the chaw, wad, or quid stays in the mouth for several hours, where it mixes with saliva and is absorbed into the bloodstream. Smokeless tobacco contains about seven times more nicotine than cigarettes, and more of it is absorbed because of the length of time the tobacco is in the mouth. It also contains a higher level of carcinogens than cigarettes.

Snuff, a form of smokeless tobacco, comes in either dry or moist form. Dry snuff is powdered tobacco mixed with flavorings, designed to be sniffed, pinched, or dipped. Moist snuff is used the same way, but it is moist, finely cut tobacco in a loose form or in a teabaglike packet. It comes in a variety of flavors. Experts believe that the flavoring of smokeless tobacco is designed to attract young users.

The Health and Economic Costs of Tobacco

Web 01 **Tobacco use affects all organs of the body and is the most preventable cause of death in our society.** Four decades after the landmark surgeon general's report on smoking, a new surgeon general's report draws four major conclusions. First, tobacco use affects all organs of the body, reducing the health of smokers. Second, quitting smoking has immediate and long-term benefits. Third, smoking cigarettes low in tar and nicotine provides no clear benefit to health. Finally, the number of diseases resulting from tobacco is much more extensive than previously thought (see Figure 1). Tobacco use is the leading cause of death in the United States, accounting for 18.1 percent of all deaths (438,000 each year). Worldwide, 2.5 to 3 million people die annually from smoking. Deaths from smoking are preventable and are linked to 7 of the 10 leading causes of death.

One way to highlight the health risks associated with smoking is to examine the health benefits associated with smoking cessation. Estimates suggest that reducing serum cholesterol to recommended levels can increase life expectancy by about one week to 6 months. In contrast, smoking cessation may increase life expectancy by 2 ½ to 4 ½ years. The earlier people quit, the more years of life they save with roughly 3 years saved for those who quit at age 60, 6 years for those who quit at age 50, and 9 years for those who quit at age 40. The most effective way to reduce health risks associated with smoking is clearly to quit; however, reducing how much one smokes also makes a difference. In one study, rates of lung cancer dropped by 27 percent among those who reduced their smoking from 20 or more to less than 10 cigarettes a day.

Web 02 **Smoking has tremendous economic costs.** In addition to the cost of human life, smoking causes more than $157 billion in annual health-related economic losses. Costs include $75 billion in direct medical costs, $81 billion in lost production, and millions in neonatal care. In addition to the costs at the societal level, there are significant financial costs for the individual, particularly with increased taxes on tobacco products. In an effort to help smokers appreciate the financial burden of smoking, the American Cancer Society has a tool on its Web site that allows the user to see how much they spend on cigarettes. For someone who smokes a pack a day for 10 years, the total is $18,250. See Web02.

The health risks from tobacco are directly related to overall exposure. In past years, tobacco companies denied there was conclusive proof of the harmful effects of tobacco products. Now, in the face of overwhelming medical evidence, tobacco officials have finally conceded that tobacco is harmful to health. It is now clear that the more you use the product (the more doses), the greater the health risk. Several factors determine the dosage: (1) the number of cigarettes smoked; (2) the length of time one has been smoking; (3) the strength (amount of tar, nicotine, etc.) of the cigarette; (4) the depth of the inhalation; and (5) the amount of exposure to other lung-damaging substances (e.g., asbestos). The greater the exposure to smoke, the greater the risk.

Brain: Increases risk of stroke

Eyes: Increases risk of cataracts two to three times

Lungs: Increases risk of lung cancer, bronchitis, emphysema, pneumonia, and asthma

Kidneys, Bladder, Pancreas: Increases risk of cancer for all and increases diabetes risk

Stomach/Abdomen: Increases risk of stomach cancer peptic ulcers and abdominal aortic aneurysm

Mouth/Throat: Increases risk of cancers of the mouth, throat, larynx, and esophagus and causes gum disease

Heart: Increases risk of coronary artery disease and atherosclerosis

Reproductive System: Increases risk of breast and cervical cancer, birth complications, unhealthy babies, and sudden death syndrome in babies of smokers

Blood: Increases risk of leukemia and decreases HDL

Figure 1 ▶ Unhealthy effects of smoking.

Carcinogens Substances that promote or facilitate the growth of cancerous cells.

Drug Any biologically active substance that is foreign to the body and is deliberately introduced to affect its functioning.

Withdrawal A temporary illness precipitated by the lack of a drug in the body of an addicted person.

Physical Dependence A drug-induced condition in which a person requires frequent administration of a drug in order to avoid withdrawal.

While risks clearly increase with the amount of exposure, recent studies suggest that even low levels of smoking have negative consequences. Many college students who smoke identify themselves as "social smokers" or "chippers." Some may view this level of smoking as safe, but even low levels of regular smoking can have significant health consequences. For example, one study found that smoking one to four cigarettes per day nearly triples the risk of death from heart disease. Social smoking may also set the stage for the development of nicotine dependence and increased use later in life. Short-term physical consequences of smoking include increased rates of respiratory infections and asthma, impairment of athletic performance, and reduced benefits and enjoyment associated with recreational exercise. Smoking also causes shortness of breath and increases in phlegm production leading to a subjectively negative state.

Cigar and pipe smokers have lower death rates than cigarette smokers but still are at great risk. Cigar and pipe smokers usually inhale less and, therefore, have less risk for heart and lung disease, but cigarette smokers who switch to cigars and pipes tend to continue inhaling the same way. As the number of cigars smoked and the depth of smoke inhalation increase, the risk for death from cigar smoking approaches that of cigarette smoking. Cigar and pipe smoke contains most of the same harmful ingredients as cigarette smoke, sometimes in higher amounts. It may also have high nicotine content, leading to no appreciable difference between cigarette and pipe/cigar smoking with respect to the development of nicotine dependence. Cigar and pipe smokers also have higher risks for cancer of the mouth, throat, and larynx relative to cigarette smokers. Pipe smokers are especially at risk for lip cancer.

Although rates of pipe smoking are relatively low, concern about cigar use has increased. Cigar smoking has become quite trendy in recent years, and many associate cigar smoking with power and influence. Perhaps as a result of positive portrayals of cigar smoking in American culture, adolescents and adults have increased their use of cigars while cigarette smoking has decreased. Efforts similar to those aimed at changing the social norm for cigarette smoking may be necessary to reduce the prevalence of cigar smoking.

Secondhand smoke poses a significant health risk. When a smoker lights up, individuals around him or her are exposed to **secondhand** smoke. Secondhand smoke is a combination of **mainstream** and **sidestream** smoke. Sidestream smoke is considered more dangerous than mainstream smoke because it contains higher concentrations of 13 carcinogens, plus other harmful substances, including nicotine, tar, and carbon monoxide. Its carbon monoxide levels are re-

Web 03

ported to be from 2 to 15 times greater than in the mainstream smoke.

Nonsmokers who must breathe secondhand smoke are, in fact, "involuntary" or "passive" smokers and can suffer serious health problems, especially if they are repeatedly exposed to tobacco smoke over long periods of time. The Environmental Protection Agency (EPA) estimated as many as 3,800 lung cancer deaths per year can be attributed to secondhand smoke. Passive smoking has also been found to increase the risk for heart attacks and asthma. Because of these effects, the EPA has classified secondhand smoke as a serious environmental problem.

Even short-term exposure to secondhand smoke can negatively impact health. One study showed that as little as 30 minutes of exposure to secondhand smoke decreases the functioning of endothelial cells in the coronary arteries, and endothelial cell function is believed to be central to the development of atherosclerosis. The researchers estimated that exposure to secondhand smoke conferred approximately 30 percent risk relative to actually smoking.

Although exposure to secondhand smoke is harmful to everyone, the risks may be particularly severe for children and adolescents. Evidence suggests that adolescents exposed to secondhand smoke are at five times the risk of developing metabolic syndrome, which increases risk for heart disease, stroke, and diabetes. Chil-

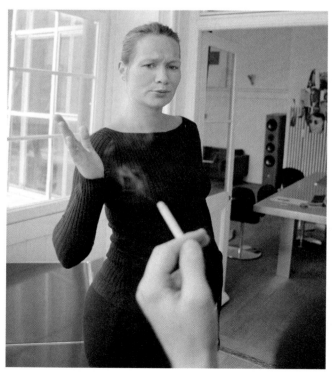

Awareness about the risks of secondhand smoke has contributed to changed social norms.

dren exposed to secondhand smoke are also at increased risk of becoming smokers themselves. One study found that secondhand smoke exposure nearly doubled the risk for becoming a smoker in adolescence, even after controlling for the number of smokers in the home. Finally, there is evidence that secondhand smoke exposure can lead to impaired academic performance. In one study, children exposed to high levels of secondhand smoke had lower test scores in reading, math, and problem solving. Thus, the risks to children and adolescents go well beyond the realm of physical health risks.

While not technically considered secondhand exposure, smoking during pregnancy can also harm a developing fetus. Smoking during pregnancy increases the risks for both short- and long-term health and behavioral consequences. Children of smoking mothers typically have lower birth weight and are more likely to be premature, both of which are risk factors for other health complications. There is also a well-established association between maternal smoking and risk for sudden infant death syndrome (SIDS). In fact, maternal smoking is the strongest known predictor of SIDS. Later in life, children of mothers who smoked during their pregnancy are at increased risk for respiratory infections and chronic asthma. In addition, these children have higher levels of behavioral problems and rates of attention-deficit disorder (ADD). It is important to note that, although in utero exposure is most harmful, significant secondhand smoke exposure can lead to many of the same detrimental effects.

The health risks of smokeless tobacco are similar to those of other forms of tobacco. Some smokers switch to smokeless tobacco because of the misconception that it is a safe substitute for cigarette, cigar, and pipe smoking. While smokeless tobacco does not lead to the same respiratory problems as smoking, the other health risks may be even greater because smokeless tobacco has more nicotine and higher levels of carcinogens. Because it comes in direct contact with body tissues, the health consequences are far more immediate than those from smoking cigarettes. One-third of teenage users have receding gums, and about half have precancerous lesions, 20 percent of which can become oral cancer within 5 years. Some of the health risks of smokeless tobacco are listed in Table 1.

The Facts about Tobacco Usage

At one time, smoking was an accepted part of our culture, but the social norm has changed. While smoking has always been a part of our culture, the industrialization and marketing in the middle of the twentieth century led to tremendous social acceptance of smoking. As odd as it may sound,

Table 1 ▶ Health Risks of Smokeless Tobacco

Smokeless tobacco increases the risk for the following:

- Oral cavity cancer (cheek, gum, lip, palate); it increases the risk by 4 to 50 times, depending on length of time used
- Cancer of the throat, larynx, and esophagus
- Precancerous skin changes
- High blood pressure
- Rotting teeth, exposed roots, premature tooth loss, and worn-down teeth
- Ulcerated, inflamed, infected gums
- Slow healing of mouth wounds
- Decreased resistance to infections
- Arteriosclerosis, myocardial infarction, and coronary occlusion
- Widespread hormonal effects, including increased lipids, higher blood sugar, and more blood clots
- Increased heart rate

cigarettes were once provided free to airline passengers when they boarded planes. The release of the surgeon general's report on smoking in 1964, aggressive and well-funded antismoking campaigns, and increases in cigarette prices have contributed to reductions in smoking in the United States. Since the 1950s, the prevalence of smoking has steadily declined from a high of 50 percent. Based on data from the National Health Interview Survey, rates of smoking in the United States have dropped from 25 percent to 20.9 percent in the past decade. The decrease from 21.6 percent to 20.9 percent between 2002 and 2004 was the largest decrease since the late 1980s. Despite these encouraging results, it appears unlikely that the national health goal of reducing the smoking rate to 12 percent by 2010 will be met. It is worth noting, however, that Utah recently became the first state to reach this goal. Although smoking among adolescents has also decreased substantially over the past decade (eighth-grade rates of daily smoking were reduced

Secondhand Smoke A combination of mainstream and sidestream smoke.

Mainstream Smoke Smoke that is exhaled after being filtered by the smoker's lungs.

Sidestream Smoke Smoke that comes directly off the burning end of a cigarette/cigar/pipe.

by over 50 percent), more recent trends are less encouraging. Among eighth graders, the percentage who reported smoking daily leveled off at 4.4 percent in 2004, and rates of use in the past 30 days actually increased slightly in 2005 to 9.3 percent.

The use of smokeless tobacco is not as prevalent as smoking, but the National Institute of Drug Abuse estimates that 22 million Americans (mostly males) have used it. Young people are also among the most frequent users. The nationwide use of smokeless tobacco among eighth to twelfth graders is 3 to 4 percent. Efforts to reduce the use of smokeless tobacco in these high-risk populations continues.

The prevalence of smoking is higher in Europe and is especially high in China. Smoking remains a global public health threat. While progress in curbing smoking is evident in the United States and other developed countries, these trends are not as apparent elsewhere. In fact, smoking rates have begun to increase in many developing countries as these populations begin to gain easier access to smoking products and advertising. With a population of over 1 billion, China is now the largest consumer of tobacco. Smoking rates among Chinese men are particularly alarming—over 60 percent are considered smokers. The popularity of smoking across the world presents a considerable challenge to the public health community because each country has its own norms and values, as well as unique policies regulating access and advertising.

Most tobacco users begin "using" during adolescence and find it hard to quit. The initiation of smoking is viewed as a pediatric problem by most public health experts. According to a report from the Centers for Disease Control and Prevention, 6,000 people every day under the age of 19 try their first cigarette. At least 3,000 adolescents a day reach adulthood (over the age of 19) as confirmed cigarette smokers. Overall, 90 percent of smokers began before the age of 19. This is the group that finds it most difficult to break the habit later in life. Smokeless tobacco use also begins early in life. Fifty percent of users report that they started before the age of 13 and early use is increasing.

Although most regular smokers begin in adolescence, a significant number start later in life, particularly during early adulthood (18–25). Smoking rates among college students are similar to rates among high school seniors (about 25 percent in the past 30 days), but rates among young adults not attending college are significantly higher (about 40 percent). Studies suggest that the same influences that lead to adolescent smoking promote smoking initiation in early adulthood.

The media play a role in promoting and preventing tobacco use. Much of the blame for tobacco use among youth is attributed to media campaigns of tobacco companies that target this age group. Substantial evidence suggests that cartoon characters, such as Joe Camel, are more effective with youth than adults. One study found that nearly a third of 3-year-olds could match Joe Camel to cigarettes. Fortunately, the Joe Camel tobacco promotion campaign has been discontinued.

Successful antitobacco campaigns have used media blitzes designed to counter tobacco campaigns that glamorize tobacco use. For example, California uses images similar to the glamorous tobacco media images but with negative health messages. In Canada, cigarettes have graphic warnings depicting the negative consequences of smoking. Examples of negative messages from California and Canada appear in Figure 2.

Legal claims against the tobacco industry have aided in antismoking campaigns. Lawsuits filed against tobacco companies have played an important role in decreased smoking rates in the United States. A landmark multistate settlement in 1998 cost the tobacco industry $246 billion. In addition, tobacco companies agreed not to market to anyone under the age of 18. These lawsuits have also had an impact on public opinions of tobacco companies. Documents uncovered from the files of tobacco companies, during litigation against

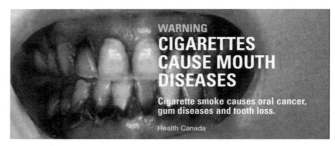

Source: Health Canada.

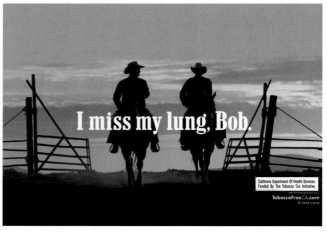

Source: TobaccoFreeCA.com.

Figure 2 ▶ Antismoking messages.

the companies, have contained incriminating evidence that has undermined the reputation of tobacco companies and contributed to an unfavorable public attitude toward the industry.

Although tobacco companies have been hit hard by legal settlements, they have escaped with considerably less damage than many expected. The impact of the multistate settlement has also been weakened by the failure of states to use the funds from the settlement to support tobacco prevention.

Public policy can affect tobacco use. As a matter of public policy, several states have passed special tax laws to fund antitobacco efforts. In addition to raising money for prevention, increased taxes are important because they have been found to be one of the most effective strategies for reducing smoking rates among youth. Public relations campaigns by several state agencies have also been very effective in reducing smoking. Four states that have aggressive antitobacco campaigns reported a 43 percent decrease in tobacco use, double that reported by other states. In addition to antitobacco media campaigns, a number of states have implemented indoor smoking bans. Twelve states have enacted indoor smoking bans, with an all-time high of 6 states enacting laws in 2005. Laws range from bans only on workplace smoking to bans that include all public facilities. The state of Washington has imposed the most restrictive ban, including areas within 25 feet of doors, windows, and vents. Including local bans by cities and counties, there are over 2,000 indoor smoking laws in the United States. In addition, Westin became the first national hotel chain to ban smoking in all hotel rooms. There is evidence that indoor smoking bans are having the desired effect. One study showed that the New York smoking ban in indoor workplaces has led to a reduction in airborne pollutants, including secondhand smoke. Immediately following the smoking ban, pollution levels in public places dropped an average of 84 percent. The smoking ban in Helena, Montana, resulted in a decrease in heart attack deaths. After the courts repealed the ban, heart attack rates went back up.

Tobacco companies are finding new ways to recruit smokers. As expected, the tobacco industry has fought back after the multistate settlement. Since that time, the industry has nearly doubled its budget for advertising and promotions, with the industry spending $22 on advertising for every $1 spent on tobacco prevention. One of the tobacco industry's most recent efforts to promote sales is to provide discounts to offset the increase in tax on tobacco products. Higher prices resulting from tax increases has been shown to be one of the strongest deterrents to teen smoking. Other marketing strategies have included the introduction of flavored cigarettes, such as Kauai Kolada

and Twista Lime. Although the industry denies that these products target teens, studies show that teen smokers are more than twice as likely to use these products as adults over the age of 19. Although not new to the market, clove cigarettes, with their distinct scent and flavor, are also disproportionately used by teenagers.

With a ban on obvious marketing to adolescents, the best legal target to whom tobacco companies can promote their products is now college students and other young adults. One approach the tobacco companies use to reach this audience is industry-sponsored parties at bars and nightclubs. In a national study of college students, nearly 1 in 10 reported attending industry-sponsored events and at least some students at nearly every campus attended. (Students who had not smoked in high school but attended industry-sponsored events where free cigarettes were provided were nearly twice as likely to begin smoking. Although the data do not allow one to determine the direction of causation, these findings are cause for concern.

Various factors influence a person's decision to begin or quit smoking. The reasons for starting smoking are varied, but strikingly similar to reasons given for using alcohol and other drugs (see Table 2). Once a person starts, he or she will typically find it difficult to quit. While a variety of smoking cessation programs are available, several studies have found that increasing the price of cigarettes is the most successful method of reducing smoking in youth.

Many young women begin smoking because they believe that it will help them control their weight and negative mood states. Some current smokers feel they are unable to quit because they fear gaining weight. The evidence shows, however, that people who smoke do not have a lower weight over the long term than nonsmokers. People who fear weight gain should not begin smoking, and those who currently smoke may need psychological help when quitting smoking to help them overcome their fears about weight gain.

Table 2 ▶ Why Young People Start Using Tobacco

- Peer influence
- Social acceptance
- Desire to be "mature"
- Desire to be "independent"
- Desire to be like their role models
- Appealing advertisements

People who smoke cigarettes tend to also use alcohol, marijuana, and hard drugs. Alcohol has often been considered a gateway to other drug use and marijuana is often thought of as a gateway to the use of other drugs, such as cocaine and heroine. Although tobacco use has been studied less extensively as a gateway drug, there is strong evidence that smoking is associated with increased risk for the use of both alcohol and illicit drugs. The combination of smoking and drinking is particularly common in college students. Results of a nationally representative study of college students indicated that 97 percent of smokers drink, compared with national averages of about 80 percent. In addition, those who drink report high levels of smoking, even for college students with rates ranging from 44 to 59 percent (compared with a national average rate of under 30 percent). The combination of alcohol use and smoking poses an even greater risk to physical health.

The addictive nature of nicotine makes it difficult to quit using tobacco. Salient examples of the power of nicotine addiction are high rates of continued use among those with serious smoking-related health consequences and low rates of success for quit attempts. In a study in 15 European countries, over half of adults who suffered from serious medical problems known to be associated with smoking (e.g., heart attack, bypass surgery) continued to smoke 1 year later. Data from the CDC found that 14.6 million adult smokers in the United States stopped for at least 1 day during the past year in an attempt to quit. Unfortunately, most of these attempts were unsuccessful. For most people, it takes many attempts before success is achieved. Withdrawal symptoms and associated cravings for nicotine are often cited reasons for failed quit attempts. Many former smokers report continued nicotine craving months and even years after quitting. The important thing is to keep trying to quit because most people will eventually succeed (45.6 million adults in the United States are former smokers).

Strategies for Action

Some techniques and strategies increase the probability of breaking the nicotine addiction. Web 08 A number of national organizations provide telephone hot lines to help those trying to quit smoking. These include the American Cancer Society (1-877-YES-QUIT), the National Cancer Institute (1-877-44U-QUIT), and the CDC (1-800-QUIT-NOW). In addition, an online smoking program sponsored by several federal agencies is now available at **www.smokefree.gov**. The U.S. Public Health Service (USPH) has published a consumer's guide to quitting smoking. It has determined that the following five factors are associated with the likelihood of success.

1. Get ready.
2. Get support.
3. Learn new skills and behaviors.
4. Get medication and use it correctly.
5. Be prepared for relapse and difficult situations.

The following are some more specific strategies that are consistent with these five basic keys to quitting:

- You must want to quit. The reasons can be for health, family, money, and so on.
- Remind yourself of the reasons. Each day, repeat to yourself the reasons for not using tobacco.
- Decide how to stop. Methods to stop include counseling, attending formal programs, quitting with a friend, going "cold turkey" (abruptly), and quitting gradually. More succeed "cold turkey" than with the gradual approach.

- Remove reminders and temptations (ashtrays, tobacco, etc.).
- Use substitutes and distractions. Substitute low-calorie snacks or chewing gum, change your routine, try new activities, and sit in nonsmoking areas.
- Do not worry about gaining weight. If you gain a few pounds, it is not as detrimental to your health as continuing to smoke.
- Get support. Try a formal "quit smoking program." Examples include "Freedom from Smoking" (American Lung Association) and "Fresh Start" (American Cancer Society). Many state, county, and local health departments, as well as colleges and universities, have programs. Seek support from friends and relatives.
- Assess your current behavior (see Lab 18A).
- Consider a "crutch." You may want to consider a product that requires a prescription, such as a nicotine transdermal patch (Zyban) or nicotine chewing gum.
- Develop effective stress-management techniques. The single most frequently cited reason for difficulty in quitting smoking is stress.
- Set up a system of rewards for your success (e.g., use the money you would have spent on cigarettes to do something nice for yourself).

The USPHS consumer guide also provides a list of questions you may want to ask yourself as you prepare to quit. This exercise may help you increase your motivation to change and decrease the likelihood of a relapse. You may want to talk about your answers with your health-care provider.

1. Why do you want to quit?
2. When you tried to quit in the past, what helped and what did not?
3. What will be the most difficult situations for you after you quit? How will you plan to handle them?
4. Who can help you through the tough times? Your family? Friends? Your health-care provider?
5. What pleasures do you get from smoking? In what ways can you still get pleasure if you quit?

The good news is that, when you quit, you may feel better right away and your body will eventually heal most of the damage. You will feel more energetic, the coughing will stop, you will suddenly begin to taste food again, and your sense of smell will return. Your lungs will eventually heal and look like the lungs of a nonsmoker. Your risk for lung cancer will return to that of the nonsmoker in about 15 to 20 years. There is life after smoking!

Online Learning Center
www.mhhe.com/corbin7e
The Online Learning Center contains a variety of Web-based resources that will help you get the most out of this book and your course. In addition to the On the Web pages, there are video activities, interactive quizzes, application assignments, and a variety of other useful study aids. Log on to the URL above to access these resources.

Technology Update
Varenicline: A Promising New Drug

Although nicotine replacement and other medications that do not include nicotine (Zyban) appear to help many who want to quit smoking, rates of success remain relatively low even with the help of medication. A promising new drug may help increase success rates. In one study, approximately 44 percent of smokers using Varenicline successfully quit smoking within 3 months while the rates for Zyban and placebo were 30 percent and 18 percent, respectively. The new drug may be available as soon as late 2006.

Web Resources

Agency for Health Care Policy and Research **www.ahcpr.gov**
Web 09 American Cancer Society **www.cancer.org**
American Heart Association **www.americanheart.org**
American Lung Association **www.lungusa.org**
Campaign for Tobacco Free Kids **www.tobaccofreekids.org**
Dr. Koop—Tackling Tobacco Abuse **www.drkoop.com/tobacco**
National Center for Chronic Disease Prevention and Health Promotion: Tobacco Information and Prevention Source **www.cdc.gov/tobacco**
Quitnet—A Free Resource to Quit Smoking **www.quitnet.org**
Surgeon general's report on smoking, 2004 **www.cdc.gov/tobacco/sgr/sgr_2004**
You Can Quit Smoking, Consumer Guide, June 2000. U.S. Public Health Service **www.surgeongeneral.gov/tobacco/consquits.htm**
You Can Quit Smoking Now **www.smokefree.gov**

Suggesting Readings

Additional reference materials for concept 18 are available at Web10.

Web 10 American Cancer Society. 2006. Tobacco product advertising and promotion fact sheet. *Quit Smoking*. Available at www.lungusa.org/site/pp.asp?c=dvLUK900E&b=44462.

Bjartveit, K., and A. Tverdal. 2005. Health consequences of smoking 1–4 cigarettes per day. *Tobacco Control* 14:315–320.
California Department of Health Services. 2004. California's adult smoking declines to historic low. *California Department of Health Services News Release* Number 04-30, May 26, http://www.dhs.ca.gov.
DiFranza, J. R., C. A. Aligne, and M. Weitzman. 2004. Prenatal and postnatal environmental tobacco smoke exposure and children's health. *Pediatrics* 113:1007–1015.
Doll, R., et al. 2004. Mortality in relation to smoking. *British Medical Journal* 328(7455):1519–1528.
Ezzati, M., and A. D. Lopez. 2003. Estimates of global mortality attributable to smoking. *Lancet* 362(9387):847–852.
Hahn, D. B., et al. 2007. *Focus on Health*. 8th ed. New York: McGraw-Hill Higher Education. Chapter 9.
Johansson, A. K., et al. 2004. How should parents protect their children from environmental tobacco smoke exposure in the home? *Pediatrics* 113(4):e291–e295.
Morbidity and Mortality Weekly Report. 2004. Cigarette smoking among adults. *Morbidity and Mortality Weekly Report* 53(20):427–431.

Office of the Surgeon General. 2004. *The Health Consequences of Smoking: A Report of the Surgeon General*. Atlanta, GA: U.S. Department of Health and Human Services.

Patterson, F., et al. 2004. Cigarette smoking practices among American college students: Review and future directions. *Journal of American College Health* 52:203–210.

Rigotti, N. A., S. E. Moran, and H. Wechsler. 2005. US college students' exposure to tobacco promotions: Prevalence and association with tobacco use. *American Journal of Public Health* 95:138–144.

Smith, S. August 20, 2006. Cigarettes pack more nicotine: State study finds a 10 percent rise over six years. *Boston Globe*.

Teague, M. L., et al. 2007. Your Health Today: Choices in a Changing Society. New York: McGraw-Hill Higher Education. Chapter 13.

U.S. Department of Health and Human Services. 2006. *The Health Consequences of Involuntary Exposure to Tobacco Smoke: A Report of the Surgeon General*. Atlanta, GA: U.S. Department of Health and Human Services, Center for Disease Control and Prevention, Coordinating Center for Health Promotions, National Center for Chronic Disease Prevention and Health Promotion, Office on Smoking and Health.

 In the News

Second Hand Smoke and Increased Nicotine in Tobacco

A new report, "The Health Consequences of Involuntary Exposure to Tobacco Smoke: A Report of the Surgeon General" establishes in detail the health dangers of secondhand smoke. If there had been question before, this report provides the scientific evidence to indicate that involuntary exposure to tobacco smoke kills. The six major conclusions of the study (see Surgeon General's Website) are abstracted below.

- Millions of Americans are exposed to secondhand smoke despite progress in tobacco control.
- Secondhand smoke causes disease and early death.
- Infants and children are especially at risk of illnesses related to secondhand smoke.
- Adult exposure to secondhand smoke is especially likely to contribute to heart disease and cancer.
- Even short exposure to secondhand smoke is dangerous.
- Eliminating secondhand smoke indoors eliminates secondhand smoking exposure but separation of smoking and nonsmoking indoor space does not

In addition to increasing spending on advertising, a new study suggests the tobacco industry might also be adding more nicotine to cigarettes. In a study of 116 brands of cigarettes assessed in 1998 and 2004, 92 brands showed an increase in the amount of nicotine that can be inhaled by a typical smoker. Only twelve brands showed a decrease with another 12 showing no significant change. Overall, the study found an average increase in nicotine content of about 10%.

Lab 18A Use and Abuse of Tobacco

Name		Section	Date

Purpose: To understand the risks of diseases (such as heart disease and cancer) associated with the use of tobacco or exposure to tobacco by-products

Procedure

1. Read the Tobacco Use Risk Questionnaire (Chart 1).
2. Answer the questionnaire based on your tobacco use or exposure.
3. Record your score and rating (from Chart 2) in the Results section.

Results

What is your tobacco risk score? [   ] (total from Chart 1)

What is your tobacco risk rating? [   ] (see Chart 2)

Chart 1 ▶ Tobacco Use Risk Questionnaire

Circle one response in each row of the questionnaire. Determine a point value for each response using the point values in the first row of the chart. Sum the numbers of points for the various responses to determine a Tobacco Use Risk score.

	Points				
Categories	**0**	**1**	**2**	**3**	**4**
Cigarette use	Never smoked		1–10 cigarettes a day	11–40 cigarettes a day	>40 cigarettes a day
Pipe and cigar use	Never smoked	Pipe— ccasional use	Cigar— infrequent daily use	Cigar or pipe— frequent daily use	Cigar—heavy use
Smoking style	Don't smoke		No inhalation	Slight to moderate inhalation	Deep inhalation
Smokeless tobacco use	Don't use	Occasional use: not daily	Daily use: one use per day	Daily Use: multiple use per day	Heavy use: repetitious, multiple use daily
Secondhand or side-stream smoke	No smokers at home or in workplace	Smokers at work-place but not at home	Smokers at home but not workplace	Smokers at home and at workplace	
Years of tobacco use	Never used	1 or less	2–5	6–10	>10

Note: Different forms of tobacco use pose different risks for different diseases. This questionnaire is designed to give you a general idea of risk associated with use and exposure to tobacco by-products.

Chart 2 ▶ Tobacco Use Risk Questionnaire Rating Chart

Rating	Score
Very high risk	16+
High risk	7–15
Moderate risk	1–6
Low risk	0

Conclusions and Implications

1. In several sentences, discuss your personal risk. If your risk is low, discuss some implications of the behavior of other people that affect your risk, including what can be done to change these risks. If your risk is above average, what changes can be made to reduce your risk?

2. In several sentences, discuss how you feel about public laws designed to curtail tobacco use. Discuss your point of view, either pro or con.

The Use and Abuse of Alcohol

Health Goals for the year 2010

- Reduce substance abuse to protect the health, safety, and quality of life for all, especially children.

- Reduce deaths and injuries caused by alcohol-related motor vehicle crashes.

- Reduce cirrhosis deaths.

- Reduce alcohol-related injuries and hospital emergency room visits.

- Reduce number of young people who ride with a driver who has been drinking alcohol.

- Increase number of young people who are alcohol free.

- Reduce binge drinking and average alcohol consumption.

- Extend legal requirements for maximum blood alcohol concentration (BAC) levels to .08 percent for drivers.

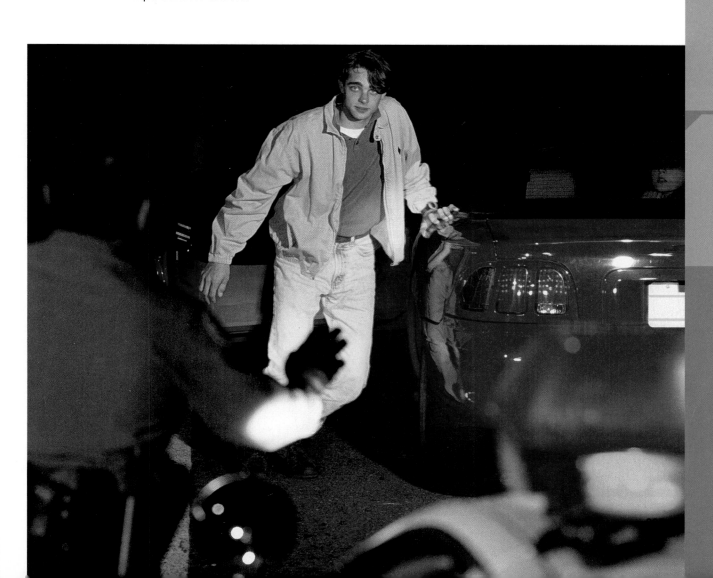

Alcohol is among the most widely used and destructive drugs and ranks high among causes of health problems and death in our culture.

Alcohol is the most widely used and destructive drug in the United States. If all of the deaths caused by this drug are counted, it is the third leading health problem and cause of early death in the United States. Only tobacco and inactivity/poor nutrition rank ahead of alcohol use. Some consider alcohol use to be the most destructive because of the devastating results of drinking and driving (or operating other vehicles) and because of the consequences of increased crime, physical and sexual abuse, and destroyed family relationships that are often associated with overindulgence in alcohol. It is estimated that about 14 million people in the United States, representing over 7 percent of the total population, meet the criteria for some type of alcohol-related diagnosis.

Alcohol and Alcoholic Beverages

Alcoholic beverages contain ethanol (ethyl alcohol), an intoxicating and addictive drug that is often misused. The active **drug** in alcoholic beverages (ethanol) is a toxic chemical, but unlike methanol (wood alcohol) and isopropyl (rubbing alcohol), it can be consumed in small doses. As a drug, it is classified as a depressant. However, this classification does not capture the full range of alcohol effects. The effects experienced by the drinker depend, in part, on whether blood alcohol concentration is rising or falling. The sedative effects of alcohol as blood alcohol levels fall are consistent with its classification as a depressant drug. In contrast, primarily stimulant effects are experienced by the user as blood alcohol concentration rises.

Humans have consumed alcoholic beverages for thousands of years. Unfortunately, many people in our culture (particularly college students) view drunkenness as a rite

of passage and an expectation. Indeed, there are more synonyms for the word *drunk* or ***intoxication*** than for any other word in the English language. This illustrates the importance we give to overconsumption. Fortunately, as people mature, they tend to reduce their consumption, as responsibilities such as work and family become more important.

Alcoholic beverages have varying concentrations of alcohol but many have similar amounts per serving. Beverages are usually served in proportions such that a drink of any one of the three categories (beer, wine, or liquor) contains the same amount of alcohol. Beer is usually served in a 12-ounce can, bottle, or mug. A typical glass of wine holds 5 ounces, and a shot of liquor is 1.5 ounces. Even though the percentage of alcohol in the beverages differs, the drinks would be equivalent in alcohol because each would contain about 15 mL of alcohol (see Figure 1).

Alcohol's effect on the body depends on many factors. Alcohol is absorbed directly into the bloodstream, primarily in the small intestine, though some absorption occurs in the mouth, esophagus, and stomach. It then concentrates in various organs in proportion to the amount of water each contains. The brain has a high water content, so much of the alcohol goes there, where it depresses the central nervous system. The rate and

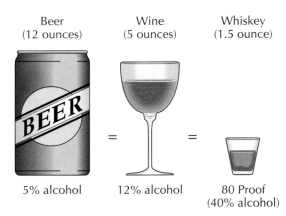

Beer (12 ounces) Wine (5 ounces) Whiskey (1.5 ounce)

5% alcohol   12% alcohol   80 Proof (40% alcohol)

Figure 1 ▶ Alcohol content of drinks.

Source: National Institute on Alcohol Abuse and Alcoholism.

magnitude of the effects on an individual depend on the drinker's level of fatigue; his or her mood; what and how much food is in the stomach; other drugs and medications consumed; body size/weight; rate of consumption; individual body chemistry and genetic predisposition; individual beliefs about the effects of alcohol; and context in which drinking occurs. In general, the more and faster one drinks, the greater the effect. Differences in effects are apparent between genders even when differences in body size are considered. One reason for this is that women have lower amounts of body water, so a given amount of alcohol will represent a greater percentage of the volume of the blood in their bloodstream. Another factor is that women have lower amounts of the enzymes needed to process alcohol. Thus, alcohol stays in the bloodstream longer before being broken down. There is also some evidence that hormone levels associated with the phases of the menstrual cycle might affect women's responses to alcohol. However, there is no clear pattern of effects, and some studies have failed to find differences associated with hormone levels.

The body cannot usually process alcohol as quickly as it is consumed. Alcohol in the bloodstream is eventually oxidized in the liver. An enzyme in the liver, called alcohol dehydrogenase (ADH), converts alcohol to acetaldehyde, which is then converted by acetate and other enzymes into carbon dioxide and water. Individuals differ with respect to their ability to metabolize alcohol, but a healthy adult takes 1 to 2 hours to metabolize one standard drink. Because the rate of alcohol consumption is typically greater than the rate at which it is processed, the alcohol concentration in the bloodstream begins to increase. The blood alcohol concentration (BAC) is measured as a percentage and is used by law enforcement officials to determine if a driver is legally intoxicated.

Studies show the risk in driving increases when the BAC is between 0.01 and 0.04 percent. A BAC of .10 percent used to be the level at which driving became illegal in most states. Due to evidence of impairment at much lower doses and the extreme social and economic costs associated with drinking and driving, all 50 states and the District of Columbia have now reduced the legal limit to .08 percent. Minnesota became the last state to adopt this standard in August 2005.

Health and Behavioral Consequences of Alcohol

Making statements about the consequences of alcohol consumption is difficult because the consequences vary depending on the amount and way in which it is consumed. The risks are also not the same for everyone. The following sections will outline the relative health risks and benefits associated with various levels of alcohol consumption.

Heavy alcohol use is associated with an increased risk for a variety of negative health outcomes. The most well-established health risk associated with alcohol consumption is liver disease. Alcohol is the leading cause of disease and death from liver dysfunction, with an estimated 2 million people suffering from alcohol-induced liver disease. Although the liver is capable of metabolizing moderate amounts of alcohol on a regular basis, persistent, heavy drinking may lead to swollen liver cells, a condition called **fatty liver.** If drinking is stopped or significantly reduced at this point, the damage to the liver is likely reversible. If drinking continues, **alcoholic hepatitis** may occur. At this point, swelling of the liver is persistent, leading to the destruction of tissue and the development of scar tissue. Due to the development of scar tissue, the body begins to have difficulty breaking down toxins. Much of this damage may still be reversible if scar tissue is not extensive. With continued heavy drinking, the individual is likely to develop **alcoholic cirrhosis,** or permanent scarring of the liver. At this point, blood flow through the liver is impaired, leading to the buildup of toxins in the body. Cirrhosis may also lead to gastrointestinal bleeding, abdominal swelling, and coughing-up of blood. Damage is not reversible at this point, though abstinence improves survival rate. Severe cases of cirrhosis necessitate liver transplant for survival.

Heavy drinking is also a risk factor for other negative health outcomes (see Figure 2, page 398). Although moderate alcohol consumption may protect against coronary heart disease (CHD) as outlined later in the concept, heavier use of alcohol may increase the risk for CHD and other cardiovascular disease. Specifically, heavy drinking is associated with increased risk for hypertension, cardiomyopathy, cardiac arrhythmia, and congestive heart failure. There is considerable evidence that alcohol consumption increases the risk for cancer, including

Drug Any biologically active substance that is foreign to the body and is deliberately introduced to affect its functioning.

Intoxication Also referred to as drunkenness; a blood alcohol level of .08.

Fatty liver Swelling of the cells of the liver.

Alcoholic Hepatitis Persistent swelling of the cells of the liver, leading to its decreased ability to break down toxins.

Alcoholic Cirrhosis Permanent scarring of the liver, resulting in reduced blood flow and the buildup of toxins in the body.

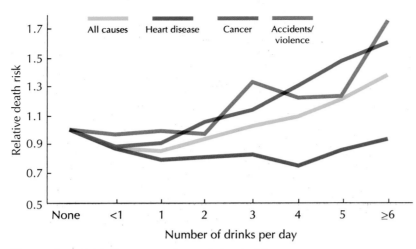

Figure 2 ▶ Alcohol consumption and death risk.
Source: American Cancer Society.

cancer of the oral cavity and pharynx, esophagus, liver, larynx, and female breast. The risk for certain types of stroke (hemorrhagic) is also increased by alcohol. With prolonged heavy use, risk for neuropsychiatric diseases increases. The most well-known neuropsychiatric disease associated with alcohol consumption is **Wernicke-Korsakoff Syndrome (WKS)**. WKS results from a thiamine deficiency that is secondary to reduced liver function and poor nutrition in alcoholics. Symptoms include confusion, disorientation, and impaired memory. Prolonged heavy drinking also increases risk for digestive diseases, including pancreatitis. There is also evidence that heavy drinking may impair immune functioning, leading to increased risk for infectious diseases, including pneumonia and tuberculosis.

In addition to increasing risk for alcohol use disorders, heavy drinking may increase risk for other psychiatric disorders that often co-occur with alcohol problems (e.g., mood and anxiety disorders). Finally, alcohol use is associated with increased risk for accidents and violence, both sources of increased morbidity and mortality. Although some of the negative outcomes associated with alcohol use require prolonged heavy use (e.g., WKS and alcoholic cirrhosis), others occur at relatively modest levels of consumption (increased risk for cancer and less severe forms of liver and cardiovascular disease). In summary, the costs associated with alcohol consumption are extensive and must be considered in relation to the potential benefits.

While heavy drinking presents many risks, moderate consumption can provide some health benefits. There is substantial evidence that moderate alcohol consumption (one drink per day for women, up to two drinks per day for men) is associated with decreased risk for coronary heart disease (CHD), Type II diabetes, and certain

types of stroke. At this point, it is not entirely clear the extent to which moderate drinking "causes" reduced risk for cardiovascular disease. It may be that moderate drinkers are at lower risk based on other characteristics, such as higher education and income, better diet, and more regular exercise. Still, mechanisms for a causal role of alcohol use in protection against CHD are plausible and have been studied extensively. There is evidence to suggest that decreased risk for CHD and stroke may be due to reductions in blood clotting and increased levels of high-density lipoproteins (HDL), or "good cholesterol." The potential mechanisms for protection against diabetes are less clear. Recent evidence suggests that moderate alcohol use may also protect against cognitive declines with aging. Although the research conducted to date has been with elderly women, researchers suggest that the benefits are likely to be similar for men.

Although the protection against health risks by moderate alcohol consumption is significant, particularly given the impact on CHD risk, it is important to keep in mind that moderate alcohol consumption may not be safe for everyone. Age, gender, health status, and a family history of alcoholism are just a few of the individual differences that contribute to the relative safety of alcohol consumption for any individual. Certain groups are best off not drinking at all, despite potential health benefits (see Table 1). It is also important to note that the pattern of drinking is as important as the absolute level. A woman who has seven drinks one time each week consumes an average of one drink per day but does not receive the same health benefits as

Table 1 ▶ People Who Should Consider Abstaining from Alcohol Use

- People under age 21 (legal age)
- Athletes striving for peak performance
- Women trying to get pregnant or who are pregnant or nursing
- Alcoholics and recovering alcoholics
- People with a family history of alcoholism
- People with a medical or surgical problem and/or on medications
- Psychiatric patients or persons experiencing severe psychosis
- People driving vehicles or operating dangerous machinery or involved in public safety
- People conducting serious business transactions or study

a woman who consumes one drink each day. Moderate consumption of alcohol can be safely incorporated into a healthy lifestyle, but heavy episodic drinking cannot.

Women appear to be especially susceptible to the negative health consequences of heavy drinking. Assuming similar levels of alcohol consumption, women are more likely to experience liver, cardiovascular, and brain damage from drinking. Alcohol also increases risk of the development of breast cancer and negatively impacts the reproductive system. Excessive alcohol use may lead to infertility, hormonal imbalance, and menstrual disturbance. Women are also more cognitively impaired by alcohol than men, which increases risk for negative behavioral outcomes, such as unprotected sexual behavior and drinking and driving. Women who are pregnant should avoid alcohol. Drinking during pregnancy can lead to fetal alcohol syndrome, which is associated with low birth weight, physical defects, mental retardation, and stunted growth.

The greatest danger of alcohol occurs when the drinker gets behind the wheel of a motor vehicle. Alcohol-related traffic crashes are the leading cause of death and spinal cord injury for young Americans. Approximately 41 percent of fatal injury traffic accidents are alcohol involved and two out of five Americans will be involved in an alcohol-related auto crash at sometime in their lives. In the United States, someone is killed in an alcohol-related crash every 30 minutes. The driver's likelihood of causing a highway accident increases significantly at a BAC of .04 percent (approximately the level reached by a 120-pound woman who has one drink in 1 hour). When BAC reaches .10 percent, the chances have increased by 600 percent. The effects of different BAC values on physical and driving performance are summarized in Table 2.

In addition to risks associated with traffic accidents, those who drink and drive face significant legal, financial, and social costs. There were approximately 1.4 million arrests for drunk driving in 2001. Many states now have mandatory license revocation laws and mandatory jail time for repeat offenders. Many states also have minimum fines for first offenders of $500 or more, and maximum penalties in some states are as high as $5,000. Although the short-term costs are significant, the long-term costs of a drunk driving arrest typically far outweigh the immediate financial burden. Having an offense on your record can lead to problems with schools, family, and future employers. Despite the potential short- and long-term costs, in a government survey 70 percent of college students reported driving while under the influence of alcohol at least once in the past year and 22 percent said they had done it five times or more. Information about alcohol policies and laws related to drunk driving is available at Web01.

Web 01

Table 2 ▶ The Effects of Blood Alcohol Concentration (BAC) on Driving Performance and Function

BAC 0.02%
- Vision is impaired: less ability to see objects in motion; less ability to monitor multiple objects.
- Attention span is lower.
- Reaction time slows.
- Less critical of own actions.

BAC 0.05–0.06%
- Inhibitions are reduced (unnecessary chances may be taken).
- Visual abilities decrease; side vision is impaired by 30%.
- Superficial feelings of relaxation.
- Judgment is the first function to be impaired.
- Braking distance is extended.
- Diminished ability to maneuver through narrow spaces.
- Coordination is impaired.
- Information processing is impaired.
- Driving performance is impaired at moderate speed.

BAC 0.08%
- Vision is seriously impaired, especially at night.
- Overconfidence in driving ability.
- Emotions are exaggerated.
- Thinking and reasoning powers are impaired.
- Less ability to concentrate.
- Judgments are dulled; driver is more careless.
- Muscle control and coordination are hindered.
- Distances are misjudged.
- Driving performance is impaired at low speeds.
- Possible steering inaccuracy.
- Driver increases the use of the accelerator and brake.

BAC .15%
- Gross motor impairment and lack of physical control.
- Blurred vision and loss of balance.
- Increased risk of hangovers.

BAC .20%
- Disorientation and difficulty waking.
- Nausea and vomiting.
- Anesthesia.
- Impaired gag reflex.
- Blackouts.

BAC .30%
- Stupor and decreased respiration.
- Loss of consciousness.

BAC .40%
- Coma.
- Death is possible, due to respiratory arrest.

Source: Mothers Against Drunk Driving.

Wernicke-Korsakoff Syndrome (WKS) A neuropsychiatric illness caused by a thiamine deficiency typically resulting from chronic alcohol dependence. Symptoms include disorientation, confusion, and memory loss.

Understanding the effects of alcohol at various blood alcohol levels and being able to estimate your own blood alcohol level can help prevent you from driving when impaired. Table 3 provides estimated BACs for men and women at various weights. Lab 19A will provide the formula necessary to calculate BAC for your precise weight. A new product from Guardian Angel™ is also available to check your BAC when you have been drinking. These small strips can be kept in your pocket and used to test your BAC before you get behind the wheel of a car. It is important to recognize that the only thing that reduces your BAC is the passage of time. Many people believe they have proven strategies to sober up, such as taking a cold shower, drinking coffee, or sleeping it off. Although these approaches may make you feel less intoxicated, they do not affect your BAC.

Alcohol Consumption and Alcohol Abuse

The prevalence of excessive alcohol consumption is a major public health challenge. After initial experimentation with alcohol, most individuals decide either to abstain or to develop a regular pattern of use. Roughly half (50.3 percent) of the U.S. population over the age of 12 reports alcohol consumption in the past 30 days. This makes alcohol the most widely used drug of abuse in this country. Most who choose to drink develop a pattern of light or moderate drinking. Although various definitions of *moderate drinking* have been proposed, the National Institute on Alcohol Abuse and Alcoholism (NIAAA) definition is perhaps the most widely used. According to the NIAAA,

moderate consumption is characterized as one drink per day or less for women and two drinks per day or less for men (see Table 4). Those who exceed these standards are often described as at-risk drinkers. Among those who are at-risk drinkers, heavy-episodic drinking (sometimes referred to as binge drinking) is common. This is generally defined as 5 or more standard alcoholic drinks consumed in a row (4 or more for women). Approximately 23 percent of the U.S. population (55 million people) report heavy-episodic drinking in the past 30 days. Thus, nearly one-half of those who drink report having five or more (four or more for women) drinks at least occasionally.

Heavy-episodic drinkers are 14 times more likely to drink and drive, and they are at increased risk for a host of negative outcomes, including motor vehicle crashes, falls, burns, drownings, and sexually transmitted diseases. The overall impact of drinking on other members of society is particularly troubling. Over 50 percent of traffic fatalities are alcohol-related. Alcohol is also the overwhelming cause of most sexual assaults (about 72 percent), family violence (about 80 percent), and child abuse (about 60 percent). Ambitious public health goals have been set for curtailing alcohol consumption in the United States, but little progress has been made. Details on the *Healthy People 2010* goals for alcohol consumption are at Web02.

Alcohol use disorders can develop over time with the repeated use of alcohol. In addition to the acute consequences of heavy-episodic drinking, those who drink at this level are at increased risk for the development of alcohol use disorders, including **alcohol abuse** and **alcohol dependence** (see Table 4 on page 401 for characteristics of these conditions). Heavy-episodic college drinkers are at 13 times greater risk for alcohol abuse and 19 times greater risk for alcohol dependence. Another term (**tolerance**) is something that many (especially men) boast about, with statements such as "I can hold my liquor." They may also ridicule others who have not developed tolerance with statements such as "You're a lightweight." The reality is that tolerance has mostly negative implications. Practically speaking, the more one develops tolerance, the more one has to drink (and spend) to get the same effects. In addition, recent evidence indicates that individuals with "innate" tolerance to alcohol's effects are at increased risk of tolerance to alcohol's developing alcohol dependence. Thus, if you are able to drink a lot without feeling the effects, by virtue of disposition or drinking experience, you should recognize that you are at high risk for alcohol use disorders. With the heavier use that comes with the development of tolerance, **withdrawal** symptoms may develop when alcohol is not administered with regularity. Withdrawal symptoms include anxiety, increased heart rate, sweating, hand tremor, nausea, and vomiting. In more severe cases, withdrawal can lead to hallucinations and grand mal seizures.

Table 3 ▶ Approximate BAC Values (%) Based on the Number of Drinks Consumed over a One-Hour Period

Number of drinks	Females		Males	
	120-Pound	180-Pound	140-Pound	200-Pound
1	.04	.03	.03	.02
2	.08	.05	.05	.04
3	.11	.08	.08	.06
4	.15	.10	.11	.08
5	.19	.13	.13	.09
6	.23	.15	.16	.11
7	.27	.18	.19	.13
8	.30	.20	.21	.15

Source: U.S. Department of Health and Human Services, Substance Abuse and Mental Health Services Administration.

Table 4 ▶ Terms and Criteria for Patterns of Alcohol Use

Term	Criteria
Moderate drinking (NIAAA)	Men: ≤2 drinks/day Women: ≤1 drink/day Over 65: ≤1 drink/day
At-risk drinking (NIAAA)	Men: >14 drinks/week or >4 drinks/occasion Women: >7 drinks/week or >3 drinks/occasion
Heavy-episodic drinking (NIAAA)	Men: 5 or more alcoholic drinks consumed in a row Women: 4 or more alcoholic drinks consumed in a row
Alcohol abuse (APA)	Maladaptive pattern of alcohol use leading to clinically significant impairment or distress, manifested within a 12-month period by one or more of the following: • Failure to fulfill role obligations at work, school, or home • Recurrent use in hazardous situations • Legal problems related to alcohol • Continued use despite alcohol-related social or interpersonal problems
Alcohol dependence (APA)	Maladaptive pattern of alcohol use leading to clinically significant impairment or distress, manifested within a 12-month period by three or more of the following: • Tolerance (either increasing amounts used or diminished effects with the same amount) • Withdrawal (withdrawal symptoms or use to relieve or avoid symptoms) • Use of larger amounts over a longer period than intended • Persistent desire or unsuccessful attempts to cut down or control use • Great deal of time spent obtaining, using, or recovering from use • Important social, occupational, or recreational activities given up or reduced • Use despite knowledge of alcohol-related physical or psychological problems

Note: NIAAA, National Institute on Alcohol Abuse and Alcoholism; APA, American Psychiatric Association. Source: O'Conner and Schottenfeld.

Age of onset of alcohol use is associated with later problems. There is considerable evidence that those who begin drinking earlier are at increased risk for the later development of alcohol-related problems, including engaging in heavy drinking, driving under the influence of alcohol, sustaining injuries related to alcohol use, and developing alcohol dependence. It may be that the effects of alcohol on the adolescent brain lead to increased risk. On the other hand, the individual characteristics of those who begin drinking early may predict later problems. For example, individuals high in impulsivity may start earlier and be more likely to have problems. Regardless, early age of onset is an important marker for later problems.

Environment also plays a role in the initiation and escalation of alcohol use. During childhood, parents play an important role in the socialization process, which includes socialization regarding alcohol use. Parents who talk to their kids about alcohol use, provide social support, and monitor their children's behavior are less likely to have children who drink excessively during adolescence. This is important because early onset of drinking increases the risk for later problems. During adolescence, peers take on a powerful role in the development of alcohol prob-

lems. One of the best predictors of adolescent alcohol use patterns is the pattern of alcohol use among their close friends. Peer influences continue into the college years, when heavy drinking becomes more normative.

College students drink more than the rest of society and are more at risk for alcohol problems than other segments of the population. The problem of college drinking has gained

Web 03

Alcohol Abuse Use of alcohol in hazardous situations or continued alcohol use in hazardous situations or despite significant negative consequences.

Alcohol Dependance Severe form of alcohol abuse that is often characterized by physical symptoms of dependence.

Tolerance The phenomenon of requiring more and more alcohol over time to achieve the desired effect.

Withdrawal Symptoms that occur when alcohol is withdrawn after a period of prolonged heavy use. Symptoms include sweating, anxiety, tremors, and seizures.

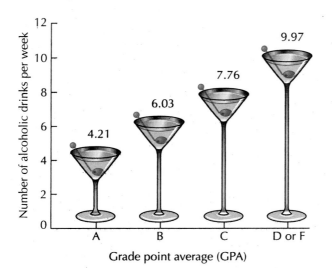

Figure 3 ▶ Average number of alcoholic drinks per week by GPA.

Source: Adapted from Core Institute.

increased attention over the past 10 years. The vast majority of college students have consumed alcohol in the past year (roughly 80 percent) and drinking among college students is a significant public health problem. It is estimated that drinking by college students is associated with 696,000 physical assaults, 599,000 injuries, 400,000 instances of unsafe sexual behavior, 97,000 sexual assaults, and 1,700 deaths annually. About 25 percent of college students report academic problems caused by drinking, including lower grades, poor performance on exams and papers, and missed classes. Grade point average has also been found to be inversely related to the amount of alcohol consumed (see Figure 3). Rates of heavy-episodic drinking are particularly high among college students, with about 43 percent reporting at least occasionally drinking at this level. Roughly 20 percent report engaging in frequent heavy-episodic drinking, defined as three or more occasions in a 2-week period. Given high rates of heavy drinking, it is not surprising that college students account for about 10 percent of all alcohol sales. One study also found that 31 percent of college students met the criteria for alcohol abuse and 6 percent met the criteria for alcohol dependence in the past 12 months.

Just as in the general population, heavy-episodic drinking is associated with increased risk for negative outcomes (see Table 5). Relative to nonheavy-episodic drinkers, occasional heavy-episodic drinkers are two to three times more likely to experience a range of negative consequences, and frequent heavy-episodic drinkers are 6 to 10 times more likely to experience the same consequences. One poll of college students showed just how prominent a role drinking plays in college life. The favorite activity reported by college students was drinking beer. About 72 percent of those polled indicated that they engaged in this activity. Working out was also popular among college students, though only 62 percent reported engaging in this activity. Even college students identify alcohol abuse as one of the

Table 5 ▶ Alcohol-Related Problems Among College Students

Problems	All students	Nonheavy-Episodic Drinkers (%)	Occasional Heavy-Episodic Drinkers (%)	Frequent Heavy-Episodic Drinkers (%)
Did something you regret	36.1	18.0	39.6	62.0
Missed a class	29.9	8.8	30.9	62.5
Drove after drinking	28.8	18.6	39.7	56.7
Forgot where you were or what you did	27.1	10.0	27.2	54.0
Argued with friends	22.5	9.7	23.0	42.6
Got behind in school work	24.1	9.8	26.0	46.3
Engaged in unplanned sexual activities	21.6	7.9	22.3	41.5
Got hurt or injured	12.4	3.9	10.9	26.6
Damaged property	10.8	2.3	8.9	22.7
Had unprotected sex	10.3	3.7	9.8	20.4

Source: Wechsler et al.

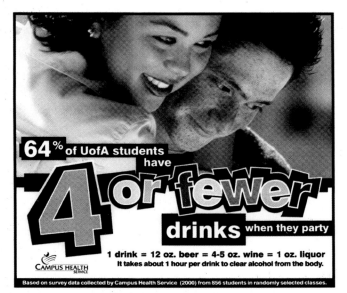

Figure 4 ▶ Knowledge of peer behavior can reduce peer pressure.
Source: University of Arizona, Campus Health Service, used by permission.

biggest problems on college campuses. A survey of college students found that 44 percent believed alcohol abuse to be the biggest problem on campus.

New strategies are being explored to curb drinking on campuses. Although increased attention to college drinking problems has led to increased education and prevention, rates of heavy use have changed little. One contributing factor may be that attention to heavy drinking has led to the perception by college students that their peers are drinking more than they actually are. Research has shown that college students routinely overestimate use by their peers and that these misperceptions are associated with increases in drinking. In theory, students drink more to keep up with what they perceive to be the norm on campus. Given these findings, prevention programs on college campuses are now trying to counter these misperceptions by looking at the high percentage of students who *do not* drink heavily. One study found that only 66.2 percent of college students reported any alcohol use in the past 30 days. Those who did report drinking had an average of 4.22 drinks over an average of 2.75 hours the last time they "partied." This amount of alcohol over this time frame would result in relatively low levels of intoxication. Figure 4 provides an example of a media campaign designed to counter misperceptions about campus drinking.

Having a family member with an alcohol problem places you at increased risk of developing a problem yourself. Experts have known for some time that the development of alcohol abuse and dependence has a ge-

netic component. Alcohol problems run in families, and it is estimated that genetics may account for as much as half of the risk for alcohol dependence. In the future, we may find out exactly how genetic differences contribute to risk, but for now we know that genetics are important. Thus, if you have a family history of alcoholism, you should be especially careful about your drinking behavior.

Beliefs about the effects of alcohol develop early and play an important role in later drinking behavior. The promotion of alcohol as a social lubricant leads to the development of positive beliefs about the effects of alcohol, referred to as alcohol expectancies. These beliefs have been shown to develop even prior to personal experience with alcohol. Media portrayals of the benefits of drinking are believed to play an important role in the development of positive alcohol expectancies. Most beer and other alcohol advertisements portray alcohol as an important part of social life that is essential to having a good time. Adolescents are bombarded with these messages from an early age. For every television commercial discouraging under-age drinking, the average teen sees approximately 86 commercials promoting alcohol, and the alcohol industry spends over $800 million annually on advertising, compared with about $30 million spent on ads designed to prevent drunk driving. Positive alcohol expectancies established during adolescence increase alcohol usage later in life.

Once drinking has begun, positive alcohol expectancies typically increase, leading to the maintenance or progression of drinking behavior. Efforts to combat unrealistic expectations about the effects of alcohol have shown promise in reducing alcohol consumption and related negative consequences. Table 6 lists some of the environmental factors that promote drinking.

Table 6 ▶ Why People Start Drinking
• Peer pressure
• Need to belong and to be accepted
• Media depiction of drinking
• Advertising depiction of drinking
• Lack of knowledge about its effects
• Easy access (especially at home)
• Absence of strong religious attachment
• Beer bonding (especially in college)
• Cultural traditions at college
• Social lubrication
• Good feelings

Strategies for Action

Determining if a problem exists is an important strategy for taking action. Moderate alcohol consumption is safe for many people and may even have some health benefits. However, many people who drink do so beyond safe levels. If you drink, experts recommend no more than one drink per day for women and no more than two drinks per day for men.

If you consume more than the recommended amount, you may have a problem. The term *alcoholism* is widely used to define individuals with alcohol problems, but this label best corresponds to alcohol dependence and therefore does not adequately define the range of alcohol-related problems depicted in Table 4. For example, one study indicated that only one of every four hazardous drinkers is alcohol dependent. The remainder would be classified as at-risk drinkers or alcohol abusers. Although the problems experienced by these hazardous drinkers may be less severe than the problems experienced by those with alcohol dependence, much of the societal costs associated with alcohol are attributable to these groups.

If you currently exceed safe levels of consumption, you can take steps to control your drinking.

- Make a list of the reasons to stop drinking or cut down.
- Set a goal for yourself and make a plan to meet that goal.
- Monitor your drinking so you know exactly when, where, and how much you are drinking.
- Use self-monitoring to identify situations that trigger strong urges to drink.
- Eliminate or limit the amount of alcohol in your home.
- Limit the amount of time you spend drinking by drinking slowly, by alternating between alcoholic and nonalcoholic drinks, or by spending less time in drinking settings, such as bars or parties.
- Practice drink refusal skills by designating certain nondrinking days. If friends offer you a drink, explain to them that you are not drinking that day. You can offer to be the designated driver on your nondrinking days.
- Don't try to keep up with your friends, and avoid drinking games that promote excessive use.
- Consult the NIAAA Web site for college students (**www.collegedrinkingprevention.gov**).

If you are giving a party at which alcohol will be served, be a responsible host.

- Encourage guests to bring a designated driver.
- Secure safe transportation for those who are intoxicated. Do not let them drive.
- Have plenty of nonalcoholic beverages and high-protein and starchy foods available for the guests.
- Tactfully remove alcoholic beverages from the hands of guests who overindulge.
- Close the bar an hour or two before the party ends.

If you think you may have a problem with alcohol, help is available. If you think you or someone you know has a problem with alcohol, a number of options are available. Self-help groups, such as Alcoholics Anonymous (AA) and Rational Recovery, are widespread in the United States. Treatment centers are also readily available. Most treatment centers focus on abstinence-based treatment, but some help nonalcohol-dependent drinkers control their drinking. The options for treating alcohol dependence have expanded in recent years.

The NIAAA conducted a multisite clinical trial demonstrating the effectiveness of 12-step programs (based on the principles of AA). This type of empirical evidence provides confidence in the effectiveness of this approach. Still, there are many for whom certain aspects of AA are poorly received. For example, there is a strong religious component to AA, which may prevent some people from seeking out AA or following through with the program.

Fortunately, there are now alternatives to 12-step programs. The multisite trial mentioned previously (Project MATCH) also demonstrated that two other behavioral programs are effective in treating alcoholism. These programs (motivational enhancement and cognitive-behavioral therapy) are just as effective as the 12-step programs and can often be implemented in a shorter period of time. They also place more emphasis on personal control over behavior. Regardless of which approach appeals to a particular person, there is now something for everyone.

Another NIAAA trial, called Project Combine, tested the individual and combined effects of a behavioral treatment and two medications (naltrexone and Acamprosate). The results suggested that both the behavioral intervention and the naltrexone were effective treatments for alcohol dependence. In contrast, Acamprosate was no better than placebo. The combination of cognitive-behavioral treatment and naltrexone did not appear any better than either approach alone. Thus, both behavioral and pharmacological treatments seem to work, giving those with alcohol problems multiple options for effective treatment.

Online Learning Center

www.mhhe.com/corbin7e

The Online Learning Center contains a variety of Web-based resources that will help you get the most out of this book and your course. In addition to the On the Web pages, there are video activities, interactive quizzes, application assignments, and a variety of other useful study aids. Log on to the URL above to access these resources.

Web Resources

Alcohol.edu **www.alcohol.edu**

Alcoholics Anonymous

Web 05   **www.alcoholics-anonymous.org**

Drinker's Check-Up **www.drinkerscheckup.com**

E-Chug **www.e-Chug.com**

My Student Body **www.mystudentbody.com**

National Clearinghouse for Alcohol and Drug Information (NCADI) **www.health.org**

National Institute on Alcohol Abuse and Alcoholism (NIAAA) **www.niaaa.nih.gov**

National Institute on Alcohol Abuse and Alcoholism (NIAAA) College Drinking Web site **www.collegedrinkingprevention.gov**

Rational Recovery **www.rational.org**

Smart Recover **www.smartrecovery.com**

Suggested Readings

Additional reference materials for Concept 19 are available at Web06.

Web 06

Anton, R. F., et al. 2006. Combined pharmacotherapies and behavioral interventions for alcohol dependence. The COMBINE study: A randomized controlled trial. *Journal of the American Medical Association* 295:2003–2017.

Hahn, D. B., et al. 2007. *Focus on Health.* 8th ed. New York: McGraw-Hill Higher Education. Chapter 8.

Hingson, R., et al. 2003. Age of first intoxication, heavy drinking, driving after drinking and risk of unintentional injury among U.S. college students. *Journal of Studies on Alcohol* 64(1):23–31.

Hingson, R., et al. 2005. Magnitude of alcohol-related mortality and morbidity among U.S. college students ages 18–24: Changes from 1998–2001. *Annual Review of Public Health* 26:257–279.

Kinney, J. 2006. *Loosening the Grip: A Handbook of Alcohol Information.* 8th ed. New York:McGraw-Hill Higher Education.

Naimi, T., et al. 2003. Binge drinking among U.S. adults. *Journal of the American Medical Association* 289:70–75.

Rehm, J., et al. 2003. The relationship of average volume of alcohol consumption and patterns of drinking to burden of disease: An overview. *Addiction* 98:1209–1228.

Stobbe, M. (Associated Press). 2006. Liquor firms violating ad ban, CDC says. *Arizona Republic,* August 25.

Task Force of the National Advisory Council on Alcohol Abuse and Alcoholism. 2005. *A Call to Action: Changing the Culture of Drinking at U.S. Colleges.* Bethesda, MD: National Institutes of Health. Available at: **www.college drinking prevention.gov.**

Teague, M. L., et al. 2007. Your Health Today: Choices in a Changing Society. New York:McGraw-Hill Higher Education. Chapter 11.

Wechsler, H., et al. 2004. Colleges respond to student binge drinking: Reducing student demand or limiting access. *Journal of American College Health* 52(4):159–168.

Technology Update
Education and Intervention Programs

A variety of Web-based alcohol assessments and education and intervention programs are available, including **www.drinkerscheckup.com**, e-Chug (**www.e-Chug.com**), **www.mystudentbody.com**, **www.alcohol.edu**, and **www. smartrecovery.com**. These sites allow users to see how their drinking compares with that of others and how their drinking is negatively impacting their lives. They are not designed for someone with alcohol dependence, though these individuals might also benefit from such sites, at least as a first step toward recovery. Primarily, these sites are designed to help those who are drinking in a problematic way to change their behavior before problems become more severe.

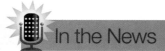 In the News

Spring Break Risks and Alcohol Ads

Spring Break is one of the most celebrated traditions among college students, but it may also be a cause for concern. Heavy drinking is common during Spring Break and may lead to a host of negative consequences, particularly for women. In an online survey commissioned by the American Medical Association, 83 percent of the women reported Spring Break involved heavier than usual drinking, and 74 percent said sexual activity was increased. More than half of the women who attended a college Spring Break trip regretted getting sick from drinking. In addition, 40 percent said they regretted blacking out or passing out, 13 percent said they had sex with more than one partner, and 10 percent said they regretted engaging in public or group sexual activity. The combination of hazardous levels of drinking and high-risk sexual behavior poses a significant risk to college women.

As discussed earlier in the concept, a contributing factor to positive expectancies about the outcomes of alcohol use is advertising by the alcohol industry. As a researcher from the CDC, Dr. Tim Naimi states, "Kids in the United States are exposed to a heck of a lot of alcohol advertising and it impacts what they drink and how much they drink." Although such messages are not supposed to be broadcast during programs primarily targeted to children, a recent study by the CDC suggests that they are, at least on the radio. Monitoring of advertising in 104 radio markets across the country for 25 brands of alcohol with high volume advetising showed that about half of the alcohol advertising aired during youth-oriented programs. The study was conducted soon after new standards were implemented so changes may have simply been slow to develop. Still, it is concerning that such a high volume of alcohol advertising is reaching youth audiences.

Lab 19A Blood Alcohol Level

Name	Section	Date

Purpose: To learn to calculate your (or a friend's) blood alcohol concentration (BAC)

Procedures

1. Assume a drink is a 12-ounce can or bottle of 5 percent beer or a 5-ounce glass (a small glass) of 12 percent alcohol (wine), or a mixed drink with a 1 ½-ounce shot glass (jigger) of 80 proof liquor.
   Case A: Assume you consumed two drinks within 40 minutes.
   Case B: Assume you consumed two drinks over a period of 1 hour and 20 minutes.
   Case C: Assume you had two six-packs of beer (12 cans) over 5 hours.
   Case D: Same as C, but, if you weigh less than 150 pounds, assume you weigh 50 pounds more than you now weigh, and, if you weigh more than 150 pounds, assume you weigh 50 pounds less.

2. Divide 3.8 by your weight in pounds to obtain your "BAC maximum per drink," or refer to Table 3 (page 400). You should obtain a number between 0.015 and 0.04 (based on one drink in 40 minutes). Use the formula below to determine BAC over time.

$$\text{Approximate BAC over time} = \frac{(3.8 \times \#\text{ of drinks})}{(\text{body weight})} - \frac{[0.01 \times (\#\text{ min.} - 40)]}{40}$$

3. After 40 minutes have passed, your body will begin eliminating alcohol from the bloodstream at the rate of about 0.01 percent for each additional 40 minutes. Multiply the number of drinks you've had by your "BAC maximum per drink" and subtract 0.01 percent from the number for each 40 minutes that have passed since you began drinking—but don't count the first 40 minutes. Compute your BAC for cases A, B, C, and D.

   Example: Case A. Mary weighs 100 pounds. $\dfrac{3.8 \times 2}{100} = \dfrac{7.6}{100} = 0.076\%$ BAC

   Case B. Mary takes 80 minutes. $0.076\% - \dfrac{[0.01 \times (80 - 40)]}{40} = 0.066\%$ BAC

4. Record your results below by writing the formula and computing the BAC for each case.

Results

Case A $\dfrac{(3.8 \times \underline{\quad}\#\text{ drinks})}{\underline{\quad}\text{ lbs}} = \underline{\quad}\%\text{BAC}$

Case B $\dfrac{(3.8 \times \underline{\quad}\#\text{ drinks})}{\underline{\quad}\text{ lbs}} - \dfrac{[0.01 \times (\underline{\quad}\#\text{ min.} - 40)]}{40} = \text{BAC } (\quad) - (\quad) = \underline{\quad}\%\text{ BAC}$

Case C $\dfrac{(3.8 \times \underline{\quad}\#\text{ drinks})}{\underline{\quad}\text{ lbs}} - \dfrac{[0.01 \times (\underline{\quad}\#\text{ min.} - 40)]}{40} = \text{BAC } (\quad) - (\quad) = \underline{\quad}\%\text{ BAC}$

Case D $\dfrac{(3.8 \times \underline{\quad}\#\text{ drinks})}{\underline{\quad}\text{ lbs}} - \dfrac{[0.01 \times (\underline{\quad}\#\text{ min.} - 40)]}{40} = \text{BAC } (\quad) - (\quad) = \underline{\quad}\%\text{ BAC}$

1. Would you (or your friend) be able to drive legally according to your state laws? Place an X over your answer.

Case A   (Yes) (No)

Case B   (Yes) (No)

Case C   (Yes) (No)

Case D   (Yes) (No)

2. Would you (or your friend) be able to drive legally if the Health Goals for the Year 2010 (.08) were put into effect? Place an X over your answer.

Case A   (Yes) (No)

Case B   (Yes) (No)

Case C   (Yes) (No)

Case D   (Yes) (No)

Conclusions and Implications: In several sentences, discuss what you have learned from doing this activity.

Lab 19B Perceptions about Alcohol Use

Name	Section Date

Purpose: To better understand perceptions about drinking behaviors

Procedures

1. Think of a person you care about. Do not identify this person on this lab report.
2. Answer each of the questions in the questionnaire below as honestly as possible, evaluating the behavior of the person you have identified. Calculate a total score and determine a rating (see Chart 1).
3. At another time, when you do not have to submit your results, you should answer the questions about yourself.
4. Answer the questions in the Conclusions and Implications section.

Results

	Never	Sometimes	Frequently	Too Often	Add Score
1. How often does the person drink?	0	1	2	3	
2. How often does the person have six or more drinks on one occasion?	0	1	2	3	
3. How often do friends of the person drink?	0	1	2	3	
4. How often has the person been unable to stop after starting to drink?	0	1	2	3	
5. How often does the person need a drink to get started in the morning?	0	1	2	3	
6. How often has the person been unable to remember previous events after drinking?	0	1	2	3	
7. How often does the person miss class or work associated with drinking?	0	1	2	3	
8. How often does the person have social or personal problems associated with drinking?	0	1	2	3	
9. How often does the person deny drinking too much (only for those who you consider to drink too much)?	0	1	2	3	

Total Score _____

Chart 1 ▶ Drinking Behavior Rating Scale

Rating	Score
Alcohol abuse*	18+
Drinking problem	12–17
Potential problem	8–11
Low risk of problem	<8

*Professional help recommended.

_____ **Rating**

409

Conclusions and Implications

1. In several sentences, discuss the drinking behavior of the person you identified. Do you think your ratings give an accurate picture of the person? Do you think the person you rated has a problem with alcohol?

2. In several sentences, discuss the drinking behavior of the person's friends. Do the friends promote drinking or not?

3. In several sentences, discuss things that you could do to help a friend or loved one solve a drinking problem.

The Use and Abuse of Other Drugs

Health Goals for the year 2010

- Reduce substance abuse to protect the health, safety, and quality of life for all, especially children.

- Reduce deaths and injuries caused by drug-related motor vehicle crashes.

- Reduce drug-induced deaths and intentional injuries from drug-related violence.

- Reduce loss of productivity in workplace and increase availability of treatment programs for drug abusers.

- Increase number of young people who stay drug free.

- Reduce steroid use among young people.

- Increase proportion of young people who disapprove of substance abuse.

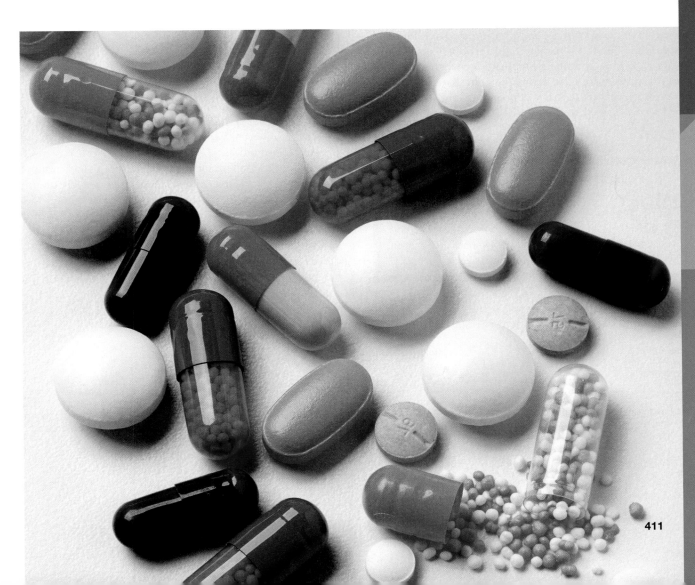

Drug abuse has serious health consequences and enormous personal, social, and economic costs.

About 36 percent of college students currently use illegal drugs annually, up from a low of 29 percent in 1991, but far below the 56.2 percent who used illicit drugs in 1980. National studies indicate that rates of illicit drug use are highest among adolescents and young adults between the ages of 16 and 25. Millions of people are arrested each year for drug offenses—including sale, distribution, and possession. This has a tremendous cost to society. This concept discusses **drug abuse** and misuse with an emphasis on the illegal, so-called street drugs.

Classification of Illicit and Prescription Drugs

Drugs can be classified in several ways, but the mood-altering, or psychoactive, drugs are the ones we hear about most. Mood-altering, or **psychoactive drugs,** may be placed in five major groups: depressants, opiate narcotics, stimulants, hallucinogens, and designer drugs. Drugs in the same group have similar effects. Narcotics, however, are actually depressants, but because the word *narcotics* is so widely used in law enforcement and

---

On the Web

www.mhhe.com/corbinweb

Web 01 Log on to this URL before reading this concept. See On the Web list of concepts. Click on the concept number you want to view. To access supplemental information, click on the number shown at each Web icon.

---

in society in general, they are generally given their own category. Each of the five categories of drugs is discussed in this concept. Their effects are classified as either physiological or psychological (primarily affecting the body versus primarily affecting behavior). The effects of drugs can vary with each individual and with different doses.

Depressant drugs include alcohol, tranquilizers, and barbiturates. Depressants come in the form of pills, liquids, and injectables (see Table 1). In small doses, they slow heart rate and respiration. In larger doses (for example, alcohol), they act as a poison and damage every organ system in the body. In large enough doses, they can dramatically depress heart rate and respiration enough to cause death, if quick intervention is not available. In terms of their effect on behavior, the user might at first feel stimulated, despite their depressant effects. Depression, loss of coordination, drop in energy level, mood swings, and confusion occur after prolonged use.

Web 01 **Opiate narcotics include heroin, codeine, morphine, and methadone.** Narcotics are either smoked, injected, sniffed, or swallowed (see Table 2, page 413). Narcotics are often used clinically to treat pain, however, heroin has no legal medical use in the United States and has a high rate of addiction. It is three times stronger than other medicinal narcotics and induces different physiological effects. Narcotics are all opium poppy derivatives or synthetics that emulate them. The *narco-* part of the word derives from the Greek word for sleep, because of its sleep-inducing properties.

Every narcotic, legal or illegal, is a potential poison. Although rare, a single dose can be fatal. Deaths related to narcotic abuse are typically caused by overdose, impurities

---

Table 1 ▶ Depressants ("Downers," Sedatives)

Examples	Physiological Effects	Psychological Effects
• Alcohol	• In small doses, slow the heart and respiration	• Initial effect: stimulation, lowered inhibitions, excited talking, sense of well-being
• Tranquilizers (e.g., Valium, Xanax, meprobamate, sleeping pills, methaqualone)	• In large doses, act as a poison and damage every organ system	• After prolonged use: depression, loss of coordination, drop in energy level, mood swings, confusion, euphoria
• Barbiturates (e.g., Mebaral, Nembutal)	• Quick sedation: vomiting; loss of motor and neurological control; combined with alcohol, can lead to coma and death	• Amnesia

Table 2 ▶ Opiate Narcotics

Examples	Physiological Effects	Psychological Effects
• Codeine • Morphine • Synthetic opiates (e.g., Vicodin, Oxycontin) • Methadone	• Narcotics: blockage of pain, chronic constipation, depressed respiration, redness and irritation of nostrils, nausea, lowered sexual drive, impaired immune system	• Narcotics: euphoria and feeling of pleasure; nontherapeutic doses may result in mental distress, such as fear and nervousness; in heavy users, drowsiness and apathy may occur
• Heroin (also called smack)	• Heroin: blood clots, bacterial endocarditis, serum hepatitis, brain abscess, HIV infection (from shared needles); in pregnant users, high risk of miscarriage, stillbirths, birth defects, toxemia, addicted babies	

Table 3 ▶ Stimulants

Examples	Physiological Effects	Psychological Effects
• Cocaine (also called coke or crack)	• Cocaine: sore throat, hoarseness, shortness of breath (leads to bronchitis and emphysema), dilated pupils, "lights" seen around objects.	• Cocaine: initial rush of energy, feeling of confidence; as it wears off: depression, moodiness, irritability, severe mental disorders • Crack: intense euphoria, then crushing depression, intense feeling of self-hate; as it wears off: depression and sadness, intense anxiety about where to get more drugs, aggressiveness, paranoia
• Amphetamines and powder methamphetamines (also called speed, crank); diet and pep pills, Ritalin	• Stimulants: excite central nervous system; increase blood pressure, respiration, and heart rate (sometimes resulting in convulsions and stroke); reduce appetite; highly addictive; overdose is fatal; with increased use: dizziness, headaches, sleeplessness; with long-term use: progressive brain damage, malnutrition	• Stimulants: initially, feeling of being invincible, alertness, excitement; with increased use: feeling of anxiety; with long-term use: hallucinations, psychosis
• Crystal methamphetamine (also called Ice)	• Ice: extreme energy, sleeplessness, seizures, flushed skin, constricted pupils	• Ice: major effect is toxic psychosis; euphoria, delusions of grandeur, feelings of invincibility, violent when provoked

of the drug, or mixing of the drug with other depressants, such as alcohol. The mixing of drugs in the same or similar categories can produce a heightened physiological effect known as synergism, or the **synergistic effect.** The combined use makes drug taking far more dangerous. The same is true among some prescription and over-the-counter drugs; when used in combination, they can be dangerous.

Stimulants include nicotine, cocaine, and amphetamines. Some effects of stimulants are described in Table 3. One of these stimulants—cocaine—comes in powder form (coke) and a rocklike form (crack). The timing and magnitude of effects of cocaine vary depending on whether it is inhaled, injected, or smoked. The low cost of crack has contributed to its abuse. Amphetamines and methamphetamines (frequently referred to as "speed") are also classified as stimulants due to their effects on the central nervous system. Stimulants are often included in diet pills to reduce appetite; others (e.g., Ritalin) are used clinically to treat attention deficit disorder.

Crystal methamphetamine (also known as ice, meth, or crystal) is a purified methamphetamine that also comes in rock form or powder. As a powder, it is usually smoked in a glass pipe or cigarette. It is a powerful stimulant, with

Drug Abuse The use of a drug to the extent that it impairs social, psychological, or physiological functioning.

Psychoactive Drug Any drug that produces a temporary change in the physiological functions of the nervous system, affecting mood, thoughts, feelings, or behavior.

Synergistic Effect The joint actions of two or more drugs that increase the effects of each.

Table 4 ▶ Hallucinogens (Psychedelics)

Examples	Physiological Effects	Psychological Effects
• Marijuana (also called pot, grass, weed, herb)	• Marijuana: long-term use: bronchitis, emphysema and lung cancer, bloodshot eyes, heart disease, infertility, sexual dysfunction, permanent memory loss (brain damage)	• Marijuana: may not hallucinate; pleasant, relaxed feeling; giddiness; self-preoccupation; less precise thinking; impaired task performance; inertia; with prolonged use: may be withdrawn and apathetic, have anxiety reactions, paranoia; eventually, decreased motivation and enthusiasm, reduced ability to absorb and integrate effectively, profoundly impaired scholastic performance
• GD-lysergic acid diethylamide (LSD, also called acid)	• LSD: changes chromosomes and may result in birth defects of babies of users; bad trips, confusion, flashback	• LSD: vivid hallucinations, feelings of overlapping/merging of the senses, expanded consciousness and mystical experiences, stimulated awareness and desire, confusion, flashback
• Phencyclidine (PCP)	• PCP: accumulates in fat cells and may remain in body longer than most drugs; impaired immune system, poor coordination, weight loss, speech problems, heart and lung failure, irreversible brain damage, convulsions, coma, death	• PCP: insensitivity to pain can lead to death; euphoria, depersonalization, hallucinations, delirium, amnesia, tunnel vision, loss of control, violent behavior
• Inhalants (solvents, aerosols, and nitrites, also known as poppers, rush)	• Inhalants: slow reaction time, headache, nausea, vomiting, seizure, brain damage, suffocation, heart attack, death, double vision, sensitivity to light, dizziness, loss of coordination, weakness, numbness; irregular heartbeat, liver and kidney failure, bone marrow damage	• Inhalants: giddiness, overexcitement, less inhibition, feelings of being all-powerful; powerfulness soon fades and leaves irritability

Table 5 ▶ Designer Drugs

Examples	Effects
Date Rape Drugs Rohypnol Gamma hydroxy butyrate (GHB) Ketamine (also called Special K)	Predominantly central nervous system depressants; Rohypnol incapacitates, may cause amnesia; GHB can cause comas, seizures, insomnia, anxiety, tremors, nausea, and sweating; Ketamine can cause delirium, amnesia, impaired motor function, high blood pressure, depression, and potentially fatal respiratory problems
3-4 methylenedioxymethamphetamine (MMDA, also called ecstasy, or X)	May cause irregular heart beat, intensified heart problems, exhaustion, liver and brain damage, nervousness, muscle tension, and dry mouth; initial feelings of calm may be followed by psychosis and/or psychological burnout

a high that lasts 8 to 30 hours. Much like crack cocaine, ice is a concentrated form of an already potent stimulant drug that is either smoked or injected. Also like crack, ice causes an intense "rush" or "flash," which is experienced as highly pleasurable. Because the effects last for only a few minutes, users need to administer the drug frequently to maintain the effects.

Drugs that cause the user to have hallucinations are called hallucinogens, or psychedelics. Among the psychedelic drugs that cause **hallucinations** are LSD, PCP, and marijuana (see Table 4). Dosages of these drugs are so potent that they are measured in micrograms (one-millionth of a gram; a gram is approximately equivalent to the weight of

Web 02

a standard paper clip). Less-known drugs in this category include mushrooms, or "shrooms," which are chewed, and peyote cactus buttons. They are used legally by some American Indians in religious rites.

Marijuana use became widespread in the 1960s; despite decreases since that time, marijuana is still the most widely used illicit drug in the United States. The active ingredient in marijuana is delta-9-tetrahydrocannabinol (THC), which leads to a range of experiences, which differ from person to person. One study indicated that the types of effects people experience may be due in part to genetic differences. Marijuana is generally smoked in a pipe, joint, or bong, though it can also be eaten and is increasingly smoked in hollowed out cigars called blunts. Blunts often contain other drugs, such as PCP, as well as marijuana.

Inhalants are sometimes classified separately from other hallucinogens because their effects are so serious. They reach the brain in seconds, and the effect lasts only a few minutes. They come in three types: (1) solvents, such as glue, gasoline, paints, paint thinner, typewriter correction fluid, lighter fluid, shoe polish, and liquid wax; (2) aerosols, such as hair spray, air fresheners, insect spray, and spray paint; and (3) nitrites, including amyl nitrite, nitrous oxide (laughing gas), and butyl nitrite (a room odorizer or liquid incense).

Designer drugs, which are made in laboratories, have many of the same properties as the drugs they simulate, such as pain relievers, anesthetics, and amphetamines. Designer drugs (see Table 5, page 414) are modifications of illegal or restricted drugs, made by underground chemists who create street drugs that are not specifically listed as controlled. They are created by changing the molecular structure of an existing drug to create a new substance. Since new drugs are being created all of the time, their potential effects are unknown. In the past, some have killed the people who have taken them, some have paralyzed people, and some have been innocuous. The people who take these drugs are human guinea pigs.

The Consequences of Drug Use

Drug use takes a human toll in terms of increased morbidity and mortality and lost productivity. In recent years, drug-related visits to the emergency room (ER) have increased. Over 600,000 drug-related visits are reported annually, with more than half due to drug overdoses. ER visits associated with cocaine, heroin, amphetamines, methamphetamine, and marijuana use have increased in recent years. Annually, over 23,500 people die of drug-induced causes, including poisonings and deaths related to prescription drug use. This does not even take into account the indirect effects of drug use on mortality, including deaths from accidents, homicides, and AIDS (acquired via intravenous drug use). Because of problems with low productivity at the worksite, a large percentage of American businesses now conduct employee drug tests. Among the problems of drug-abusing employees are more frequent absences, erratic performance, increased violence and stealing, bad judgment, and increased accidents, many of which endanger others.

Drug use also has significant economic costs. The economic costs of illicit drug abuse are estimated at approximately $180 billion a year. Approximately 22.5 million people abuse or are dependent on illicit drugs, but most of the national economic burden is not related to treatment (3 percent). More than half of the costs are associated with drug-related crime. Figure 1 illustrates the portion of societal costs resulting from factors such as law enforcement expenditures, social programs, and reduced productivity.

Drug use can lead to significant legal problems, resulting in jail time and substantial fines. State laws regarding the possession and sale of illicit drugs vary considerably, and penalties within states vary based on the amount of the drug, the type of drug, and the type of offense (possession, sales, or production). Penalties for the possession of small amounts are the least severe, with penalties for the sale or production of large amounts the most severe. Still, the penalties for the possession of even small amounts of illicit drugs are substantial. In most states, the maximum jail time for possession ranges from 6 months to a year for marijuana and from 1 to 7 years for cocaine, methamphetamine, and ecstasy. In addition, fines between $500 and $1,000 for marijuana and between $5,000 and $25,000 for other illicit drugs are typical of most states. For the sale of illicit drugs, maximum jail time in most states ranges between 1 and 8 years for marijuana and between 5 and 25 years for cocaine, methamphetamine, and ecstasy. Fines typically range between $5,000 and $25,000 for marijuana and between $10,000 and $100,000 for other illicit drugs.

Use and Abuse of Drugs

Drug use generally begins with cigarette smoking and alcohol use. Of course, most people who smoke or drink will not go on to use illegal drugs, but it is rare for people who do not smoke or drink to use illegal drugs. The average age for starting to smoke cigarettes is 12; for

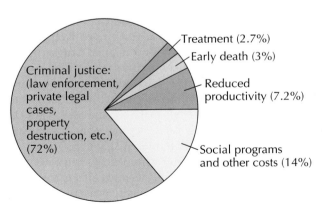

Figure 1 ▶ The estimated cost of drug abuse (percentage of total costs).
Source: National Institute on Drug Abuse.

Hallucinations Imaginary things seen, felt, or heard or things seen in a distorted way.

alcohol and marijuana about 13. In general, the younger a person is when he or she starts using drugs, including nicotine and alcohol, the more likely that person is to use illegal drugs and the more likely he or she is to become physically dependent on drugs.

Web 03 **The reasons people give for using drugs are similar to the reasons given for using alcohol and tobacco.** Typically, the reasons people give when asked why they use drugs or how they got started include the following:

- Peer pressure (i.e., "Everyone is doing it," even though most people aren't using drugs)
- It makes young people feel more "adult"
- "I just wanted to see what it was like (to experiment)"
- To have fun
- "It makes me feel good"
- As a rebellion against parents or authority
- To cope with pressure/stress
- To take a risk (thrill seeking)

Web 04 **Some risk factors make one more likely to develop drug abuse or dependence on drugs.** Drug-related behaviors and attitudes are associated with risk for abuse and dependence on drugs. The criteria for abuse and dependence parallel the criteria previously outlined in Concept 19. With drugs, the potential for **addiction** depends on genetic vulnerability, the type of drug used, the method of administration used, attitudes toward drug use, peer group use, expectations regarding drug effects, and ease of access. Genetics accounts for as much as 50 percent of alcohol and nicotine addiction and the same is likely true for other drugs of abuse. This does not mean that one is destined to become an addict; the remaining 50 percent is within your control. Some drugs are more addictive than others, so dependence on narcotics and sedatives is more likely than dependence on hallucinogens or designer drugs (though addiction to these substances occurs as well). The route of administration also affects risk for addiction. For example, the likelihood of becoming addicted to cocaine is much higher if it is smoked as crack than if it is inhaled as powder. People who believe drug use is acceptable and affiliate with others with similar views are more likely to use drugs and to develop problems. Those who believe drugs will have strong positive effects and few negative effects are also at greater risk, especially if they use drugs as a way to cope with stress. People who live in areas where drugs are readily available are also at increased risk.

The use of most illicit drugs has leveled or decreased in the past decade. In the United States, rates of illicit drug use peaked in the 1970s, followed by sharp decreases during the 1980s and smaller increases during the early 1990s. Although these trends are observed at the population level, they are not present for all groups. In particular, college students and young adults have continued to show small increases in illicit drug use during the past 10 years (See Figure 2). In addition, recent declines have not been observed across all drug types. Among adolescents and young adults, the use of prescription narcotics and sedatives (barbiturates) has increased in recent years. In fact, the nonmedical use of prescription psychotherapeutic drugs is now the second most common form of drug use (not including alcohol and tobacco), trailing only marijuana in overall prevalence. Rates of illegal use of narcotic pain medications (e.g., Vicodin, Oxycontin) and tranquilizers (e.g., Valium, Xanax) is particularly high. Such high rates of use of these drugs is of particular concern, given that they are highly addictive. Young adults, including college students, have also shown increased rates of use of powder cocaine, amphetamine, crystal methamphetamine, and tranquilizers during the past 10 years. Although recent trends in ecstasy (MDMA) use show decreases, large increases were observed during the mid to late 1990s. Finally, inhalant use, which had been decreasing among

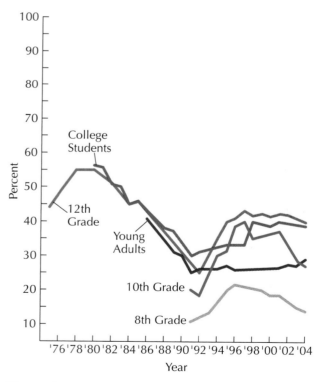

Figure 2 ▶ Trends in annual prevalence of an illicit drug use index across five populations.

Notes: Use of "any illicit drugs" includes any use of marijuana, LSD, other hallucinogens, crack, other cocaine, or heroin, or any use which is not under a doctor's orders of other opiates, stimulants, barbiturates, methaqualone (excluded since 1990), or tranquilizers.

Source: National Institute on Drug Abuse.

adolescents for many years, has shown an upswing in use over the past several years. In summary, although trends over the past decade are encouraging, continued increases among young adults and overall increases in prescription drug misuse are cause for concern.

The development of new drugs and "generational forgetting" contribute to the maintenance of drug use in the United States. New drugs are always being manufactured, and new ways of administering old drugs often lead to a resurgence in use. Club drugs provide examples of new drugs and crack cocaine and crystal methamphetamine are examples of old drugs that became popular in new forms. When these new drugs become available, information about their benefits is generally spread immediately by word of mouth. In contrast, the risks associated with use are often unknown until the drug has been used for a number of years. This gives new drugs a period of time to become popular before information that might deter their use is available. Ecstasy is a good example of this phenomenon. Fortunately, public campaigns to provide information about risks by the National Institute on Drug Abuse and other agencies helped curb levels of use relatively quickly. Ecstasy use has been on the decline for the past several years in all age groups. In addition to the introduction of new drugs, there seems to be a "generational forgetting" of the risks associated with older drugs that leads to a resurgence in their use after years of reduced prevalence. Increases in the use of drugs that have been decreasing or stable for a period of time are first identified in the youngest users. Increases in usage are then noted in other (older) age groups as the young users age. Reductions in perceptions of risk associated with the use of drugs often precede escalation in rates of use.

Marijuana is the most widely used drug in the United States and is associated with a host of physical health and social consequences. In a survey, nearly 15 million Americans, or roughly 6 percent of people over the age of 12, reported the use of marijuana in the past month (see Figure 3). Although many believe it is a relatively safe drug, and some favor decriminalization or legalization, a number of risks are associated with marijuana use. With respect to health, chronic marijuana use leads to many of the negative consequences associated with cigarette smoking, including cardiovascular disease and lung cancer. One study showed that marijuana use also increases risk for stroke. Another study found that marijuana use leads to nearly a five-fold increase in acute risk for a heart attack, especially among those with existing cardiovascular risk. Marijuana use is also associated with impaired cognitive abilities. Short-term marijuana use leads to a reduction in IQ scores. Long-term marijuana use leads to impairments in attention, memory, and

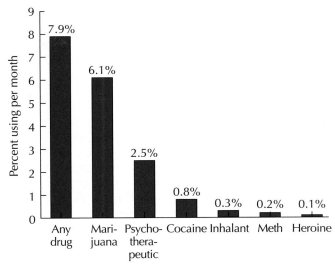

Figure 3 ▶ Illicit drug use among persons 12 and older, by drug (% per month).

Source: Substance Abuse and Mental Health Services Administration.

learning. Although the debate is ongoing regarding the addictive (physical dependence) potential of marijuana, it is clear that one can become psychologically addicted to the drug. Psychological dependence is characterized by craving for the drug and continued use despite negative consequences.

Stimulants, including cocaine and methamphetamine, are the second most commonly used illicit drugs. Cocaine and methamphetamine are both stimulant drugs, and they share a number of other characteristics. First, both come in powder form as well as more concentrated crystal (ice) or rock (crack) forms. Crack cocaine was one of the most abused drugs in the United States during the peak rates of use in the early to mid 1980s, and crystal methamphetamine was at the center of the more recent but less dramatic increase in illicit drug use in the early 1990s. Crack and ice also share the characteristic of being highly addictive. Because the high associated with using these drugs is intense and short-lived, patterns of repeated use are developed quickly, leading to rapid development of dependence. Both drugs are also known to damage dopamine neurons in the brain and lead to a host of short- and long-term health consequences. Short-term effects that occur after the initial high include irritability, anxiety, and paranoia. In terms of long-term risk, cocaine and methamphetamine use lead to increased risk for stroke, respiratory problems (including respiratory failure), irregular heartbeat, and heart attacks.

Addiction A drug-induced condition in which a person requires frequent administration of a drug in order to avoid withdrawal; also referred to as physical dependence.

Ice has added risks associated with its production. It is produced in clandestine laboratories from relatively inexpensive and easily attainable products. Although inexpensive, it is also highly dangerous to produce. The chemicals used to manufacture ice are highly volatile, leading to a high incidence of fires and explosions.

The continued use of club drugs is a concern, given the strong evidence of their harmful effects. Club drugs include ecstasy (MDMA), Rohypnol, GHB, Ketamine, DOM, DOB, and NEXUS. Ecstasy, a hallucinogen, is inhaled, injected, or swallowed. The drug was initially popular at all-night dance parties called raves, but its use has expanded beyond the club scene. Ecstasy alters brain levels of serotonin, negatively impacts memory, and affects the brain regions that regulate sleep, mood and learning. The negative effects of ecstasy may last as long as 7 years. Dealers often pass off other drugs, such as paramethoxyamphetamine (PMA), as ecstasy and they are even more dangerous.

Rohypnol and GHB are predominately central nervous system depressants, like the other sedative drugs described previously. Because these drugs are odorless, colorless, and tasteless, they can be added to food or beverages without the consumer detecting their presence. Because of these properties, Rohypnol and GHB are known as drug-assisted assault or date-rape drugs. In addition to incapacitating the user, these drugs lead to anterograde amnesia, or the inability to remember events that occur after consumption. Thus, victims often do not remember events that occur after they unknowingly take these drugs. Women should be especially careful not to leave their drinks unattended or to accept drinks from strangers. In response to this threat, the U.S. Congress passed legislation in 1996 to increase penalties for drug-assisted sexual assaults.

Inhalant use poses a serious risk to physical health, including risk for sudden death. Those who use inhalants are at risk for what is known as "sudden sniffing death." Sniffing inhalants can lead to irregular and rapid heart rhythms that can cause heart failure and rapid death. This can occur from a single episode of sniffing in an otherwise healthy adolescent. Inhalant use can also lead to premature death via a number of other mechanisms, including asphyxiation, suffocation, convulsions and seizures, coma, and choking. Other negative effects of inhalant use include muscle weakness, disorientation, and depression.

Misuse and abuse of prescription and over-the-counter (OTC) drugs have become an increasing problem. Prescription drugs are often used inappropriately. Examples include using prescriptions written for other people and using medicines for purposes other than prescribed. Users may also obtain prescription drugs without prescriptions via the Internet. A survey of nearly 150 Internet sites showed that 90 percent required no prescription to purchase drugs (including depressants, stimulants, and opiates). Most provided no method of preventing purchases by children. Among the more commonly abused prescription drugs among college students are Ritalin, Valium, Xanax, Percoset, Vicodin, and Oxycontin. Oxycontin, sometimes called "hill billy heroin," is a painkiller that has received much attention because of its misuse by celebrities and its link to many deaths nationwide. Another trend is the misuse of nonprescription cough remedies, especially among youth. Dextromethorphan, also called DXA, is the active ingredient in more than 120 cough remedies, including Robitussin, Coricidin, and Vicks NyQuil. Overdoses of DXA have resulted in considerable numbers of emergency room visits, with patients having a variety of symptoms.

Accidental misuse is another common problem. Examples of unwitting misuse of drugs include taking a medicine twice, accidentally using a medicine taken from a medicine cabinet at night in the dark, taking the wrong medicine from unlabeled bottles, and using outdated medicines. Another cause of unintentional misuse is taking multiple medications that negatively interact with one another. Thus, it is important to understand the nature of all the medications you are taking (including supplements, prescription drugs, and OTC drugs) and how they interact. Steps such as labeling properly, using daily pill containers, and destroying outdated medicine can reduce the accidental misuse of drugs. Although attention to the misuse of prescription medication has generally been restricted to the use of psychoactive substances, inappropriate use of antibiotics has also become a cause for concern. Although there is no risk for addiction to antibiotics, there is concern about the development of resistance. For this reason, physicians have become more conservative in prescribing antibiotics.

Women who are pregnant, are nursing, or want to get pregnant should avoid drug use, including many prescription drugs. The most recent results of the National Pregnancy Healthy Survey, conducted by the National Institute on Drugs Abuse (NIDA), estimated that 5.5 percent of the 4 million women who give birth each year in the United States used illegal drugs while they were pregnant. Taking drugs during pregnancy can result in various conditions:

- Premature separation of the placenta from the womb and hemorrhage, threatening the lives of both the baby and the mother
- Miscarriage resulting from increased blood pressure, causing uterine contractions. Birth defects also occur.
- Decreased oxygen to the baby and possible fetal stroke
- Low birth weight and shorter babies
- Babies born addicted
- Increased risk of sudden infant death syndrome (SIDS)
- Increased risk for learning disabilities, as well as delayed motor, speech, and language development

Strategies for Action

The best way to avoid problems associated with drug use is not to try illegal drugs and to be careful in the use of legal drugs. The information presented in this concept clearly indicates that starting to take a drug for reasons other than managing your own good health increases the risk of taking more drugs in the future. Most readers of this book have already made the decision not to take illegal drugs and will follow the guidelines presented earlier concerning how to avoid misusing legal drugs. Nevertheless, most people will take medication at sometime in their lives. Be continually aware of what you are taking and why. Monitor the use of medications to be sure that you are using them as directed and not with other medications that may result in dangerous synergistic effects.

Learning skills to cope with problems and stress is also essential (see Concept 17). Making responsible decisions is another skill that needs to be acquired. Knowing the effects and risks of drugs should help you to make more responsible decisions. To combat peer pressure, the ability to clearly and effectively say no is necessary. Be assertive. And finally, you need to choose friends whose values support, rather than undermine, your own.

People who have a problem with drugs typically will need help to develop skills and personal characteristics to quit using them. For people with a problem, the first step is recognizing that help is needed. In Lab 20A, you will have the opportu-

nity to evaluate the behavior of a friend or loved one to determine if the person needs help. If a person needs help, he or she needs to talk to someone who can be trusted, perhaps a friend or relative. You may be able to help the person seek help from a referral source, such as an employee assistance program, a family or university physician or hospital, or your city or county health department. These sources help get the person into a treatment program or support group. Some of the better-known, nationwide programs include Alcoholics (or Narcotics or Cocaine) Anonymous and Al-Anon Family Groups. The web addresses in the Web Resources section can also aid you in finding information and assistance. Another option is to look in the yellow pages of the telephone book for programs operated by public and private agencies. Still another possibility is to call a hot line, and someone will direct you to help in your area. Three of these include

- National Institute on Drug Abuse (NIDA) Hotline (1-800-662-HELP)
- Cocaine Helpline (1-800-COCAINE)
- Just Say No International (1-800-258-2766)

At a later time, it would be wise to answer the questions in Lab 20A for yourself rather than for a friend or loved one. This will allow you to determine if you need help.

Online Learning Center

www.mhhe.com/corbin7e
The Online Learning Center contains a variety of Web-based resources that will help you get the most out of this book and your course. In addition to the On the Web pages, there are video activities, interactive quizzes, application assignments, and a variety of other useful study aids. Log on to the URL above to access these resources.

Web Resources

Drug Free Resource Net **www.drugfreeamerica.org**
National Center for Addiction and Substance Abuse (Columbia University) **www.casacolumbia.org**
National Clearinghouse for Alcohol and Drug Information **www.health.org**
National Institute on Drug Abuse **www.nida.nih.gov**

Technology Update
Ecstasy and Hyperthermia

The greatest acute risk associated with ecstasy (MDMA) use is hyperthermia. This consequence can be particularly dangerous when strenuous activity (e.g., dancing) is undertaken after consuming the drug. Body temperatures as high as 109°F have been reported and can lead to multiple organ failure and death. To date, the only treatment available in these cases has been to apply ice or refrigeration blankets. However, a study of mice found that a compound called nantenine is able to block or reverse the hyperthermic effects of ecstasy. Although not yet tested in humans, this compound could be a life saver in cases of malignant hyperthermia resulting from ecstasy use.

National Drug Publications and Public Service Announcements
www.drugabuse.gov/NIDA_Notes/NNIndex.html
www.drugabuse.gov/researchreports/researchindex.html
www.drugabuse.gov/drugpages/PSAhome.html
Substance Abuse and Mental Health Services Administration
www.samhsa.gov

Suggested Readings

Web 09

Additional reference materials for Concept 20 are available at Web08.

Barrett, S., et al. 2007. *Consumer Health: A Guide to Intelligent Decisions.* 8th ed. New York: McGraw-Hill Higher Education. Chapter 18.

Fields, R. 2007. *Drugs in Perspective.* 6th ed. New York: McGraw-Hill.

Hahn, D. B., et al. 2007. *Focus on Health.* 8th ed. New York: McGraw-Hill Higher Education. Chapter 7.

ImpacTeen Illicit Drug Team. 2002. *Illicit Drug Policies: Selected Laws from the 50 States.* Berrien Springs, MI: Andrews University.

Johnston, L. D., et al. 2006. *Monitoring the Future National Results on Adolescent Drug use: Overview of Key Findings, 2004.* (NIH Publication No. 06-5882). Bethesda, MD: National Institute on Drug Abuse.

Ksir, C. J., et al. 2008. *Drugs, Society, and Human Behavior.* 12th ed. New York: McGraw-Hill Higher Education.

National Center on Addiction and Substance Abuse. 2004. *You've Got Drugs! Prescription Drug Pushers on the Internet.* New York: National Center on Addiction and Substance Abuse. Available at **www.casacolumbia.org**.

National Institute on Drug Abuse. 2005. *National Institute on Drug Abuse Research Report Series: Inhalant Abuse* (NIH Publication No. 05-3818). Rockville, MD: U.S. Department of Health and Human Services, National Institutes of Health.

Office of National Drug Control Policy. 2004. *The Economic Costs of Drug Abuse in the United States, 1992–2002.* Washington, DC: Executive Office of the President (Publication No. 207303).

Solowij, N., et al. 2002. Cognitive functioning of long-term heavy cannabis users seeking treatment. *Journal of American Medical Association* 287(9):1123–1131.

Substance Abuse and Mental Health Services Administration. 2005. *Overview of Key Findings from the 2004 National Survey on Drug Use and Health* (Office of Applied Studies, NSDUH Series H-27, DHHS Publication No. SMA 05-4061). Rockville, MD: Department of Health and Human Services.

Teague, M. L., et al. 2007. *Your Health Today: Choices in a Changing Society.* New York: McGraw-Hill Higher Education. Chapter 11.

Wilson, H. T. 2008. *Annual Editions: Drugs, Society and Behavior.* 22nd ed. New York: McGraw-Hill Higher Education.

 In the News

Prescription Pain Medications

Data from the 2004 National Household Survey on Drug Use and Health showed that the class of drugs with the largest number of new users was nonmedical use of prescription narcotics. Although Oxycontin has garnered most of the media attention, the misuse of prescription pain medications is not restricted to this drug. In fact, Oxycontin was only the fourth most common prescription pain medication used among new initiates. Percoset, Darvocet, and Vicodin all ranked ahead of Oxycontin, with nearly half of new prescription pain medication abusers reporting the use of Vicodin.

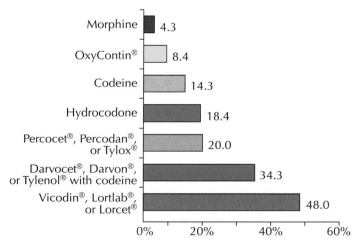

Figure 4 ▶ Specific Types of Pain Relievers Used during the Past Year among Initiates of Nonmedical Use of Pain Relievers 2004.

Source: Substance Abuse Mental Health Services Administration.

Lab 20A Use and Abuse of Other Drugs

Name	Section	Date

Purpose: To evaluate a friend or family member's behavior and potential for becoming an abuser of drugs; if this report is submitted to an instructor, be sure *not* to identify by name the person you are evaluating

Procedure: Answer these questions to determine if the person you are evaluating is an abuser of medications. Place an X over the answer that applies.

A. Prescription Drug Abuse

(Yes) (No) 1. Does he/she take more medicine than prescribed per dosage?

(Yes) (No) 2. Does he/she feel more nervous than ever when the medicine wears off?

(Yes) (No) 3. Does he/she hoard medicine?

(Yes) (No) 4. Does he/she gulp pills?

(Yes) (No) 5. Does he/she hide the amount of medicine taken from friends, family, or his/her doctors?

(Yes) (No) 6. Does his/her doctor know he/she has other doctors, and does the doctor have a list of all the medications he/she is taking from all sources (dentist, family physician, specialists)?

The more questions to which you answered "yes," the more likely he/she is to be a drug abuser.

B. Risk Factors for Becoming Addicted

(Yes) (No) 1. Have any members of his/her family ever abused drugs?

(Yes) (No) 2. Was he/she abused as a child, or did he/she go through other trauma during childhood?

(Yes) (No) 3. Is he/she now undergoing unusual stress or mental pain?

(Yes) (No) 4. Does he/she have easy access to drugs?

(Yes) (No) 5. Has he/she used or does he/she use drugs recreationally?

(Yes) (No) 6. If he/she has used or now uses drugs recreationally, did or does he/she choose the fastest method of getting a hit?

The more "yes" answers, the greater his/her risk of addiction. (Remember that alcohol is a drug, too.)

C. Signs and Symptoms That a Problem with Drugs Exists

(Yes) (No) 1. Does he/she use drugs as an escape or to cope with a stressful situation?

(Yes) (No) 2. Does he/she become depressed easily?

(Yes) (No) 3. Does he/she use drugs the first thing in the morning?

(Yes) (No) 4. Has he/she ever tried to quit and resumed using again?

(Yes) (No) 5. Does he/she do things under the influence of a drug that he/she would not normally do?

(Yes) (No) 6. Has he/she had any drug-related "close calls" with the police or any arrests?

(Yes) (No) 7. Does he/she think a party or social gathering isn't fun unless drugs are served?

(Yes) (No) 8. Does he/she feel proud of an increased tolerance to drugs?

(Yes) (No) 9. Does he/she use drugs when alone?

(Yes) (No) 10. Has or does he/she use a wide variety of drugs?

(Yes) (No) 11. Is he/she constantly thinking about being high?

(Yes) (No) 12. Does he/she avoid people or places that oppose usage?

(Yes) (No) 13. Has his/her friends, family, teachers, or employer expressed concern about his/her use?

(Yes) (No) 14. Is his/her usage causing him/her to neglect responsibilities?

(Yes) (No) 15. Has he/she ever had blackouts or lack of memory of drug use or other events?

(Yes) (No) 16. Has he/she stolen to get money for drugs?

(Yes) (No) 17. Has he/she seriously considered that he/she might have a drug problem?

The more "yes" answers, the more likely he/she is to have a serious problem with drugs.

Results

A. Does he/she abuse prescription drugs?   (Yes) (No)
   (Questions A: 1–6)

B. Is he/she at considerable risk for addiction?   (Yes) (No)
   (Questions B: 1–6)

C. Does he/she have a serious problem with drugs?   (Yes) (No)
   (Questions C: 1–17)

Conclusions and Implications: In several sentences, discuss a plan of action that could be taken by a person who has a problem with the misuse of over-the-counter drugs, prescription drugs, or illegal drugs. Discuss specific things you could do to help a person with a problem. At some point, you may want to answer the questions about yourself.

Preventing Sexually Transmitted Infections

Health Goals for the year 2010

- Promote responsible sexual behaviors, to prevent sexually transmitted infections (STIs) and their complications.

- Reduce incidence of chlamydia, gonorrhea, syphilis, genital herpes, human papillomavirus (HPV), pelvic inflammatory disease (PID), and hepatitis B.

- Reduce incidence of and death from human immunodeficiency virus (HIV) and acquired immune deficiency syndrome (AIDS).

- Increase proportion of young people who abstain from sexual intercourse, use condoms during sexual activity, and avoid risky sexual behaviors.

- Increase STI screening and treatment.

- Via television programming, increase positive messages relating to responsible sexual behavior.

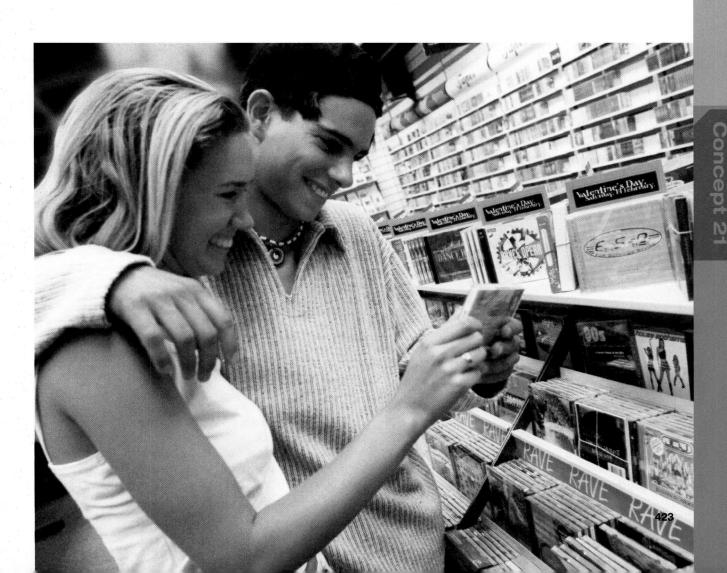

Safe sex and sound information about sexually transmitted infections are important to health and wellness.

The sexual experience is an interpersonal one that influences our actions and behaviors. It is basic to family life and fundamental to the reproduction of the human species. Approached responsibly, the human sexual experience contributes to wellness and quality of life in many ways. When approached irresponsibly, it can result in disease and personal and interpersonal suffering. Learning and adopting safe sex practices are important aspects of a healthy lifestyle. Safe sex is critical for avoiding unwanted pregnancies and for reducing risks for various infections and diseases. This concept will provide information about the symptoms, causes, and treatments of various infections and diseases transmitted through sexual contact.

The term *sexually transmitted disease (STD)* has been commonly used to refer to these conditions, but there has been a recent move toward the use of the broader term **sexually transmitted infection (STI)**. Although STIs lead to disease in many cases, typically a period of infection occurs prior to the emergence of disease symptoms. HIV/AIDS is a good example, as one can be infected for many years before signs of disease begin to occur. In other cases, STIs never result in identifiable disease symptoms. Human papillomavirus (HPV) is a good example. Although HPV can lead to cervical cancer in women, most women infected with HPV will never experience disease symptoms. Because *STI* better captures the range of outcomes, this term will be used throughout the remainder of the concept.

General Facts

The healthy sexual experience can contribute to wellness in many ways. Because human sexual experience is interpersonal, it is a social one. It affects many more people than a sexual partner. Personal beliefs have much to do with the feelings that participants have toward

---

the sexual experience; thus, spiritual wellness is influenced. Because the sexual experience is often emotionally charged, emotional wellness is also affected. Clearly, intellectual decisions are made concerning the experience, so intellectual well-being is a factor to consider as well. The sexual act is a physical experience that can be pleasurable but that has many long-lasting physical consequences. All five wellness dimensions are involved in decisions concerning participation in, the meaningfulness of, and the long-term consequences of the sexual experience. The healthy sexual experience requires sensitive and thoughtful consideration of the consequences.

Decisions concerning sexual behavior have lifelong consequences. Positive consequences of a sexual experience include pleasure, childbearing, and an enriched, happy family life. Negative lifelong consequences can include unwanted pregnancy, emotional and physical stress, and strained social relationships, among others. Unsafe sex also takes a toll in disease and death for large numbers of people worldwide.

Unsafe sexual activity can result in disease, poor health, and much pain and suffering. Until the 1940s, STIs were a leading cause of death. The discovery of penicillin and other antibiotics, and improved public health practices, lowered the death rate from STIs, but they remained a significant health problem. In 1991, STIs became 1 of the 10 leading causes of death in the United States, principally because of the high death rate from **acquired immune deficiency syndrome (AIDS)** caused by the **human immunodeficiency virus (HIV)**. STIs have since dropped from the top 10 list, primarily because of the effectiveness of recently developed drugs in reducing the death rate from HIV/AIDS.

HIV/AIDS

Of all the STIs, HIV/AIDS poses the greatest health threat to the world. Health experts indicate that we are in the midst of a worldwide HIV/AIDS epidemic. Many experts say that the AIDS epidemic has become larger than the plague was. Each year, about 40,000 people in the United States are infected with HIV, and over 1 million are already infected. Worldwide, the problem is even more profound, with about 11,000 people infected each day and a total of 40 million

---

On the Web

www.mhhe.com/corbinweb

Web 01 ☞ Log on to this URL before reading this concept. See On the Web list of concepts. Click on the concept number you want to view. To access supplemental information, click on the number shown at each Web icon.

people currently living with HIV. The problem of HIV/ AIDS is particularly bad in Sub-Saharan Africa. The rate of HIV infection among adults in Botswana, for example, is over 33 percent. International health agencies and foundations have been working to address the gap in awareness and the limited access to treatments in these parts of the world. See Web01 for more information.

Women and minorities are populations in which the incidence of HIV/AIDS is increasing disproportionately. What was once thought to be a disease of males, especially gay men, is now increasingly a female condition. New cases among women are 27 percent in the United States and 50 percent worldwide. The proportion of heterosexuals with HIV is also higher for women (75 percent) than men (33 percent). Approximately 51 percent of all new infections are among African Americans and nearly 20 percent are among Hispanics. Among women with HIV, 64 percent are African American.

HIV attacks the immune system and can lead to AIDS. A test of **serostatus** can indicate if a person is seropositive. When a person tests seropositive for HIV, it means that a blood test has indicated the presence in the body of the HIV. HIV invades the body's immune system cells, even killing them. This results in damage to the immune system and the body's ability to fight infections. One of the principal problems is that HIV causes immune suppression by directly invading and killing **CD4+ helper cells.** When too many of these cells (also called **T helper cells**) are destroyed, the body cannot fight **opportunistic infections** effectively.

When T cell counts are low and the **viral load** is high, the immune system can no longer function properly, thereby making the seropositive person more susceptible to various types of diseases and disorders. **Antibodies** in the blood that normally fight infections are ineffective in stopping the HIV from invading the body. Though it is not clear exactly why HIV affects the immune system as it does, the stages of HIV are better understood than in the past. First, HIV infects the body. Over time, white blood cells are damaged, and antibodies become ineffective. Depending on the time elapsed and individual variance in the progression of the disease, AIDS may develop or no symptoms may appear. After HIV enters the body, it takes several months before enough antibodies are developed to be able to detect its presence. Newer tests detect a portion of the HIV virus known as P24.

An individual has AIDS when he or she is infected with HIV and develops various opportunistic diseases because of impairment of the immune system. Examples of opportunistic diseases associated with AIDS are pneumonia, tuberculosis, **Kaposi's sarcoma,** yeast infections, and cervical cancer. Other symptoms include fatigue, swollen glands, rashes, weight loss, and loss of appetite. Once one

receives a diagnosis of AIDS, this diagnosis is maintained even if the individual becomes nonsymptomatic. In other words, one cannot move from AIDS back to HIV-positive status without AIDS.

There are two mechanisms for most HIV transmission. The two primary mechanisms responsible for the transmission of HIV are sexual activity and contact with infected blood (needle sharing). Among men, the greatest number of new cases result from men having sex with men, though a significant number of cases result from heterosexual sex. Among women, risk of transmission is most frequent in heterosexual sex. Worldwide, 75 percent of all AIDS cases are transmitted by heterosexual sex.

More than 25 percent of new cases are a result of injecting drugs with contaminated needles, and most of the rest of the cases are among people who combine these risk factors. Some cases are transmitted from HIV-infected mothers to children during childbirth. As many as 20 percent of mothers have not been tested for HIV. This is of

Sexually Transmitted Infection (STI) An infection for which a primary method of transmission is sexual activity.

Acquired Immune Deficiency Syndrome (AIDS) An HIV-infected individual is said to have AIDS when he or she has developed certain opportunistic infections (for example, pneumonia, tuberculosis, yeast infections, or other infections) or when his or her CD4+ cell count drops below 200.

Human Immunodeficiency Virus (HIV) A virus that causes a breakdown of the immune system among humans, resulting in the body's inability to fight infections. It is a precursor to AIDS.

Serostatus A blood test indicating the presence of antibodies the immune system creates to fight disease. A seropositive status indicates that a person has antibodies to fight HIV and is HIV positive.

CD4+ Helper Cells (T Helper Cells) Cells that protect against infections and activate the body's immune response. HIV kills these cells, so a high count usually means better health.

Opportunistic Infections Infections that typically do not affect healthy people, but may lead to diseases in people whose immune systems have been compromised.

Viral Load The level of virus (HIV) in the blood.

Antibodies Bodies in the bloodstream that react to overcome bacterial and other agents that attack the body.

Kaposi's Sarcoma A type of cancer evidenced by purple sores (tumors) on the skin.

concern, since one dose of the drug nevirapine has been shown to be effective in reducing mother-to-child transmission. At least one study has shown that cesarean delivery can reduce the risk of mother-to-baby transmission if the mother is seropositive. Recent evidence has also led to the recommendation that infected mothers consider alternatives to breast-feeding.

Those with other STIs, such as herpes and syphilis, have a greater risk of HIV transmission than those who do not have these conditions. Eight percent of HIV cases in one recent study were a result of oral sex. If future studies verify this finding, it suggests that oral sex may be a more risky behavior than previously thought.

HIV is not spread through the air or in saliva, sweat, or urine. It does not spread by hugging, sharing foods or beverages, or casual kissing. Contact with phones, silverware, or toilet seats does not cause the spread of HIV.

HIV must invade the blood in order for a person to become infected. People who had blood transfusions prior to 1985 had an increased risk of HIV transmission, but since that time the safety of the blood supply has increased dramatically.

The risk of acquiring HIV/AIDS is reduced if exposure to HIV and to the methods of transmission is avoided. Experts from the National Institutes of Health have concluded that HIV transmission could be reduced if legislative barriers to needle exchange programs were lifted, if greater emphasis were given to youth education programs about HIV/AIDS, if greater funding were available for the treatment of people who abuse drugs, and if educational efforts among high-risk populations were increased. Worldwide, the money expended on treatment far exceeds the amounts spent on prevention. Experts suggest that, if we are to meet national and international health goals, more effort and money will need to be spent on prevention. Taking personal responsibility for reducing risky behaviors is important for prevention on a personal level. Increasing awareness of and education about these risks is important for national and international prevention. Steps that can be taken to lower your risk of HIV infection are presented in Table 1.

Early detection is critical for controlling the spread of AIDS. Awareness of infection (early identification) and proper counseling can help prevent spread of HIV to others and enhance the effect of treatment. One study found that routine HIV screening would be cost-effective when compared with screening for other health problems, such as diabetes and high-blood pressure. Testing for HIV and other STIs can be either confidential or anonymous. When a test is confidential, there is a written record of the test results, but there is also assurance that this information will be kept private by the health-care provider. An anonymous test is one for which there is no written record such that the re-

Web 02

Table 1 ▶ Factors Associated with Reducing Risk for HIV/AIDS

- Abstain from sexual activity.
- Limit sexual activity to a noninfected partner. A lifetime partner who has never had sex with other people and has never used injected drugs (other than medically administered) is the only safe partner.
- Avoid sexual activity or other activity that puts you in contact with another person's semen, vaginal fluids, or blood.
- Use a new condom (latex) every time you have sex, especially with a partner who is not known to be safe. Know how to use it properly.
- Use a water-based lubricant with condoms because petroleum-based lubricants increase risk for condom failure.
- Abstain from risky sexual activity, such as anal sex and sex with high-risk people (prostitutes, people with HIV or other STIs).
- Do not inject drugs.
- Never share a needle or drug paraphernalia.
- Get tested for STIs, and seek proper treatment.
- Use a condom or dental dam when engaging in oral sex.
- Talk with your partner about his or her and your own sexual history before initiating sexual behavior.
- Remember that condoms are for STI prevention as well as pregnancy prevention. Even if your partner is using another form of birth control, use condoms if your partner has not been tested or you do not know his or her sexual history.

sults cannot be connected to your name or other identifiable information. There are clinics throughout the country that provide both confidential and anonymous (in most states) testing at no cost. See Web02 for information on testing.

In the past, HIV tests required blood samples and had to be completed in the presence of a health-care provider. In addition, the wait for test results lasted for weeks. Much has changed in the past decade. There are now self-testing kits that can be mailed to labs for analysis so the individual does not have to see a health-care provider. Some of these tests are noninvasive, requiring the user to use a swab to collect cells from the inside of the mouth. There are also tests that provide results with 99 percent accuracy in as little as 20 minutes. Although these rapid HIV tests currently must be completed in the presence of a health-care provider or mailed to a lab to obtain results, the FDA is considering permitting such tests to be sold over-the-counter. This would allow people to test themselves for HIV and get results in less than 30 minutes.

Early identification can also lead to longer life (average of 1 ½ years) for the infected person. Many have become free of detectable amounts of HIV as long as they continue the treatments. Nondetectable levels of HIV among those infected, however, does not prevent transmission, though there is less risk of transmission for those with low blood virus levels. Apparently virus "reservoirs" exist that allow transmission even when drugs have reduced HIV to undetectable levels.

There is no cure for AIDS but treatments have improved. For those infected with HIV/AIDS, there is no known cure. However, treatments have been developed to suppress or slow the progress of the disease process. Understanding how the drugs used to treat HIV/AIDS work requires an understanding of the process by which HIV attacks the body. First, the virus must enter T cells in the body. Once HIV enters these cells, HIV RNA is translated into DNA through a process called reverse transcription. Once the HIV RNA has been converted, an enzyme called integrase facilitates the integration of HIV DNA into the host DNA of the cell. The HIV DNA is then able to generate new protein sequences necessary to create new copies of the virus. In the final step, the HIV protein called protease separates the protein sequence into its component parts so these proteins can combine to form new viruses.

The medications used to treat HIV/AIDS interfere at different points in the process. Fusion inhibitors are a class of drugs that operate in the first step of the process by interfering with the virus's ability to enter the host cell. Reverse transcriptase inhibitors disrupt reverse transcription so that HIV RNA cannot be converted into DNA or integrated into the DNA of the host cell. Finally, protease inhibitors interfere with the protease enzyme, which prevents the HIV DNA from being separated into its component parts. This prevents the development of new viruses within the host cell. Because mutations can occur in the replication process, no single drug is effective in preventing the spread of the virus. Thus, drugs from multiple classes are typically combined to disrupt the process at multiple steps. Such combinations are referred to as highly active antiretroviral therapy (HAART), or the "HIV cocktail."

The specific combination of drugs selected for a given individual depends on factors such as the person's readiness for treatment, the potential for adherence, the person's willingness to take many pills, the severity of the infection, the potential for adverse drug effects, other existing illnesses, and potential interactions with other drugs. A limitation of the combination treatments is that a number of different drugs need to be taken in a specific sequence. A three drug "cocktail" has been the most common treatment but the FDA recently approved a new "once a day" pill for treating HIV. This new drug (Atripla) includes all three drugs in one tablet (Sustiva, Viread and Emtriva). The advent of this new medication greatly simplifies the treatment and is considered to be a big forward step by experts. However, the recent discovery of new strains of HIV have caused concern among public health officials. More than a few of the new strains are resistant to one or more of the classes of anti-HIV drugs. People with resistant strains have fewer available treatment options. Resistant strains are now being passed from those who are currently HIV positive to those previously not infected.

Although drug therapies offer hope, they also contribute to a host of undesirable side effects. Medications used to treat HIV have some negative consequences. Some of the many side effects include nausea, diarrhea, gastrointestinal symptoms, liver abnormalities, defects in blood fat metabolism, premature bone thinning, insulin abnormalities, inflammation of the pancreas, nerve damage, and death. In addition, the person can develop immunity to these drugs. This is particularly problematic for patients who have been on the drugs for a long time. Fortunately, a new class of medications, called maturation inhibitors, is currently under development. These drugs have shown promise in fighting HIV/AIDS in patients who are resistant to other medications.

The search for a vaccine for HIV is well underway, though no vaccine is currently available. More than 100 vaccines have been tested in humans or animals and 16 vaccines are currently undergoing clinical trials in the U.S. and abroad. Although a vaccine that prevents initial infection with HIV is the ultimate goal, researchers have not yet found a vaccine that triggers the production of antibodies (the mechanism of action for most vaccines), and some fear it will not be possible. The most promising vaccine currently undergoing clinical trials is a combination of three genes that are administered via an adenovirus (common cold virus). The genes trick the body into believing it has been infected, resulting in an effective immune response. Researchers are also hopeful that vaccines will be effective in preventing those already infected with HIV from developing AIDS and will prolong the life span of those who develop AIDS. Newly developed vaccines have shown promise in prolonging life in monkeys with simian immunodeficiency virus (SIV)—officials believe similar vaccines may be effective in humans. These studies also identified a marker for the efficacy of vaccines that can provide evidence of immune benefits in a period of only a few months. If this marker works similarly in humans, it could significantly speed the process of identifying an effective vaccine in humans.

Many people with HIV do not know they are infected. The Centers for Disease Control and Prevention (CDC) estimates that about 30 percent of those with HIV are unaware that they are infected. In a sample of about

19,000 AIDS patients, two of five people tested positive for HIV within a year of being diagnosed with AIDS. Even in a sample of people at high risk for HIV, about 30 percent reported that they had not been tested. This complicates efforts to achieve national and international health goals because treatment is often delayed and those who are unaware of their HIV status may transmit the virus unknowingly. Public health efforts have begun to focus more on this problem, stressing the need for more prevention targeting those who may be unknowingly transmitting HIV.

Other Sexually Transmitted Infections

STIs infect about 15 million people each year. Although HIV is the deadliest of the sexually transmitted infections, it is not among the most common in the United States. Table 2 lists some of the most common STIs in terms of both incidence (new cases) and prevalence (cumulative number of cases). Although rates of human papillomavirus (HPV) have not been well studied because the vast majority of those infected are unaware that they are infected, it is estimated that over 50 percent of sexually active adults will be infected with HPV at some point in their lifetime. Thus, HPV is by far the most common STI. Of the STIs that are tracked by the CDC, **chlamydia** has been the most commonly reported for the past decade. With improved methods of screening and efforts by the CDC and other agencies to increase screening, rates of identified cases have increased dramatically in the past 25 years despite the fact that most experts believe that rates of infection are not increasing. Gonorrhea was the most commonly

reported STI until the early 1990s and is now the second most common. Rates of gonorrhea infection in the United States have decreased dramatically over the past 25 years. Syphilis rates are much lower and have remained more stable during the last quarter century. Rates peaked in the early 1990s and then decreased significantly during the remainder of the decade. Unfortunately, rates began to rise again in 2000, a trend that continued through the first half of the decade. Figure 1 provides a graphic depiction of the rates of common STIs and AIDS and trends over the past 25 years.

Chlamydia is a common STI but it is often difficult to detect. About 3 million new cases of chlamydia are reported in the United States each year. Chlamydia, however, is known as the "silent" STI because about three-fourths of infected women and about half of infected men have no symptoms. If symptoms do occur, it is typically in the first three weeks following infection. For men who experience symptoms, the most common are discharge from the penis and a burning sensation when urinating. Common symptoms in women include abnormal vaginal discharge, a burning sensation when urinating, lower abdominal or back pain, pain during intercourse, and bleeding between menstrual periods. If chlamydia is left untreated, the health consequences of chlamydia can be extensive, particularly for women. The disease has been linked to increased risk of **pelvic inflammatory disease (PID),** as well as a number of other secondary health problems, including urethritis, cervicitis, ectopic pregnancy, infertility, and chronic pelvic pain. As a result of the high levels of risk for women, guidelines from the U.S. Preventive Services Task Force suggest that sexually active women under the age of 25 undergo routine screening for chlamydia. Fortunately, chlamydia is very treatable, and its long-term health consequences can be prevented if the in-

Table 2 ▶ Rankings of Incidence and Prevalence of Common STIs		
STI	**Rank of Incidence (Number of New Cases of the Condition)**	**Rank of Prevalence (Number of People with Condition)**
Chlamydia	2	3
Gonorrhea	4	4
Hepatitis B	5	5
Herpes	3	1
Human papillomavirus (HPV)	1	2
Syphilis	6	6

Source: Cates et al.

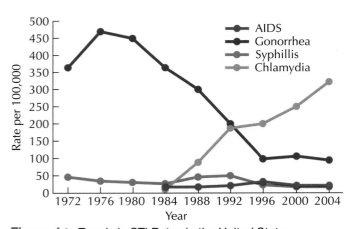

Figure 1 ▶ Trends in STI Rates in the United States.
Based on data from the annual CDC Sexually Transmitted Disease Surveillance reports and HIV/AIDS Surveillance reports.

fection is identified quickly. Treatment with antibiotics can clear up the infection within a week to 10 days.

Early detection is critical for effective treatment of gonorrhea. **Gonorrhea** is a bacterial infection that can be treated with modern antibiotics if detected early. However, recent strains of the gonorrhea organism have become resistant to antibiotics, due to widespread overuse. This has caused concern among public health officials, since some cases are quite difficult to treat.

Sexual activity is the principal method of disease transmission. Penile and vaginal gonorrhea are the most common types. Symptoms usually occur within 3 to 7 days after bacteria enter the system. Among men, the most common symptoms are painful urination and penile drip or discharge. Symptoms are less apparent among women, though painful urination and vaginal discharge are not uncommon. Other types of gonorrhea often have fewer symptoms. Chills, fever, painful bowel movements, and sore throat are the most common.

Early detection by a culture or smear test at the site or sites of sexual contact is how the disease is diagnosed. Early cure is especially important for females because gonorrhea can lead to pelvic inflammatory disease, which can result in infertility.

Hepatitis B is considered to be an STI. Like other STIs, hepatitis B (HPB) is typically spread through unprotected sex with an infected partner, IV drug use, or transmission from an infected mother to her baby. Although rare, HPB can be spread through blood transfusion or any other contact with infected blood. Symptoms of HPB include jaundice, fatigue, abdominal pain, loss of appetite, and nausea. Among those chronically infected with the virus, chronic liver disease typically develops, leading to premature death in 15 to 25 percent of cases. Fortunately, a vaccine for HPB has been available since 1982, and rates have decreased since then from an average of 260,000 cases to an average of 60,000 cases in 2004.

Of all STIs, genital herpes is among the most commonly spread because of a lack of awareness of infection. **Genital herpes,** one of the most commonly reported STIs, is caused by the herpes simplex virus (HSV). Although fewer new cases of genital herpes are reported annually than cases of HPV and chlamydia, the number of individuals currently infected is much higher. This is because chlamydia is treatable and HPV typically goes away on its own. In contrast, once someone contracts genital herpes, he or she will always carry the virus. HSV is a family of many viruses that can produce various disorders in humans, such as shingles and chicken pox. HSV Type 1 is often called lip or oral herpes because it causes cold sores and fever blisters on the lips and the mouth. HSV Type 2 is often referred to as the STI type because it is known to cause genital lesions. These lesions or blisters on the penis, vagina, or cervix usually occur 2 to 12 days after infection and typically last a week to a month. Swollen glands and headache may also occur.

Though Type 2 HSV is generally referred to as the STI type, it is now known that both Types 1 and 2 HSV can cause genital sores. No cure exists for genital sores caused by HSV, though some prescription drugs can help treat the disease symptoms. Episodic antiviral therapy is taken at the first sign of an outbreak and suppressive antiviral therapy is taken daily to prevent outbreaks from occurring. HSV can remain dormant in the body for long periods of time and, as a result, symptoms can recur at any time, especially after undergoing stress or illness.

Genital herpes is especially contagious when the blisters are present. Condom use or abstinence from sexual activity when symptoms are present can reduce the risk of transmission of the disease. Although genital herpes is less infectious when there are no symptoms present, the infection can still be spread to other partners. In addition, although condoms provide some protection, they are not totally effective in preventing infection because they do not cover all genital areas. Herpes is more dangerous for women than men because of the association between genital herpes and cervical cancer and the risk of transmitting the disease to the unborn.

The human papillomavirus (HPV) is a very common STI in young people. An estimated 6.2 million people become infected with HPV each year, making this STI the most commonly transmitted. HPV is responsible for the development of genital warts, but most people do not develop them and are therefore unaware that they are infected. Although the disease is asymptomatic in the short term, it leads to significantly increased risk for cervical cancer in women. In fact, HPV is the leading cause of cervical cancer. Certain strains of HPV are particularly dangerous, accounting for approximately 80 percent of cases of cervical cancer. The risk for cervical cancer is compounded for women with a history of HPV and chlamydia. One

---

Chlamydia A bacterial infection, similar to gonorrhea, that attacks the urinary tract and reproductive organs.

Pelvic Inflammatory Disease (PID) An infection of the urethra (urine passage), which can lead to infertility among women.

Gonorrhea A bacterial infection of the mucous membranes, including the eyes, throat, genitals, and other organs.

Genital Herpes A viral infection that can attack any area of the body but often causes blisters on the genitals.

study suggests that the combination of HPV and chronic use of birth control pills also compounds the level of risk. Women with a history of chlamydia and/or women who have used birth control pills for five or more years should consider being tested for HPV, due to the combined risk associated with these factors.

Although a vaccine is now available for HPV (see Technology Update on page 432), there is no available treatment for those already infected. Fortunately, rates of cervical cancer are quite low in the United States due to routine use of Pap tests. Regular Pap tests can identify cell changes that are caused by HPV before they become cancerous. These cell changes can be treated to prevent the development of cervical cancer. Thus, although there is no treatment for HPV, the health risks associated with HPV are largely preventable.

Syphilis is another serious but less commonly contracted STI. **Syphilis** was a serious national health problem in the 1940s, when it was 10 times more prevalent than it is now. STIs showed a dramatic increase during the 1970s and 1980s. Fortunately, progress toward the national health goal of reducing the number of syphilis cases has been made. Syphilis was the first STI for which national control measures were initiated. Reported cases of syphilis declined 84 percent nationwide during the 1990s. CDC reports that syphilis continues to have a disproportionate effect on African Americans and people living in the South.

Like gonorrhea, syphilis is a bacterial infection that can be effectively treated with antibiotics. The symptoms of syphilis include **chancre** sores that generally appear at the primary site of sexual contact, then change from a red swelling to a hardened ulcer on the skin. Even if not treated, the sores disappear after 1 to 5 weeks. It is important to get treatment even after this primary phase of the disease because the disease is still present and contagious. After several weeks or longer, secondary symptoms occur, such as a rash, loss of hair, joint pain, sore throat, and swollen glands. Even after these symptoms go away, untreated syphilis lingers in a latent phase. Serious health problems may result, including blindness, deafness, tumors, and stillbirth.

Early detection is important and can be diagnosed from chancre discharge or a blood test several weeks after the appearance of chancres. There is an association between syphilis and the spread of HIV. Apparently, the presence of chancres greatly increases the risk of transmitting HIV during sexual activity.

Some lesser known STIs are significant health problems. **Pubic crab lice, chancroid,** and **genital warts** are examples of lesser known but prevalent STIs. Some general information about these diseases is presented in Table 3. There are also a number of vaginal infections that can be sexually transmitted, including bacterial vaginosis (BV) and trichomoniasis.

Table 3 ▶ Facts about Lesser Known STIs

Genital Warts (Condylomas)

- Comprise approximately 5 % of all reported STIs
- Are most prevalent in ages 15 to 24
- Are caused by the human papillomavirus (HPV)
- Are hard and yellow or gray on dry skin
- Are soft and pink, red or dark on moist skin
- Are treated by the prescription drug Podophyllin

Pubic Crab Lice

- Are pinhead-sized insects (parasites) that feed on the blood of the host
- Are transmitted by sexual contact and/or contact with contaminated clothes, bedding, and other washable items
- Have symptoms that include itching, but some people have no symptoms
- Can be controlled by using medicated lotion and shampoos and by washing contaminated bedding, and so on
- Do *not* transmit other STIs

Chancroid

- Is caused by bacteria
- Is more commonly seen in men than in women, particularly uncircumcised males
- Have symptoms including one or more sores or raised bumps on the genitals
- Can result in progressive ulcers occurring on the genitals; sometimes the ulcers persist for weeks or months
- Can be successfully treated with certain antibiotics

Syphilis An infection, caused by a corkscrew-shaped bacteria, that travels in the bloodstream and embeds itself in the mucous membranes of the body, including those of the sexual organs.

Chancre A sore or lesion commonly associated with syphilis.

Pubic Crab Lice Lice that attach themselves to the base of pubic hairs.

Chancroid A bacterial infection resulting in sores or ulcers on the genitals; different from chancres associated with syphilis.

Genital Warts Warts, caused by a virus, that grow in the genital/anal area (also called condyloma).

The first step in prevention is to recognize the risk; young people are especially at risk for STIs. Nearly two-thirds of all STIs occur in people under the age of 25. Both teens and college students are at high risk. In Lab 21A, you will have the opportunity to evaluate the risk of a friend or loved one. You may also want to evaluate your own risk using the STI Risk Questionnaire. Probable reasons for the high risk among young people are

- Perceived immortality. Many teens feel that disease is something that happens to other people, not to them.
- Risky sexual activity. Evidence suggests that teens and young adults often do not follow the STI guidelines presented earlier in this concept.
- Instant gratification. Many young people believe that sex should be spontaneous. They also fear what their partner might say if he or she is prepared to have sex and has protection available.
- Inability to talk about sexual issues. It is difficult for most young people to truly communicate with each other about commitments and protection.

College students are at risk for HIV and other STIs due to the practice of serial monogamy. Many college students are sexually active, yet most do not use condoms on a consistent basis. This is, in part, due to perceptions that they are in committed relationships and, therefore, are at low risk for infection. Such perceptions are problematic for several reasons. First, college students typically define a regular partner as someone they have been with for as little as 1 month, with most defining a regular partner as someone they have been with for less than 6 months. Second, most college students do not get tested on a regular basis, if at all. Third, when students perceive that they are in a committed relationship, the likelihood of condom use decreases dramatically. This is particularly true when an alternative form of birth control, primarily birth control pills, is being used. The common result is unprotected sexual intercourse between two people who have known one another for a relatively short period of time and who are unaware of their own and each other's STI status. Many students go through multiple committed relationships during the college years. This type of serial monogamy places college students at increased risk for HIV and other STIs, even though they may not believe that they are engaging in high-risk behavior.

Oral sex puts individuals at risk for STIs. Although oral sex puts individuals at much lower risk for contracting STIs than do vaginal and anal sex, this behavior is not without risk. In particular, oral sex significantly increases risk for the two most commonly reported types of STIs, chlamydia and gonorrhea. Although the level of risk for HIV transmission is quite low, cases of HIV infection from oral sex have been reported. Research evidence shows that adolescents perceive this behavior to be very low risk, and most indicate that they have not "had sex" with someone if they have had only oral sex. There is concern that such perceptions will lead to increased rates of unprotected oral sex. Although trends in the behavior have only recently been assessed in large samples, there is some evidence that these concerns are warranted. A study of trends in oral sex among adolescents (15–19) between 1995 and 2002 found an increase in receptive oral sex for male adolescents who had never engaged in sexual intercourse. In this group, rates increased from 15.4 percent in 1995 to 20.7 percent in 2002.

The methods for preventing other STIs are the same as those for preventing HIV. The factors associated with reduced risk for HIV/AIDS presented in Table 1 are also important in preventing other STIs. The only true way to be protected against STIs is to have sex with a mutually exclusive partner who has never had sex with anyone else or has tested negative for all STIs. Even condoms, the primary form of protection against STIs, are not fail safe.

Another method of prevention that may be available in the future is the use of topical microbicides. A microbicide is a topical preparation (foam, gel, or cream) that is applied vaginally or anally to prevent infection. These products are primarily being developed to target HIV, but evidence shows they could also be effective in preventing other STIs. Several topical microbicides are currently undergoing clinical trials, but it may be several years before they become available.

Regular screening and notification of partners who may be infected can reduce the spread of STIs. Regular screening for sexually transmitted infections can reduce rates of new infections. In addition, because many STIs are treatable with antibiotics, catching them early can reduce the negative health consequences associated with infection. For those who are sexually active with partners of unknown STI status, yearly testing is a good idea. Even more frequent testing may be appropriate for those at very high risk (e.g., IV drug users and those previously diagnosed with an STI). When an individual is identified with a sexually transmitted infection, it is important that he or she notify his or her sexual partners so they can also receive treatment. This helps reduce the spread of the infection. One approach tested in clinical trials is called expedited partner therapy. When a partner of an infected person is identified, but chooses not to seek direct medical help (for privacy), medication is dispensed to the infected person to provide to the partner. Thus, partners of the identified individual do not have to seek medical care directly. Although this approach is relatively new, there is evidence of positive outcomes, at least among heterosexual adults with chlamydia and gonorrhea.

Hot lines are available to help people who want information concerning STIs, such as HIV/AIDS. National AIDS toll-free hotlines that allow callers to retain anonymity are available on page 432.

Online Learning Center

www.mhhe.com/corbin7e
The Online Learning Center contains a variety of Web-based resources that will help you get the most out of this book and your course. In addition to the On the Web pages, there are video activities, interactive quizzes, application assignments, and a variety of other useful study aids. Log on to the URL above to access these resources.

National AIDS and STI hotlines

AIDS hotline (English): 1-800-342-AIDS (2437)
AIDS hotline (Spanish): 1-800-344-SIDA (7432)
CDC STD (STI) hotline: 1-800-232-4636
  (information for many STIs)

Web Resources

American Social Health Association STD/STI Center
  www.ashastd.org
Web 06 CDC Center for STD Prevention
  www.cdc.gov/nchstp/od/nchstp.html
CDC—Division of Sexually Transmitted Diseases
  www.cdc.gov/nchstp/dstd/dstd.html
Cells Alive! Human Immunodeficiency Virus
  www.cellsalive.com/hiv5.htm
HIV Vaccine Trials Network **www.hvtn.org/**
Institute of Human Virology **www.ihv.org/**
National Institute of Allergy and Infectious Diseases
  www.niaid.nih.gov
National Institutes of Health Aids Information
  http://aidsinfo.nih.gov/
The Office of HIV/AIDS Policy
  www.surgeongeneral.gov/aids

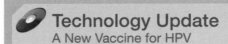

Technology Update
A New Vaccine for HPV

In June of 2006, the FDA announced the approval of the first vaccine for preventing cervical cancer. The vaccine, called Gardasil, works by preventing precancerous genital lesions and genital warts due to human papillomavirus (HPV). According to a spokesperson for the FDA, "This vaccine is a significant advance in the protection of women's health in that it strikes at the infections that are the root cause of many cervical cancers." It should be noted that the vaccine is not effective for those who became infected with HPV prior to receiving the vaccine. Although it protects against most forms of HPV, the vaccine does not protect against less common forms of HPV (see FDA website). It is estimated that widespread use of HPV vaccines could reduce cervical cancer rates by 70 percent. In July of 2006, the Advisory Committee on Immunization Practices (ACIP) unanimously recommended immunization for all girls and women ages 11–26. It also recommended (but did not require) the future immunization of all 11- and 12-year old girls.

Suggested Readings

Additional reference materials for Concept 21 are available at Web07.
Web 07 Centers for Disease Control and Prevention. 2005. *HIV/AIDS Surveillance Report, 2004*. Vol. 16. Atlanta, GA: U.S. Department of Health and Human Services.
Centers for Disease Control and Prevention. 2005. *Sexually Transmitted Disease Surveillance, 2004*. Atlanta, GA: U.S. Department of Health and Human Services.
Centers for Disease Control and Prevention. 2006. *HPV: Common Infection. Common Reality.* Available at **www.cdc.gov/std/hpv/common–infection/ HPVBrochureCleared–Online.pdf.**
Chesson, H. W., et al. 2004. The estimated direct medical cost of sexually transmitted diseases among American youth. *Perspectives on Sexual and Reproductive Health* 36(1):11–19.
Hamann, B. P. 2007. *Disease: Identification, Prevention and Control* 3rd ed. New York: McGraw-Hill Higher Education.

 In the News

Contraceptive Use and Risk for Sexually Transmitted Infections.

Depo Provera (a form of birth control that is injected into the arm or buttocks once every 3 months) has recently been linked to increased risk for gonorrhea and chlamydia. One study found that women using Depo Provera had three to four times higher risk for these two common STIs. An important implication of these results is that women who are using birth control need to continue to use condoms to protect themselves from STIs. In other news about pregnancy prevention, a recent study reported that the controversial "morning after" pill does not appear to increase high risk sexual behavior or rates of STIs. After an FDA advisory council in 2003 overwhelmingly supported the approval of the Plan B pill without a prescription, the acting director went against the advice of the panel. The concern has been that wider availability of the drug could lead to increased promiscuity and decreased use of protection against sexually transmitted infections. However, a new study published in the *Journal of the American Medical Association* found no evidence to support these concerns.

Lab 21A Sexually Transmitted Infection Risk Questionnaire

Name		Section	Date

Purpose: To help you understand the risks of contracting a sexually transmitted infection.

Procedure

1. Read the Sexually Transmitted Infection Risk Questionnaire.
2. Answer the questionnaire based on information about someone you know who might be at high risk of contracting an STI.
3. Record the scores in the Results section for the person for whom the questionnaire was answered but do *not* include the person's name on the lab sheet. Use the scores to make a rating (Chart 2) and draw conclusions.
4. You may also wish to answer the questionnaire based on your own information but do *not* record your personal results on the lab sheet. Use these scores strictly for your own personal information.

Chart 1 ▶ Sexually Transmitted Infection Risk Questionnaire

Directions: Mark an X over one response in each row of the questionnaire. Determine a point value for each response using the values in the circles. Sum the numbers of points for the various responses to determine an STI risk score.

Categories	**Points**				
	0	**1**	**3**	**5**	**8**
Feelings about prevention	Able to talk with future partner about STIs (0)	Finds it hard to discuss STIs with a possible partner (1)			
Behaviors	Never engages in sexual activity (0)		Sexual activity with one partner, well known to him or her (3)	Sexual activity with one partner, not well known to him or her (5)	Sexual activity with multiple partners and/or high-risk individuals (8)
Behavior of friends	Most friends do not engage in unsafe sexual activity (0)	Many friends engage in unsafe sexual activity (1)			
Contraception	Not sexually active (0)	Would use condom to prevent STI (1)		Would sometimes use condom to prevent STI (5)	Would never use condom to prevent STI (8)
Other	Does not use drugs (0)				Uses injected drugs in unsafe manner (8)

Chart 2 ► Risk Questionnaire Rating Chart

Rating	Score
High risk	9+
Above average risk	7–8
Moderate risk	4–6
Low risk	0–3

Results

What is the person's STI risk score? _____ (Total from STI Risk Questionnaire)

What is the person's STI rating? _____ (See STI Risk Questionnaire Rating Chart.)

Conclusions and Implications: Of course, risk varies with different types of STIs. However, this questionnaire will give you an idea of an individual's "general" risk for most STIs. Answer the following questions about the risk of the person you scored and rated.

1. In several sentences, explain which STI you think this person should be especially concerned about. Why?

2. What specific recommendations would you have for the person for whom you filled out this questionnaire?

Cancer, Diabetes, and Other Health Threats

Health Goals for the year 2010

- Reduce cancer cases, as well as illness, disability, and death from it.
- Increase rate of cancer screening.
- Increase cancer survivors (5 years or more).
- Increase diabetes screening and education.
- Prevent and reduce death from diabetes and disabilities associated with diabetes.
- Decrease incidence of depression.
- Increase healthy days.
- Increase screening and availability of medical treatment for a variety of health threats.
- Eliminate health disparities.
- Improve air quality, ensure safe water, and reduce environmental waste and hazards.
- Reduce unintentional injuries (focus on head and spinal cord) from all sources, including firearms; drowning; pedestrian, bicycle, and auto accidents; and fires.
- Reduce violence and abuse.
- Reduce the proportion of people who experience regular sadness or unhappiness.

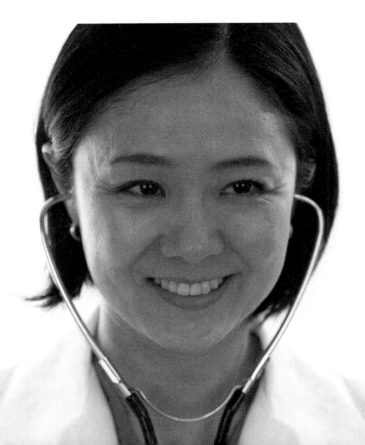

Many health problems that cause pain, suffering, and premature death are associated with unhealthy lifestyles.

Each year, many deaths and much pain and suffering could be prevented by altering lifestyles associated with various diseases and health threats. Heart disease, the leading cause of death; stroke (third leading cause of death); and osteoporosis were discussed in the concept on health benefits of physical activity (Concept 4), so they will not be discussed here. Among the conditions that are discussed in this concept are cancer, diabetes, bronchitis/emphysema, injuries, diabetes mellitus, and emotional disorders (including suicide). As noted in Concept 4, cancer is second only to heart disease among the leading causes of death. Heart disease causes more deaths for people of all ages, but cancer is the leading cause of death for people 75 years of age and younger. Cancer deaths have decreased in recent years but new cases have remained steady. Diabetes, injuries, and suicide all rank among the top 10 leading causes of death in our society.

Cancer

Cancer is a group of more than 100 different diseases. According to the American Cancer Society, cancer is a group of many different conditions characterized by abnormal, uncontrolled cell growth that will ultimately invade the blood and lymph tissues and spread throughout the body if not treated. Throughout the human body, new cells are constantly being created to replace older ones. For reasons unknown, abnormal cells sometimes develop capable of uncontrolled growth. **Benign tumors** are generally not considered to be cancerous because a protective membrane restricts their growth to a specific area of the body. Treatment is important because any tumor can interfere with normal bodily functioning. Once removed, a benign tumor typically will not return.

Malignant tumors are called **carcinomas** because they are capable of uncontrolled growth that can cause death to tissue. Malignant cells invade healthy tissues, de-plete them of nutrition, and interfere with a multitude of tissue functions. In the early stages of cancer, malignant tumors are located in a small area and can be more easily treated or removed. In advanced cancer, the cells invade the blood or lymph systems and travel throughout the body **(metastasize).** When this occurs, cancer becomes much more difficult to treat. In Concept 4, a brief illustration of the progression of cancer was presented. Figure 1 provides an illustration of the stages in the spread of cancer. The figure illustrates how an abnormal cell can divide to form a primary tumor (a), get nourishment from new blood vessels (b), invade the blood system (c), and escape to form a new (secondary) tumor (d). The four stages of cancer range from I to IV, with I being the early stage and IV being most advanced. The early stage is characterized by containment only in the layers of cells where they developed. When cancer spreads beyond the original layers (see Figure 1), it is considered to be invasive and is rated at a higher stage. Early detection is very important in the treatment and cure of cancer. One method of detecting a tumor is to take a **biopsy** of suspicious lumps in the breasts, testicles, or other parts of the body.

Cancer is not only a leading killer but a cause of much suffering. One of every four deaths in the United States is caused by some form of cancer. Slightly more than one in three women and slightly less than one in two men will have cancer at sometime in his or her life. It is the cause of much suffering and accounts for a large portion of the money spent on health care. There are over 100 forms of cancer, but four of them (sometimes referred to as the Big 4) account for more than half of all illness and death (see Figure 2). Because of the high incidence of these types of cancers (lung, colon-rectal, breast, and prostate) they are discussed in more detail here. In addition, three forms of cancer for which college students have relative high risk are also discussed (skin, ovary, and uterus). While some forms of cancer are equally threatening to both sexes (e.g., lung and colon-rectal), others are more specific to one sex or the other (see Figure 2). It is also important to note that incidence rates are different than death rates. Skin cancer is an example of a form of cancer that is high in incidence (fifth for men and sixth for women) but relatively low in death rate (not in the top 10 for men or women). This is because it can be treated with early detection and steps can be taken to prevent it. In Lab 22A you will have the opportunity to assess your risk for the major forms of cancer.

On the Web
www.mhhe.com/corbinweb

Web 01 Log on to this URL before reading this concept. See On the Web list of concepts. Click on the concept number you want to view. To access supplemental information, click on the number shown at each Web icon.

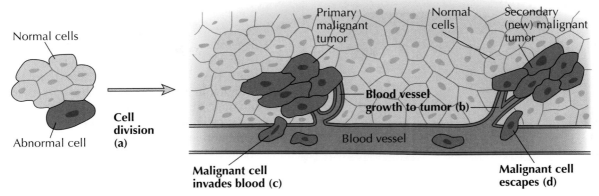

Figure 1 ▶ The spread of cancer (metastasis).

Cancer Type

Deaths Rank/%	Incidence Rank/%	Cancer Type
1. 31%	2. 31%	lung/bronchus
2. 10%	3. 10%	colon/rectal
3. 9%	1. 33%	prostate
4. 6%	10. 2%	pancreas
5. 4%	9. 3%	leukemia
6. 4%	*	liver
7. 4%	*	esophagus
8. 3%	6. 4%	non-Hodgkin lymphoma
9. 3%	4. 6%	urinary/bladder
10. 3%	7. 3%	kidney
*	5. 5%	skin
*	8. 3%	oral

Men   **Women**

Deaths Rank/%	Incidence Rank/%	Cancer Type
1. 26%	2. 31%	lung/bronchus
2. 15%	1. 10%	breast
3. 10%	3. 33%	colon/rectal
4. 6%	10. 2%	pancreas
5. 6%	8. 3%	ovary
6. 4%	*	leukemia
7. 3%	5. 4%	non-Hodgkin lymphoma
8. 3%	4. 6%	uterine
9. 2%	*	multiple myeloma
10. 2%	*	brain/nerve
*	6. 4%	skin
*	7. 3%	thyroid
*	9. 2%	urinary/bladder

Figure 2 ▶ Cancer incidence and death by site and sex (percent).

Source: American Cancer Society.

Breast Cancer

Web 02

Breast cancer is the most prevalent form of cancer among women, but lung cancer causes more deaths. This is partly due to improved early diagnosis of breast cancer resulting from screening and more effective treatments. Though not as common among men, both men and women should do regular screening for breast cancer. Like colon-rectal and lung cancers, breast cancer is most prevalent among African Americans and least prevalent among Asians and Hispanics (more than twice as frequent).

Benign Tumors Slow-growing tumors that do not spread to other parts of the body.

Malignant Tumor (Carcinoma) *Malignant* means "growing worse." A malignant tumor is one that is considered to be cancerous and will spread throughout the body if not treated.

Metastasize The spread of cancer cells to other parts of the body.

Biopsy The removal of a tissue sample that can be checked for cancer cells.

Mammograms X rays of the breast.

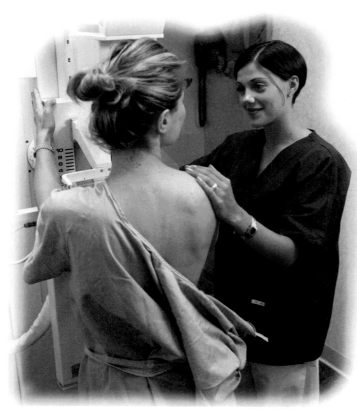

Cancer risk can be reduced by periodic medical tests and self-screening.

Symptoms include lumps and/or thickening or swelling of the breasts. In many cases, lumps are present before they can be detected with self-exams. This is one reason for regular **mammograms** (breast X rays). Breast pain may also exist but is more often a symptom of benign tumors. Risk becomes greater as you grow older. Other risk factors include sex (females have higher risk), family history of disease, early menstruation, hormone supplementation, use of oral contraceptives, late childbirth or no children, excessive use of alcohol, poor eating habits, and sedentary living. The discovery of a breast cancer "gene" provides a possible explanation of the hereditary risks. Research has demonstrated that both breast implantation and hormone replacement therapy may increase risk of breast cancer (see Web02). Because a number of factors influence breast cancer risk, it is important to follow appropriate screening procedures to detect the possible presence of the disease.

Early detection steps include regular self-exams of the breasts (see Lab 22B), breast exams by a physician, and regular mammograms. However, there is some debate among experts as to the frequency with which women should have a mammogram. Currently, the American Cancer Society (ACS) recommends that "women age 40 and older should have a screening mammogram every year, and should continue to do so for as long as they are in good health." In one study, only about two-thirds of college-educated women, most of whom had insurance, actually had a mammogram as frequently as once every 2 years. It should also be noted that there is evidence that digital mammography may be more effective than traditional film mammography. Digital mammography is still quite rare but will no doubt become more common in the future. The breast cancer screening guidelines currently recommended by the ACS are summarized in Table 1.

Standard treatments for breast cancer include lumpectomy (removal of the tumor and surrounding lymph nodes), mastectomy (removal of breast and surrounding lymph nodes), chemotherapy, radiation, and/or hormone therapies. Tamoxifen, or other drugs, may be prescribed for those at high risk.

Colon-Rectal Cancer

Colon-rectal cancers are the second leading overall killers because they affect men and women equally. There has been a consistent but small decline in colon-rectal cancer among men and women over the past two decades. Like lung cancer, risk is highest among African Americans. Whites have slightly less risk. Risk among Asians and Hispanics is less than half that of blacks. Lifestyle risk factors include diet, use of alcohol, family history, physical activity patterns, and smoking (see Lab 22A). A high-fiber diet and physical activity can decrease the risk. It is most common among those over 50 years of age. When caught early, 90 percent of colon-rectal cancers can be cured.

Symptoms include cramping in the lower stomach, change in the shape of the stool, urge to have a bowel movement when there is no need to have one, and blood in the stool. Because observable blood in the stool could indicate an advanced problem, do regular screenings, including a fecal blood test (see Table 1). Other screening tests include a barium enema, a sphygmoidoscopy, and a colonoscopy. A six-sample stool test (fecal blood test) done in the home has been shown to be better than the one-sample test done in a doctor's office. Also, the colonoscopy has been shown to be more effective than the sigmoidoscopy because it checks the entire colon for polyps rather than the lower one-third. A study of women showed that polyps often occur higher in the colon and go undetected by a sigmoidoscopy. The colonoscopy test is therefore viewed as the most accurate by the ACS.

All of the tests are designed to detect either the presence of polyps that can turn into cancer or polyps (or cancers) that are bleeding. Any or all of the tests may be recommended by a physician, especially after age 50.

Table 1 ▶ Cancer Screening Guidelines

Test or Procedure	Sex	Age	Frequency
General Cancer Related Checkup			
Exam for cancers of the thyroid, prostate, ovaries or testes, lymph nodes, mouth, and skin	Men and women	20–39	Every 3 years
Breast Cancer			
Breast self-exam	Women	20	Every month
Breast exam by physician, including mammogram	Women	20–39	Every 3 years
	Women	40+	Every year
Colon-Rectal Cancer[a]			
Fecal occult blood test	Men and women	50+	Every year
Sigmoidoscopy	Men and women	50+	Every 5 years
Barium enema	Men and women	50+	Every 5 to 10 years
Colonoscopy	Men and women	50+	Every 10 years
Lung			
X ray (chest)	Men and women	Any age	If other symptoms exist
Prostate			
Digital rectal exam and PSA test	Men (normal risk)	50+	Yearly
	Men (high risk)	45+	Yearly[b]
Testes			
Self-exam	Men	20+	Monthly
Uterus/Cervix			
Pelvic exam and PAP test	Women	Sexually active	Yearly
Endometrial	Women		
Screening and biopsy	Women at risk	35+	With risk or symptoms
Skin Cancer			
Self-exam	Men and women	Any age	Monthly
Exam by physician	Men and women	Any age	With symptoms

[a]Frequency varies based on tests done and test results; all tests may not be necessary.

The frequency of screening recommended by the ACS is shown in Table 1.

Studies show that the frequency of screening should vary, depending on symptoms and heredity. For example, people with a family history of colon-rectal cancer and those who have found a polyp in previous exams should schedule a procedure more frequently than listed in Table 1. People who smoke and drink should also begin screening earlier. Polyps can occur as many as 8 years earlier among this group than among nonsmokers and nondrinkers.

Several innovations in testing for colon cancer are being pioneered. One is a probe-free colonoscopy that uses either two-dimensional or three-dimensional CT scans. The 3-D version may be more effective than the colonoscopy and is much less invasive. It does involve radiation exposure equal to that of a chest X ray, however. Another test, the APC gene test, offers promise for the future. It involves examination of stool samples for damaged genes that trigger cancer. The most common treatments are surgery for cancer or polyp removal, radiation, and/or chemotherapy.

Lung Cancer

Web 04 ▶ Lung cancer is the leading cause of cancer death in men and women. Lung cancer rates have dropped in the past decade and this has been attributed, in part, to declines in smoking. In the past decade, smoking rates among youth and young adults have increased, however, suggesting that lung cancer deaths may increase in the years ahead. Incidence and death rates are much higher among African Americans than whites, with considerably lower rates among Asians and Hispanics.

By far, the greatest risk factor for lung cancer is smoking. Environmental tobacco smoke (ETS) has been shown to be a potent risk factor. According to the American Cancer Society, nonsmoking spouses of smokers have a 30 percent greater risk of developing lung cancer than do spouses of nonsmokers. A number of other carcinogens, including radon, asbestos, and pollution, have been linked to lung cancer, so nonsmokers can also get lung cancer.

Symptoms of lung cancer include persistent cough, chest pain, recurring pneumonia or bronchitis, and sputum (spit) streaked with blood. Lung cancer can spread to other organs and tissues before symptoms are evident, so it is important to pay attention to possible symptoms rather than to disregard them.

Early detection steps include monitoring for symptoms, chest X rays, and analyses of sputum samples. Standard treatments include radiation and chemotherapies.

Prostate Cancer

Web 05 ▶ Prostate cancer is one of the most common forms of cancer in men. Estimates suggest that men have about a 17 percent chance of being diagnosed with prostate cancer in their lifetime. Deaths from prostate cancer account for 10 percent of all cancer deaths in men (3 percent of total deaths). The death rate among African Americans is five times higher than among Asians, more than three times higher than Hispanics and more than twice as high as whites.

Risks of prostate cancer increase dramatically after the age of 50, so current guidelines recommend that men begin annual screening between the ages of 45 and 50. Symptoms of prostate cancer are urination problems (weak or interrupted stream, inability to start or stop, pain, high frequency of urination at night and/or presence of blood

in the urine). Early detection techniques include a digital rectal exam by a physician (to detect an enlarged prostate gland) and a prostate-specific antigen (PSA) blood test. A PSA threshold of 4 nanograms per milliliter was previously used as an indicator of potential risk but other screening criteria are now being used. Research suggests that year-to-year changes in PSA are a better predictor, even if the score is lower than 4. A single PSA test misses as many as 15 percent of cancers, so regular testing is advised. A new "autoantibody signatures" test has promise for the future. If future research verifies early findings, this test may be used instead of, or in addition to, the PSA test. Preliminary studies with the new test show that it identifies 82 percent of cancers correctly.

Current treatment for prostate cancer have been shown to be highly effective, and death rates due to prostate cancer have decreased. Initiation of treatment early in the disease process is critical for good results. The primary treatment options include surgery to remove the prostate, radiation and chemotherapy, and the implantation of radioactive "seeds" into the prostate to kill the tumor.

Uterine and Ovarian Cancers

Web 06 ▶ Combined, uterine and ovarian cancers account for 10 percent of all cancer cases and 7 percent of all deaths among women. Uterine cancer is of two different types: cervical cancer occurs when cancers develop in the cervix, or opening to the uterus, and endometrial cancer occurs when a tumor develops in the inner wall of the uterus. Ovarian cancer occurs when a cancer develops in an ovary. Symptoms of ovarian cancer include abdominal swelling and digestive disturbances. Vaginal bleeding can be a symptom of either uterine or ovarian cancer. Other vaginal discharge may be a symptom of uterine cancer.

The most important risk factor for cervical cancer is infection by human papillomavirus (HPV), a sexually transmitted infection. As noted in Concept 21, the FDA recently approved a "cervical cancer" vaccine (Gardasil) that acts to prevent precancerous genital lesions and genital warts due to HPV among those not previously infected. While it is not effective against all forms of HPV, it is effective against the most common forms implicated in most cervical cancers. For more information on the vaccine and recommendations for its use, refer to page 432 in Concept 21.

Other risk factors include having sex at an early age, having sex with many partners, and a history of smoking. The other form of uterine cancer, endometrial cancer, is less common and has a different mechanism of causation. The known risk factors, such as early menarche, late menopause, infertility, and obesity, are all associated with increased exposure to estrogen during the life span. Other risks include obesity and a high-fat diet. Risk fac-

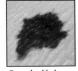

A. Asymmetry

One half does not match other half

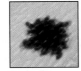

B. Border Irregularity

Ragged or notched edges

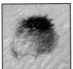

C. Color

Color uneven shades of tan, brown, or black and sometimes red, white or blue

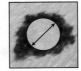

D. Diameter

Diameter larger than 1/4 inch (diameter of a pencil eraser)
Note: some cancers can be smaller

Figure 3 ▶ The ABCD rule for skin cancer self-examination.

tors for ovarian cancer include age, family history, and lack of pregnancy during the lifetime. One study showed that risk is considerably higher among those who have taken estrogen-progestin therapy, especially those who have taken it for 10 years or more. Those who have had breast cancer or who are at high risk for breast cancer have a relative high risk for ovarian cancer.

A periodic and thorough pelvic exam is the best method of screening for cervical and ovarian cancers. A **PAP test** is an important part of the exam for detecting cervical cancer. This test—named for Dr. George Papanicolaou, who pioneered it—involves taking scrapings (samples) from the cervix and analyzing them under a microscope. Liquid-based PAP testing (sometimes referred to as ThinPrep) has been shown to improve detection of cancers and precancerous cells. This test also allows testing for HPV from the same sample. Some home PAP smear kits are available, but these have not been found to provide accurate information. Women should begin having annual PAP tests after becoming sexually active or after turning 21.

Treatments include surgery to remove one or both of the ovaries and fallopian tubes (depending on age) and/or removal of the uterus (hysterectomy). Radiation therapy and chemotherapy are other options.

Skin Cancer

Each year, more than 1 million people get basal or squamous cell cancer. This curable form is not included in the overall incidence statistics in Figure 2. **Melanoma,** on the other hand, is a deadly cancer if not treated early. Melanoma is 10 times more frequent in whites than African Americans. Unlike many other forms of cancer, it is not necessarily a disease of older adults. Young people who do not take preventive measures are at risk.

Symptoms include darkly pigmented growths, changes in size or color of moles, changes in other nodules on the skin, skin bleeding or scaliness, and skin pain. The principal risk factor is exposure to ultraviolet light, such as sun exposure. Excessive sun exposure is common among college students. Some feel that tanning lights are safe,

but research has shown the opposite. Other risk factors include family history, pale skin, exposure to pollutants, and radiation.

Early detection is essential to treatment, so regular screening is important. Screening techniques include self-exams of the skin followed by a physician's exam of suspicious lesions. The American Cancer Society recommends that you follow the ABCD rule for self-exams (see Figure 3). *A* is for asymmetry; does one-half of a growth look different than the other half? *B* is for border irregularity; are the edges notched, rugged, or blurred? *C* is for color; is the color uniform, not varying in shades of tan, brown, and black? *D* is for any lesion with a diameter greater than 6 millimeters (about ⅜ inch). Beware of sudden or progressive growth of any lesion.

Nonmalignant basal and squamous cell cancers can be treated in a doctor's office using freezing, heat, or laser procedures. These milder forms of cancer have become more common among younger people in recent years. They occur on the head and neck in 90 percent of cases; however, with the increase in total body exposure and tanning practices, they are now much more common on other parts of the body. Once you have had one of these cancers, your risk of having another is high. Treatment for early melanoma involves the removal of affected cells and surrounding lymph tissues. Advanced cases require chemo and/or radiation therapies. Immunotherapy is another option.

Important preventive measures include limiting exposure to the sun or tanning devices, reducing exposure during midday hours (10 a.m. to 4 p.m.), covering the skin when exposed to the sun (hat, long pants, long-sleeve shirts, high collars on shirts, sunglasses), and using sunscreen (sun protection factor, or SPF, 15 or higher). Those with a history of severe sunburn as a child should be especially careful.

The ACS uses the slogan "Slip, Slop, Slap and Wrap" to encourage safe practices in the sun: slip on a shirt, slop on sunscreen, slap on a hat, and wrap on sunglasses to protect your eyes. Some rules for using sunscreen can help you use it more effectively. Apply it 20 to 30 minutes before going outside, apply it generously (a palmful),

PAP Test A test of the cells of the cervix to detect cancer or other conditions.

Melanoma Cancer of the cells that produce skin pigment.

Web 07

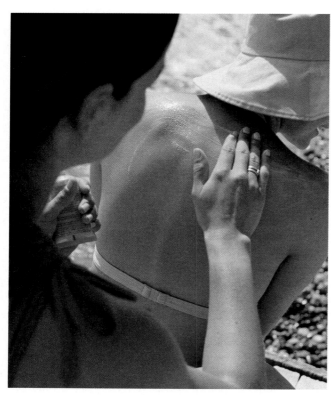

Using sunscreen can protect the skin and reduce the risk of skin cancer.

cover all body parts, and reapply every 2 hours and after swimming, sweating heavily, or using a towel.

There is some debate over the sunscreen SPF number that should be used. Some experts recommend sunscreens with an SPF higher than 15, especially for those who are at risk for skin cancer. Experts also recommend sunscreen with ingredients that give maximum protection against both types of ultraviolet rays (UVA and UVB). Chemical blocks, such as benzophenone and octocrylene, are effective in blocking UVB rays and mexoryl is effective in blocking UVA rays. Physical blocks are good for people with allergies to chemicals. They contain substances, such as zinc oxide and titanium dioxide, that reflect UVA and UVB rays.

Many factors are associated with increased risk for cancer; unhealthy lifestyles are among them. The malfunction of genes that control cell growth and development is responsible for all cancers. Five to 10 percent of cancers result from an inherited faulty gene. While genetics can't be altered, cancer is known to be influenced by a variety of lifestyle and environmental factors (see Figure 4). Dietary factors and tobacco collectively account for over 65 percent of overall cancer risk. Many of the recommendations for cancer prevention in Table 2 reflect the importance of minimizing exposure to **carcinogens.**

Other contributors to cancer risk include geophysical entities, such as radon and radiation; pollution; and various industrial products (e.g., polychlorinated biphenyls [PCBs] produced in making plastics and asbestos). These compounds are considered to be carcinogens because exposure to them causes cancer. Avoiding exposure to or consumption of carcinogens reduces risk for cancer.

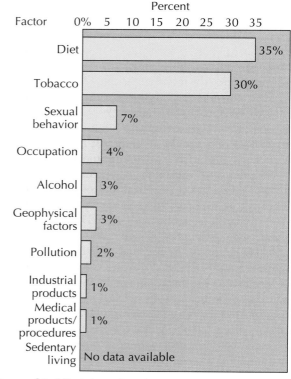

Figure 4 ▶ Lifestyle and environmental cancer risk factors.

Factor	Percent
Diet	35%
Tobacco	30%
Sexual behavior	7%
Occupation	4%
Alcohol	3%
Geophysical factors	3%
Pollution	2%
Industrial products	1%
Medical products/ procedures	1%
Sedentary living	No data available

Table 2 ▶ Strategies for Preventing Cancer

- Eat a healthy diet: reduce fat to less than 30%, avoid junk food, and eat green and yellow vegetables.

- Eliminate tobacco use: cigarettes and smokeless tobacco.

- Perform regular activity: be fit and avoid obesity.

- Reduce sun and ultraviolet light exposure: use sunscreen, wear protective clothing, avoid excess sun and tanning lights.

- Do regular self-screening and medical testing.

- Avoid carcinogens in food (such as sodium nitrate in bacon) and in other sources (such as insecticides).

- If you drink alcohol, do so in moderation.

- Avoid breathing polluted air.

- Avoid excessive X rays.

Web 08 **Many forms of cancer can now be effectively treated.** Many people have lived long, healthy lives after breast, skin, and many other forms of cancer. These people die from other causes and some would consider them to be "cured." Still, what constitutes a cure is illusive. The 5-year survival rate for all forms of cancer is 62 percent. Though people who survive for 5 years after detection may not be considered cured, the high survival rate illustrates that cancer can be treated even for those with inherited faulty genes.

Because of the prevalence of cancer, the chances are high that someone you know and care about will get cancer in your lifetime. It is important that you learn to help others who have cancer, as well as those who have survived cancer. There is evidence that some cancer survivors have problems after initial treatment. The National Academy of Sciences has prepared a booklet to help cancer survivors (see Web08).

Web 09 **Medical consultation is essential when considering hormone replacement therapy.** For years, hormone replacement therapy (HRT) was prescribed to women by medical doctors to help reduce the symptoms of menopause, prevent loss of bone density, and reduce risk for heart disease. However, it has been known for some time that administering hormones increases the risk for some forms of cancer. Recent evidence suggests that HRT is not effective in reducing heart disease, and it increases the risk for blood clots. Some experts still support HRT as a method of relieving menopausal symptoms, such as hot flashes, sleep disturbances, fatigue, poor concentration, and disruption of work and recreational activities, though other experts have challenged these benefits. Studies such as those reported here consider group risk rather than individual risk. The risk for increased disease from HRT is relatively small, compared with other risk factors. Nevertheless, small risks add up over time. Most experts agree that each case should be considered individually, with each patient and doctor weighing all risks and benefits before choosing a course of action. For those who do not continue HRT, alternate methods of preventing bone loss and reducing postmenopausal symptoms should be discussed with their physician.

Recognizing early warning signals can help reduce the risk of cancer. The acronym CAUTION will help you remember these early warning signs. Look for the following:

C	=	Changes in bowel or bladder habits
A	=	A sore that does not heal
U	=	Unusual bleeding or discharge
T	=	Thickening or lump (e.g., breast)
I	=	Indigestion or difficulty swallowing
O	=	Obvious change in a wart or mole
N	=	Nagging cough or hoarseness

Diabetes

Several classifications of diabetes cause health risk for many individuals. Glucose, a source of energy, is a sugar in the blood. Diabetes mellitus, typically referred to as diabetes, is a disease that occurs when the blood sugar is abnormally high. Normally, glucose levels range from 50 to 100 mg per 100 ml of blood based on a Fasting Plasma Glucose Test (FPG). According to the American Diabetes Association (ADA) **pre-diabetes** exists when blood glucose levels range from 101–125 and diabetes exist when blood glucose levels regularly exceed 125 using the FPG test. An oral glucose tolerance test can also be used to detect diabetes, but different values are used to indicate its prevalence. The ADA recommends the FPG test because it is "easier, faster, and less expensive to perform."

There are as many as 30 different reasons for high blood sugar, therefore diabetes is really many different diseases not just one. There is no cure for diabetes, however, with proper medical treatment and healthy lifestyle modifications, the condition can be managed effectively.

Insulin, a hormone produced by the pancreas, regulates the glucose in the blood. When a person's body fails to produce adequate insulin and the individual needs to take insulin (oral or injection) to regulate blood glucose levels, he or she is said to have **Type I diabetes.** About 5 percent of all diabetics have Type I diabetes, and this condition is typically diagnosed before the age of 30.

Type II diabetes (fasting blood glucose >126) is typically noninsulin dependent and can often be controlled with significant lifestyle changes and drugs other than insulin. Nearly 95 percent of all diabetics have Type II diabetes. Nearly 21 million people have been diagnosed with diabetes and more than 6 million are diabetic and do not know it. Type II diabetes was referred to as adult-onset diabetes in the past because it was a disease that occurred later in life. In the past decade, children and adolescents have begun to develop the disease. This development

---

Carcinogens Substances that tend to produce a tumor or cancer.

Insulin A hormone that regulates blood sugar levels.

Type I Diabetes A chronic metabolic disease characterized by high blood sugar (glucose) levels associated with the inability of the pancreas to produce insulin; also called insulin-dependent diabetes mellitus (IDDM) or juvenile-onset diabetes.

Type II Diabetes A chronic metabolic disease characterized by high blood sugar, usually not requiring insulin therapy; also called noninsulin dependent diabetes mellitus (NIDDM) or adult-onset diabetes.

is closely tied to the epidemic of obesity among youth, thought to be caused primarily by excessive caloric intake and sedentary living.

According to the ADA, before people develop diabetes, they almost always have a condition referred to as pre-diabetes. This condition was formerly known as impaired glucose tolerance, but the name was changed to help focus attention on the seriousness of the problem of this condition. Recent research has shown that pre-diabetes can result in long-term damage to the body similar to that of diabetes. People who do screening and take steps to control pre-diabetes can delay or even prevent the development of Type II diabetes. A third and relatively rare form of diabetes is referred to as gestational diabetes mellitus. This occurs when high blood sugar levels occur in pregnant women previously not known to have diabetes. This condition is present in about 3 percent of all pregnancies, can have implications for the fetus, and may or may not result in a diabetic state after pregnancy. Other forms of diabetes are rare.

People have a familial predisposition to Type I and Type II, though the predisposition is greater for Type I diabetes. Some people with Type II diabetes do not produce enough insulin to regulate their blood sugar levels. More commonly, they are insensitive to insulin, so the body cannot effectively regulate blood sugar.

Diabetes and related conditions are a leading cause of death in our society. As noted in Web 10 Concept 1, diabetes is the sixth leading cause of death, and it is a leading killer in other Western nations, including Canada. People with diabetes have a shortened life span, as well as many short-term and long-term complications associated with the disease. People must recognize their illness because proper medication and changes in lifestyle can greatly reduce the complications of the disease and the death rate associated with it.

African Americans and Native Americans are especially at risk for diabetes. Not only is the death rate higher among these groups but so are the health problems associated with the disease. Unlike heart disease and cancer that have shown recent decreases in incidence, the incidence of diabetes has increased in the last decade with little progress being made in accomplishing national health goals for this disease.

Diabetes is associated with other health problems. People with diabetes have an increased risk for additional health problems. For example, diabetes is considered to be a risk factor for heart disease and high blood pressure. Diabetics have a higher rate of kidney failure (including the need for kidney transplants and kidney dialysis), a high incidence of blindness, and a high incidence of lower limb amputation. Women with diabetes also have a high rate of pregnancy complications. A national health goal is to increase the rate of diagnosis and to increase the number of diabetics who get regular blood lipid assessments, blood pressure checks, and eye examinations.

Lifestyle changes can help reduce the symptoms and complications associated with diabetes. National health goals for the year 2010 reflect lifestyle changes that can help reduce health problems associated with diabetes:

- Reduce overweight (fatness) in the general population. Reducing body fat is probably the most significant way to reduce the incidence of diabetes in our society.
- Increase daily physical activity. Regular exercise expends calories and is one way to help reduce overfatness. It also helps regulate blood sugar levels and helps body cells become more sensitive to insulin.
- Reduce dietary fat intake, increase intake of complex carbohydrates, and decrease total caloric intake. Particularly important is the value of a sound diet in reducing body fatness.

As noted in Concept 13, the incidence of overweight and obesity has not decreased but rather increased to an all time high of 66 percent overweight and 30 percent obese as of 2006. Health experts suggest that diabetes is a big problem that will get bigger in the future, especially if more children and adults do not alter their activity and eating patterns to reduce the incidence of overweight and obesity in western society.

Screening for pre-diabetes and diabetes is essential for diagnosis and treatment. Early Web 11 diagnosis as a result of attention to the symptoms can expedite treatment. Guidelines recommend screening for pre-diabetes and diabetes using either of two blood tests: a fasting plasma glucose (FPG) test, which measures levels of glucose in the blood after an overnight fast, or a 2-hour **oral glucose tolerance test (OGTT),** which includes the FPG test but also tests glucose levels 2 hours after a person drinks a standard glucose solution. Guidelines recommend regular screening beginning at age 45. Because African Americans, Hispanics, Asians, American Indians, and Pacific Islanders have especially high risk, some experts recommend testing at age 30 or earlier for these groups. Others with diabetes risk factors and those with a BMI over 25 should also consider testing at an earlier age.

Once diabetes is recognized, adherence to a treatment program is essential to prevent related conditions. Controlling weight, eating properly, and performing regular exercise can help prevent the symptoms of Type II diabetes, in particular. In addition to these strategies, adherence to a regular medication schedule and stress management are important. However, if symptoms such as nausea, fatigue, weakness, excessive thirst, and loss of weight occur, as they often do in Type I diabetics, or, if blurred vision, numbness of the limbs, and skin or gum infections occur, medical help should be sought. Type I diabetics typically test blood samples regularly and self-administer insulin as needed.

Other Health Threats

Injuries are a major cause of death and suffering. Not only are injuries the fifth leading cause of death among people of all ages, but they also claim more lives than chronic and infectious diseases among people aged 40 and younger. According to the U.S. Public Health Service, the major causes of injuries are motor vehicle crashes, falls, poisoning, drowning, and residential fires.

Injuries also account for much pain and suffering. Of all hospital stays, one in six results from a nonfatal injury. Injury rates are higher among males than females, and they are quite high among ethnic and racial minority groups. In the past decade, the number of deaths caused by unintentional injuries and by work-related injuries has decreased.

Changes in lifestyles can reduce injury rates. A major conclusion of the Public Health Service is that the prevention of injuries requires the combined efforts of many fields, including health, education, transportation, law, engineering, architecture, and safety science.

The second major conclusion of the Public Health Service is that alcohol is "intimately associated" with the causes and severity of injuries. Other lifestyle behaviors are also associated with reducing injury incidence, and some of the steps that can be taken to reduce these injuries are listed in Table 3.

Prompt emergency medical care is critical for saving lives. Paramedics and emergency medical teams work hard to provide emergency medical service (EMS) when needed. Emphasis is placed on reducing the average time required to reach the majority of residents in different areas. Where you live can have a lot to do with whether you get good medical treatment. A survey of medical directors in the nation's 50 largest cities conducted over an 18-month period shows that treatment effectiveness for those needing emergency medical care varies, depending on where you live. In many cities, the EMS responses were slow and less than effective. The study estimates that about 1,000 lives a year could be saved with more effective systems. Figure 5 provides information concerning which of the 50 cities had the most effective EMS, according to the survey (see page 446).

Improved occupational safety could help reduce injury rates. Many of the nation's health goals focus on improving occupational safety, especially among construction, health-care (e.g., nurses), farm, transportation, and mine workers.

Many mental disorders pose threats to health and wellness. The health goals for the nation identify suicide, schizophrenia, and depression as the most serious mental disorders needing attention. Although the Public Health Service uses the term *mental disorders,*

Table 3 ► Steps to Reduce Injuries
Reduce Motor Vehicle Accidents
• Do not drive while under the influence of alcohol.
• Use shoulder seat belts and air bags.
• Reduce driving speed.
• Use motorcycle helmets.
• Increase safety programs for pedestrians and cyclists.
• Establish more effective licensing for very young and older drivers.
Improve Home and Neighborhood Environments
• Require safety controls on handguns.
• Require sprinkler systems in homes with high risk of fire.
• Increase presence of functional smoke detectors in homes.
• Increase injury and poison education in schools.
• Wear effective safety gear in sports.
• Improve pool and boat safety education.
• Learn cardiopulmonary resuscitation.
• Properly mark poisons and prescription drugs.
• Require childproof packaging for poisons and prescription drugs.

they are sometimes called emotional disorders. Other common mental disorders are panic disorders, alcohol and other drug problems, personality disorders, and phobias.

Mental disorders result in loss of life, injury, and inability to function, and they cost the public millions of dollars annually. Nearly 1 in 4 adults suffers from a diagnosed mental disorder that limits the ability to function effectively and requires special assistance. Depression and other mood disorders affect nearly 1 in 10 people, and anxiety disorders affect about 1 in 5. These disorders cost $150 billion annually, primarily from loss of productivity. The most serious outcome of mental disorders is suicide (30,000 annually).

Pre-diabetes A condition in which fasting blood glucose levels are higher than normal but not high enough to be clinically diagnosed as diabetes.

Oral Glucose Tolerance Test (OGTT) A test used to diagnose diabetes. It consists of a blood sugar measurement following the ingestion of a standard amount of sugar (glucose) after a period of fasting.

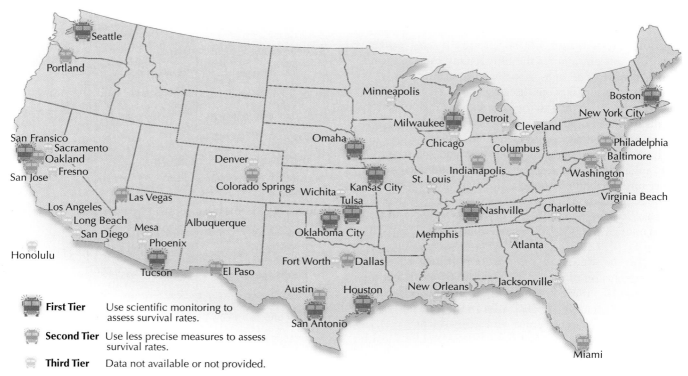

First Tier   Use scientific monitoring to assess survival rates.

Second Tier   Use less precise measures to assess survival rates.

Third Tier   Data not available or not provided.

Figure 5 ▶ Emergency medical treatment effectiveness in major cities.
Source: USA Today EMS survey.

Reducing the incidence of suicide and serious injury from suicide attempts is an important national health goal. Progress has been made in reducing suicide but it is still far too common. Women are about three times more likely to attempt suicide than men, but men are four times more likely to complete a suicide attempt. Among male teenagers, it is the second leading cause of death, and male teenagers with antisocial personality disorders are especially susceptible.

Depression is closely associated with suicide, as are alcohol and other drug abuse. Inability to cope with stressful life events may contribute to suicide. Examples of precipitating events are divorce, separation, loss of a loved one, unemployment, and financial setbacks.

The best chance for reducing suicides appears to be early detection and treatment of mental disorders such as depression. Professional help should be sought, and as many concerned people as possible should be recruited to help the suicidal individual seek professional assistance. Experts suggest that threats of suicide must be taken seriously.

Depression, a common mental disorder, can usually be treated effectively. Most people occasionally feel depressed or sad. This type of depression is usually not a mental disorder. People with clinical depression (classified as a mental disorder) have chronic feelings of guilt, hopelessness, low self-esteem,

Web 12

and dejection. They might have trouble sleeping, loss of appetite, lack of interest in social activities, lack of interest in sex, and inability to concentrate.

Among the lifestyle changes that can help relieve symptoms are exercising regularly, increasing social contact, setting realistic goals, using stress-management techniques (see Concept 17), and removing oneself from situations that contribute to depression. These changes, however, may need to be accompanied by professional therapy and/or medication.

Sleep disorders can often be helped by lifestyle changes. Sleep disorders, especially insomnia (long-term problems with sleep), can result in depression and other dysfunctions. Physiological problems in the brain can cause sleep disorders, but they are often a result of depression, stress, chronic pain, or abuse of alcohol or other drugs. Some sleep disorders require professional help; however, you can take action to prevent insomnia. Creating a healthy sleeping environment, avoiding excessive caffeine or alcohol, exercising regularly and establishing a regular routine for sleeping can help avoid sleep disorders.

Various health threats put the public's health at risk. The health threats outlined in *Healthy People 2010* are too numerous to be dealt with in depth in this text. More information concerning such health threats as chronic kidney disease, hepatitis, asthma, and arthritis can be found at the *Healthy People 2010* Web site and in the *Web Resources* section.

Adhering to sound medical advice is important for disease prevention and treatment. Many of the conditions described in this concept, especially cancer and diabetes, can be managed or cured with early diagnosis and proper treatment. Many people ignore early warning signs or symptoms, hoping that problems go away on their own. Some people fear disease and avoid medical advice because of this fear. An important key to good health is to note any irregularities in your health and to seek expert advice when needed. Establishing a regular habit of getting scheduled checkups and/or health screens is a part of a healthy lifestyle because it helps ensure that your health is where it should be. Periodic checks can also help detect early signs of heart disease, cancer, diabetes, and other health threats and this allows for more effective treatment. These checks become increasingly important with advancing age because people become vulnerable to a wider array of chronic conditions.

The Cooper Clinic in Dallas, Texas, specializes in preventive medical care. A staff physician (Dr. Tedd Mitchell) has categorized the types of reasons people give for

Table 4 ▶ Types of People Who Avoid Medical Checkups
• *Gamblers*. These people do not think about their health until a serious problem occurs.
• *Martyrs*. These people are so busy taking care of others that they fail to take care of themselves.
• *Economists*. These people think the cost of preventive exams is too high for the benefits received.
• *Shamans*. These people buy in on the latest health fad and self-diagnose, while avoiding regular medical care.
• *Informers*. These people have an ax to grind with health-care professionals and avoid health care for this reason.
• *Queens of denial (Cleopatra syndrome)*. These people do not believe something could be wrong with them or do not want to know if there is.
• *Busy bees*. These people feel they are too busy to take the time to get regular medical care.

not seeing a doctor or getting a regular medical checkup. See Table 4. According to Dr. Mitchell, "there is no good reason to avoid your annual visit to the doctor."

Strategies for Action

Self-assessments and regular medical exams can help you determine if you need help with various health problems. Just as the fitness assessments you completed earlier in this book helped you build a profile that will help you improve your fitness, regular self-assessments can help you identify and prevent common health problems. Regular medical exams that include the tests outlined in Table 1 as well as those described in other sections of this concept will help you identify problems that can be treated and cured with early diagnosis. In Lab 22A, you will have the opportunity to assess your cancer risk. In Lab 22B, you will learn to do self-exams to help

you resist breast and testicular cancer. Web addresses for self-assessments are provided in Lab 22B.

Staying current with new health information can help you identify and get treatment for health problems. Information about various health problems changes rapidly as new methods of treatment and prevention become available. It is important to learn ways to stay current on health topics. Addresses for the Web sites of reputable health organizations that will help you stay abreast of current information are included in *Web Resources*.

Online Learning Center

www.mhhe.com/corbin7e
The Online Learning Center contains a variety of Web-based resources that will help you get the most out of this book and your course. In addition to the On the Web pages, there are video activities, interactive quizzes, application assignments, and a variety of other useful study aids. Log on to the URL above to access these resources.

Web Resources

American Cancer Society **www.cancer.org**
American Diabetes Association **www.diabetes.org**
Web 13 Environmental Protection Agency **www.epa.gov**
Healthy People 2010 **www.health.gov/healthypeople**
National Cancer Institute **www.nci.nih.gov**
National Center for Environmental Health
   www.cdc.gov/nceh
National Center for Health Statistics **www.cdc.gov/nchs**
National Institute of Mental Health (NIMH)
   www.nimh.nih.gov

Suggested Readings

Additional reference materials for Concept 22 are available at Web14.

American Diabetes Association. 2006. *Diabetes by the Numbers for 2006.* Available at **www.diabetes.org**.

D'Amico, A. U., et al. 2004. Preoperative PSA velocity and the risk of death from prostate cancer after radical prostatectomy. *New England Journal of Medicine* 351(2):125–135.

Edwards, B. K., et al. 2005. Annual report to the nation on the status of cancer. *Journal of the National Cancer Institute* 97(19):1407–1427.

Hallstrom, A., and I. P. Ornato. 2004. Public-access defibrillators and survival after out-of-hospital cardiac arrest. *New England Journal of Medicine* 351(7):637–646.

Hamann, B. P. 2007. *Disease: Identification, Prevention and Control.* 3rd ed. New York: McGraw-Hill Higher Education.

Hewitt, M., et al. 2006. *From Cancer Patient to Cancer Survivor: Lost in Transition.* Washington, DC: National Academies Press.

Hoyert, D. L., H. Kung, and B. L. Smith. 2005. Deaths: Preliminary data for 2003. *National Vital Statistics Reports* 53(15):1–32.

National Cancer Institute. 2005. Cancer Trends Progress Report—2005 Update. Washington, DC: National Cancer Institute. Available at **http://progressreport.cancer.gov/highlights.asp**

Pisano, E., et al. 2006. Utilization of screening mammography in New Hampshire. *Cancer* 104(8):1726–1732.

Rubin, R. 2005. Vaccine prevents cervical cancer. *USA Today.* October 7.

U.S. Preventive Services Task Force. 2006. Genetic risk assessment and BRCA mutation testing for breast and ovarian cancer susceptibility: Recommendation statement. *Annals of Internal Medicine* 143(5):355–361.

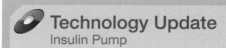

Technology Update
Insulin Pump

The insulin pump is a recent technological advancement that allows diabetics to get daily doses of insulin without injections. The device is a battery-operated pump combined with a computer chip and an insulin reservoir inside a small plastic case about the size of a pedometer. A plastic tube runs from the reservoir to a "cannula," which is inserted under the skin, typically in the abdominal region. The computer chip is programmed to cause the pump to send regular doses of insulin as needed. It is not totally automatic, however; users have to regulate the dose based on factors such as eating and exercise habits. The reservoir can hold enough doses to last several weeks. The insulin pump reduces the need for insulin injections and has been shown to be useful in children.

In the News

Decline in Cancer Deaths

A report from the National Cancer Institute (2005) indicates that the death rate from cancer in the United States continues to decline. Cancer death rates have been declining since 1990, and results from the most recent report suggest that rates will continue to decline in the years ahead. The single biggest factor in the drop in cancer deaths is the decline in Americans who use tobacco products. Early detection and better treatments were also cited in the report as key contributing factors to the decline. The effects were most notable for breast cancer, which has continued to exhibit declines in deaths for the past 10 years.

A troubling aspect of the report is that the racial divide in cancer risks and prognosis continues. Black women have a 30 percent higher death rate from breast cancer than white women, and black men are twice as likely to die from prostate cancer than white men. Overall cancer death rates are 18 percent higher among black women than white women and 40 percent higher among black men than white men. Poverty was shown to be a critical component in cancer survival because it influences both the risk of developing the disease and the quality of treatment. To close the gap in death rates across minority groups, it is necessary to close the gaps in access to cancer prevention, screening, and treatment.

Lab 22A Determining Your Cancer Risk

Name	**Section** **Date**

Purpose: To become aware of your risk for various types of cancer

Procedures

1. Answer the questions in the six-part questionnaire for the various forms of cancer.
2. Record the number of "yes" answers for each form of cancer in the Results section.
3. Use Chart 1 to determine ratings and record the ratings in the Results section.
4. Answer the questions in the Conclusions and Implications section.

Results: Mark an X over your answer to each question.

Skin Cancer Risk Factors

Do you frequently work or play in the sun for long periods of times?	Yes	No
Do you work or have you worked near industrial exposure (coal mine, radioactivity)?	Yes	No
Do you have a family history of skin cancer?	Yes	No
Do you have fair skin?	Yes	No

Lung Cancer Risk Factors

Do you smoke?	Yes	No
Do you work or have you worked near industrial exposure (coal mine, radioactivity)?	Yes	No
Do you have a family history of cancer?	Yes	No
Do you work in a place that allows smoking, such as a bar, or live in a home with smokers?	Yes	No

Colon-rectal Cancer Risk Factors

Do you eat poorly, abuse alcohol, or smoke?	Yes	No
Are you African American or over 50?	Yes	No
Do you have a family history of colon or rectal cancer?	Yes	No
Have you noticed blood in your stool?	Yes	No

Breast Cancer Risk Factors

Do you have a family history of breast cancer?	Yes	No
Are you sedentary, do you eat poorly, or do you abuse alcohol?	Yes	No
Are you a female over 35 who has not had children?	Yes	No
Have you ever detected lumps or cysts in your breasts?	Yes	No

Uterine/Cervical Cancer Risk Factors* (Females)

Do you regularly have bleeding between periods?	Yes	No
Is your body fat level high?	Yes	No
Did you have early intercourse and multiple sexual partners?	Yes	No
Have you had viral infections of the vagina such as HPV?	Yes	No

Prostate Cancer Risk Factors (Males)

Do you eat a high-fat or low-fiber diet?	Yes	No
Are you a male over 50 years of age or African American?	Yes	No
Have you had a regular PSA test?	Yes	No
Has a digital rectal exam shown an enlargement of the prostate?	Yes	No

*Because of the personal nature of several questions, do not record results if turned in to an instructor.

Cancer Type	Score	Rating
Breast		
Uterine/cervical (women)*		
Colon-rectal		
Skin		
Lung		
Prostate (men)		

*Do not record results if handed in to an instructor.

Chart 1 ▶ Cancer Risk Ratings

Rating	Score
High risk	4
Relatively high risk	3
Lower risk	2
Low risk	0–1

Conclusions and Implications: In several sentences, discuss the type or types of cancer for which you are at greatest risk and why. Also, discuss the lifestyles you could modify to reduce your risk.

Lab 22B Breast and Testicular Self-Exams

Name	**Section**	**Date**

Purpose: To learn to do breast or testicular self-exams

Procedures

1. If you are female, read the procedures for breast self-exams. Note: Males should also be aware of abnormal lumps in their breasts.
2. If you are male, read the procedures for testicular self-exams.
3. After reading the directions, perform the self-exam.
4. If you find lumps or nodules, contact a physician.
5. This procedure should be done monthly. The breast exam is best done a day or two after the end of menstrual flow. For this lab, it can be done at any time.
6. It is not necessary to record your results here. Do answer the questions in the Conclusions and Implications section.

Testicular Self-Exam (Men)

1. Using both hands, grasp one testicle between the thumb and first finger.
2. Roll the testicle gently with the thumb and first finger, feeling for lumps or nodules.
3. Examine the other testicle using the same procedure.
4. If you find a lump or nodule, consult a physician. Note: a lump or nodule may not be a result of disease but this can only be determined by a physician.
5. For more details concerning a testicular self-exam, see Web15.

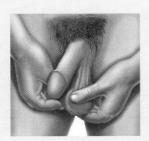

Breast Self-Exam (Women and Men)

1. Lie down on your back. Place a pillow or towel under one shoulder and place your arm overhead.
2. With the opposite hand, gently move the fingers over the breast. Use a circular motion (see picture) to probe for lumps, starting in a large circle and continuing to probe in smaller and smaller circles. Examine every part of your breast, including your nipple. A band of firm tissue along the lower part of the breast is normal. If you have questions, consult your physician.
3. Finally, squeeze each nipple gently between the thumb and first finger. If you notice blood or clear discharge, contact a physician.

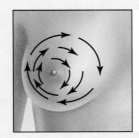 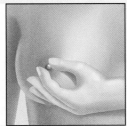

4. Repeat on the other breast. If you notice any lumps, report it to a physician.
5. Periodic exams before a mirror can be helpful. With the arms above the head, look for any changes in the breast (from your normal). Repeat with the hands on the hips—flex the chest muscles. Again look for any changes from normal.
6. For more details concerning a breast self-exam, see Web16.

Conclusions and Implications: In several sentences, discuss the effectiveness of the procedure you performed. Do you think that the directions provided were adequate for you to perform the self-exam effectively? Do you think you will perform this self-exam on a regular basis? Do you believe that the screening procedures described in the lab are effective? Why or why not? What could be done to motivate you and others to do regular self-exams?

Additional Self-Exam Information

Several national health agencies maintain Web sites that include detailed breast and testicular self-exam information. These sites contain both written and pictorial descriptions of both self-exam procedures. For more information, visit the sites listed below.

American Cancer Society
   www.cancer.org

Mayo Clinic
   www.mayohealth.org

National Cancer Institute
   www.nci.nih.gov

Evaluating Fitness and Wellness Products: Becoming an Informed Consumer

Health Goals for the year 2010

- Increase number of college and university students who receive information on priority health-risk behaviors.

- Improve health literacy and increase access to public health information.

- Increase health communication activities that include research and evaluation.

- Increase adoption and maintenance of appropriate daily physical activity.

- Increase proportion of people who meet national dietary guidelines.

- Promote healthy and safe communities.

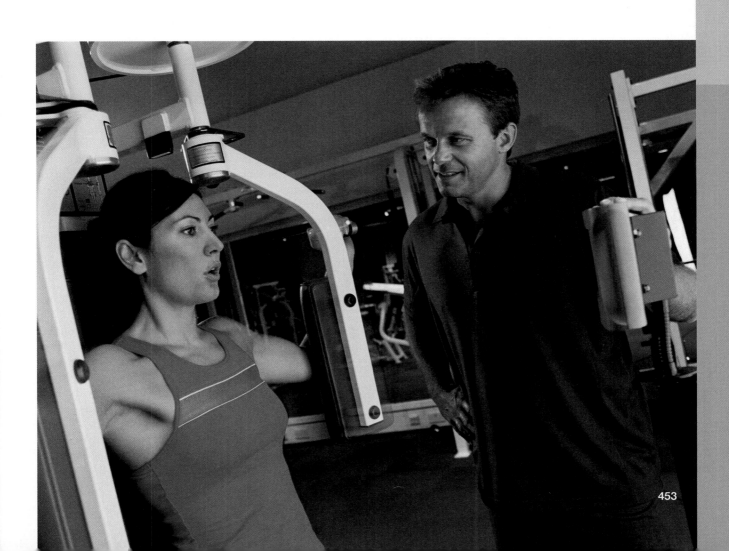

"Let the buyer beware" is a good motto for the consumer seeking advice or planning a program for developing or maintaining fitness, health, or wellness.

People have always searched for the fountain of youth and an easy, quick, and miraculous route to health and happiness. In current society, this search often focuses on fitness, nutrition, weight loss, or appearance. A variety of products are available that promise weight loss, improved health, or improved fitness with little or no effort. The sale of these products can typically be classified as either quackery or fraud, since most do not work.

The dictionary definition of *quack* is "a pretender of medical skill" or "one who talks pretentiously without sound knowledge of the subject discussed." These definitions imply that the promotion of quackery involves deliberate deception, but quacks often believe in what they promote. A consumer watchdog group called Quackwatch defines quackery more broadly as "anything involving overpromotion in the field of health." This definition encompasses questionable ideas as well as questionable products and services. The word *fraud* is reserved for situations in which deliberate deception is involved. This concept discusses common myths and provides important guidelines to help you be a more informed consumer of fitness, health, and wellness products.

Quacks and Quackery

Quacks can be identified by their unscientific practices. Some of the ways to identify quacks, frauds, and rip-off artists are to look for these clues:

Web 01

- They do not use the scientific method of controlled experimentation, which can be verified by other scientists.
- To a large extent, they use testimonials and anecdotes to support their claims rather than scientific methods.

> **⊕ On the Web**
> www.mhhe.com/corbinweb
> Web 01 Log on to this URL before reading this concept. See On the Web list of concepts. Click on the concept number you want to view. To access supplemental information, click on the number shown at each Web icon.

There is no such thing as a valid testimonial. Anecdotal evidence is no evidence at all.

- They have something to sell and they advise you to buy something you would not otherwise have bought.
- They claim everyone can benefit from the product or service they are selling. There is no such thing as a simple, quick, easy, painless remedy/tonic or other concoction that is effective for ailments or conditions for which medical science has not yet found a remedy.
- They promise quick, miraculous results. A perfect, no-risk treatment does not exist.
- Their claims for benefits cover a wide variety of conditions.
- They may offer a money-back guarantee. A guarantee is only as good as the company.
- They may claim the treatment or product is approved by the FDA. Note: federal law does not permit the mention of the FDA in any way that suggests marketing approval.
- They may claim the support of experts, but the experts are not identified.
- The ingredients or materials in the product may not be identified.
- They may claim there is a conspiracy against them by "bureaucrats," "organized medicine," the FDA, the American Medical Association (AMA), and other experts and governmental bodies. Never believe a doctor who claims the medical community is persecuting him or her or that the government is suppressing a wonderful discovery.
- Their credentials may be irrelevant to the area in which they claim expertise.
- They use scare tactics, such as "If you don't do this, you will die of a heart attack."
- They may appear to be a sympathetic friend who wants to share a new discovery with you.
- They may quote from a scientific journal or another legitimate source, but they misquote or quote out of context to mislead you; they may also mix a little bit of truth with a lot of fiction.
- They may cite research or quote from individuals or institutions that have questionable reputations for scientific truth.
- They may claim it is a new discovery (usually it is said to have originated in Europe). There is never a great medical breakthrough that debuts in an obscure mag-

azine or tabloid. No secret cures or magic formulas have been recognized by the scientific community, a picture on the cover of *Time* magazine, nomination for a Nobel Prize, and so on.

- The product or organization named is often similar to that of a famous person or creditable institution (e.g., the Mayo diet had no connection with the Mayo Clinic).
- They often sell products through the mail, which does not allow you to examine the product personally.

Experts have a good education, have a good scientific base, and meet other professional criteria. Unlike quacks, experts base their work on the scientific method. Some characteristics of professional experts are an extended education, an established code of ethics, membership in well-known associations, involvement in the profession as an intern before obtaining credentials, and a commitment to perform an important social service. Some experts require a license. Examples of experts in the fitness, health, and wellness area are medical doctors, nurses, certified fitness leaders, physical educators, registered dietitians, physical therapists, and clinical psychologists. In most cases, you can check if a person has the credentials to be considered an expert before obtaining his or her services. Some things that can be done to determine a person's expertise include

- Determining where the person obtained his or her education and the nature of the degree and/or certification
- Checking with the person's professional association or with a government board, licensing agency, or certifying agency to see if there are any complaints against the person; for example, you can check with the medical board in your state to check complaints against physicians
- Checking if the person has the credentials to provide the service you are seeking; for example, a registered dietician is qualified to give nutrition advice but not medical advice

You can reduce your susceptibility to quackery by being an informed consumer. The three key characteristics that predispose people to health-related quackery are a concern about appearance, health, or performance; a lack of knowledge; and a desire for immediate results. Understanding the principles of exercise and nutrition presented in this book will help you know when something sounds "too good to be true."

When evaluating health-related products or information, carefully consider the quality of your source. Common sources of misinformation are magazines, health food stores, and TV infomercials. These entities all have an economic incentive in promoting the purchase and use of exercise, diet, and weight loss products. Because of freedom of speech laws, it is legal to state opinion

through these media. Note, however, that few companies make claims on product labels, since this is false advertising. Follow these additional guidelines to avoid being a victim of quackery:

- Read the ad carefully, especially the small print.
- Do not send cash; use a check, money order, or credit card so you will have a receipt.
- Do not order from a company with only a post office box, unless you know the company.
- Do not let high-pressure sales tactics make you rush into a decision.
- When in doubt, check out the company through your Better Business Bureau (BBB).

Scientific research is a systematic search for truth. Occasionally, companies will mention that their product or program has been scientifically tested, but this does not necessarily mean that the results were positive. Even if a study did show positive results, the study may have been flawed. An article in a prominent scientific journal documented that results of studies, especially small studies that are not well controlled, are often found to be wrong or the effects are not as large as originally thought. The media often highlight the results of novel or unusual findings, and this leads some people to conclude that experts simply "can't make up their minds." In actuality, scientists typically take a cautious approach with any new finding and wait for other studies to confirm the results. It is usually the press that overstates the value of one study, not the experts. It takes a body of evidence to determine the effectiveness of a medicine, a supplement, or a health product of any kind. One study is better than none at all, but several supporting studies are necessary to support the use of a product.

Beware also of news reports that denounce established evidence based on a single study or "preliminary research." With accumulating evidence, even the most established beliefs may change. But it takes many confirming studies to provide the best evidence. Consider this before making quick consumer judgments.

Physical Activity and Exercise Equipment

There is no easy way to get the benefits from physical activity. Contrary to the hype from some fitness commercials and products, the benefits associated with regular activity require real effort maintained over time. Advertisements for some fitness devices claim that 10 minutes on their product is as good as 30 minutes on another product—this is simply not true. The benefits of any activity depend on the relative intensity and duration, not on the equipment. Some products promise to enhance metabolism in the same way as exercise, and

Web 02

these are just stimulants that have little or no effect on energy expenditure and certainly no effect on fitness.

Claims for many forms of exercise are overstated or unsubstantiated. New exercise programs or routines are often promoted as the complete answer for total fitness or a **panacea** for health. Claims for Hatha Yoga suggest it will help you lose weight, trim inches, strengthen glands and organs, or cure health problems, such as the common cold or arthritis. Hatha Yoga can be useful in reducing stress, promoting relaxation, and improving flexibility, but the other claims are overstated.

Similar hype may be used for promoting new pieces of exercise equipment. Each piece of equipment claims to be fun, easy to use, and more effective than other forms of exercise. The benefits from exercise are dependent on the relative intensity and duration of the activity—and whether it is done regularly over time. The best form of exercise is clearly the one that you are willing and able to do.

Contrary to claims, passive exercises do not provide any benefits for fitness or weight loss. For exercise to be beneficial, the work must be done by contracting skeletal muscles. A variety of **passive exercise** forms have been promoted to try to reduce the effort required to perform regular exercise. Some passive devices have value for people with special needs, when used by a qualified person, such as a physical therapist. However, passive devices sold for use by the general public are ineffective. The goal of sellers is to convince people that there is an effortless way to exercise—there is not. The fallacies associated with many past forms of passive exercise, such as fat rolling machines (purported to break up and redistribute fat), seem obvious today but new approaches come out all the time with different marketing and promotions. The list that follows highlights some of the common forms of passive exercise.

- *Vibrating belts.* These wide canvas or leather belts are driven by an electric motor, causing loose tissue of the body part to shake. They have no beneficial effect on fitness, fat, or figure. They are potentially harmful to the back and if used on the abdomen (especially if used by women during pregnancy, during menstruation, or while an IUD is in place).
- *Vibrating tables and pillows.* Contrary to advertisements, these passive devices (also called toning tables) will not improve posture, trim the body, reduce weight, or develop muscle **tonus.**
- *Continuous passive motion (CPM) tables.* The motor-driven CPM table, unlike the vibrating table, moves body parts repeatedly through a range of motion. Tables are designed to do such things as passively extend the leg at the hip joint and raise the upper trunk in a sit-up like motion. Advocates claim that the tables remove cellulite, increase circulation and oxygen

flow, and eliminate excess water retention. All of these claims are false. Hospitals and rehabilitation centers use a similar machine to maintain range of motion in the legs of knee surgery patients, maintain integrity of the cartilage, and decrease the incidence of blood clots. Certainly, a healthy person has nothing to gain from using such a device.
- *Motor-driven cycles and rowing machines.* Like all mechanical devices that do the work for the individual, these motor-driven machines are not effective in a fitness program. They may help increase circulation, and some may even help maintain flexibility, but they are not as effective as active exercise. *Nonmotorized cycles and rowing machines* are good equipment for use in a fitness program.
- *Massage.* Whether done by a certified or licensed massage therapist or by a mechanical device, massage is passive, requiring no effort on the part of the individual. It can help increase circulation, induce relaxation, prevent or loosen adhesions, retard muscle atrophy, and serve other therapeutic uses when administered in the clinical setting for medical reasons. However, massage has no useful role in a physical fitness program and will not alter your shape. There is no scientific evidence that it can hasten nerve growth, remove subcutaneous fat, or increase athletic performance. Some athletes (e.g., cyclists) find that it aids in recovery from exercise.
- *Magnets.* The law requires magnets marketed with medical claims to obtain clearance from the Food and Drug Administration (FDA). To date, the FDA has not approved the marketing of any magnets for medical use, and sellers making medical claims for magnets are in violation of the law.
- *Electrical muscle stimulators.* Neuromuscular electrical stimulators cause the muscle to contract involuntarily. In the hands of qualified medical personnel, muscle stimulators are valuable therapeutic devices. They can

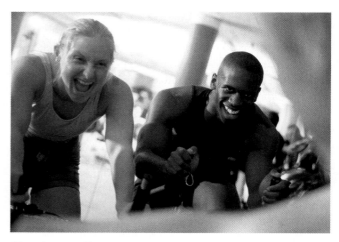

Changing your lifestyle, rather than quick solutions, is the key to health, fitness, and wellness.

increase muscle strength and endurance selectively and aid in the treatment of edema. They can also help prevent atrophy in a patient who is unable to move, and they may decrease muscle spasms, but in a healthy person they do not have the same value as exercise. The Federal Trade Commission (FTC) has filed false advertising claims against several firms that market exercise stimulators that promise to build *"six-pack abs"* and tone muscles without exercise. These devices, worn over the abdomen, are heavily advertised in infomercials and have been shown to be ineffective and potentially hazardous to health. Electrical stimulators placed on the chest, back, or abdomen can interfere with the normal rhythm of the heart, even for normally healthy people. For those with heart, gastrointestinal, orthopedic, kidney, and other health problems, such as epilepsy, hernia, and varicose veins, they can be especially dangerous. Beware of spas and clinics that use these devices and make claims of fitness enhancement for healthy people.

- *Weighted belts.* Claims have been made that these belts reduce waists, thighs, and hips when worn for several hours under the clothing. In reality, they do none of these things and have been reported to cause physical harm. However, when used in a progressive resistance program, wristlet, anklet, or laced-on weights can help produce an overload and, therefore, develop strength or endurance.

- *Inflated, constricting, or nonporous garments.* These garments include rubberized inflated devices (sauna belts and sauna shorts) and paraphernalia that are airtight plastic or rubberized. Evidence indicates that their girth-reducing claims are *unwarranted*. If exercise is performed while wearing such garments, the exercise, not the garment, may be beneficial. You cannot squeeze fat out of the pores, nor can you melt it.

- *Body wrapping.* Some reducing salons, gyms, and clubs advertise that wrapping the body in bandages soaked in a magic solution will cause a permanent reduction in body girth. This so-called treatment is pure quackery. Tight, constricting bands can temporarily indent the skin and squeeze body fluids into other parts of the body, but the skin or body will regain its original size within minutes or hours. The solution is usually similar to epsom salts, which can cause fluid to be drawn from tissue. The fluid is water, not fat, and is quickly replaced. Body wrapping may be dangerous to your health; at least one fatality has been documented.

Home exercise equipment can be helpful, but care should be used when selecting and purchasing equipment. Many types of home exercise equipment are available on the market. Because they are often expensive, care should be used when making a decision. To determine if a piece of equipment is worthwhile, ask yourself the following four questions. Do you need it? Will you use it? Does it work? Does it work for you? For it to be a worthwhile purchase, the answer to all four questions should be yes. Many people wonder about the relative advantages and disadvantages of different pieces of equipment. The answer to the question "What is the best piece of exercise equipment?" is "the equipment you will use."

It is best to buy your equipment from reputable dealers or companies. When considering several models of the same type of device, remember that you get what you pay for. Higher-end models may last longer and may promote more use, since they may be quieter or feel better to use than lower-priced models. Consult an expert if you want to know more about the quality and effectiveness of various products. Individuals with a college degree in physical education, physical therapy, or kinesiology should be able to give you good advice.

The use of hand weights and wrist weights while walking, running, dancing, or bench-stepping can increase the energy expended but requires caution. Various devices have been marketed for increasing the energy expenditure in activities such as walking, running, and other forms of aerobic exercise. Examples include wrist, arm, or ankle weights and small, hand-held weights. Step benches are another device that can be used to increase energy expenditure for aerobic exercise.

The practice of carrying weights is controversial. Carrying weights (not more than 1 to 3 pounds) while doing aerobic dance, walking, and other aerobic activities has been shown to increase energy expenditure, but the effect is negligible unless the arms are pumped (bending the elbow and raising the weight to shoulder height and then extending the elbow as the arm swings down). When the arms are pumped, the energy output is comparable to a slow jog. Some experts caution that pumping the arms using weight can increase the risk for injury and suggest that the benefit of added energy expenditure is not worth the added risk for injury. Also, gripping weights while exercising can cause an increase in blood pressure.

Those who choose to use weights while doing aerobic activity are at less risk for injury if they use wrist weights rather than hand-held weights. Arm movements should be limited to a range of motion below the shoulder level.

Panacea A cure-all; a remedy for all ills.

Passive Exercise Exercise in which no voluntary muscle contraction occurs; an outside force moves the body part with no effort by the person.

Tonus The most frequently misused and abused term in fitness vocabularies. Tonus is the tension developed in a muscle as a result of passive muscle stretch. Tonus cannot be determined by feeling or inspecting a muscle. It has little or nothing to do with the strength of a muscle.

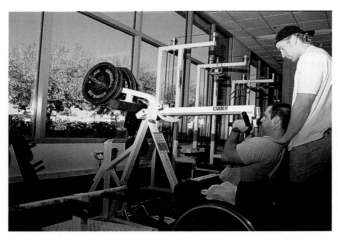

Visit a health club before you join.

Coronary patients and people with shoulder or elbow joint problems, such as arthritis, are advised not to use hand or wrist weights. Ankle weights are not recommended because they may alter your gait pattern in a way that is stressful to the knees.

Health and Fitness Clubs

Health and fitness clubs provide access to equipment and support, but it is important to consider a number of factors before deciding to join. The first question to ask yourself is whether access to the facility is essential for you to begin or maintain your exercise program. The second question is whether the facility is convenient enough for you to access regularly. The distance of the gym from home or work will greatly influence your potential use of the facility. If you are serious about joining a club, consider the following points:

- Determine the qualifications of the personnel, especially of the individual responsible for your program. Is he or she an expert, as defined previously?
- Observe staff conduct to determine if they are available and efficient in day-to-day operations.
- Check to see if your membership can be sold or transferred to another person if you move. Check to see if you can cancel the contract if you prove you are moving outside the community.
- Choose a no-contract or monthly payment option if it is available so you can change your mind. Be prepared to resist options for long-term contracts.
- Check for hidden costs associated with membership (e.g., costs for testing, use of personal training).
- Do not be swayed by promises of quick results.
- Check the equipment to be sure that it is up to date and well maintained.
- Check for cleanliness. How often do you see the staff cleaning?

- Check to see if quack products are sold and pushed to clients. If so, it does not speak well of the professionalism of the staff.
- Check to see if unproven products, such as supplements, are sold or pushed to gain income.
- Check to see that towels are provided to wipe machines after use and that weights are replaced after use. If not, it is a good indication that supervision is not adequate.
- Check to see if rules are posted. For example, is there a time limit for using machines and is there a dress code?
- Speak with other members to get an insider's perspective on how they have been treated.
- Make a trial visit to the establishment during the hours when you would normally expect to use the facility to determine if it is open, if it is overcrowded, and if you would enjoy the company of the other patrons.
- Make certain the club is a well-established facility that will not disappear overnight.
- Check its reputation with the Better Business Bureau. Be aware, however, that the BBB can only tell you if complaints have been made against a company. It does not endorse companies and may lack information on new companies.
- Investigate programs offered by the YMCA/YWCA, local colleges and universities, and municipal park and recreation departments. These agencies often have excellent fitness classes at lower prices than commercial establishments and usually employ qualified personnel.

Body Composition

Getting rid of cellulite does not require a special exercise, diet, cream, or device, as some books and advertisements insist. Cellulite is ordinary fat with a fancy name. You do not need a special treatment or device to get rid of it. In fact, it has no special remedy. To decrease fat, reduce calories and do more physical activity.

Spot-reducing, or losing fat from a specific location on the body, is not possible. When you do physical activity, calories are burned and fat is recruited from all over the body in a genetically determined pattern. You cannot selectively exercise, bump, vibrate, or squeeze the fat from a particular spot. If you are flabby to begin with, local exercise can strengthen the local muscles, causing a change in the contour and the girth of that body part, but exercise affects the muscles, not the fat on that body part. General aerobic exercises are the most effective for burning fat, but you cannot control where the fat comes off.

Surgically sculpting the body with implants and liposuction to acquire physical beauty will not give you physical fitness and may be harmful. Rather than doing it the hard way, an increasing number of people are having their *"love handles"* removed surgically and fake calf and pectoral muscles implanted to improve their physique. Liposuction is not a weight loss technique but, rather, a contouring procedure. Like any surgery, it has risks. There are risks for infection, hematoma, skin slough, and other conditions, and there have been fatalities.

Muscle implants give a muscular appearance, but they do not make you stronger or more fit. The implants are not really muscle tissue but, rather, silicon gel or saline, such as that used in breast implants or a hard substitute. Some complications can occur, such as infection and bleeding, and some physicians believe that calf implants may put pressure on the calf muscles and cause them to atrophy. A better way to improve physique and fitness is to engage in proper exercise.

Nutrition

Diets are a major source of quackery. Basic guidelines for sound eating were described in Concepts 14 and 15. Beware of diets that do not follow these guidelines. Diets that emphasize one nutrient at the expense of others (unbalanced diets), diets that require the purchase of special products, especially products that make claims inconsistent with established guidelines, and diets that are proposed by people lacking sound credentials should be avoided.

It is not true that, if a little of something is "good," more is "better." The marketing of nutrition products often relies on convincing people that additional vitamins, minerals, or enzymes are beneficial. It is true that deficiencies of certain compounds may be harmful, but extra amounts don't always provide added protection or improved health. The myth that vitamin C can cure the common cold is based on the fact that deficiencies of vitamin C can lead to scurvy. The same hype is used to sell consumers many other unnecessary supplements. For example, protein supplements are marketed with convincing (and honest) claims that the body needs amino acids to form muscle. The hidden truth is that the body cannot store or use more than it needs.

Beware of energy drinks with "boosts" sold at health bars in fitness clubs. Health bars often sell food and drinks of various types. Some drinks contain "boosts" consisting of a tablespoon or two of a food supplement. Health clubs that sell drinks with supplements are susceptible to the claim that they are selling products for financial gain rather than the best interests of clients. Even if supplements are effective, which most are not, taking one dose in a drink would be ineffective and a waste of money.

Current legislation does not protect food supplement customers. There are many types of supplements, including vitamins, minerals, herbals (also called botanicals), amino acids, and products made from other sources (e.g., shellfish parts, shark cartilage, and cattle and horse parts). The passage of the Dietary Supplements Health and Education Act in 1994 shifted the burden of providing assurances of product effectiveness from the FDA to the food supplement industry, which really means it shifted to you—the consumer. Food supplements are typically not considered to be drugs, so they are not regulated. Unlike drugs and medicines, food supplements need not be proven effective or even safe to be sold in stores. To be removed from stores, they must be proven ineffective or unsafe. This leaves consumers vulnerable to false claims. Many experts suggest that quackery has increased significantly since 1994, when the act was passed.

More than one-half of American adults are unaware that food supplements are unregulated by the FDA or any other governmental agency. Because they are unregulated, there is no guarantee that a supplement contains the ingredients it claims to contain. Further, many have been shown to contain contaminants. Even when a supplement is what it claims to be, the effects can vary widely from one person to another. Many supplements have dangerous interactions with prescribed and over-the-counter medicines and can be very dangerous.

In spite of the problems associated with lack of supplement regulations, one study indicated that nearly half of Americans routinely take supplements and slightly more than half believe in the value of the supplements. Interestingly, 44 percent believe that physicians know little or nothing about supplements.

Most adults (80 percent) believe that the FDA should review supplements before they are offered for sale. More than 60 percent believe that there are not enough rules to ensure purity and accurate dosage. A similar number of adults want more regulation on advertising claims. More than a few critics point out that self-regulation within the industry has not worked well. They suggest that the public would have more confidence in supplements if the FDA were watching out for their best interests. Table 1 (p. 460) presents some questions that should be asked about food supplements.

Consumers should review the evidence carefully before using supplements. In 2006 a review panel of the National Institutes of Health (NIH) prepared a report concerning vitamins/minerals and chronic disease prevention. The report noted the value of some vitamin and mineral supplements while not recommending others. It endorsed folic acid supplements for women of childbearing age, calcium and vitamin D to protect against osteoporosis for postmenopausal women,

Table 1 ▶ Questions and Comments about Food Supplements

Questions	Comments
Does the government regulate this product to be sure that it is safe and effective?	Since 1994, food supplements can be sold without proof that they are effective. The government does not test food supplements to ensure effectiveness or safety. The FDA must prove the product to be harmful or ineffective to remove it from the market. It is much harder to prove a product ineffective than to provide evidence that it is effective.
Do claims for the supplement have supporting evidence?	The evidence should be based on research with normal people, not evidence based on a population of subjects who have medical problems or nutritional deficiencies. Third-party information often cites research out of context or refers to weak studies that use inappropriate research techniques.
What are the active ingredients?	If the active ingredient really works, research will show its effectiveness. Of course, if it works, then it is much like a medicine and has similar side effects. Sellers of supplements often suggest the product works but that it has no side effects that are associated with medicines. Both cannot be true. For example, Cholestin is a variety of red yeast—a natural product. It contains lovastatin, the same active ingredient in medicines for lowering cholesterol. Though the product works, it has been banned by the FDA as an over-the-counter supplement because it has the same active ingredient as medicine and has the same side effects. The regulation of this product by the FDA has been challenged in the courts by the supplement industry. The decision of the courts will have consequences for future regulation of supplements.
What are the possible side effects and risks of taking the supplement?	As noted above, if a product works as well as a medicine, it probably has the same side effects. If you know the active ingredient, you will know more about the side effects.
Are there possible interactions associated with taking the supplement?	When you take a medicine, consult a physician or pharmacist about drug interactions. Supplements may interact with other supplements or medicines.
What are the long-term effects of taking the supplement?	Because supplements are not regulated, there has been little research about long-term effects of products. For example, melatonin is a hormone that is used for insomnia. Hormones have strong effects on the body and little is known about melatonin's long-term effects. Consider alternative solutions to long-term use of an unstudied supplement.
Are you sure the product is what it claims to be and that the size of the dose is appropriate?	U.S. Pharmacopeia (USP) is a private, nonprofit organization that tests vitamins, minerals, and other supplements to assure quality and purity as well as appropriate size and strength of a standard unit of the product (dose size and strength). The USP label ensures that the product is what it says it is. As many as two or three dozen herbal products are currently being evaluated to determine appropriate dose size. Products with the USP label that fail to meet standards will be removed from stores. Without the USP label, you are at the mercy of the company that produces the product. Since food supplements were deregulated in 1994, numerous deaths have been attributed to supplements containing contaminants.
Who makes the product?	In the absence of regulations, the reputation of the company that makes the product is crucial. Have complaints been made against the company? Have there been health problems with their products? How long has the company been in business? Large pharmaceutical companies are beginning to sell supplements because of the high profit margin. The fact that a product is from a large drug company may ensure that a product is what it is supposed to be, but it does not ensure that the product is effective.
Is the cost worth the potential benefits?	The costs of dietary supplements are typically quite high. For example, protein supplements may cost as much as $1.00 a gram. The cost per gram of good food, such as protein in a chicken breast, is typically a few cents per gram. Most experts suggest that even the most effective supplements have relatively small effects at a high cost.
Is the source of your information about the supplement reliable and accurate?	Avoid verbal information about products, especially information from the seller. Be wary of third-party literature or research in obscure journals. Be wary of those who discredit sound medical advice or inormation from reulatory agencies, such as the FDA.

and several other supplements for those with an eye condition called macular degeneration. The board found that there was not enough evidence to support taking a daily multivitamin. The board did not suggest, however, that those already taking a multivitamin stop doing it and did not find evidence that daily multivitamins are harmful. The review board did take a position against beta-carotene (a form of vitamin A), saying there was no evidence that it is effective. Also, board members warned against taking very high levels of vitamins and minerals (megadoses), noting that they are not beneficial and can be dangerous.

Many other supplements, such as herbals, have not been as well studied. Part of the problem is that there are thousands of products and few resources to support studies. Herbals are made from one plant or plant parts, or a mixture of plants and plant parts. Herbs are sometimes assumed to be safer or better than other supplements because they are purported to be "natural". However, a large percentage of medicines are extracted from plants. The fact that it "comes from nature" does not mean that it is safe. One herbal on which there is considerable evidence is ephedra, which was removed from the market in 2004 after 155 deaths and thousands of adverse reactions from it. It was widely used in weight loss supplements.

Saw Palmetto is another herbal supplement. It is widely used as a preventive for prostate cancer and there were preliminary studies supporting its use. Echinacea is an herbal widely used to reduce symptoms of the common cold; however, one large study did not support its use.

Some supplements are not made from plants. Glucosamine, for example, is made from shellfish and chrondroitin is made from the cartilage of sharks and/or cattle. Glucosamine and chrondroitin are two of the most widely used supplements other than vitamins and minerals. They are often used to relieve symptoms and pain from osteoarthritis. Results of one large clinical trial suggested that the two supplements, taken together or separately, were no more effective than a placebo; however, a small group of people who had moderate to severe pain did experience some relief from the use of the supplements.

The effectiveness of supplements is in question. Also in question is the safety of supplement use. Some of the problems that you should be aware of when considering the use of supplements are described in Table 2.

The cost of supplements is substantial. Since the Dietary Supplements Health and Education Act was passed in 1994, the annual sales of food supplements nearly tripled, totaling more than $20 million each year. In addition to dollar costs, there are costs to people who experience health problems associated with the use of some supplements.

Table 2 ▶ Problems Associated with Supplements
Postsurgical problems, including bleeding, irregular heartbeat, and stroke—examples: echinacea, ephedra, ginkgo, kava, St. John's wort, ginseng
Dangerous interactions with medicines—examples: ephedra, St. John's wort (interact with birth control pills and HIV pills)
FDA warnings concerning unsubstantiated claims about herbs added to foods, such as energy bars and water—examples: ginkgo, ginseng, echinacea
Allergic and other physiological reactions; negative effect on decision making—example: GHB
Known ill effects to health—examples: comfrey (kidneys), kava (liver), ephedra (multiple deaths)
Recall because of dangerous effects associated with contamination—examples: PC SPES, Lipokinetix
Action by the FTC because of deceptive advertisements—examples: Exercise in a Bottle, Fat Trapper
Banned by several sporting groups, including the International Olympic Committee, NCAA, and NFL—examples: steroids, androstendione, ephedra (illegal in doses above 10 mg), THC
Contents may not be what they appear to be and dosage information is unknown—example: the government does not guarantee contents of supplements and there is little evidence concerning dosage for most supplements

Over the past few years, the FDA has received thousands of complaints of adverse events (resulting in approximately 200 deaths). An editorial in a leading national newspaper suggests that "troubling side effects mount" and that "putting customers' health at risk is a high price to pay for a free market in diet supplements." Among the adverse effects reported are lead poisoning, nausea, vomiting, diarrhea, abnormal heart rhythm, fainting, impotence, and lethargy. Over a 6-year period, 2,621 adverse events were reported to the FDA and 184 resulted in death. Also, one study showed that 15 to 20 percent

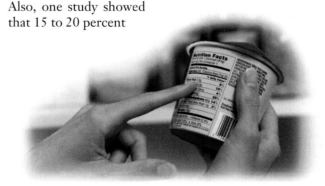

Reading labels and product information can help you be an informed consumer.

of over 1,600 supplements tested included substances that would cause a positive test for drugs banned by sports organizations.

Be wary of claims made for supplements. The Dietary Supplements Health and Education Act has had at least one positive effect. Food supplement labeling must now be truthful. Claims concerning disease prevention, treatment, or diagnosis must be substantiated in order to appear on the product. Unfortunately, the act did not limit false claims if they are not on the product label. The result has been the removal of claims from labels in favor of claims on separate literature, often called third-party literature, because the label makes no claims and the seller (the second party) makes no written claims. Rather, the seller provides claims in literature by other people (a third party). The literature is distributed separately from the product, thus allowing sellers to make unsubstantiated claims for products. Also, the law does not prohibit unproven verbal claims by salespeople. Many medical experts feel that "alternative treatments" should be subjected to the same type of rigorous scientific testing used to evaluate other medicines. However, as things currently stand, it is up to the consumer to make decisions about the safety and effectiveness of food supplements, so it is especially important to be well informed.

Other Consumer Information

Saunas, steam baths, whirlpools, and hot tubs provide no significant health benefits, and guidelines must be followed to ensure safety. Baths do not melt off fat; fat must be metabolized. The heat and humidity from baths may make you perspire, but it is water, not fat, oozing from the pores.

The effect of such baths is largely psychological, although some temporary relief from aches and pains may result from the heat. The same relief can be had by sitting in a tub of hot water in your bathroom. The following guidelines and precautions should be considered when using a sauna, steam bath, whirlpool, or hot tub:

- Take a soap shower before and after entering.
- Do not wear makeup or skin lotion or oil.
- Wait at least an hour after eating before bathing.
- Cool down after exercise before entering the bath.
- Drink plenty of water before or during the bath.
- Do not wear jewelry.
- Do not sit on a metal stool; do sit on a towel.
- Do not drink alcohol before bathing.
- Get out immediately if you become dizzy; feel hot, chilled, or nauseous; or get a headache.
- Get approval from your physician if you have heart disease, low or high blood pressure, a fever, kidney disease, or diabetes; are obese; are pregnant or think you might be pregnant; or are on medications (especially anticoagulants, stimulants, or tranquilizers).
- Limit use for the elderly and for children.
- Do not exercise in a sauna or steam bath.
- Skin infections can be spread in a bath; make certain it is cleaned regularly and that the hot tub or whirlpool has proper pH and chlorination.
- Follow appropriate guidelines:
  Sauna: should not exceed 190°F (88°C) and duration should not exceed 10 to 15 minutes
  Steam bath: should not exceed 120°F (49°C) and duration should not exceed 6 to 12 minutes
  Whirlpool/hot tub: should not exceed 100°F (37°C) and duration should not exceed 5 to 10 minutes

Having a good tan is often associated with being fit and looking good, but getting tanned can be risky. Tanning salons may claim their lamps are safe because they emit only UV-A rays, but these rays can age the skin prematurely making it look wrinkled and leathery. They may also increase the cancer-producing potential of UV-B rays and cause eye damage. Since there is no warning sign of redness, overdosing can occur. Thirty minutes of exposure to UV-A can suppress the immune system. Tanning devices can also aggravate certain skin diseases. The Food and Drug Administration (FDA) advises against the use of any suntan lamp. It is dangerous to use tanning accelerator lotions with the lamps because they can promote burning of the skin. Tanning pills are an even worse choice. They can cause itching, welts, hives, stomach cramps, and diarrhea and can decrease night vision. Tanning in the sun is also hazardous because it damages the skin, making it age prematurely, and it is a cause of skin cancer.

Books, Magazines, and Articles

Not all books provide scientifically sound, accurate, and reliable information. Some material is published on the basis of how popular, famous, or attractive the author is or how sensational or unusual his or her ideas are. Very few movie stars, models, TV personalities, and Olympic athletes are experts in biomechanics, anatomy and physiology, exercise, and other foundations of physical fitness. Having a good figure or physique, being fit, or having gone through a training program does not, in itself, qualify a person to advise others.

After reading the facts presented in this book, you should be able to evaluate whether or not a book, a magazine, or an article on exercise and fitness is valid, reliable, and scientifically sound. To assist you further, however, 10 guidelines are listed in Lab 23A.

The Internet

Not all Web sites provide scientifically sound, accurate, and reliable information. Nearly three-fourths of all teens and young adult computer users seek health information on the Web. The leading topics of information are cancer, diabetes, sexually transmitted infections, and weight control. A health goal for the nation—as outlined in *Healthy People 2010*—is to increase the proportion of households with access to the Internet, with the intent of making reliable health information available to as many people as possible. The Internet has made an almost unlimited amount of health information accessible; it has also been the source of much misinformation and even fraud.

The FTC is charged with making sure that advertising claims for products are not false or misleading. Several years ago the FTC initiated "Operation Cure-All" in an effort to help "clean up" Web sites that provide false information. You can file a complaint with the FTC at the "cure-all" Web site if you find incorrect or misleading information on the Web (**www.ftc.gov/cureall**). In spite of the FTC efforts, there is still much health misinformation on the Web, leading one FTC official to suggest that "miracle cures, once thought to have been laughed out of existence, have now found a new medium . . . on the Internet". Clearly,

Internet users must be careful in selecting Web sites for obtaining fitness, health, and wellness information. One of the most useful rules is to consult at least two or more sources to confirm information. Getting confirmation of information from non-Web sources is also a good idea.

You can follow some general rules when you use the Web to obtain fitness, health, and wellness information. In general, government Web sites are good sources that contain sound information prepared by experts and based on scientific research. Government sites typically include ".gov" as part of the address. Professional organizations and universities can also be good sources of information. Organizations typically have ".org" and universities typically have ".edu" as part of the address. However, caution should still be used with organizations because it is easy to start an organization and obtain an ".org" Web address. Your greatest trust can be placed in the sites of stable, credible organizations (see *Web Resources* in this book). The great majority of Web sites promoting health products have ".com" in the address because these are commercial sites, which are in business to make a profit. Thus, they are more inclined to contain information that is suspect or totally incorrect, although some ".com" sites contain good information—for example, those listed at the end of each concept of this book. Nevertheless, it is important to evaluate all information with special care.

Strategies for Action

Being a good consumer requires time, information, and effort. With time and effort, you can gain the information you need to make good decisions about the products and services you purchase. In Lab 23A, you will evaluate an exercise device, a food supplement, a magazine article, or a Web site. In Lab 23B, you will evaluate a health/wellness or fitness club. Taking the time to investigate a product will help you save money and help you avoid making poor deci-

sions that affect your health, fitness, and wellness. When you are making decisions about products or services, it is a good idea to begin your investigation well in advance of the day when a decision is to be made. Salespeople often suggest that "this offer is only good today." They know that people often make poor decisions when under time pressure, and they want you to make a decision today so that they will not lose a sale.

Online Learning Center

www.mhhe.com/corbin7e
The Online Learning Center contains a variety of Web-based resources that will help you get the most out of this book and your course. In addition to the On the Web pages, there are video activities, interactive quizzes, application assignments, and a variety of other useful study aids. Log on to the URL above to access these resources.

Web Resources

Agency for Health Care Policy and Research
www.ahcpr.gov
AMA Health Insight **www.ama-assn.org**
American Dietetics Association **www.eatright.org**
American Psychological Assocation, Psychology Matters
www.psychologymatters.org
Center for Science in the Public Interest **www.cspinet.org**
Federal Trade Commission **www.ftc.gov**
Food and Drug Administration **www.fda.gov**
Healthfinder **www.healthfinder.gov**
Medwatch **www.fda.gov/medwatch/**

National Center for Complementary and Alternative
    Medicine **http://nccam.nih.gov**
National Council against Health Fraud **www.ncahf.org**
Office of Dietary Supplements **http://ods.od.nih.gov**
Quackwatch **www.quackwatch.org**
U.S. Consumer Information Center **www.pueblo.gsa.gov**

Suggested Readings

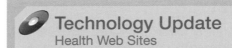

Additional reference materials for Concept 23 are available at Web10.

Web 10

Barrett, S., et al. 2007. *Consumer Health: A Guide to Intelligent Decisions*. 8th ed. New York: McGraw-Hill Higher Education.

Clegg, D.O., et al. 2006. Glucosamine, chondroitin sulfate, and the two in combination for painful knee osteoarthritis. *New England Journal of Medicine* 354(8):795–808.

Drazen, J. M. 2003. Inappropriate advertising of dietary supplements. *New England Journal of Medicine* 348(9):777–778.

Fontanarosa, P. B., et al. 2003. The need for regulation of dietary supplements—Lessons from ephedra. *Journal of the American Medical Association* 289(12):1568–1570.

Ioannidis, J. P. A. 2005. Contradicted and initially stronger effects in highly cited clinical research. *Journal of the American Medical Association* 29(2):218–228.

Krone, C. 2004. Nutritional supplements: Friend or foe? *New Zealand Medical Journal* 117(1196):U937–U945.

Markel, H. 2005. Why America needs a strong FDA. *Journal of the American Medical Association* 294(19):2489–2491.

Radley, D.C., et al. 2006. Off-label prescribing among office-based physicians. *Archives of Internal Medicine* 166(9):1021–1026.

Strom, B.L. 2006. How the US drug safety system should be changed. *Journal of the American Medical Association* 295(17):2072–2075.

Technology Update
Health Web Sites

Some new Web site servers may help consumers make better health decisions:

- Medwatch, a Web site of the FDA, is a good source of consumer information; it includes safety alerts for drugs, product recall advisories, changes in drug safety labeling, warnings and safety information about dietary supplements, and health advisories concerning medical devices (**www.fda.gov/medwatch**).

- The American Psychological Association has developed a Web site called Psychology Matters: Psychological Applications in Daily Life (www.psychologymatters.org). This Web site offers sound advice concerning "how to be a wise consumer of psychological research."

- The National Institutes of Health has a National Center for Complementary and Alternative Medicine. Its purpose is to conduct research and provide consumers with the most recent scientific information on these topics (**http://nccam.nih.gov**).

- Google, the popular Web search engine, has developed several new health-related Web products. Google-Health is a search enhancement that is designed as a portal to assist in searches of health-related topics. At the time this book went to press Google-Health was not online but it will be available soon.

Tekin, K. A., and L. Kravitz. 2004. The growing trend of ergogenic aids and supplements. *ACSM's Health and Fitness Journal* 8(2):15–18.

In the News

Consumer Health Issues

There are many news stories related to consumer health issues. Some of the more recent are listed below:

- A major national supplement company sold a product purported to increase height, breast size, and penis size. The company was found guilty of selling pills that do not work as advertised. The company took in more than $77 million. Of the money recovered, most will go to lawyers. Approximately $4 million will go to refunds to consumers.

- In 2005, Representative Steven Israel introduced Tim Fagen's law in Congress. The legislation, named after a patient who took bogus medicine, is aimed at cracking down on fake medicines. If signed into law, it will be harder for fake medicines to be sold and will increase the penalties for those who sell them.

- Hi Health, a major supplier of supplements, was fined by the FTC ($450,000) for false and misleading claims for one of its supplements. The product (Ocular Nutrition) was advertised frequently on a national radio news show. No studies have confirmed the effectiveness of the product.

Consumer Health Digest provides articles about health products and health quackery. To get a free online subscription send a blank e-mail to chdigest-subscribe@ssr.com.

Lab 23A Practicing Consumer Skills: Evaluating Products

Name	**Section**	**Date**

Purpose: To evaluate an exercise device, a book, a magazine article, an advertisement, a food supplement, or a Web site

Procedures

1. Evaluate an exercise device, a book, an article, a newspaper or magazine advertisement, a food supplement or a Web site. Place an X in the circle by the item you choose to evaluate. Attach a copy if you evaluate an advertisement.
2. Read each of the 10 evaluation factors for the item you selected. Place an X in the circle by the factors that describe the item you are evaluating.
3. Total the number of X marks to determine a score for the item being evaluated. The higher the score, the more likely it is to be safe and/or effective.
4. Answer the questions in the Conclusions and Implications section.

Results

Directions: Place an X in the circle by the product you evaluated. Place an X over the circle by each true statement. Provide information about the product in the space provided.

Exercise Device

○ 1. The exercise device requires effort consistent with the FIT formula.

○ 2. The exercise device is safe and the exercise done using the device is safe.

○ 3. There are no claims that the device uses exercise that is effortless.

○ 4. Exercise using the device is fun or is a type that you might do regularly.

○ 5. There are no claims using gimmick words, such as *tone, cellulite, quick,* or *spot fat reduction.*

○ 6. The seller's credentials are sound.

○ 7. The product does something for you that cannot be done without it.

○ 8. You can return the device if you do not like it (the seller has been in business for a long time).

○ 9. The cost of the product is justified by the potential benefits.

○ 10. The device is easy to store or you have a place to permanently use the equipment without storing it.

Exercise Device

Name of device: _____
_____
_____

Description and manufacturer:
_____
_____
_____

○ **Advertisement**

Source: _____
_____

○ **Book or Article**

Author(s): _____
_____
_____

Journal article or book title: _____
_____
_____

Journal name or name of publisher:
_____
_____

Date of publication: _____
_____
_____

Book/Article/Advertisement

○ 1. The credentials of the author are sound. He or she has a degree in an area related to the content of the book or magazine.*

○ 2. The facts in the article are consistent with the facts described in this book.

○ 3. The author does not claim "quick" or "miraculous" results.

○ 4. There are no claims about the spot reduction of fat or other unfounded claims.

○ 5. The author/advertisement is not selling a product.

○ 6. Reputable experts are cited.

○ 7. The article does not promote unsafe exercises or products.

○ 8. New discoveries from exotic places are not cited.

○ 9. The article/advertisment does not rely on testimonials by nonexpert, famous people.

○ 10. The author/advertisement does not make claims that the AMA, the FDA, or another legitimate organization is trying to suppress information.

*Not applicable for advertisement.

Food Supplement

1. The seller is not the prime source of product information.

2. The seller has been in business for a long time and has a good reputation.

3. There is scientific evidence of product effectiveness.

4. There is clear evidence about the side effects of the active ingredients.

5. The long-term effectiveness and safety of the product are cited.

6. You are sure of the content of the product.

7. You have information that the manufacturer is reputable.

8. The known benefits are worth the cost.

9. There is evidence that you can get benefits from this product that cannot be obtained from good food.

10. There are no claims that use quack words or claims about conspiracies against the product by reputable organizations.

Food Supplement

Name: _____

_____

_____

Purported benefit: _____

_____

_____

Manufacturer/seller: _____

_____

_____

Dose and active ingredient: _____

_____

_____

Web Site

Web address: _____

_____

_____

Type of information provided: ____

_____

_____

Organization or person responsible for information: _____

_____

_____

Web Site

1. The site does not sell products associated with information provided.

2. The provider is a person, an organization (org), or a governmental agency (gov) with a sound reputation.

3. The site does not use quack words.

4. The site does not try to discredit well-established organizations or governmental agencies.

5. The site does not rely on testimonials, celebrities, or people with unknown credentials.

6. The site is well regarded by experts, and has a high rating at http://navigator.tufts.edu.

7. The site has a history of providing good information.

8. The site provides complete information that is documented by research.

9. No claims of quick cures or miracle results are made.

10. The site provides information consistent with information provided in this text.

Conclusions and Implications

Total the number of Xs for the device, book/magazine, advertisement, food supplement, or Web site: [   ]

In several sentences, give your assessment of the product. Did it score well? Would you use/buy the product? Explain.

Lab 23B Evaluating a Health/Wellness or Fitness Club

Name	**Section**	**Date**

Purpose: To practice evaluating a health club (various combinations of the words *health, wellness,* and *fitness* are often used for these clubs)

Procedures

1. Choose a club and make a visit.
2. Listen carefully to all that is said and ask lots of questions.
3. Look carefully all around you as you are given the tour of the facilities; ask what the exercises or the equipment does for you or ask leading questions, such as "Will this take inches off my hips?"
4. As soon as you leave the club, rate it, using Chart 1. Space is provided for notes in Chart 1.

Chart 1 ▶ Health Club Evaluation Questionnaire

Directions: Place an X over a "yes" or "no" answer. Make notes as necessary.

	Yes	No	Notes
1. Were claims for improvement in weight, figure/physique, or fitness realistic?	○	○	
2. Was a long-term contract (1 to 3 years) encouraged?	○	○	
3. Was the sales pitch high-pressure to make an immediate decision?	○	○	
4. Were you given a copy of the contract to read at home?	○	○	
5. Did the fine print include objectionable clauses?	○	○	
6. Did they ask you about medical readiness?	○	○	
7. Did they sell diet supplements as a sideline?	○	○	
8. Did they have passive equipment?	○	○	
9. Did they have cardiovascular training equipment or facilities (cycles, track, pool, aerobic dance)?	○	○	
10. Did they make unscientific claims for the equipment, exercise, baths, or diet supplements?	○	○	
11. Were the facilities clean?	○	○	
12. Were the facilities crowded?	○	○	
13. Were there days and hours when the facilities were open but would not be available to you?	○	○	
14. Were there limits on the number of minutes you could use a piece of equipment?	○	○	
15. Did the floor personnel closely supervise and assist clients?	○	○	
16. Were the floor personnel qualified experts?	○	○	
17. Were the managers/owners qualified experts?	○	○	
18. Has the club been in business at this location for a year or more?	○	○	

Results

1. Score the chart as follows:

   A. Give 1 point for each "no" answer for items 2, 3, 5, 7, 8, 10, 12, 13, and 14 and place the score in the box.

   Total A [ ]

   B. Give 1 point for each "yes" answer for items 1, 4, 6, 9, 11, and 18 and place the score in the box.

   Total B [ ]

   Total A and B above and place the score in the box.

   Total A and B [ ]

   C. Give 1 point for each "yes" answer for items 15, 16, and 17 and place the score in the box.

   Total C [ ]

2. A total score of 12–15 points on items A and B suggests the club rates at least fair, compared with other clubs.

3. A score of 3 on item C indicates that the personnel are qualified and suggests that you could expect to get accurate technical advice from the staff.

4. Regardless of the total scores, you would have to decide the importance of each item to you personally, as well as evaluate other considerations, such as cost, location, and personalities of the clients and the personnel, to decide if this would be a good place for you or your friends to join.

Conclusions and Implications: In several sentences, discuss your conclusion about the quality of this club and whether you think it would fit your needs if you wanted to belong.

Toward Optimal Health and Wellness: Planning for Healthy Lifestyle Change

Health Goals for the year 2010

- Increase quality and years of healthy life.
- Increase healthy days.
- Eliminate health disparities.
- Increase adoption and maintenance of appropriate daily physical activity.
- Promote health by improving dietary factors and nutritional status.
- Promote healthy and safe communities.
- Promote availability of high-quality health information.
- Increase availability of health care and counseling for mental health problems.
- Avoid destructive behaviors.

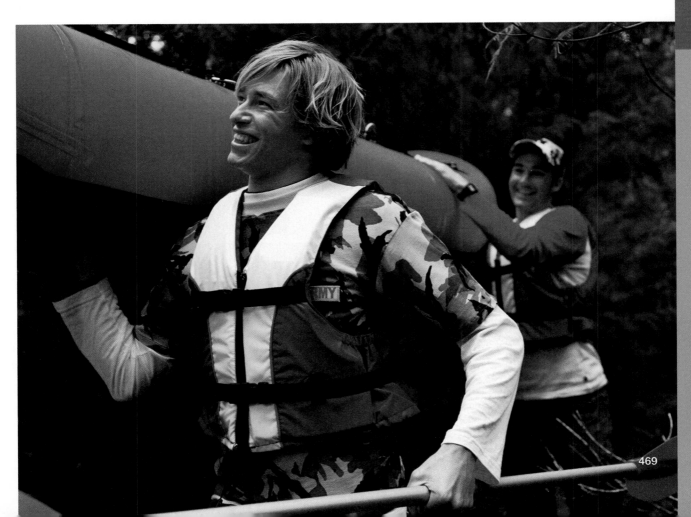

In addition to healthy lifestyles, other factors such as heredity, health care, the environment, and personal actions and interactions, contribute to good health, wellness, and fitness.

The two primary health goals for the nation for the year 2010 are increasing the quality and years of life and eliminating health disparities so that all people can attain and maintain lifelong health, wellness, and fitness. In the first concept in this book, you were introduced to a model that explained the many factors that influence health, wellness, and fitness (see Figure 1). The focus of this book has been on changing factors over which you have control. For this reason, much of the discussion has centered on changing lifestyles because it impacts health, wellness, and fitness more than any of the other factors. Still, other factors are important. In this final concept, the focus is on providing additional strategies for action related to the "changeable" factors in the model.

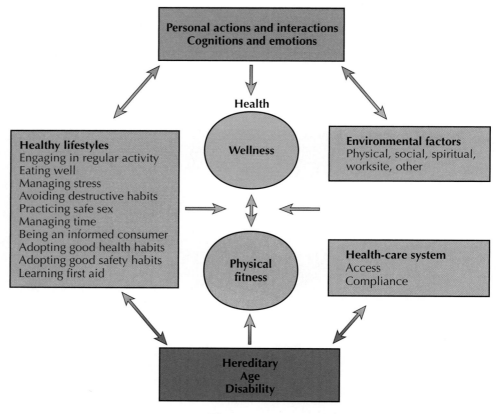

Figure 1 ▶ Factors influencing physical fitness, health, and wellness.

On the Web
www.mhhe.com/corbinweb

Web 01 Log on to this URL before reading this concept. See On the Web list of concepts. Click on the concept number you want to view. To access supplemental information, click on the number shown at each Web icon.

Strategies for Action

Consider strategies for taking advantage of your heredity. You are aware that heredity is a factor that affects all aspects of fitness as well as your health and wellness. You can use several strategies to overcome negative predispositions and to take advantage of positive ones:

- *Learn about your family history.* If members of your family have had specific diseases or health problems, make sure you inform your physician. Investigate to see if the conditions might affect you.
- *Take action to diminish risk factors for which you have a predisposition.* For example, if you have a family history of Type II diabetes, do regular activity, eat well, and keep your body fat level in the good fitness zone.
- *Take advantage of your hereditary strengths.* Self-assessments can help you see where you have strength and account for weaknesses. Build on your strengths and find ways to compensate for your weaknesses. For example, people who have fewer fast-twitch muscle fibers will probably not be great sprinters but often have more slow-twitch fibers, which favor endurance performances, such as distance running.

Web 01 **Consider strategies for using the health-care system effectively.** Consider the information in Table 1 concerning health care. Do a self-assessment of your current use of health care (see Lab 24A). Develop a plan using some of the following strategies (see Lab 24B):

- *Get periodic medical exams.* Do not wait until something is wrong before you seek medical advice. After

Table 1 ▶ Facts about Personal Physicians and Health Insurance

- More women than men have a regular physician.
- More than half of young men have no personal doctor.
- Three times more women than men have visited a doctor in the past year.
- Women are more aware of health issues than men.
- Nearly half of men wait a week or more to see a doctor when ill.
- Many men see sickness as "unmanly."
- Married men see doctors more frequently than single men because their wives prompt them.
- Lack of health insurance results in fewer doctor's visits, less frequent health screening, and less access to prescribed medicine.

40 years of age, a yearly preventive physical exam is recommended. Younger people should have an exam at least every 2 years. Mammograms for women and prostate tests (PSA) for men are recommended. Breast and testicular self-exams are also important.

- *Get medical insurance.* Find a way to get health insurance. Young people who save money by avoiding the payment of insurance premiums are placing themselves (and families) at risk.
- *Immunize.* Pneumonia and the flu are the sixth leading cause of death. With immunization, death, hospitalization, and loss of healthy days decrease dramatically.
- *Investigate and then identify a regular doctor or doctors.* Check with other physicians you know and trust for referrals. Check with your state medical board and national directories (e.g., Directory of Board Certified Medical Specialists, www.abms.org) for specialist certifications or fellowships.
- *Investigate and then choose an emergency care center and a hospital.* Choose an accredited emergency center near your home and a hospital that is accredited and grants privileges to your personal doctors.
- *Be there, or have others present, when those you care about are in the hospital.* Medical mistakes cause nearly 100,000 unnecessary deaths each year. According to the National Patient Safety Foundation (www.npsf.org), watching staff to ensure good hygiene, asking about medications and treatments, and telling a nurse or doctor if things look wrong can help eliminate mistakes. Learn the nurses' routines so you know how to find them when necessary.
- *Ask questions.* Do not be afraid to speak up. Prepare questions for doctors and other medical personnel. The American College of Surgeons suggests several questions before surgeries: What are the reasons for the surgery? Are there alternatives? What will happen if I don't have the procedure? What are the risks? What are the long-term effects and problems? How will the procedure impact my quality of life and future health?
- *If you have doubts about medical advice, get a second opinion.* As many as 30 percent of original diagnoses are incorrect or differ from second opinions. Do not be afraid you will offend your doctor by getting another opinion. Good doctors encourage second opinions.
- *Communicate with your physician.* Prepare a list of all medications and supplements that you take and make all physicians aware of them. Share records of past medical treatments.
- *Read drug inserts or ask your doctor or pharmacist about them.* The FDA recently simplified drug inserts to help you understand them and to help your doctor prescribe better.

- *Become familiar with the symptoms of common medical problems.* If symptoms persist, seek medical help. Many deaths can be prevented if early warning signs of medical problems are heeded.
- *If medical advice is given, comply.* People commonly stop taking medicine when symptoms stop rather than taking the full amount of medicine prescribed.
- *Be cautious when using the Internet for health information.* If you use the Internet for health information, be sure to use reliable Web sites (see Concept 23). Seek information from more than one source.
- *Make your wishes for health care known.* Have a medical power of attorney. This document spells out the treatments you desire in the case of severe illness. Without such a document, your loved ones may not be able to make decisions consistent with your wishes. Be sure your loved ones have a similar document so that you can help them carry out their wishes.

Consider strategies for improving your environment. Consider the information in Table 2 when trying to improve environments related to wellness.

Web 02

- *Strategies for interacting with the physical environment.* Avoid polluted environments, such as smoke-filled establishments; choose a living location low in pollution; keep your home free of pollutants (regularly check filters, avoid use of toxic products); and seek out environments that are conducive to physical activity (see Concept 6) and healthy eating (see Concept 15).
- *Strategies for the social environment.* Find a social community that accommodates your personal and family needs; get involved in community affairs, including those that affect the environment; build relationships with family and friends; provide support for others so that their support will be there for you when you need it; use time-management strategies to help you allocate time for social interactions.
- *Strategies for the spiritual environment.* Pray, meditate, read spiritual materials, participate in spiritual discussions, find a place to worship, provide spiritual support for others, seek spiritual guidance from those with experience and expertise, keep a journal, experience nature, honor relationships, help others.
- *Strategies for the intellectual environment.* Make decisions based on sound information, question simple solutions to complex problems, seek environments that stimulate critical thinking.
- *Strategies for the work environment.* Choose a job that has a healthy physical environment, including adequate space, lighting, and freedom from pollution (tobacco smoke), as well as a healthy social, spiritual, and intellectual environment and one that has a worksite wellness program led by professionals.

- *Strategies for finding an environment that supports healthy lifestyles.* Choose a place to live that is near parks and playgrounds and has sidewalks, bike paths, jogging trails, and swimming facilities; join a gym or health club; avoid environments that limit choices to fast food and food with empty calories; find a social environment that reinforces healthy lifestyles.

Consider strategies for adopting healthy lifestyles. Statistics show that more than half of early deaths are caused by unhealthy lifestyles. For this reason, changing lifestyles is the focus of this book. We emphasized priority healthy lifestyles such as being regularly active, eating well, managing stress, avoiding destructive behaviors, and practicing safe sex because they are factors over which we have some control and, if adopted, they have considerable impact on health, wellness, and fitness. Other healthy lifestyles not emphasized in this book are described in Table 3.

- *Use the six steps to help you plan lifestyle programs.* In Concept 2 you learned about the six steps involved in planning for healthy lifestyle change. The labs at the end of this concept are designed to help you create plans for a variety of lifestyles using the six steps. Lab24A helps you assess many of the factors that influence health, wellness, and fitness so that you can identify areas in which you especially need to prepare lifestyle change plans. Lab 24B is designed to help you prepare plans for making lifestyle change from the list presented in Figure 1 (e.g., eating well, managing stress). Lab 24C is designed to help you plan a personal physical activity program.
- *Use self-management skills.* Learning and using self-management skills, discussed in Concept 2 and throughout the book, can help you adopt and maintain healthy lifestyles.
- *Formal steps can become less formal with experience.* Few of us will go through life doing formal fitness assessments every month, writing down goals weekly, or self-monitoring activity daily. However, the more a person does self-assessments, the more he or she is aware of personal fitness status. This awareness reduces the need for frequent testing. For example, a person who does regular heart rate monitoring knows when he or she is in the target zone without counting heart rate every minute. A person who has frequently used skinfold measures to self-assess fatness can develop a good sense of body fatness with less frequent measurements. The same is true of other self-management skills. With experience, you can use the techniques less formally.

Consider your cognitions and emotions when planning strategies for action. Much of the information in this book is designed to help you make good decisions about health, wellness, and fitness. Using the guidelines presented

Table 2 ▶ Environmental Factors Influencing Health, Wellness, and Fitness

Physical Environment

The physical environment in which you live has both direct and indirect effects on your health and wellness. Some examples are:

- *Pollution.* Air pollution (increased ozone, hydrocarbons, and particulates) and water pollution both have negative effects on health. Smoking in public places is a source of pollution.
- *Urban sprawl and population growth.* Sprawl reduces opportunities for healthy lifestyles, such as walking and biking, and increases the need for auto travel. Population growth results in greater housing density and can result in less community and home safety. Urban growth places great demands on sanitation systems and contributes to land pollution.

Social Environment

A healthy social environment offers opportunities for friendly interactions in a supportive environment, including the following:

- *Sense of community.* Being a part of the greater community is important to social and mental health.
- *Opportunities for supportive personal relationships.* We all need friendly personal interactions. Support by others, especially family members, can help in managing stress and in adopting healthy lifestyles.
- *Time availability.* We tend to take time for what we think is important. Social interactions require that time be spent with other people.
- *Removal from abusive environments.* If relationships become abusive, you may have to remove yourself and others at risk and seek help from others.

Spiritual Environment

A positive environment provides each person with opportunities to find spiritual fulfillment. Some examples are:

- *Opportunities for spiritual development.* Reading spiritual materials, prayer, meditation, and discussions with others (of similar and dissimilar beliefs) all provide opportunities to clarify and solidify spiritual beliefs.
- *Access to spiritual community and leadership.* Finding a community for worship and/or spiritual support has been shown to be comforting and a path to fulfillment for many. Spiritual fulfillment may benefit from consultation with those with experience and expertise.

Intellectual Environment

Environments that foster learning and sound critical thinking are important to intellectual wellness. Factors to consider include:

- *Access to accurate information.* Whether the source is formal education or self-learning, access to accurate information is essential. Of course, good information is beneficial only if used.
- *Stimulation for effective thinking.* Sometimes we can become lazy, failing to evaluate information effectively. Seeking environments that stimulate critical thinking is important.

Work Environment

The work environment is a combination of the physical, social, intellectual, and spiritual environments. Factors that lead to a healthy work environment include:

- *Healthy physical and social environment.* A healthy work environment includes an adequate, well-lit, pollution-free workspace and reasonable work hours. Good relationships with bosses and co-workers and adequate work breaks are key elements of a healthy social work environment.
- *Opportunity and support for healthy lifestyles.* Many companies have worksite wellness programs, which include opportunities for physical activity and other healthy lifestyle change. Programs that have quality professional leadership have been shown to reduce absenteeism, reduce health-care costs, and increase job satisfaction.

Environment Supporting Healthy Lifestyles

Environments that promote healthy lifestyles can enhance health and wellness. Factors to consider include:

- *Active environments.* If we are to promote healthy lifestyles at home, work, and school, it is important to create environments that encourage active lifestyles. Examples include providing safe, open recreational areas and worksite wellness programs.
- *People working together.* Changes designed to promote healthy lifestyles require the efforts of many people. Cooperative efforts by groups with well-defined goals are most likely to be successful. Many communities have created health coalitions to create these environments.

---

throughout this book and using self-management skills can help you make good decisions. As noted in Concept 1, it is also important to consider your emotions when making decisions. Consider these guidelines:

- *Collect and evaluate information before you act.* Become informed before you make important decisions. Get information from good sources and consult with others you trust.
- *Emotions are important to making certain decisions but should not be used instead of good decision-making processes.* Fear and anger are two emotions that can affect your judgment and influence your ability to make decisions. Even love for another person can influence your actions. Get control of your emotions, or seek guidance

from others you trust, before making important decisions in emotionally charged situations.

- *Resist pressure to make quick decisions when there is no need to decide quickly.* Sales people often press for a quick decision to get a sale. Take some time to think before making a quick decision that may be based on emotion rather than critical thinking. Of course, some decisions must be made when emotions are charged (e.g., medical care in an emergency) but, when possible, delaying a decision can be to your advantage.
- *Use stress-management techniques to help you gain control when you must make decisions in emotionally charged situations.* Practice stress-management techniques (see Concepts 16 and 17) so that you can use them effectively when needed.

Table 3 ► Other Healthy Lifestyles	
Lifestyle	**Examples**
Adopting good personal health habits. Many of these habits, important to optimal health, are considered to be elementary because they are often taught in school or in the home at an early age. In spite of their importance, many adults regularly fail to adopt these behaviors.	• Brushing and flossing teeth • Regular bathing and hand washing • Adequate sleep • Care of ears, eyes, and skin
Adopting good safety habits. Unintentional injuries cost Canadians about $8.7 billion per year and, in the United States, the cost of injury and violence is $224 billion a year. Thousands of people die each year and thousands more suffer disabilities or problems that detract from good health and wellness. Not all accidents can be prevented, but we can adopt habits to reduce risk.	• *Automobile accidents.* Wear seat belts, avoid using the phone while driving, do not drink and drive, and do not drive aggressively. • *Water accidents.* Learn to swim, learn CPR, wear life jackets while boating, do not drink while boating. • *Others.* Store guns safely, use smoke alarms, use ladders and electrical equipment safely, and maintain cars, bikes, and motorcycles properly.
Learning first aid. Many deaths could be prevented and the severity of injury could be reduced if those at the sites of emergencies were able to administer first aid.	• Learn cardiopulmonary resuscitation (CPR). • Learn the Heimlich maneuver to assist people who are choking. • Learn basic first aid.

Web 03 **Consider strategies for taking action and benefiting from interactions.** In the end, it is what you do that counts. You can learn everything there is to know about fitness, health, and wellness, but, if you do not take action and take advantage of your interactions with people and your environments, you will not benefit (see Figure 1). The following are some strategies for taking action and interacting effectively:

- *Plan your actions and interactions.* Use the information in this book to plan your actions. Seek environments that produce positive interactions. People who plan are not only more likely to act but also more likely to act effectively.
- *Put your plans into action.* Do not put off until tomorrow what you can do today. For good plans to be effective, they must be implemented. Actions and interactions that influence various dimensions of wellness are described in Table 4 (page 475).
- *Honor your beliefs and relationships.* Actions and interactions that are inconsistent with basic beliefs and that fail to honor important relationships can result in reduced quality of life.
- *Seek the help of others and provide support for others who need your help.* As already noted, support from friends, family, and significant others can be critical in helping you achieve health, wellness, and fitness. Get help. Do what you can to be there for others who need your help.
- *Consider using professional help.*

Most colleges have programs through their health centers that provide free, confidential assistance or referral. Many businesses have employee assistance programs (EAP). The programs have counselors who will help you or your family members find help with a particular problem.

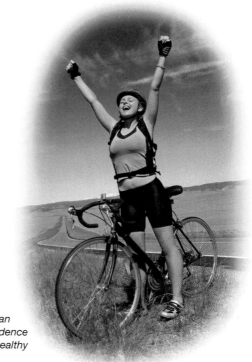

Making lifestyle changes, such as becoming more physically active, can improve your confidence and lead to other healthy lifestyle changes.

Many other programs and support groups are available to help you change your lifestyle. For example, most hospitals and many health organizations have hot lines that provide you with referral services for establishing healthy lifestyles.

Consider your personal beliefs and philosophy when making decisions. Though science can help you make good decisions and solve problems, most experts tell you that there is more to it than that. Your personal

Table 4 ▶ Actions and Interactions that Influence Wellness	
Dimension of Wellness	**Influential Factors**
Physical wellness	Pursuing behaviors that are conducive to good physical health (being physically active and maintaining a healthy diet)
Social wellness	Being supportive of family, friends, and co-workers and practicing good communication skills
Emotional wellness	Balancing work and leisure and responding proactively to challenging or stressful situations
Intellectual wellness	Challenging yourself to continually learn and improve in your work and personal life
Spiritual wellness	Praying, meditating, or reflecting on life
Total wellness	Taking responsibility for your own health

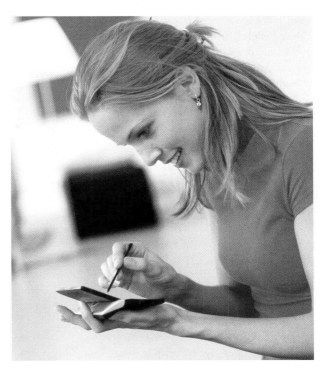

Good planning and a positive attitude can help in making lifestyle changes.

philosophy and beliefs play a role. The following are factors to consider:

- *Clarify your personal philosophy and consider a new way of thinking.* The determination of whether a person is healthy, well, or fit is often subjective. Many make comparisons with other people, and such comparisons often result in setting personal standards impossible to achieve. Achieving the body fat of a model seen on television is not realistic or healthy for most people. Expecting to be able to perform as a professional athlete is not something most of us can achieve. It is for this reason that the standards for health, wellness, and fitness in this book are based on health criteria rather than comparative criteria. As you began your study on this book, you were introduced to the HELP philosophy. Adhering to this philosophy can help you adopt a new way of thinking. This philosophy suggests that each person should use health (H) as the basis for making decisions rather than comparisons with others. This is something that everyone (E) can do for a lifetime (L). It allows each of us to set personal (P) goals that are realistic and possible to attain.

- *Allow for spontaneity.* The reliance on science emphasized in this book can help you make good choices. But if you are to live life fully you sometimes must allow yourself to be spontaneous. In doing so, the key is to be consistent with your personal philosophy so that your spontaneous actions will be enriching rather than a source of future regret.

- *Believe that you can make a difference.* As noted previously, you make your own choices. Though heredity and several other factors are out of your control, the choices that you make are yours. Believing that your actions make a difference is critical to taking action and making changes when necessary, allowing you to be healthy, well, and fit for a lifetime.

Online Learning Center

www.mhhe.com/corbin7e
The Online Learning Center contains a variety of Web-based resources that will help you get the most out of this book and your course. In addition to the On the Web pages, there are video activities, interactive quizzes, application assignments, and a variety of other useful study aids. Log on to the URL above to access these resources.

Web Resources

Web 04

American Association of Retired Persons Health Guide **www.aarp.org/health/healthguide**
American Board of Medical Specialties **www.abms.org**
American College Health Association **www.acha.org**
American Dietetics Association **www.eatright.org**
Cleveland Clinic Second Opinion **www.eclevelandclinic.org**

Healthfinder **www.healthfinder.gov**
Healthy People 2010 **www.health.gov/healthypeople**
Mayo Clinic **www.mayoclinic.com**
National Patient Safety Foundation **www.npsf.org**
Research America **www.researchamerica.org**
U.S. Consumer Information Center **www.pueblo.gsa.gov**
World Health Organization **www.who.int**

Suggested Readings

Web 05

Additional reference materials for Concept 24 are available at Web05.

Banks, J., et al. 2006. Disease and disadvantage in the United States and in England. *Journal of the American Medical Association* 295(17):2037–2045.

Brennan, T. A., et al. 2006. Health industry practices that create conflicts of interest: A policy proposal for academic medical centers. *Journal of the American Medical Association* 295(4):429–433.

Lasser, K. E., et al. 2006. Access to care, health status, and health disparities in the United States and Canada: Results of a cross-national population-based survey. *American Journal of Public Health*. Published online May 30, ahead of print.

Leape, L. L., and D. M. Berwick. 2006. Five years after to err is human: What have we learned? *Journal of the American Medical Association*. 293(19):2384–2390.

Roizen, M. F., and M. C. Oz. 2006. *You: The Smart Patient: An Insider's Handbook for Getting the Best Treatment*. New York: Free Press.

Snyder, C. R., and S. J. Lopez. 2006. *Positive Psychology: The Scientific and Practical Exploration of Human Strengths*. Thousand Oaks, CA: Sage Publications.

Taylor, S. 2006. *Health Psychology*. 6th ed. New York: McGraw-Hill.

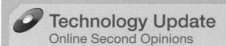

Technology Update
Online Second Opinions

Earlier in this concept, you were encouraged to get a second opinion when facing medical problems. The Cleveland Clinic, a well-respected medical institution, has begun offering online medical services. Among them is a system for getting online second opinions. *MyConsult®* allows you to get a second opinion for over 600 life-threatening or life-altering diagnoses online. This service is available to anyone who has a computer and is especially useful to people who live in remote locations or who do not have access to medical facilities near their homes. For more information, access **www.eclevelandclinic.org**.

In the News

Health News

The following are bits of information regarding important health issues in the news.

- *Adults are emphasizing prevention.* A national poll indicates that 82 percent of people are taking steps to prevent health problems later in life. Being active, eating well, and getting medical attention lead the list (see www.researchamerica.org for more information).

- *Evidence indicates that simple steps can prevent health problems.* Infections can be prevented by hand washing but many adults do not wash regularly. Most adults (more than 90 percent) say that they wash their hands after using a public rest room, but a recent observational study indicated that only 83 percent really do. Men are less likely to wash than women.

- *Evidence indicates it is best to stay at home when sick.* Most companies (62 percent) urge employees to stay at home when they are sick to prevent spreading sickness to others. Forty percent of employees say they have gotten the flu at work. Still, 40 percent of employees say they feel pressure to go to work when sick.

- *Health status in the U.S. is lower than in Canada and Great Britain.* In spite of recent encouraging health statistics in the United States, the rate of chronic disease (e. g., diabetes, high blood pressure) in the United States is higher than in Canada and Britain. One study suggests that universal insurance in Canada may be one reason. Similar results were not found for Britain.

- *Music players may lead to increases in hearing loss.* Researchers fear an epidemic of hearing loss in the future. The popularity of iPod and other MP3 devices has increased the risks for hearing loss. Maximum volume on one of these devices is 120 decibels, equal to a live concert or sporting event and just lower than a jet engine or sound of a gun shot.

Lab 24A Assessing Factors That Influence Health, Wellness, and Fitness

| Name | | Section | | Date | |

Purpose: To assess the factors that relate to health, wellness, and fitness

Chart 1 ▶ Assessment Questionnaire: Factors That Influence Health, Wellness, and Fitness

Factor	Very True	Somewhat True	Not True At All	Score
Heredity				
1. I have checked my family history for medical problems.	③	②	①	
2. I have taken steps to overcome hereditary predispositions.	③	②	①	
			Heredity Score =	
Health Care				
3. I have health insurance.	③	②	①	
4. I get regular medical exams and have my own doctor.	③	②	①	
5. I get treatment early, rather than waiting until problems get serious	③	②	①	
6. I carefully investigate my health problems before making decisions.	③	②	①	
			Health-Care Score =	
Environment				
7. My physical environment is healthy.	③	②	①	
8. My social environment is healthy.	③	②	①	
9. My spiritual environment is healthy.	③	②	①	
10. My intellectual environment is healthy.	③	②	①	
11. My work environment is healthy.	③	②	①	
12. My environment fosters healthy lifestyles.	③	②	①	
			Environment Score =	
Lifestyles				
13. I am physically active on a regular basis.	③	②	①	
14. I eat well.	③	②	①	
15. I use effective techniques for managing stress.	③	②	①	
16. I avoid destructive behaviors.	③	②	①	
17. I practice safe sex.	③	②	①	
18. I manage my time effectively.	③	②	①	
19. I evaluate information carefully and am an informed consumer.	③	②	①	
20. My personal health habits are good.	③	②	①	
21. My safety habits are good.	③	②	①	
22. I know first aid and can use it if needed.	③	②	①	
			Lifestyles Score =	
Personal Actions and Interactions				
23. I collect and evaluate information before I act.	③	②	①	
24. I plan before I take action.	③	②	①	
25. I am good about taking action when I know it is good for me.	③	②	①	
26. I honor my beliefs and relationships.	③	②	①	
27. I seek help when I need it.	③	②	①	
			Personal Actions/Interactions Score =	

Procedures

1. Answer each of the questions in Chart 1 on page 477. Consider the information in this concept as you answer each question.
2. Calculate the scores for heredity (sum items 1 and 2), health care (sum items 3–6), environment (sum items 7–12), lifestyles (sum items 13–22), and actions/interactions (sum items 23–27).
3. Determine ratings for each of the scores using the Rating Chart.
4. Record your scores and ratings in the Results chart. Record your comments in the Conclusions and Implications section.

Results

Factor	Score	Rating
Heredity		
Health care		
Environment		
Lifestyles		
Actions/interactions		

Rating Chart

Factor	Healthy	Marginal	Needs Attention
Heredity	6	4–5	Below 4
Health care	11–12	9–10	Below 9
Environment	16–18	13–15	Below 13
Lifestyles	26–30	20–25	Below 20
Actions/interactions	13–15	10–12	Below 10

Conclusions and Implications

1. In the space below, discuss your scores for the five factors (sums of several questions) identified in Chart 1. Use several sentences to identify specific areas that need attention and changes that you could make to improve.

2. For any individual item on Chart 1, a score of 1 is considered low. You might have a high score on a set of questions and still have a low score in one area that indicates a need for attention. In several sentences, discuss actions you could take to make changes related to individual questions.

Lab 24B Planning for Improved Health, Wellness, and Fitness

Name		Section	Date

Purpose: To plan to make changes in areas that can most contribute to improved health, wellness, and fitness

Procedures

1. Experts agree that it is best not to make too many changes all at once. Focusing attention on one or two things at a time will produce better results. Based on your assessments made in Lab 24A, select two areas in which you would like to make changes. Choose one from the list related to environments and health care and one related to lifestyle change. Place a check by those areas in Chart 1 in the Results section. Because Lab 24C is devoted to physical activity, it is not included in the list. You may want to make additional copies of this lab for future use in making other changes in the future.

2. Use Chart 2 to determine your Stage of Change for the changes you have identified. Since you have identified these as an area of need, it is unlikely that you would identify the stage of maintenance. If you are at maintenance, you can select a different area of changes that would be more useful.

3. In the appropriate locations, record the change you want to make related to your environment or health care. State your reasons, your specific goal(s), your written statement of the plan for change, and a statement about how you will self-monitor and evaluate the effectiveness of the changes made. In Chart 3, record similar information for the lifestyle change you identified.

Results

Chart 1 ▶

Check one in each column.

Area of Change	✔	Area of Change	✔
Health insurance		Eating well	
Medical checkups		Managing stress	
Selecting a doctor		Avoiding destructive habits	
Physical environment		Practicing safe sex	
Social environment		Managing time	
Spiritual environment		Becoming a better consumer	
Intellectual environment		Improving health habits	
Work environment		Improving safety habits	
Environment for lifestyles		Learning first aid	

Chart 2 ▶

List the two areas of change identified in Chart 1. Make a rating using the diagram at the right.

Identified Area of Change	Stage of Change Rating
1.	
2.	

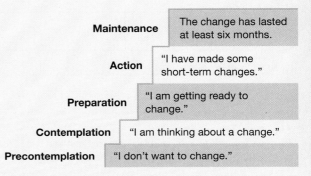

Maintenance — The change has lasted at least six months.

Action — "I have made some short-term changes."

Preparation — "I am getting ready to change."

Contemplation — "I am thinking about a change."

Precontemplation — "I don't want to change."

Note: Some of the areas identified in this lab relate to personal information. It is appropriate not to divulge personal information to others (including your instructor) if you choose not to. For this reason, you may choose not to address certain problems in this lab. You are encouraged to take steps to make changes independent of this assignment and to consult privately with your instructor to get assistance.

Chart 3 ▶ Making Changes for Improved Health, Wellness, and Fitness

Describe First Area of Change (from Chart 1)	**Describe Second Area of Change (from Chart 1)**
Step 1: State Reasons for Making Change	**Step 1: State Reasons for Making Change**

Step 2: Self-Assessment of Need for Change
List your stage from Chart 2.

Step 2: Self-Assessment of Need for Change
List your stage from Chart 2.

Step 3: State Your Specific Goals for Change
State several specific and realistic goals.

Step 3: State Your Specific Goals for Change
State several specific and realistic goals.

Step 4: Identify Activities or Actions for Change
List specific activities you will do or actions you will take to meet your goals.

Step 4: Identify Activities or Actions for Change
List specific activities you will do or actions you will take to meet your goals.

Step 5: Write a Plan; Include a Timetable
Expected start date:

Expected finish date:

Days of week and times: list times below days.

Mon.	Tue.	Wed.	Th.	Fri.	Sat.	Sun.

Location: where will you do the plan?

Step 5: Write a Plan; Include a Timetable
Expected start date:

Expected finish date:

Days of week and times: list times below days.

Mon.	Tue.	Wed.	Th.	Fri.	Sat.	Sun.

Location: where will you do the plan?

Step 6: Evaluate Your Plan
How will you self-monitor and evaluate to determine if the plan is working?

Step 6: Evaluate Your Plan
How will you self-monitor and evaluate to determine if the plan is working?

Lab 24C Planning Your Personal Physical Activity Program

Name	Section	Date

Purpose: To establish a comprehensive plan of lifestyle physical activity and to self-monitor progress in your plan (note: you may want to reread the concept on planning for physical activity before completing this lab)

Procedures

Step 1. Establishing Your Reasons

In the spaces provided below, list several of your principal reasons for doing a comprehensive activity plan.

1.	4.
2.	5.
3	6.

Step 2. Identify Your Needs Using Fitness Self-Assessments and Ratings of Stage of Change for Various Activities

In Chart 1, rate your fitness by placing an X over the circle by the appropriate rating for each part of fitness. Use your results obtained from previous labs or perform the self-assessments again to determine your ratings. If you took more than one self-assessment for one component of physical fitness, select the rating that you think best describes your true fitness for that fitness component. If you were unable to do a self-assessment for some reason, check the "No Results" circle.

Chart 1 ▶ Rating for Self-Assessments

	Rating				
Health-Related Fitness Tests	High-Performance Zone	Good Fitness Zone	Marginal Zone	Low Zone	No Results
1. Cardiovascular: 12-minute run (Chart 6, page 127)	○	○	○	○	○
2. Cardiovascular: step test (Chart 2, page 125)	○	○	○	○	○
3. Cardiovascular: bicycle test (Chart 5, page 127)	○	○	○	○	○
4. Cardiovascular: walking test (Chart 1, page 125)	○	○	○	○	○
5. Cardiovascular: swim test (Chart 7, page 128)	○	○	○	○	○
6. Flexibility: sit-and-reach test (Chart 1, page 168)	○	○	○	○	○
7. Flexibility: shoulder flexibility (Chart 1, page 168)	○	○	○	○	○
8. Flexibility: hamstring/hip flexibility (Chart 1, page 168)	○	○	○	○	○
9. Flexibility: trunk rotation (Chart 1, page 168)	○	○	○	○	○
10. Strength: isometric grip (Chart 3, page 204)	○	○	○	○	○
11. Strength: 1 RM upper body (Chart 2, page 203)	○	○	○	○	○

Chart 1 ▶ Rating for Self-Assessments, *continued*

Health-Related Fitness Tests	Rating				
	High-Performance Zone	Good Fitness Zone	Marginal Zone	Low Zone	No Results
12. Strength: 1 RM lower body (Chart 2, page 203)	○	○	○	○	○
13. Muscular endurance: curl-up (Chart 4, page 204)	○	○	○	○	○
14. Muscular endurance: 90-degree push-up (Chart 4, page 204)	○	○	○	○	○
15. Muscular endurance: flexed arm support (Chart 5, page 204)	○	○	○	○	○
16. Fitness rating: skinfold (Chart 1, page 293)	○	○	○	○	○
17. Body mass index (Chart 7, page 295)	○	○	○	○	○

Skill-Related Fitness and Other Self-Assessments	Rating				
	High-Performance Zone	Good Fitness Zone	Marginal Zone	Low Zone	No Results
1. Agility (Chart 1, page 267)	○	○	○	○	○
2. Balance (Chart 2, page 268)	○	○	○	○	○
3. Coordination (Chart 3, page 268)	○	○	○	○	○
4. Power (Chart 4, page 269)	○	○	○	○	○
5. Reaction time (Chart 5, page 269)	○	○	○	○	○
6. Speed (Chart 6, page 270)	○	○	○	○	○
7. Fitness of the back (Chart 2, page 244)	○	○	○	○	○
8. Posture (Chart 2, page 247)	○	○	○	○	○

Summarize Your Fitness Ratings Using the Results Above	Rating				
	High-Performance Zone	Good Fitness Zone	Marginal Zone	Low Zone	No Results
Cardiovascular	○	○	○	○	○
Endurance	○	○	○	○	○
Strength	○	○	○	○	○
Flexibility	○	○	○	○	○
Body fatness	○	○	○	○	○
Skill-related fitness	○	○	○	○	○
Posture and fitness of the back	○	○	○	○	○

Rate your stage of change for each of the different types of activities from the physical activity pyramid. Make an X over the circle beside the stage that best represents your behavior for each of the five types of activity in the lower three levels of the pyramid. A description of the various stages is provided below to help you make your ratings.

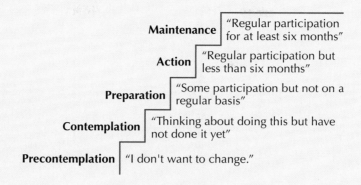

Maintenance "Regular participation for at least six months"

Action "Regular participation but less than six months"

Preparation "Some participation but not on a regular basis"

Contemplation "Thinking about doing this but have not done it yet"

Precontemplation "I don't want to change."

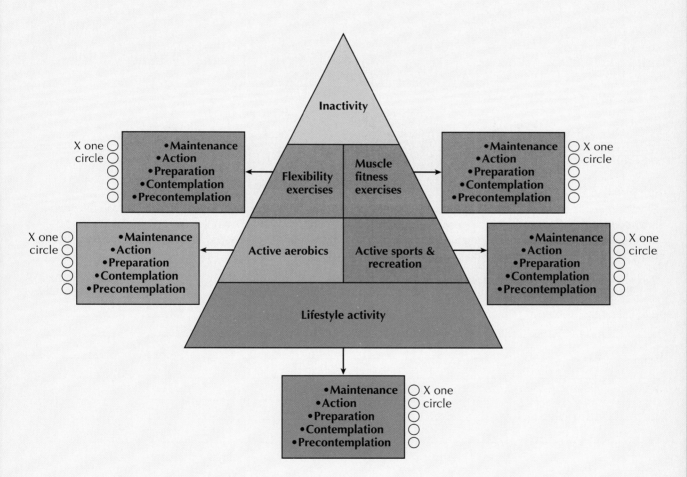

In step 1, you wrote down some general reasons for developing your physical activity plan. Setting goals requires more specific statements of goals that are realistic and achievable. For people who are at the contemplation or preparation stage for a specific type of activity, it is recommended that you write only short-term physical activity goals (no more than 4 weeks). Those at the action or maintenance level may choose short-term goals to start with or, if you have a good history of adherence, choose long-term goals (longer than 4 weeks). Precontemplators are not considered because they would not be doing this activity.

Step 3. Set Specific Goals

Chart 2 ▶ Setting Goals

Physical Activity Goals. Place an X over the appropriate circle for the number of days of the week and the number of weeks for each type of activity. Write the number of exercises or activities you plan in each of the five areas.

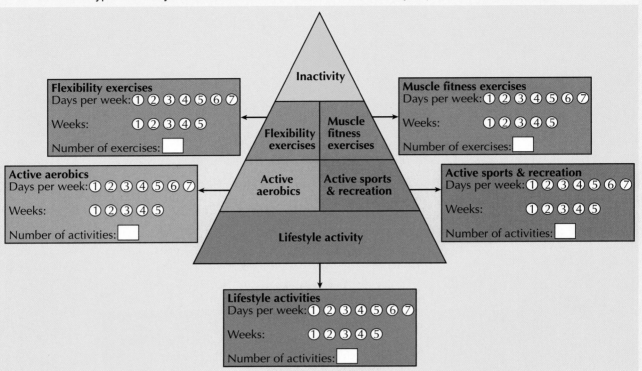

Physical Fitness Goals (for People at Action or Maintenance Only). Write specific physical fitness goals in the spaces provided below. Indicate when you expect to accomplish the goal (in weeks). Examples include improving the 12-minute run to a specific score, being able to perform a specific number of push-ups, attaining a specific BMI, and being able to achieve a specific score on a flexibility test.

Part of Fitness	Description of Specific Performance	Weeks to Goal

Step 4. Selecting Activities

In Chart 3, indicate the specific activities you plan to perform from each area of the physical activity pyramid. If the activity you expect to perform is listed, note the number of minutes or reps/sets you plan to perform. If the activity you want to perform is not listed, write the name of the activity or exercise in the space designated as "Other." For lifestyle activities, active aerobics, and active sports and recreation, indicate the length of time the activity will be performed each day. For flexibility, muscle fitness exercises, and exercises for back and neck, indicate the number of repetitions for each exercise.

Chart 3 ▶ Lifetime Physical Activity Selections

✔	Lifestyle Activities	Min./Day	✔	Active Aerobics	Min./Day	✔	Active Sports and Recreation	Min./Day
	Walking			Aerobic exercise machines			Basketball	
	Yard work			Bicycling			Bowling	
	Active housework			Circuit training or calisthenics			Golf	
	Gardening			Dance or step aerobics			Karate/judo	
	Social dancing			Hiking or backpacking			Mountain climbing	
	Occupational activity			Jogging or running (or walking)			Racquetball	
	Wheeling in wheelchair			Skating/cross-country skiing			Skating	
	Bicycling to work or store			Swimming			Softball	
	Other:			Water activity			Skiing	
	Other:			Other:			Soccer	
	Other:			Other:			Volleyball	
	Other:			Other:			Other:	
	Other:			Other:			Other:	
	Other:			Other:			Other:	
	Other:			Other:			Other:	

✔	Flexibility Exercises	Reps/Sets	✔	Muscle Fitness Exercises	Reps/Sets	✔	Exercises for Back and Neck	Reps/Sets
	Calf stretch			Bench or seated press			Back saver stretch	
	Hip and thigh stretch			Biceps curl			Single knee to chest	
	Sitting stretch			Triceps curl			Low back stretch	
	Hamstring stretch			Lat pull down			Hip/thigh stretch	
	Back stretch (leg hug)			Seated rowing			Pelvic tilt	
	Trunk twist			Wrist curl			Bridging	
	Pectoral stretch			Knee extension			Wall slide	
	Arm stretch			Heel raise			Pelvic stabilizer	
	Other:			Half-squat skiing			Neck rotation	
	Other:			Lunge			Isometric neck exercise	
	Other:			Toe press			Chin tuck	
	Other:			Crunch or reverse curl			Trapezius stretch	
	Other:			Other:			Other:	
	Other:			Other:			Other:	
	Other:			Other:			Other:	

Step 5. Preparing a Written Plan

In Chart 4, place a check in the shaded boxes for each activity you will perform for each day you will do it. Indicate the time of day you expect to perform the activity or exercise (Example: 7:30 to 8 A.M. or 6 to 6:30 P.M.). In the spaces labeled "Warm-Up Exercises" and "Cool-Down Exercises," check the warm-up and cool-down exercises you expect to perform. Indicate the number of reps you will use for each exercise.

Chart 4 ▶ My Physical Activity Plan

✔ Monday	Time	✔ Tuesday	Time	✔ Wednesday	Time
Lifestyle activity		Lifestyle activity		Lifestyle activity	
Active aerobics		Active aerobics		Active aerobics	
Active sports/rec.		Active sports/rec.		Active sports/rec.	
Flexibility exercises*		Flexibility exercises*		Flexibility exercises*	
Muscle fitness exercises*		Muscle fitness exercises*		Muscle fitness exercises*	
Back/neck exercises*		Back/neck exercises*		Back/neck exercises*	
Warm-up exercises		Warm-up exercises		Warm-up exercises	
Other:		Other:		Other:	

✔ Thursday	Time	✔ Friday	Time	✔ Saturday	Time
Lifestyle activity		Lifestyle activity		Lifestyle activity	
Active aerobics		Active aerobics		Active aerobics	
Active sports/rec.		Active sports/rec.		Active sports/rec.	
Flexibility exercises*		Flexibility exercises*		Flexibility exercises*	
Muscle fitness exercises*		Muscle fitness exercises*		Muscle fitness exercises*	
Back/neck exercises*		Back/neck exercises*		Back/neck exercises*	
Warm-up exercises		Warm-up exercises		Warm-up exercises	
Other:		Other:		Other:	

✔ Sunday	Time	✔ Warm-Up Exercises	Reps	✔ Cool-Down Exercises	Reps
Lifestyle activity		Walk or jog 1–2 min.		Walk or jog 1–2 min.	
Active aerobics		Calf stretch		Calf stretch	
Active sports/rec.		Hamstring stretch		Hamstring stretch	
Flexibility exercises*		Leg hug		Leg hug	
Muscle fitness exercises*		Sitting side stretch		Sitting side stretch	
Back/neck exercises*		Zipper		Zipper	
Warm-up exercises		Other:		Other:	
Other:		Other:		Other:	

*Perform the specific exercises you checked in Chart 3.

Step 6. Keeping Records of Progress and Evaluating Your Plan

Make copies of Chart 4 (one for each week that you plan to keep records). Each day, make a check by the activities you actually performed. Include the times when you actually did the activities in your plan. Periodically check your goals to see if they have been accomplished. At some point, it will be necessary to reestablish your goals and create a revised activity plan.

Results

After performing your plan for a specific period of time, answer the question in the space provided.

How long have you been performing the plan?

Conclusions and Implications

1. In several sentences, discuss your adherence to the plan. Have you been able to stick with the plan? If so, do you think it is a plan you can do for a lifetime? If not, why do you think you are unable to do your plan?

2. In several sentences, discuss how you might modify your plan in the future.

3. In several sentences, discuss your goals for your program. Do you think you will meet your goals? Why or why not?

Appendix A
Metric Conversion Charts

Chart 1 ▶ Traditional/Metric Measurement Conversions

	Metrics to Traditional	Traditional to Metrics
Length	centimeters to inches: cm × .39 = 1 in.	inches to centimeters: in. × 2.54 = cm
	meters to feet: m × 3.3 = ft.	feet to meters: ft. × .3048 = m
	meters to yards: m × 1.09 = yd.	yards to meters: yd. × 0.92 = m
	kilometers to miles: km × 0.6 = mi.	miles to kilometers: mi. × 1.6 = km
Weight (Mass)	grams to ounces: g × 0.0352 = oz.	ounces to grams: oz. × 28.41 = g
	kilograms to pounds: kg × 2.2 = lb.	pounds to kilograms: lb. × 0.45 = kg
Volume	milliliters to fluid ounces: ml × 0.03 = fl. oz.	fluid ounces to milliliters: fl. oz. × 29.573 = ml
	liters to quarts: l × 1.06 = qt.	quarts to liters: qt. × 0.95 = l
	liters to gallons: l × 0.264 = gal.	gallons to liters: gal. × 3.8 = l

Chart 2 ▶ 12-Minute Run Test (Scores in Meters)

	Men (Age)			
Classification	17–26	27–39	40–49	50+
High-performance zone	2,880+	2,560+	2,400+	2,240+
Good fitness zone	2,480–2,779	2,320–2,559	2,240–2,399	2,000–2,239
Marginal zone	2,160–2,479	2,080–2,319	2,000–2,239	1,760–1,999
Low zone	<2,160	<2,080	<2,000	<1,760

	Women (Age)			
Classification	17–26	27–39	40–49	50+
High-performance zone	2,320+	2,160+	2,000+	1,840+
Good fitness zone	2,000–2,319	1,920–2,159	1,840–1,999	1,680–1,839
Marginal zone	1,840–1,999	1,680–1,919	1,600–1,839	1,520–1,679
Low zone	<1,840	<1,680	<1,600	<1,520

Chart 3 ▶ 12-Minute Swim Rating Chart (Scores in Meters)

	Men (Age)			
Classification	17–26	27–39	40–49	50+
High-performance zone	644+	598+	552+	506+
Good fitness zone	552–643	506–597	460–551	413–505
Marginal zone	460–551	414–505	368–459	322–412
Low zone	<460	<414	<368	<322

	Women (Age)			
Classification	17–26	27–39	40–49	50+
High-performance zone	552+	506+	460+	414+
Good fitness zone	460–551	414–505	367–459	321–413
Marginal zone	367–459	321–413	276–366	230–320
Low zone	<367	<321	<276	<230

Chart 4 ▶ Isometric Strength Rating Scale (kg)

Classification	Men			Women		
	Left Grip	Right Grip	Total Score	Left Grip	Right Grip	Total Score
High-performance zone	57+	61+	118+	34+	39+	73+
Good fitness zone	45–56	50–60	95–117	27–33	32–38	59–72
Marginal zone	41–44	43–49	84–94	20–26	23–31	43–58
Low zone	<41	<43	<84	<20	<23	<43

Suitable for use by young adults between 18 and 30 years of age. After 30, an adjustment of 0.5 of 1 percent per year is appropriate because some loss of muscle tissue typically occurs as you grow older.

Chart 5 ▶ Power Rating Scale

Classification	Men	Women
Excellent	68 cm+	60 cm+
Very good	53–67 cm	48–59 cm
Good	42–52 cm	37–47 cm
Fair	31–41 cm	27–36 cm
Poor	<32 cm	<27 cm

Chart 6 ▶ Reaction Time Rating Scale

Classification	Score in Inches	Score in Centimeters
Excellent	>21	>52
Very good	19″–21	48–52
Good	16″–18 ¾	41–47
Fair	13″–15 ¾	33–40
Poor	<13	<33

Chart 7 ▶ Speed Rating Scale

Classification	Men		Women	
	Yards	Meters	Yards	Meters
Excellent	24+	22+	22+	20+
Very good	22–23	20–21.9	20–21	18–19.9
Good	18–21	16.5–19.9	16–19	14.5–17.9
Fair	16–17	14.5–16.4	14–15	13–14.4
Poor	<16	<14.5	<14	<13

Appendix B

Calorie, Fat, Saturated Fat, Cholesterol, and Sodium Content of Selected Fast-Food Items

Burger King	Calories	Total Fat	Sat. Fat	Chol.	Sodium
Hamburger	320	14	7	45	530
Whopper Jr.	410	23	8	50	520
Whopper	680	39	13	80	940
Chicken sandwich	660	39	11	70	1,330
Double cheeseburger	570	34	19	110	1,020
Bacon double cheeseburger	780	47	19	105	1,390
Double whopper	920	57	22	150	1,020
Double whopper with cheese	1,020	65	27	170	1,460
Fries (small—2.25 oz.)	230	11	60	0	530
Fries (medium—4 oz.)	360	18	10	0	690
Fries (large—5.5 oz.)	500	25	13	0	940
Fries (king—6 oz.)	600	30	16	0	1,140
Onion rings (medium—3.5 oz.)	320	16	8	0	460
Onion rings (king—5.5 oz.)	550	27	13	0	N/A
Coca-Cola classic (small—16 oz.)	160	0	0	0	N/A
Coca-Cola classic (med.—22 oz.)	230	0	0	0	N/A
Coca-Cola classic (large—32 oz.)	330	0	0	0	N/A
Coca-Cola classic (king—42 oz.)	430	0	0	0	N/A
Shake (medium—14 oz.)	460	8	5	30	320
Apple pie	340	14	6	0	470
Sundae pie	310	18	15	10	140

Taco Bell	Calories	Total Fat	Sat. Fat	Chol.	Sodium
Chicken fiesta burrito	370	12	4	35	1,000
Bean burrito	370	12	4	10	1,080
Chili cheese burrito	330	13	5	24	900
Chicken burrito supreme	410	16	6	45	1,120
Steak burrito supreme	420	16	6	35	1,140
7-layer burrito	520	22	7	25	1,270
Grilled stuft chicken burrito	690	29	8	70	1,900
Grilled stuft steak burrito	690	30	8	60	1,970
Chicken chalupa nacho cheese	350	19	5	25	640
Chicken chalupa baja	400	24	5	40	660
Beef chalupa nacho cheese	370	22	6	25	740
Steak chalupa baja	400	24	6	30	680
Chicken gordita supreme	300	13	5	45	530
Steak gordita supreme	300	14	5	35	550
Beef gordita supreme	300	14	5	35	550
Chicken soft taco	190	7	3	35	480
Beef soft taco	210	10	4	30	570
Steak soft taco	280	17	4	35	630
Taco supreme	260	16	6	40	350
Double decker taco supreme	420	21	8	40	760
Pintos and cheese	180	8	4	15	640
Nachos	320	18	4	5	560
Nachos supreme	440	24	7	35	800
Nachos bell grande	760	39	11	35	1,300
Chicken quesadilla	540	30	12	80	1,270
Taco salad with salsa	850	52	14	70	2,250
Shake (large—32 oz.)	1,010	29	19	115	530
Cola (small—16 oz.)	100	0	0	0	10
Cola (medium—20 oz.)	130	0	0	0	10

McDonald's	Calories	Total Fat	Sat. Fat	Chol.	Sodium
Hamburger	280	10	4	30	590
Fillet o-fish	470	26	5	50	890
Crispy chicken	550	27	5	50	1,180
Cheeseburger	330	14	6	50	830
Quarter pounder	430	21	8	70	840
Big Mac	590	34	11	85	1,090
Quarter pounder with cheese	590	30	13	95	1,310
French fries (small—2.5 oz.)	210	10	3	0	140
French fries (medium—5 oz.)	450	22	8	0	290
French fries (large—6 oz.)	540	26	9	0	350
French fries (supersize—7 oz.)	610	29	10	0	390
Grilled chicken caesar salad	100	3	2	40	240
Garden salad	100	6	3	75	120
Chef salad	150	8	4	95	740
Caesar dressing	150	13	3	10	400
Thousand island dressing	130	9	2	15	350
Honey mustard	160	11	2	15	260
Coca-Cola classic (small—16 oz.)	150	0	0	0	N/A
Coca-Cola classic (med.—21 oz.)	210	0	0	0	N/A
Coca-Cola classic (large—32 oz.)	310	0	0	0	N/A
Coca-Cola classic (supersize—42 oz.)	410	0	0	0	N/A
Shake (small—14 oz.)	360	9	6	40	230
Hot fudge sundae	340	12	9	30	170
McFlurry	610	22	14	75	250
Shake (large—32 oz.)	1,010	29	19	115	530

Wendy's	Calories	Total Fat	Sat. Fat	Chol.	Sodium
Grilled chicken sandwich	300	7	2	55	740
Spicy chicken sandwich	410	14	3	65	1,280
Chicken breast fillet sandwich	430	16	3	55	750
Chicken club sandwich	470	20	5	65	940
Jr. cheeseburger	310	12	6	45	800
Jr. cheeseburger deluxe	350	16	6	45	800
Jr. bacon cheeseburger	380	19	7	55	870
Classic single with everything	410	19	7	70	920
Big bacon classic	580	30	12	100	1,460
Classic double with everything	760	45	19	175	1,730
Classic triple with everything	1,030	65	29	245	2,280
Chicken nuggets	230	16	3	30	470
French fries (small—3 oz.)	270	13	4	0	90
French fries (med.—5 oz.)	420	20	6	0	130
French fries (biggie—5.5 oz.)	470	23	7	0	150
French fries (great biggie—6.5 oz.)	570	27	8	0	180
Plain baked potato	310	0	0	0	30
Chili	210	7	3	30	800
Broccoli and cheese potato	470	14	3	5	470
Bacon and cheese potato	530	17	4	25	820
Cola (small—16 oz.)	100	0	0	0	10
Cola (med.—20 oz.)	130	0	0	0	10
Cola (biggie—32 oz.)	210	0	0	0	20
Frosty (small)	170	4	3	20	100
Frosty (large)	330	8	5	35	200

Jacobson, M. F. and Hurley, J.

Appendix C
Calorie Guide to Common Foods

Beverages

Coffee (black)	0
Coke (12 oz.)	137
Hot chocolate, milk (1 cup)	247
Lemonade (1 cup)	100
Limeade, diluted to serve (1 cup)	110
Soda, fruit-flavored (12 oz.)	161
Tea (clear)	0

Breads and Cereals

Bagel (1 half)	76
Biscuit (2" × 2")	135
Bread, pita (1 oz.)	80
Bread, raisin ($^1/_2$" thick)	65
Bread, rye	55
Bread, white enriched ($^1/_2$" thick)	68
Bread, whole-wheat ($^1/_2$" thick)	67
Bun (hamburger)	120
Cereals, cooked ($^1/_2$ cup)	80
Corn flakes (1 cup)	96
Corn grits (1 cup)	125
Corn muffin (2$^1/_2$" diam.)	103
Crackers, graham (1 med.)	28
Crackers, soda (1 plain)	24
English muffin (1 half)	74
Macaroni, with cheese (1 cup)	464
Muffin, plain	135
Noodles (1 cup)	200
Oatmeal (1 cup)	150
Pancakes (1–4" diam.)	59
Pizza (1 section)	180
Popped corn (1 cup)	54
Potato chips (10 med.)	108
Pretzels (5 small sticks)	18
Rice (1 cup)	225
Roll, plain (1 med.)	118
Roll, sweet (1 med.)	178
Shredded wheat (1 med. biscuit)	79
Spaghetti, plain cooked (1 cup)	218
Tortilla (1 corn)	70
Waffle (4$^1/_2$" × 5")	216

Dairy Products

Butter, 1 pat (1$^1/_2$ tsp.)	50
Cheese, cheddar (1 oz.)	113
Cheese, cottage (1 cup)	270
Cheese, cream (1 oz.)	106
Cheese, Parmesan (1 tbsp.)	29
Cheese, Swiss natural (1 oz.)	105
Cream, sour (1 tbsp.)	31
Frozen custard (1 cup)	375
Frozen yogurt, vanilla (1 cup)	180
Ice cream, plain (prem.) (1 cup)	350
Ice cream soda, choc. (large glass)	455
Ice milk (1 cup)	184
Ices (1 cup)	177
Milk, chocolate (1 cup)	185
Milk, half-and-half (1 tbsp.)	20
Milk, malted (1 cup)	281
Milk, skim (1 cup)	88
Milk, skim dry (1 tbsp.)	28
Milk, whole (1 cup)	166
Sherbet (1 cup)	270
Softserve cone (med.)	335
Whipped topping (1 tbsp.)	14
Yogurt (1 cup)	150

Desserts and Sweets

Cake, angel (2" wedge)	108
Cake, chocolate (2" × 3" × 1")	150
Cake, plain (3" × 2$^1/_2$")	180
Chocolate, bar	200–300
Chocolate, bitter (1 oz.)	142
Chocolate, sweet (1 oz.)	133
Chocolate, syrup (1 tbsp.)	42
Cocoa (1 tbsp.)	21
Cookies, plain (1 med.)	75
Custard, baked (1 cup)	283
Donut (1 large)	250
Gelatin, dessert (1 cup)	155
Gelatin, with fruit (1 cup)	170
Gingerbread (2" × 2" × 2")	180
Jams, jellies (1 tbsp.)	55
Pie, apple ($^1/_7$ of 9" pie)	345
Pie, cherry ($^1/_7$ of 9" pie)	355
Pie, chocolate ($^1/_7$ of 9" pie)	360
Pie, coconut ($^1/_7$ of 9" pie)	266
Pie, lemon meringue ($^1/_7$ of 9" pie)	302
Sugar, granulated (1 tsp.)	27
Syrup, table (1 tbsp.)	57

Fruit

Apple, fresh (med.)	76
Applesauce, unsweetened (1 cup)	184
Avocado, raw ($^1/_2$ peeled)	279
Banana, fresh (med.)	88
Cantaloupe, raw ($^1/_2$, 5" diam.)	60
Cherries (10 sweet)	50
Cranberry sauce, unsweetened (1 tbsp.)	25
Fruit cocktail, canned (1 cup)	170
Grapefruit, fresh ($^1/_2$)	60
Grapefruit juice, raw (1 cup)	95
Grape juice, bottled ($^1/_2$ cup)	80
Grapes (20–25)	75
Nectarine (1 med.)	88
Olives, green	72
Olives, ripe (10)	105
Orange, fresh (med.)	60
Orange juice, frozen diluted (1 cup)	110
Peach, fresh (med.)	46
Peach, canned in syrup (2 halves)	79
Pear, fresh (med.)	95
Pears, canned in syrup (2 halves)	79
Pineapple, crushed in syrup (1 cup)	204
Pineapple ($^1/_2$ cup fresh)	50
Prune juice (1 cup)	170
Raisins, dry (1 tbsp.)	26
Strawberries, fresh (1 cup)	54
Strawberries, frozen (3 oz.)	90
Tangerine (2$^1/_2$" diam.)	40
Watermelon, wedge (4" × 8")	120

Meat, Fish, Eggs

Bacon, drained (2 slices)	97
Bacon, Canadian (1 oz.)	62
Beef, hamburger chuck (3 oz.)	316
Beef pot pie	560
Beef steak, sirloin or T-bone (3 oz.)	257
Beef and vegetable stew (1 cup)	185
Chicken, fried breast (8 oz.)	210
Chicken, fried (1 leg and thigh)	305
Chicken, roasted breast (2 slices)	100
Chili, with meat (1 cup)	510
Chili, with beans (1 cup)	335
Egg, boiled	77
Egg, fried	125
Egg, scrambled	100
Fish and chips (2 pcs. fish; 4 oz. chips)	275
Fish, broiled (3" × 3" × $^1/_2$")	112
Fish stick	40
Frankfurter, boiled	124
Ham (4" × 4")	338
Lamb (3 oz. roast, lean)	158
Liver (3" × 3")	150
Luncheon meat (2 oz.)	135
Pork chop, loin (3" × 5")	284
Salmon, canned (1 cup)	145
Sausage, pork (4 oz.)	510

Shrimp, canned (3 oz.)	108	**Sauces, Fats, Oils**		Cauliflower (1 cup)	25
Tuna, canned ($^1/_2$ cup)	185	Catsup, tomato (1 tbsp.)	17	Carrot, raw (med.)	21
Veal, cutlet (3" × 4")	175	Chili sauce (1 tbsp.)	17	Carrots, canned (1 cup)	44
		French dressing (1 tbsp.)	59	Celery, diced raw (1 cup)	20
Nuts and Seeds		Margarine (1 pat)	50	Coleslaw (1 cup)	102
Cashews (1 cup)	770	Mayonnaise (1 tbsp.)	92	Corn, sweet, canned (1 cup)	140
Coconut (1 cup)	450	Mayonnaise-type (1 tbsp.)	65	Corn, sweet (med. ear)	84
Peanut butter (1 tbsp.)	92	Vegetable, sunflower, safflower oils		Cucumber, raw (6 slices)	6
Peanuts, roasted, no skin (1 cup)	805	(1 tbsp.)	120	Lettuce (2 large leaves)	7
Pecans (1 cup)	752			Mushrooms, canned (1 cup)	28
Sunflower seeds (1 tbsp.)	50	**Soup, Ready-to-Serve** (1 Cup)		Onion, raw (med.)	25
		Bean	190	Onions, French fried (10 rings)	75
Sandwiches (2 Slices of White Bread)		Beef noodle	100	Peas, field ($^1/_2$ cup)	90
Bologna	214	Cream	200	Peas, green (1 cup)	145
Cheeseburger (small McDonald's)	300	Tomato	90	Pickles, dill (med.)	15
Chicken salad	185	Vegetable	80	Pickles, sweet (med.)	22
Egg salad	240	**Vegetables**		Potato, baked (med.)	97
Fish fillet (McDonald's)	400	Alfalfa sprouts ($^1/_2$ cup)	19	Potato, French fried (8 sticks)	155
Ham	360	Asparagus (6 spears)	22	Potato, mashed (1 cup)	185
Ham and cheese	360	Bean sprouts (1 cup)	37	Radish, raw (small)	1
Hamburger (small McDonald's)	260	Beans, green (1 cup)	27	Sauerkraut, drained (1 cup)	32
Hamburger, Burger King Whopper	600	Beans, lima (1 cup)	152	Spinach, fresh, cooked (1 cup)	46
Hamburger, Big Mac	550	Beans, navy (1 cup)	642	Squash, summer (1 cup)	30
Hamburger (McDonald's Quarter		Beans, pork and molasses (1 cup)	325	Sweet pepper (med.)	15
Pounder)	420	Broccoli, fresh, cooked (1 cup)	60	Sweet potato, candied (small)	314
Peanut butter	250	Cabbage, cooked (1 cup)	40	Tomato, cooked (1 cup)	50
Roast beef (Arby's Regular)	425			Tomato, raw (med.)	30

Note: The listing of foods above is intended as only a quick reference. The MyPyramid Web site provides a way to obtain detailed reports on the calorie content of your diet. Students are encouraged to consult the MyPyramid Web site at **www.mypyramid.gov**.

Appendix D

Calories of Protein, Carbohydrates, and Fats in Foods

Food No./Food Choice	Total Calories	Protein Calories	Carbohydrate Calories	Fat Calories	Food No./Food Choice	Total Calories	Protein Calories	Carbohydrate Calories	Fat Calories
Breakfast					*Lunch*				
1. Scrambled egg (1 lg.)	111	29	7	75	1. Hamburger (reg. FF[1])	255	48	120	89
2. Fried egg (1 lg.)	99	26	1	72	2. Cheeseburger (reg. FF)	307	61	120	126
3. Pancake (1-6)	146	19	67	58	3. Doubleburger (FF)	563	101	163	299
4. Syrup (1 T[4])	60	0	60	0	4. $1/4$ lb. burger (FF)	427	73	137	217
5. French toast (1 slice)	180	23	49	108	5. Doublecheese burger (FF)	670	174	134	362
6. Waffle (7-inch)	245	28	100	117	6. Doublecheese baconburger (FF)	724	138	174	340
7. Biscuit (medium)	104	8	52	44	7. Hot dog (FF)	214	36	54	124
8. Bran muffin (medium)	104	11	63	31	8. Chili dog (FF)	320	51	90	179
9. White toast (slice)	68	9	52	7	9. Pizza, cheese (slice FF)	290	116	116	58
10. Wheat toast (slice)	67	14	52	6	10. Pizza, meat (slice FF)	360	126	126	108
11. Peanut butter (1 T)	94	15	11	68	11. Pizza, everything (slice FF)	510	179	173	158
12. Yogurt (8 oz. plain)	227	39	161	27	12. Sandwich, roast beef (FF)	350	88	126	137
13. Orange juice (8 oz.)	114	8	100	6	13. Sandwich, bologna	313	44	106	163
14. Apple juice (8 oz.)	117	1	116	0	14. Sandwich, bologna-cheese	428	69	158	201
15. Soft drink (12 oz.)	144	0	144	0	15. Sandwich, ham-cheese (FF)	380	91	133	156
16. Bacon (2 slices)	86	15	2	70	16. Sandwich, peanut butter	281	39	118	124
17. Sausage (1 link)	141	11	0	130	17. Sandwich, PB and jelly	330	40	168	122
18. Sausage (1 patty)	284	23	0	261	18. Sandwich, egg salad	330	40	109	181
19. Grits (8 oz.)	125	11	110	4	19. Sandwich, tuna salad	390	101	109	180
20. Hash browns (8 oz.)	355	18	178	159	20. Sandwich, fish (FF)	432	56	147	229
21. French fries (reg.)	239	12	115	112	21. French fries (reg. FF)	239	12	115	112
22. Donut, cake	125	4	61	60	22. French fries (lg. FF)	406	20	195	191
23. Donut, glazed	164	8	87	69	23. Onion rings (reg. FF)	274	14	112	148
24. Sweet roll	317	22	136	159	24. Chili (8 oz.)	260	49	62	148
25. Cake (medium slice)	274	14	175	85	25. Bean soup (8 oz.)	355	67	181	107
26. Ice cream (8 oz.)	257	15	108	134	26. Beef noodle soup (8 oz.)	140	32	59	49
27. Cream cheese (T)	52	4	1	47	27. Tomato soup (8 oz.)	180	14	121	45
28. Jelly (T)	49	0	49	0	28. Vegetable soup (8 oz.)	160	21	107	32
29. Jam (T)	54	0	54	0	29. Small salad, plain	37	6	27	4
30. Coffee (cup)	0	0	0	0	30. Small salad, French dressing	152	8	50	94
31. Tea (cup)	0	0	0	0	31. Small salad, Italian dressing	162	8	28	126
32. Cream (T)	32	2	2	28	32. Small salad, bleu cheese	184	13	28	143
33. Sugar (t)	15	0	15	0	33. Potato salad (8 oz.)	248	27	159	62
34. Corn flakes (8 oz.)	97	8	87	2	34. Cole slaw (8 oz.)	180	0	25	155
35. Wheat flakes (8 oz.)	106	12	90	4	35. Macaroni and cheese (8 oz.)	230	37	103	90
36. Oatmeal (8 oz.)	132	19	92	21	36. Beef taco (FF)	186	59	56	71
37. Strawberries (8 oz.)	55	4	46	5	37. Bean burrito (FF)	343	45	192	106
38. Orange (medium)	64	6	57	1	38. Meat burrito (FF)	466	158	196	112
39. Apple (medium)	96	1	86	9	39. Mexican rice (FF)	213	17	160	36
40. Banana (medium)	101	4	95	2	40. Mexican beans (FF)	168	42	82	44
41. Cantaloupe (half)	82	7	73	2	41. Fried chicken breast (FF)	436	262	13	161
42. Grapefruit (half)	40	2	37	1	42. Broiled chicken breast	284	224	0	60
43. Custard pie (slice)	285	20	188	77	43. Broiled fish	228	82	32	114
44. Fruit pie (slice)	350	14	259	77	44. Fish stick (1 stick FF)	50	18	8	24
45. Fritter (medium)	132	11	54	67	45. Fried egg	99	26	1	72
46. Skim milk (8 oz.)	88	36	52	0	46. Donut	125	4	61	60
47. Whole milk (8 oz.)	159	33	48	78	47. Potato chips (small bag)	115	3	39	73
48. Butter (pat)	36	0	0	36	48. Soft drink (12 oz.)	144	0	144	0
49. Margarine (pat)	36	0	0	36					

The principal reference for the calculation of values used in this appendix was the *Nutritive Value of Foods*, published by the United States Department of Agriculture, Washington, DC, Home and Gardens Bulletin, No. 72, although other published sources were consulted, including Jacobson, M., and S. Fritschner. *The Fast-Food Guide* (an excellent source of information about fast foods). New York: Workman.

Notes:

1. FF by a food indicates that it is typical of a food served in a fast food restaurant.
2. Your portions of foods may be larger or smaller than those listed here. For this reason, you may wish to select a food more than once (e.g., two hamburgers) or select only a portion of a serving (i.e., divide the calories in half for a half portion).
3. An oz. equals 28.35 grams.
4. T = tablespoon and t = teaspoon.

Food No./Food Choice	Total Calories	Protein Calories	Carbohydrate Calories	Fat Calories
49. Apple juice (8 oz.)	117	1	116	0
50. Skim milk (8 oz.)	88	36	52	0
51. Whole milk (8 oz.)	159	33	48	78
52. Diet drink (12 oz.)	0	0	0	0
53. Mustard (t)	4	0	4	0
54. Catsup (t)	6	0	6	0
55. Mayonnaise (T)	100	0	0	100
56. Fruit pie	350	14	259	77
57. Cheesecake (slice)	400	56	132	212
58. Ice cream (8 oz.)	257	15	108	134
59. Coffee (8 oz.)	0	0	0	0
60. Tea (8 oz.)	0	0	0	0

Dinner

Food No./Food Choice	Total Calories	Protein Calories	Carbohydrate Calories	Fat Calories
1. Hamburger (reg. FF)	255	48	120	89
2. Cheeseburger (reg. FF)	307	61	120	126
3. Doubleburger (FF)	563	101	163	299
4. $\frac{1}{4}$ lb. burger (FF)	427	73	137	217
5. Doublecheese burger (FF)	670	174	134	362
6. Doublecheese baconburger (FF)	724	138	174	412
7. Hot dog (FF)	214	36	54	124
8. Chili dog (FF)	320	51	90	179
9. Pizza, cheese (slice FF)	290	116	116	58
10. Pizza, meat (slice FF)	360	126	126	108
11. Pizza, everything (slice FF)	510	179	173	158
12. Steak (8 oz.)	880	290	0	590
13. French fried shrimp (6 oz.)	360	133	68	158
14. Roast beef (8 oz.)	440	268	0	172
15. Liver (8 oz.)	520	250	52	218
16. Corned beef (8 oz.)	493	242	0	251
17. Meat loaf (8 oz.)	711	228	35	448
18. Ham (8 oz.)	540	178	0	362
19. Spaghetti, no meat (13 oz.)	400	56	220	124
20. Spaghetti, meat (13 oz.)	500	115	230	155
21. Baked potato (medium)	90	12	78	0
22. Cooked carrots (8 oz.)	71	12	59	0
23. Cooked spinach (8 oz.)	50	18	18	14
24. Corn (1 ear)	70	10	52	8
25. Cooked green beans (8 oz.)	54	11	43	0
26. Cooked broccoli (8 oz.)	60	19	26	15
27. Cooked cabbage	47	12	35	0
28. French fries (reg. FF)	239	12	115	112
29. French fries (lg. FF)	406	20	195	191
30. Onion rings (reg. FF)	274	14	112	148
31. Chili (8 oz.)	260	49	62	148
32. Small salad, plain	37	6	27	4
33. Small salad, French dressing	152	8	50	94
34. Small salad, Italian dressing	162	8	28	126
35. Small salad, bleu cheese	184	13	28	143
36. Potato salad (8 oz.)	248	27	159	62
37. Cole slaw (8 oz.)	180	0	25	155
38. Macaroni and cheese (8 oz.)	230	37	103	90
39. Beef Taco (FF)	186	59	56	71
40. Bean burrito (FF)	343	45	192	106
41. Meat burrito (FF)	466	158	196	112
42. Mexican rice (FF)	213	17	160	36
43. Mexican beans (FF)	168	42	82	44
44. Fried chicken breast (FF)	436	262	13	161

Food No./Food Choice	Total Calories	Protein Calories	Carbohydrate Calories	Fat Calories
45. Broiled chicken breast	284	224	0	60
46. Broiled fish	228	82	32	114
47. Fish stick (1 stick FF)	50	18	8	24
48. Soft drink (12 oz.)	144	0	144	0
49. Apple juice (8 oz.)	117	1	116	0
50. Skim milk (8 oz.)	88	36	52	0
51. Whole milk (8 oz.)	159	33	48	78
52. Diet drink (12 oz.)	0	0	0	0
53. Mustard (t)	4	0	4	0
54. Catsup (t)	6	0	6	0
55. Mayonnaise (T)	100	0	0	100
56. Fruit pie (slice)	350	14	259	77
57. Cheesecake (slice)	400	56	132	212
58. Ice cream (8 oz.)	257	15	108	134
59. Custard pie (slice)	285	20	188	77
60. Cake (slice)	274	14	175	85

Snacks

Food No./Food Choice	Total Calories	Protein Calories	Carbohydrate Calories	Fat Calories
1. Peanut butter (1 T)	94	15	11	68
2. Yogurt (8 oz. plain)	227	39	161	27
3. Orange juice (8 oz.)	114	8	100	6
4. Apple juice (8 oz.)	117	1	116	0
5. Soft drink (12 oz.)	144	0	144	0
6. Donut, cake	125	4	61	60
7. Donut, glazed	164	8	87	69
8. Sweet roll	317	22	136	159
9. Cake (medium slice)	274	14	175	85
10. Ice cream (8 oz.)	257	15	108	134
11. Softserve cone (reg.)	240	10	89	134
12. Ice cream sandwich bar	210	40	82	88
13. Strawberries (8 oz.)	55	4	46	5
14. Orange (medium)	64	6	57	1
15. Apple (medium)	96	1	86	9
16. Banana (medium)	101	4	95	2
17. Cantaloupe (half)	82	7	73	2
18. Grapefruit (half)	40	2	37	1
19. Celery stick	5	2	3	0
20. Carrot (medium)	20	3	17	0
21. Raisins (4 oz.)	210	6	204	0
22. Watermelon (4" × 6" slice)	115	8	99	8
23. Chocolate chip cookie	60	3	9	48
24. Brownie	145	6	26	113
25. Oatmeal cookie	65	3	13	49
26. Sandwich cookie	200	8	112	80
27. Custard pie (slice)	285	20	188	77
28. Fruit pie (slice)	350	14	259	77
29. Gelatin (4 oz.)	70	4	32	34
30. Fritter (medium)	132	11	54	67
31. Skim milk (8 oz.)	88	36	52	0
32. Diet drink	0	0	0	0
33. Potato chips (small bag)	115	3	39	73
34. Roasted peanuts (1.3 oz.)	210	34	25	151
35. Chocolate candy bar (1 oz.)	145	7	61	77
36. Choc. almond candy bar (1 oz.)	265	38	74	164
37. Saltine cracker	18	1	1	16
38. Popped corn	40	7	33	0
39. Cheese nachos	471	63	194	214

Canada's Food Guide to Healthy Eating

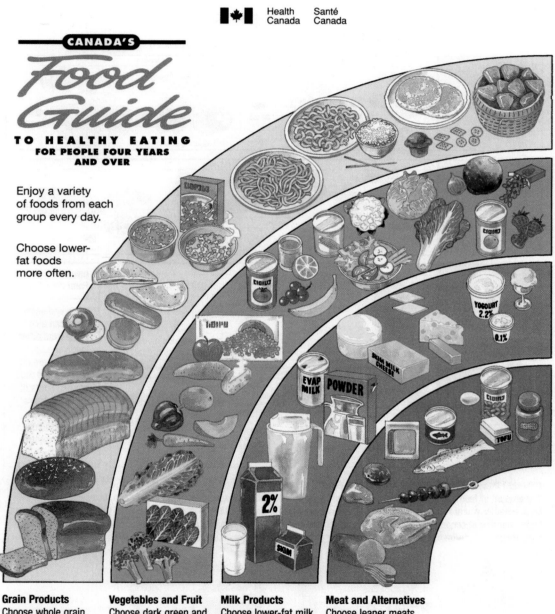

Health Canada — Santé Canada

CANADA'S

Food Guide

TO HEALTHY EATING
FOR PEOPLE FOUR YEARS
AND OVER

Enjoy a variety
of foods from each
group every day.

Choose lower-
fat foods
more often.

Grain Products
Choose whole grain
and enriched
products more often.

Vegetables and Fruit
Choose dark green and
orange vegetables and
orange fruit more often.

Milk Products
Choose lower-fat milk
products more often.

Meat and Alternatives
Choose leaner meats,
poultry and fish, as well
as dried peas, beans
and lentils more often.

Canada

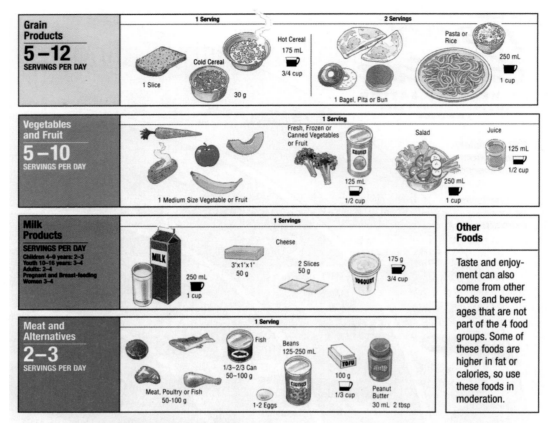

Different People Need Different Amounts of Food

The amount of food you need every day from the 4 food groups and other foods depends on your age, body size, activity level, whether you are male or female and if you are pregnant or breast-feeding. That's why the Food Guide gives a lower and higher number of servings for each food group. For example, young children can choose the lower number of servings, while male teenagers can go to the higher number. Most other people can choose servings somewhere in between.

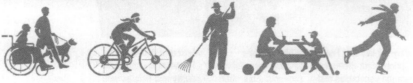

Consult *Canada's Physical Activity Guide to Healthy Active Living* to help you build physical activity into your daily life.

Enjoy eating well, being active and feeling good about yourself. That's VITALIT

© Minister of Public Works and Government Services Canada, 1997
Cat. No. H39-252/1992E   ISBN 0-662-19648-1
No changes permitted. Reprint permission not required.

Selected References

This list includes references new to the seventh edition of *Concepts of Fitness and Wellness*. For a complete listing of all references, visit the book's Online Learning Center at **www.mhhe.cm/corbin7e**.

ACSM. 2006. ACSM's Guidelines for Exercise Testing and Prescription. (7th ed.). Philadelphia: Lippencott, Williams & Wilkins.

Ahrens. R.W. and Snider, J. (2005). Alcohol manufacturers send their ads to college. *USA Today*, November 17.

Almond, C. S. D. et al. 2005. Hyponatremia among runners in the Boston Marathon. New *England Journal of Medicine*. 352(15):1550–1556.

American College Health Association. (2006). American College Health Association – *National College Health Assessment: Reference Group Data Report Fall 2005*. Baltimore, MD: American College Health Association.

American Health Association. 2005. American Heart Association Guidelines for Cardiopulmonary Resuscitation and Emergency Cardiovascular Care. *Circulation*. 112 (24 supplement):IV 1–203 (a series of articles).

American Heart Association. 2005. *Metabolic Syndrome*. Dallas, TX: American Heart Association. Available at www.americanheart.org/presenter. jhtml?identifier=4756

American Medical Association. (2006). Sex and intoxication among women more common on spring break according to AMA poll. Available at http://www.ama-assn.org/ama/pub/category/16083.html Accessed June, 6, 2006.

American Social Health Association. Fact Sheet on Herpes. Accessed online at http://www.ashastd.org/pdfs/Herpes_factsheet.pdf

Asplund, C. A. and D. L. Brown. 2005. The Running Shoe Prescription: Fit for Performance. The Physician and Sportsmedicine. 33(1):17–24.

Banks, J. et al. 2006. Disease and disadvantage in the United States and in England. Journal of the American Medical Association. 295(17):2037–2045.

Barrett, S. et al. 2007. Consumer Health: A Guide to Intelligent Decisions (8th ed.). New York: McGraw-Hill Higher Education. Chapter 18.

Becklake, M.R., Ghezzo, H., and Ernst, P. (2005). Childhood predictors of smoking in adolescence: A follow-up study of Montreal schoolchildren. *Canadian Medical Association Journal* 173:377–379

Bjartveit, K. and Tverdal, A. (2005). Health consequences of smoking 1–4 cigarettes per day. Tobacco Control 14:315–320.

Brannon, L. and J. Feist. 2006. Health Psychology - An Introduction to Behavior and Health 5th ed. Stamford, CT: Wadsworth.

Brennan, T. A. et al. 2006. Health industry practices that create conflicts of interest: A policy proposal for academic medical centers. *Journal of the American Medical Association*. 295(4):429–433.

Breslow, L. 2006. Health measurement in the third era of health. American Journal of Public Health. 96 (1):17–19.

Brown, W. J. et al. 2006. 10,000 steps Rockhampton: Evaluation of whole community approach to improving population levels of physical activity. Journal of Physical Activity and Health. 3(1):1–14.

Brownson, R. C. et al., 2005. Declining rates of physical activity in the United States: what are the contributors? Annual Review of Public Health. 26:421–443.

Bry, S. A. and H. A. Born. 2004. Transition to university and vigorous physical activity: Implications for health and psychological well-being. *Journal of American College Health*. 52(4):181–188.

Burgard, M. and Gallagher, K. I. 2006. Self-monitoring: Influencing effective behavior change in your clients. ACSM's Health and Fitness Journal. 10(1):14–19

Carney, P. A. et al. 2005. Utilization of screening mammography in New Hampshire. *Cancer*. 104(8):1726–1732.

Centers for Disease Control and Prevention. (2005). HIV/AIDS Surveillance Report, 2004. Vol. 16. Atlanta, GA: US Department of Health and Human Services.

Centers for Disease Control and Prevention. (2005). Sexually Transmitted Disease Surveillance, 2004. Atlanta, GA: U.S. Department of Health and Human Services.

Centers for Disease Control and Prevention. (2006). Expedited Partner Therapy in the Management of Sexually Transmitted Diseases. Atlanta, GA: US Department of Health and Human Services.

Centers for Disease Control and Prevention. Adult participation in recommended levels of physical activity—United States, 2001 and 2003 (2005). MMWR Morbidity and Mortality .Weekly.Report. (54):208–1212.

Chenoweth, D. et al. 2006. The cost of sloth: Using a tool to measure the cost of physical activity. ACSM's Health and Fitness Journal. 10(2):8–13.

Christou, D. D. et al. 2005. Fatness is a better predictor of cardiovascular disease risk factor profile than aerobic fitness in healthy men. Circulation. 111(15):1904–1914.

Clarke, B. 2006. 5 and 10K Training. Champaign. IL: Human Kinetics.

Clegg, D. O. et al. 2006. Glucosamine, chondroitin sulfate, and the two in combination for painful knee osteoarthritis. New England Journal of Medicine. 354(8):795–808.

Corbin, C. B. et al. 2004. Making sense of multiple physical activity recommendations. In Corbin, et al. Toward a Better Understanding of Physical Fitness and Activity, Selected Topics, Volume II. Scottsdale, AZ: Holcomb Hathaway Publishers, pp. 37–46.

Corbin, C. B., et al. 2004. Definitions: Health, Fitness and Physical Activity. In Corbin, et al. Toward a Better Understanding of Physical Fitness and Activity, Selected Topics, Volume II. Scottsdale, AZ: Holcomb Hathaway Publishers.

Corbin, C. B., et al. 2004. Toward a uniform definition of wellness: A commentary. In Corbin, et al. Toward a Better Understanding of Physical Fitness and Activity, Selected Topics, Volume II. Scottsdale, AZ: Holcomb Hathaway Publishers.

Crespo, C. J. 2005. Physical activity in minority populations: Overcoming a health challenge. President's Council on Physical Fitness and Sports Research Digest. 6(2):1–8.

Dannenberg, A. C., et al. 2005. Assessing the walkability in the workplace: A new audit tool. American Journal of Health Promotion. (5):39–44.

Department of Health and Human Services. 2005. Summary of health statistics for US adults: National Health Interview Survey. Vital and Health Statistics. 10 (228):1–282.

Federal Interagency Forum on Age-Related Statistics. 2004. Older Americans 2004: Key Indicators of Well-Being. Washington, DC: United States Government Printing Office. Also available at http://www.agingstats.gov/chartbook2004/default.htm

Flegal, K.M. et al. 2006. Excess deaths associated with underweight, overweight, and obesity. Journal of the American Medical Association. 293(15):1861–1867.

Frank, L. D., et al. 2005. Linking objectively measured physical activity with objectively measured urban form: findings from SMARTRAQ. American Journal of Preventive Medicine. 28 (2 Suppl):117–125.

Giddings, S. S. et al. 2005. American Heart Association; American Academy of Pediatrics. Dietary recommendations for children and adolescents: A guide for practitioners: Consensus statement of the American Heart Association. Circulation. 112, 2061–2075.

Gorman, C. and A. Park. 2005. New Heart Scanning Technology Could Save Your Life. Time 166(10):58–71.

Green, P. and Skinner, D. (2005). Does time management training work? An evaluation. International Journal of Training and Development 9: 124 139.

Greenberg, J. S. 2006. Comprehensive Stress Management (9th ed.). New York: McGraw-Hill.

Gulati, M. et al. 2005. The Prognostic value of a nomogram for exercise capacity in women. New England Journal of Medicine. 353(5):468–475.

Hahn, D. B. et al. 2007. Focus on Health (8th ed.). New York: McGraw-Hill Higher Education, Chapter 7.

Halpern-Felsher, B.L. et al. (2005). Oral versus vaginal sex among adolescents: Perceptions, Attitudes, and Behavior. Pediatrics 115:845–851.

Hamann, B. P. 2007. Disease: Identification, Prevention and Control (3rd. ed.). New York: McGraw-Hill Higher Education.

Harper, D.M. (2006). Sustained efficacy up to 4.5 years of a bivalent L1 virus-like particle vaccine against human papillomavirus types 16 and 18: follow-up from a randomised control trial. Lancet 367:1247–1255.

Helliker, K. (2006). Online counsel, discreet advice for drink woes. The Arizona Republic, March 12.

Hills, A. P. et al., 2006. Validation of the intensity of walking for pleasure in obese adults. Preventive Medicine. 42(1):47–50.

Howard, B.V., Manson, J.E., Stefanick, M.L., Beresford, S.A., Frank, G., Jones, B. et al. 2006. Low fat dietary pattern and weight change over 7 years. Journal of the American Medical Association, 295(1):39–49

Hultquist, C. N. et al. 2005. Comparison of walking recommendations in previously inactive women. Medicine and Science in Sport and Exercise. 37(4):676–683.

Humpel, N. et al., 2004. Changes in neighborhood walking are related to changes in perceptions of environmental attributes. Annals of Behavioral Medicine. 27(1):60–67.

Iestra, J.A. et al. (2005). Effect size estimates of lifestyle and dietary changes on all-cause mortality in coronary artery disease patients: A systematic review. Circulation 112:924–934.

Ioannidis, J. P. A. 2005. Contradicted and initially stronger effects in highly cited clinical research. American Medical Association. 29(2):218–228.

Johnston, L.D. et al. (2006). Monitoring the Future National Results on Adolescent Drug Use: Overview of Key Findings (NIH Publication No. 06-5882). Bethesda, MD: National Institute on Drug Abuse.

Jones, A. Y., Dean, E., & Scudds, R. J. (2005). Effectiveness of a community-based Tai Chi program and implications for public health initiatives. Arch Phys. Med Rehabil., 86, 619–625.

Jurca, R. 2005. Assessing cardiorespiratory fitness without performing exercise testing. American Journal of Preventive Medicine. 29(3):185–193.

Jurca, R. et al. 2005. Physical activity and nontraditional CHD risk factors. President's Council on Physical Fitness and Sports Research Digest. 6(4):1–8.

Kinney, J. 2006. Loosening the Grip: A Handbook of Alcohol Information (8th ed.). New York: McGraw-Hill Higher Education.

Koch, W. (2005). 39% live in areas limiting smoking: Six more states pass restrictions in 2005. USA Today, December, 2005.

Kraemer, W. et al. 2005. Progression and resistance training. President's Council on Physical Fitness and Sports Research Digest. 6(3):1–8.

Ksir, C. J. et al. 2008. Drugs, Society, and Human Behavior (12th ed.). New York: McGraw-Hill Higher Education.

Kuiper, N. et al. (2005). State-specific prevalence of cigarette smoking and quitting among adults - United States, 2004. Morbidity and Mortality Weekly Reports 54:1124–1127.

Kuk, J.L. et al. 2006. Visceral fat is an independent predictor of all-cause mortality in men. Obesity Research 14:336–341.

Kushi, L. H., et al. (2006). American Cancer Society Guidelines on Nutrition and Physical Activity for Cancer Prevention: Reducing the Risk of Cancer With Healthy Food Choices and Physical Activity CA Cancer J Clinicians. 56(5):254–281

Lasser, K. E. et al. 2006. Access to care, health status, and health disparities in the United States and Canada: Results of a cross-national population-based survey. American Journal of Public Health. Published online May 30, ahead of print.

Leape, L. L. and D. M. Berwick. 2006. Five years after to err is human: What have we learned? Journal of the American Medical Association. 293(19): 2384–2390.

Levine JA, Lanningham-Foster LM, McCrady SK, Krizan AC, Olson LR, Kane

PH, Jensen MD, Clark MM. Interindividual variation in posture allocation: possible role in human obesity. Science 307:584–586, 2005.

Lichtenstein, A.H. et al. 2006. Diet and lifestyle recommendations Revision 2006. A Scientific Statement from the American Heart Association. Nutrition Committee. Circulation, 114:82–96

Manore, M. M. 2006. A nutritionist's view" Feeding the active male and female: Part III. *ACSM's Health and Fitness Journal.* 10(1):26–28.

Mao, C. et al. (2006). Efficacy of human papillomavirus-16 vaccine to prevent cervical intraepithelial neoplasia: A randomized controlled trial. Obstetrics and Gynecology 107:18–27.

Markel, H. 2005. Why America needs a strong FDA. Journal of the American Medical Association. 294(19)2489–2491.

Mattapallil, J.J. et al. (2006). Vaccination preserves CD4 memory T cells during acute simian immunodeficiency virus challenge. *Journal of Experimental Medicine* 203:1533–1541.

Mitchell, T. (2005). New hope for smokers: A promising new drug may help those who want to quit. *USA Today*, Dec. 23.

Montain, S. J. et al. 2006 Exercise associated hyponatraemia: quantitative analysis to understand the aetiology. *British Journal of Sports Medicine.* 40:98–105.

Moudon, A.V et al. 2006. Operational definitions of walkable neighborhood: Theoretical and empirical insights. Journal of Physical Activity and Health. 3(S1):S99–117.

Murtagh, E. M. et al., 2005. The effects of 60 minutes of brisk walking per week, accumulated in two different patterns, on cardiovascular risk. *Preventive Medicine.* 41(1):92–97.

Naimi, T.S. et al. (2005). Cardiovascular risk factors and confounders among nondrinking and moderate-drinking U.S. adults. *American Journal of Preventive Medicine* 28:369–373.

National Institutes of Health. 2006. Multivitamin/mineral supplements and chronic disease prevention: A draft report. Available online at http://consensus.nih.gov/2006/MVMDRAFT051706.pdf

National Institutes of Health. 2006. Multivitamin/mineral supplements and chronic disease prevention: A draft report. Available online at http://consensus.nih.gov/2006/MVMDRAFT051706.pdf

Noakes, T. D. 2006. Sports drinks: Prevention of "voluntary dehydration" and development of exercise-associated hyponatremia. Medicine & Science in Sports & Exercise. 38(1):193

O'Keefe, E. J. and D. S. Berger. 2007. Self-management for College Students: The ABC Approach (3rd ed.). Hyde Park, NY: Partridge Hill Publishers.

Ogden, C.L. et al., 2006 Prevalence of overweight and obesity in the United States, 1999–2004. Journal of the American Medical Association 293(13):1549–1555.

Peterson, J. et al. 2006. Differential effects of active living on quality of life at various levels of income. *Health Education Research.* 21(1):146–56.

Radley, D. C. et al. 2006. Off-label prescribing among office-based physicians. *Archives of Internal Medicine.* 166(9):1021–1026.

Raine, T.R. et al. (2005). Direct access to emergency contraception through pharmacies and effect on unintended pregnancy and STIs: A randomized controlled trial. *Journal of the American Medical Association* 293:54–62.

Rankinen, T. and Bouchard, C. 2004. Dose-response issues concerning relations between regular physical activity and health. In Corbin, et al. *Toward a Better Understanding of Physical Fitness and Activity, Selected Topics, Volume II.* Scottsdale, AZ: Holcomb Hathaway Publishers, pp. 73–80.

Riebe, R. et al. 2005. Long-term maintenance of exercise and healthy eating behaviors in overweight adults. Preventive Medicine. 40(6):769–778.

Roizen, M. F. and M. C. Oz. 2006. You The Smart Patient: An Insider's Handbook for Getting the Best Treatment. New York: Free Press.

Romas, J. A. and M. Sharma. 2007. Practical Stress Management: A Comprehensive Workbook for Managing Change and Promoting Health (4th ed.). San Francisco: Benjamin Cummings.

Sallis, J. F., et al. 2005. An Ecological Approach to Creating Active Living Communities. *Annual Review of Public Health.*

Sanders, G.D. et al. (2005). Cost-effectiveness of screening for HIV in the era of highly active antiretroviral therapy. *New England Journal of Medicine* 352:570–585.

Schmidt, R. & Lee, T. 2005. Motor Control and Learning, 4th ed. Champaign. IL: Human Kinetics.

Sherman, K.J. et al., 2005. Comparing yoga, exercise, and a self-care book for chronic low back pain: a randomized, controlled trial. Annals of Internal Medicine 143(12):849–56.

Shiner, J. et al. 2005. Integrating low-intensity plyometrics into strength and conditioning programs. Strength and Conditioning Journal 27(6):10–20.

Shrier, I. 2004. Does Stretching Improve Performance?: A Systematic and Critical Review of the Literature. Clinical Journal of Sport Medicine: Volume 14(5):267–273

Shrier, I. 2005. An intervention program to reduce hamstring injuries. Physician & Sportsmedicine. 33(12):8–8.

Shrier, I. 2005. An intervention program to reduce hamstring injuries. Physician & Sportsmedicine. 33(12):8–8.

Snyder, C. R. and S. J. Lopez. 2006. Positive Psychology: The Scientific and Practical Exploration of Human Strengths. Thousand Oaks, CA: Sage Publications.

Stampfer, M.J. et al. (2005). Effects of moderate alcohol consumption on cognitive function in women. *The New England Journal of Medicine* 352:245–253.

Stefanick, M. L. et al. 2006. Effects of conjugated equine estrogens on breast cancer and mammography screening in postmenopausal women with hysterectomy. *Journal of American Medical Association.* 295(14):1647–1657.

Stockdale, M.S., Dawson-Owens, H.L., and Sagrestano, L.M. (2005). Social, attitudinal, and demographic correlates of adolescent vs college-age tobacco use initiation. *American Journal of Health Behavior* 29:311–323.

Strom, B. L. 2006. How the US drug safety system should be changed. *Journal of the American Medical Association.* 295(17):2072–2075.

Strong, W. B. et al. et al. 2005. Evidence based physical activity for school-age youth. Journal of Pediatrics, 146(6), 732–737.

Taiwo, B.O. et al. (2005). Cost-effectiveness of screening for HIV. *New England Journal of Medicine* 352:2137–2139

Teague, M. L. et al. 2007. Your Health Today: Choices in a Changing Society. New York: McGraw-Hill Higher Education, Chapter 13.

The Center on Alcohol Marketing and Youth (2005). *Alcohol industry "responsibility" advertising on television, 2001 to 2003: Executive Summary.* Washington DC: Center on Alcohol Marketing and Youth.

Tudor-Locke et al., 2005. How many days of pedometer monitoring predict weekly physical activity in adults? Preventiv Medicine, 40(3):293–298.

Tullya, M. A., et al. 2005 Brisk walking, fitness, and cardiovascular risk: A randomized controlled trial in primary care. *Preventive Medicine*. 41(2):622–628.

U. S. Department of Health and Human Services. 2004. Bone Health and Osteoporosis: A Report of the Surgeon General. Rockville, MD: U.S.D,H.H.S., Office of Surgeon General.

U. S. Department of Health and Human Services. 2006. The Health Consequences of Involuntary Exposure to Tobacco Smoke: A Report of the Surgeon General. Atlanta, GA: U. S. Department of Health and Human Services, Centers for Disease Control and Prevention, Coordinating Center for Health Promotions, National Center for Chronic Disease prevention and Health Promotion, Office on Smoking and Health.

United Nations (2006). Report on the Global AIDS Epidemic: Executive Summary. Geneva, Switzerland: Joint United Nations Programme on HIV/AIDS.

Weitzman, E.R. and Chen, Y.Y. (2005). The co-occurrence of smoking and drinking among young adults in college: National survey results from the United States. *Drug and Alcohol Dependence* 80:377–386.

Weitzman, M. et al. (2005). Tobacco smoke exposure is associated with metabolic syndrome in adolescents. *Circulation* 112:862–869.

Wilson, H. T. 2008. Annual Editions: Drugs, Society and Behavior (22nd ed.). New York: McGraw-Hill Higher Education

Winker, M. A. et al. 2000. Guidelines for medical and health information on the internet. Log on to www.ama-assn.org, use keywords internet guidelines.

World Health Organization. 2005. World Health Report 2005: Make Every Mother and Child Count. Geneva: World Health Organization. Available at www.who.int/whr/en

Credits

Concept 1

CO1: © Dennis Welsh/PunchStock; p. 3, Figure 1: World Health Organization, www.who.int/inf-pr-2000/en/pr2000-life.html and National Center for Health Statistics www.cdc.gov/nchs/pressroom/05facts/lifeexpectancy.htm; p. 3: © JLP/Jose L. Pelaez/Corbis; p. 7, Figure 5: Body composition: © Charles B. Corbin; Flexibility: © D. Berry/PhotoLink/Getty Images; Strength: © Javier Pierini/Getty Images; Cardiovascular fitness: © Karl Weatherly/Getty Images; Muscular endurance: © PhotoLink/Getty Images; p. 8, Figure 6: Agility: © PhotoDisc/Getty Images; Balance: © PhotoDisc/Getty Images; Coordination: © Karl Weatherly/Getty Images; Power: © Ryan McVay/Getty Images; Reaction time: © Royalty-Free/PunchStock; Speed: © PhotoDisc/Getty Images; p. 10: © Jonathan Nourok/The Image Bank/Getty Images; p. 12, Table 3: National Center for Health Statistics, www.cdc.gov (leading causes of death); p. 13, Table 4: Mokdad, A.H., et al. 2004. "Actual Causes of Death in the United States." *Journal of the American Medical Association* 291(10):1238–1246; p. 13: © BananaStock/PunchStock.

Concept 2

CO2: © Brian Bailey/Stone/Getty Images; p. 25: © LWA-Stephen Welstead/Corbis; p. 29: © Royalty-Free/PunchStock; p. 30: © Royalty-Free/PunchStock; p. 31: © Jon Feingersh/Corbis; p. 33: © Jose Luis Pelaez, Inc./Corbis; p. 34: Data for Technology Update from VidaOne, Inc.

Concept 3

CO3: © Karl Weatherly/Getty Images; p. 44: © Tom & Dee Ann McCarthy/Corbis; p. 45, Table 1: American College of Sports Medicine. *ACSM's Guidelines for Exercise Testing and Prescription.* 6th ed. Philadelphia: Lippincott, Williams & Wilkins, 2000; p. 47: © Mark Ahn; p. 49, Table 4: National Oceanic and Atmospheric Administration, www.ncdc.noaa.gov/oa/climate/research/heatstress/index.html; p. 49: © Royalty-Free/Corbis; p. 50, Table 5: National Weather Service, www.nws.noaa.gov/om/windchill/windchillglossary.shtml, 2001; p. 51: © 2005 Dennis Welsh/PunchStock.

Concept 4

CO4: © John Kelly/The Image Bank/Getty Images; p. 67, Table 1: National Cholesterol Health Education Program; p. 69, Table 2: National Institutes of Health, www.nhlbi.nih.gov/health/dci/Diseases/Hbp/HBP_WhatIs.html; p. 75: © Geoff Manasse/Photodisc Red/Getty Images; p. 76: © Lori Adamski Peek/Getty Images/Stone; p. 81, Lab 4A: Adapted from CAD Risk Assessor, William J. Stone. Reprinted by permission.

Concept 5

CO5: © Randy M. Ury/Corbis; p. 89: © Bob Winsett/Corbis; p. 90, Table 1: National Health Interview Survey, http://www.cdc.gov/nchs/about/major/nhis/released200609.htm.

Concept 6

CO6: © Jim Cummins/Corbis; p. 102, gardening: © Brand X Pictures; p. 102, walkers: Cara Sherman; inset (pedometer): Courtesy of New Lifestyles, Inc.; p. 104, Table 5: Tudor-Locke, C. 2004. How many steps/day are enough? Preliminary pedometer indices for public health. *Sport Medicine.* 34(1):1–8; p. 105: © Jim Cummins/Getty Images.

Concept 7

CO7: © PhotoDisc/Getty Images; p. 116, Figure 3: Adapted from Blair, S.N., et al. "Influences of Cardiorespiratory Fitness and Other Precursors on Cardiovascular Disease and All-Cause Mortality in Men and Women." 1996. *Journal of the American Medical Association.* 276(3):205; p. 119, Figure 5: © Creatas Images/PunchStock; p. 119, Figure 6: © PhotoDisc/Getty Images; p. 122: Courtesy of Polar(r); p. 125, Chart 1: Adapted from the *One-Mile Walk Test* with permission from the author, James M. Rippe, M.D.; p. 125, Chart 2: Data from Kasch F.W., and Boyer, J.L. *Adult Fitness: Principles and Practices.* Palo Alto, CA: Mayfield Publishing Co., 1968; pp. 126–127, Charts 3, 4, and 5: Astrand, P.O., and Rodahl, K. *Textbook of Work Physiology.* New York: McGraw-Hill, 1986; pp. 127–128, Charts 6 and 7: Cooper, K.H. *The Aerobics Program for Total Well-Being.* Toronto: Bantam Books, 1982; p. 129, Chart: Borg, G. "Psychological Bases of Perceived Exertion." 1982. *Medicine and Science in Sports and Exercise.* 14:377.

Concept 8

CO8: © PhotoDisc/PunchStock; p. 137, Figure 3: Data from Sporting Goods Manufacturers Association Survey, www.sgma.org; p. 138: © Leland Bobbe/Getty Images/Stone; p. 140: © PhotoDisc/Getty Images; p. 141, Table 2: Data from Sporting Good Manufacturers Survey, www.sgma.org; p. 142, Table 3: Data from Sporting Good Manufacturers Survey, www.sgma.org.

Concept 9

CO9: © Royalty-Free/Corbis; p. 152: © Benelux Press/Taxi/Getty Images; p. 153: © PhotoDisc/Getty Images; p. 157, Figure 4: Shier, D., Butler, J, and Lewis, R. *Hole's Human Anatomy and Physiology.* 8th ed. New York: McGraw-Hill, 2002; p. 158: © Charles B. Corbin; pp. 162–163, Table 3: Muscle illustrations 1, 3–5, 7, and 8 adapted from McKinley, M., and O'Loughlin, V.D. *Human Anatomy.* New York: McGraw-Hill, 2006, pp. 327–359. Muscle illustrations 2 and 6 adapted from Saladin, K.S. *Anatomy and Physiology: The Unity of Form and Function.* 4th ed. New York: McGraw-Hill, 2007, p. 347; pp. 164–165, Table 4: Muscle illustrations 1–3, 5–8 adapted from McKinley, M., and O'Loughlin, V.D. *Human Anatomy.* New York: McGraw-Hill, 2006, pp. 385–390. Muscle illustration 4 adapted from Saladin, K.S. *Anatomy and Physiology: The Unity of Form and Function.* 4th ed. New York: McGraw-Hill, 2007, p. 373; p. 166, Table 5: Muscle illustration 1 adapted from Saladin, K.S. *Anatomy and Physiology: The Unity of Form and Function.* 4th ed. New York: McGraw-Hill, 2007, p. 363. Muscle illustrations 2 and 4 adapted from McKinley, M., and O'Loughlin, V.D. *Human Anatomy.* New York: McGraw-Hill, 2006, pp. 360–362.

Concept 10

CO10: © Javier Pierini/Getty Images; p. 175, Figure 1: Shier, D., Butler, J., and Lewis, R. *Hole's Human Anatomy and Physiology.* 8th ed. New York: McGraw-Hill, 2002; p. 177: © PhotoDisc/PunchStock; p. 180: © Mark Ahn; p. 181: Royalty-Free/Corbis; p. 182: © BananaStock/PunchStock; p. 189: Courtesy of Fitness Quest; pp. 192–193, Table 6: Muscle illustrations 1–8 adapted from McKinley, M., and O'Loughlin, V.D. *Human Anatomy.* New York: McGraw-Hill, 2006, pp. 327–378; pp. 194–195, Table 7: Muscle illustrations 1 and 7 adapted from Saladin, K.S. *Anatomy and Physiology: The Unity of Form and Function.* 4th ed. New York: McGraw-Hill, 2007, pp. 344 and 373. Muscle illustrations 2–6 and 8 adapted from McKinley, M., and O'Loughlin, V.D. *Human Anatomy.* New York: McGraw-Hill, 2006, pp. 326–385; pp. 196–197, Table 8: Muscle illustrations 1–3 and 5–8 adapted from McKinley, M., and O'Loughlin, V.D. *Human Anatomy.* New York: McGraw-Hill, 2006, pp. 326–378. Muscle illustration 4 adapted from Saladin, K.S. *Anatomy and Physiology: The Unity of Form and Function.* 4th ed. New York: McGraw-Hill, 2007, p. 344; p. 198, Table 9: Muscle illustrations 1–3 adapted from McKinley, M., and O'Loughlin, V.D. *Human Anatomy.* New York: McGraw-Hill, 2006, p. 347. Muscle illustration 4 adapted from Saladin, K.S. *Anatomy and Physiology: The Unity of Form and Function.* 4th ed. New York: McGraw-Hill, 2007, p. 344; p. 201, Chart 1: Reprinted with permission from the *Journal of Physical Education, Recreation & Dance,* January 1993, p. 89. *JOPERD* is a publication of the American Alliance for Health, Physical Education, Recreation and Dance, 1900 Association Drive, Reston, VA 22091; p. 202: © Charles B. Corbin.

Concept 11

CO11: © Ryan McVay/Getty Images; p. 222: © Charles B. Corbin; p. 225: © MediaX 96, Inc.; pp. 228–234, Table 4: Muscle illustrations 1–3, 5–7, 12–13, and 15 adapted from McKinley, M., and O'Loughlin, V.D. *Human Anatomy.* New York: McGraw-Hill, 2006; pp. 326–389. Muscle illustrations 4, 8–11, and 14 adapted from Saladin, K.S. *Anatomy and Physiology: The Unity of Form and Function.* 4th ed. New York: McGraw-Hill, 2007, pp. 344, 369, and 373; p. 235, Table 5: Muscle

Index

C